Primary Healthcare and Family Medicine

Primary Healthcare and Family Medicine

Edited by **Kelly Ward**

Callisto Reference
New York

Published by Callisto Reference,
106 Park Avenue, Suite 200,
New York, NY 10016, USA
www.callistoreference.com

Primary Healthcare and Family Medicine
Edited by Kelly Ward

International Standard Book Number: 978-1-63239-751-5 (Hardback)

Printed in China.

Contents

Preface

Primary healthcare is a field dedicated to making essential healthcare accessible to every individual across the globe. Family medicine is a specialty under the umbrella of primary healthcare. Together they are pushing the boundaries of the traditional healthcare system. This book focuses on the goals, concepts and principles of primary healthcare and family medicine. It brings forth the diverse approaches in this area and their applications in the modern times. It outlines the processes and studies that are constantly contributing towards the evolution of this field. With state-of-the-art inputs by acclaimed experts of this field, this book targets students and healthcare and public health professionals.

Various studies have approached the subject by analyzing it with a single perspective, but the present book provides diverse methodologies and techniques to address this field. This book contains theories and applications needed for understanding the subject from different perspectives. The aim is to keep the readers informed about the progress in the field; therefore, the contributions were carefully examined to compile novel researches by specialists from across the globe.

Indeed, the job of the editor is the most crucial and challenging in compiling all chapters into a single book. In the end, I would extend my sincere thanks to the chapter authors for their profound work. I am also thankful for the support provided by my family and colleagues during the compilation of this book.

Editor

1

Reasons for inpatients not to seek clarity at Dr George Mukhari Academic Hospital, Pretoria

Authors:
Langalibalele H. Mabuza[1]
Olufemi B. Omole[2]
Indiran Govender[1]
John V. Ndimande[1]

Affiliations:
[1]Department of Family Medicine and Primary Health Care, University of Limpopo (Medunsa Campus), South Africa

[2]Department of Family Medicine, University of the Witwatersrand, South Africa

Correspondence to:
Langalibalele Mabuza

Email:
honeymanyosi@gmail.com

Postal address:
PO Box 222, Medunsa, 0204, South Africa

Background: Healthcare practitioners should provide patients with information regarding their clinical conditions. Patients should also feel free to seek clarity on information provided. However, not all patients seek this clarity.

Objectives: To explore the reasons inpatients gave for not seeking clarity on information that was received but not understood.

Methods: This was a qualitative arm of a larger study, titled 'Are inpatients aware of the admission reasons and management plans of their clinical conditions? A survey at a tertiary hospital in South Africa', conducted in 2010. Of the 264 inpatients who participated in the larger study, we extracted the unstructured responses from those participants (n = 152) who had indicated in the questionnaire that there was information they had not understood during their encounter with healthcare practitioners, but that they had nonetheless not sought clarity. Data were analysed thematically.

Results: Themes that emerged were that inpatients did not ask for clarity as they perceived healthcare practitioners to be 'too busy', aloof, non-communicators and sometimes uncertain about patients' conditions. Some inpatients had unquestioning trust in healthcare practitioners, whilst others had experiences of bad treatment. Inpatients had poor self-esteem, incapacitating clinical conditions, fear of bad news and prior knowledge of their clinical conditions. Some inpatients stated that they had no reason for not seeking clarity.

Conclusion: The reasons for not seeking clarity were based on patients' experiences with the healthcare practitioners and their perceptions of the latter and of themselves. A programme should be developed in order to educate inpatients on effective communication with their healthcare practitioners.

Les raisons pour lesquelles les patients internes de l'hôpital Dr George Mukhari Academic, à Pretoria, ne demandent pas d'explications concernant leur état

Présentation: Les professionnels de la santé devraient fournir à leurs patients des informations concernant leur état clinique. Les patients devraient également se sentir libres de demander des explications quant aux informations qui leurs sont fournies. Cependant, tous les patients ne le font pas.

Objectifs: Étudier les raisons fournies par les patients pour expliquer le fait qu'ils ne demandent pas d'explications concernant les informations reçues mais non comprises.

Méthodes: Cette étude constitue un volet qualitatif d'une étude de plus grande envergure, intitulée « Les patients internes ont-ils conscience des raisons de leur admission et des plans de prise en charge de leur état clinique ? Étude réalisée dans un hôpital tertiaire en Afrique du Sud », réalisée en 2010. Sur les 264 patients internes qui ont participé à l'intégralité de l'étude, nous avons extrait les réponses non structurées des participants (n = 152) qui avaient indiqué dans le questionnaire qu'ils n'avaient pas compris certaines informations fournies lors de leurs échanges avec les professionnels de la santé, et n'avaient néanmoins pas demandé d'explications. Les données ont été analysées par thème.

Résultats: Les thèmes qui en sont ressortis étaient que si les patients internes n'avaient pas demandé d'explications, c'est parce qu'ils avaient le sentiment que les professionnels de la santé étaient « trop occupés », distants, communiquaient mal, et parfois n'étaient pas certains de l'état des patients. Certains patients avaient une confiance aveugle en eux, mais d'autres avaient déjà été mal traités. Les patients internes avaient une piètre estime d'eux-mêmes, souffraient d'un état clinique débilitant, avaient peur d'entendre de mauvaises nouvelles ou connaissaient déjà leur état clinique. Certains patients ont affirmé qu'ils n'avaient aucune raison de demander des explications.

Conclusion: Les raisons pour lesquelles les patients internes ne demandaient pas d'explications s'appuyaient sur leurs expériences avec les professionnels de la santé et leur perception de ces derniers et de leur propre personne. Il conviendrait d'élaborer un programme visant à éduquer les patients internes afin de leur permettre de mieux communiquer avec les professionnels de la santé.

Introduction

Countries world-wide have adopted and adapted The Patients' Rights Charter which seeks to address comprehensive healthcare for patients.[1,2,3,4] Although a patient's right to access information has been assured in each country's charter, the realisation of this ideal is in the hands of individual healthcare institutions.

It is the right of every patient whose clinical condition warrants admission to a healthcare institution to be made aware of the clinician's working diagnosis, the reason for the admission and the inherent risks of non-admission. Once in the ward, the patient needs to be updated constantly with regard to the management plan, including the estimated length of hospital stay, investigative procedures, medication and any operative procedures envisaged. It has been shown in patients with tuberculosis that raising awareness about the patient's condition improves patient cooperation with healthcare practitioners[5] and guides them toward realistic expectations with regard to the healthcare team's abilities.[6] On the other hand, patients who receive poor communication from their physicians have been found to have a 19% higher risk of non-adherence to treatment, compared with those who received adequate communication.[7]

Acquisition of information by a patient is the responsibility of both the healthcare practitioner and the patient.[5] A balance is required between the responsibility of the healthcare practitioner to inform patients and the responsibility of the patients to seek information and clarification where the latter did not understand what was said. The healthcare practitioner can only be guided by the patient to areas that require emphasis and clarification. This has been found to occur in a balanced healthcare practitioner–patient relationship[8] and such effective communication has been found to improve patient health outcomes.[9] Patient engagement with healthcare practitioners about their health conditions has been found to benefit patients as they take charge of their own health.[10,11,12] However, anecdotal evidence suggests that patients do not always seek clarification on health issues from their healthcare practitioners, for a variety of reasons. The fact that patients do not engage with their healthcare practitioners so as to seek clarification about their clinical conditions prompted the authors to conduct a study amongst inpatients at Dr George Mukhari Academic Hospital (DGMAH). This study sets out to explore the reasons given by inpatients for not seeking clarity on information received from their healthcare practitioners.

Contribution to field

It has been established that effective communication with patients improves patient adherence to management.[7] For patients to adhere, they must understand the information given and to understand, they need clarity. However, patients are often reluctant to engage with healthcare practitioners in a conversation about their clinical condition, no matter how little they understand.[13] The reasons for this have not been explored, thus this article seeks to bridge that gap.

Research method and design

Design

This study was the qualitative arm of the study titled 'Are inpatients aware of the admission reasons and management plans of their clinical conditions? A survey at a tertiary hospital in South Africa', conducted from 6–17 December 2010 on 264 patients.

Setting

The study was conducted at DGMAH, a tertiary hospital located about 30 km north of the city of Tshwane (Pretoria). It serves as the training hospital for health sciences students at the University of Limpopo (Medunsa Campus). It comprises 39 wards which are clustered according to clinical disciplines. The hospital is a 1550-bedded hospital, with an average daily bed occupancy rate of 65.5% (982 inpatients) at the time of the study.

Sampling

The study population comprised all inpatients at the time of the study excluding those in the paediatric ward, psychiatric ward, labour ward, burns unit and intensive care wards. These wards were excluded because of the difficulty associated with obtaining informed consent from these patients. There were 27 remaining wards after these exclusions, with an average of 31 patients in each. Accordingly, that amounted to a study population of 837.

At a confidence level of 95% and a confidence interval of 0.05, the sample size from the study population mentioned above worked out to 264.[14] Since the sample size represented 32% of the total study population, the number of patients from each ward was calculated *pro rata* using this percentage. The patients were selected using a systematic sampling method; for example, in a ward with 25 patients we selected eight patients (32%), where the first patient was selected by throwing a dice and every third patient thereafter was selected from the list in the ward patient register. If a patient declined participation, or was clinically or mentally unstable, they were excluded and the next patient in the patient register was given the option to participate.

Apart from collecting sociodemographic information and other structured answers, the questionnaire focused on patients' perceptions and views on issues pertaining to awareness of the reasons for their admissions and management plan. One of these questions was:

> You have stated that you have the responsibility as a patient to ask for clarity where you did not understand what you were told. You have also stated that there was something about your illness and/or condition which when you were informed you did not understand. What would you say led you not to seek this clarity?

Participants' unstructured responses to this question were extracted. There were 152 respondents for this question.

Data collection methods

A questionnaire was developed *de novo* by the researchers, subjected to peer review by an independent researcher and a statistician and then piloted in a nearby 158-bedded hospital. It was translated from English into Setswana and isiZulu (the predominant languages spoken at the research setting) and then back-translated into English to ensure the accuracy of the translation. Each consenting patient was given a questionnaire by one of the five research assistants to complete in their preferred language. Privacy was ensured by conducting the data collection session with curtains drawn around the patient's bed. The research assistant was present for each patient to assist with clarification of any question on the questionnaire. The responses to the semi-structured questionnaire given in the local languages were translated into English through the services of an expert in Linguistics.

Data analysis

After initial analysis of the participants' responses and themes developed therefrom, the findings of this study were subjected to researcher triangulation amongst the four researchers. Group consensus on themes and categories was also achieved at a group meeting. An independent senior researcher did a peer review and acted as a 'devil's advocate', challenging the research team to provide evidence for their interpretations and the conclusions drawn, based on the data.[15] The research team subjected the data to an iterative process, whereby the data were visited and revisited, connecting them with emerging insights and progressively refining the focus of understanding.[16] In this way, data gathered were analysed using thematic analysis.[17] Member checking to authenticate the study findings through eliciting feedback from the participants[18] was not performed because of a high patient turnover in a number of the wards in which the study was conducted.

Trustworthiness

To ensure trustworthiness of the study findings, the principles of credibility, dependability, confirmability and transferability were followed.[19] To ensure data credibility, the research team checked the data entry of each questionnaire to ensure its correctness. Furthermore, the study findings were subjected to peer review by a senior researcher who was not part of the study.[19] With regard to dependability, we looked at the range of experience (variability) rather than the average experience of all the participants.[20] Therefore, each participant's response was considered when grouping the data categories into themes. Confirmability was ensured by non-involvement of the research team in data collection, as well as by researcher triangulation so as to achieve objectivity in data collection and reporting.[19] Transferability was ensured by providing a thick description of the study to allow evaluation regarding how well the study conclusions can be applied to other similar settings.[21]

Results

We identified seven healthcare practitioner-related and five patient-related themes (see Table 1). These are presented below with supporting quotations where applicable.

Healthcare practitioner-related themes

Theme 1: Healthcare practitioners were perceived to be too busy

The inpatients reported that they were attended to by healthcare practitioners who appeared to be very busy during the ward rounds, moving speedily from one patient to another. Information would be given through the nurse interpreter without eliciting questions from the patient to test their understanding of the information given:

> 'It was hard enough to ask questions initially because he seemed really busy, so…I just chose not to ask anything again'. (Female, aged 13–20, with tertiary education)

> 'Nurses don't want to explain anything to patients. Always busy'. (Female, aged 13–20, with secondary education)

Theme 2: Experiences of bad treatment

Healthcare practitioners were perceived to be ill-disposed toward the inpatients. This perception affected the inpatients' willingness to engage the healthcare practitioners about their clinical conditions:

> 'Here in this hospital it isn't easy, as the nurses treat us so bad, so you end up not able to ask anything'. (Male, aged 51–60, with secondary education)

> 'The nurses are so impatient with us and it is sad because we need their help. What they say goes. We don't even have a chance to ask anything without being snapped at'. (Female, aged 21–30, with tertiary education)

This perception led some patients to pretend they understood all the information they received, as they saw no benefit in engaging the healthcare team any further:

> 'How can you ask anything about your condition when they don't even care if you're cold and need help to bath, so I'll just pretend to be fine….You just don't receive proper help and care'. (Male, aged 41–50, with secondary education)

Theme 3: Patients forbidden to ask questions

Some patients reported that they were advised not to ask questions, whilst others were told that the healthcare

TABLE 1: List of themes.

A. Healthcare practitioner-related themes	B. Patient-related themes
1. Healthcare practitioners were perceived to be too busy	1. Notion that healthcare practitioners held patients in low esteem
2. Experiences of bad treatment	2. Incapacitating clinical condition
3. Patients forbidden to ask questions	3. No reason for not asking
4. Healthcare practitioners were perceived to be aloof from patients	4. Patients' fear of bad news
5. Unquestioning trust in health care practitioners	5. Patients already knew their conditions
6. Language barrier	-
7. Healthcare practitioners were feared by patients	-
8. The healthcare practitioner appeared uncertain about the patient's condition	-

practitioners knew better and that they were not to be bothered with questions:

> 'It's as if they are pressing you or stopping you from asking questions. They tell you that they know better so you shouldn't ask any questions'. (Male, aged 31–40, with secondary education)

> 'Doctor X tells us that he's a doctor and he knows best so we shouldn't bother him with questions and that's not right because it's my body and my condition. I'm the one in pain and need answers and assurance'. (Female, aged 31–40, with secondary education)

Theme 4: Healthcare practitioners were perceived to be aloof

The patients reported that healthcare practitioners were inaccessible because they did not communicate with patients, but rather amongst themselves:

> 'They are so distant that you end up keeping quiet and sometimes when you respect someone a lot you end up having to keep quiet when you shouldn't'. (Female, aged 21–30, with tertiary education)

> 'Doctors just discuss among themselves'. (Female, aged 21–30, with secondary education)

> 'It's not that I'm slandering their name but they hardly ever tell us anything so it's up to them if they tell us anything'. (Male, aged > 60, with secondary education)

Patients also found it difficult to approach the healthcare practitioners, who were perceived to be distant:

> 'Negative, unapproachable health workers'. (Male, aged 51–60, with secondary education)

Theme 5: Unquestioning trust in the healthcare workers

Some inpatients saw healthcare practitioners, specifically medical doctors, as knowing what they were doing. Some inpatients reported that they saw no reason to understand what the doctors were doing and others reported that they had a good relationship with the healthcare workers:

> 'I just thought that my doctor knows best and indeed I'm happy about how I'm treated by all the doctors and nurses'. (Female, aged 51–60, with primary education)

> 'Sometimes I don't understand what the doctors or nurses say but I don't ask because I trust that they know what they are doing and it is for my own good'. (Male, aged 41–50, with no formal education)

> 'I wait for doctors to tell me how I am progressing, although I do not understand, at times I do not find my understanding necessary. They know what they are doing'. (Male, aged 31–40, with secondary education)

Where doctors did not give information, some patients assumed that the doctors had a reason for not telling them anything:

> 'I assumed that what they do not tell, I do not need to know'. (Female, aged 21–30, with primary education)

Theme 6: Language barrier

There were language barriers to effective communication. Patients reported that the healthcare practitioners spoke in English, sometimes using medical jargon:

> 'I was unable to ask because the doctor was speaking in English – there was no one to translate, that's why I didn't seek clarity'. (Female, aged 41–50, with no formal education)

> 'Medical terminology – most of the time doctors make use of big terms'. (Male, aged 21–30, with secondary education)

Theme 7: Fear of inconveniencing healthcare practitioners

Some patients indicated that they were fearful of the healthcare practitioners. Others worried about their questions being seen as 'stupid'. This led them to refrain from seeking clarity where the healthcare practitioner's explanation was not understood:

> 'I feel scared to ask doctors who appear to have a lot on their plates. I am even afraid to raise my concerns'. (Female, aged 51–60, with primary education)

Theme 8: The healthcare practitioner appeared uncertain about the patient's condition

Some patients indicated that they thought the healthcare practitioner was not sure of the patient's condition. These were the cases where the healthcare practitioner mentioned a few possibilities for the patient's condition and indicated that they were still investigating:

> 'Doctors do not give me a direct answer, it's like they are also uncertain of my condition'. (Female, aged 21–30, with secondary education)

In some cases, patients found themselves confused by the various versions (sometimes conflicting) of their condition that were presented to them by different healthcare practitioners:

> 'Different doctors are telling me different things, so I no longer ask where I do not understand, I'm just confused'. (Male, aged 21–30, with tertiary education)

Patient-related themes

Theme 1: Notion that healthcare practitioners held patients in low esteem

The notion by patients that the healthcare practitioners held them in low esteem caused some patients to refrain from asking for clarity when it was necessary for them to do so. That notion was brought about by their perception that healthcare practitioners did not regard them as being worthy of consideration as they did not engage with the patients during their ward rounds. Furthermore, that notion led the patients to hesitate, as they were worried that their questions would be labelled as 'stupid':

> 'How can you ask anything when they don't take you into consideration?'. (Male, aged 21–30, with secondary education)

> '[*Doctors*] they'll think you are stupid if you ask certain things'. (Male, aged 21–30, with secondary education)

Theme 2: Incapacitating clinical conditions

Some of the reasons given by patients for not asking questions about their clinical conditions related to the incapacity induced by the clinical conditions themselves:

> 'I was too weak to talk'. (Male, aged 41–50, with tertiary education)

'At first I was distraught that I had to deliver quickly so my stress was too much…'. (Female, aged 31–40, with secondary education)

Theme 3: No reason for not asking

It was noted that sometimes the inpatients could not give reasons for not asking for clarity – it just had not crossed their minds:

'It didn't cross my mind to ask questions on their instructions to take the medicine'. (Female, aged > 60, with secondary education)

Theme 4: Patients' fear of bad news

Some of the patients were reluctant to ask questions for fear of hearing bad news which would cause them distress:

'I was afraid of seeking clarity on my diagnosis in fear that my condition may be serious'. (Female, aged 13–20, with secondary education)

Theme 5: Patients already knew their conditions

Some patients indicated that they had already known about their clinical conditions before admission (some had been informed by their family doctors):

'I didn't seek clarity because I knew before I was admitted'. (Male, aged 31–40, with no formal education)

Ethical considerations

Ethical approval was obtained from the MEDUNSA Research Ethics Committee (MREC) of the University of Limpopo (Clearance Certificate Number: MCREC/M/24/2008:IR). Permission to conduct the study on site was granted by the Chief Executive Officer (CEO) of the DGMAH. Ethical principles of confidentiality, justice and autonomy were ensured throughout the study. Personal details were not included on the questionnaires so as to ensure anonymity.

Discussion

This study sought to explore the reasons given by inpatients for not seeking clarity on information received from healthcare practitioners on their clinical conditions. As far as the authors could ascertain, this was the first study in a healthcare institution in South Africa to examine this issue. The themes that emerged were related, on the one hand, to the inpatients' perceptions of healthcare practitioners and, on the other hand, to the inpatients' perceptions of themselves.

The perception that inpatients had that doctors and nurses were often rushed, contributed significantly to their not seeking clarity on the information they were given. As studies have shown, patients are reluctant to inconvenience the doctors that they perceive to be busy by delaying them with clarification questions.[12,16] However, this approach disempowers patients and renders them passive partners in the management of their own clinical conditions.[22] The partnership with patients in the management of their conditions has been shown to be vital in patient care.[23]

Apart from doctors, nurses could also been seen as a source of information for patients. Nurses are perceived to spend more time with patients than doctors. That said, studies have shown that they spend less than 40% of their time 'by the bedside' of patients.[24,25] In our study, patients reported nurses as being 'too busy' to be consulted for clarification of information given to patients during the ward rounds. Nursing duties are multiple; besides taking ward rounds with doctors and other healthcare team members, they also have administrative tasks. These duties compete with direct patient care.[19] Furthermore, in South Africa the patient to nursing ratio is unfavourable for prolonged interaction with patients in public healthcare institutions.[26]

The finding that inpatients were 'told not to ask questions' goes against the *Batho Pele* ('Putting People First') Principles[27] advocated by the South African government toward improved accountability and efficiency in service delivery. The South African National Patients' Rights Charter states that the patient has the right to be 'attended to by only clearly identified health care providers'.[3] Because of this right, any patient has the option to take the matter up with relevant hospital authorities on the identified healthcare practitioner. Withdrawing from interaction all together by 'pretending to be fine' should be discouraged,

Furthermore, inpatients perceived healthcare practitioners to be 'distant' from their patients. Healthcare practitioners need to be conscious of their body language when dealing with patients.[28] The inpatients observed doctors discussing 'amongst themselves' and not with the patients. Thus, the message received by the inpatients was that the doctors were distancing themselves from the patients. The patients then adopted the attitude of 'so it is up to them if they want to tell us anything'. That discouraged patients from asking anything of the doctors, even if they had overhead something they would have liked to have had explained. Such a tarnished relationship augurs badly for patient healthcare.[17] Moreover, because the doctors were perceived to be unwilling to reach out to patients, they were regarded as 'unapproachable' – once again at patient's expense.

It is common practice in South Africa for healthcare practitioners who do not speak the patient's first language to make use of nurse interpreters.[29] This has its own problems, in that the translation is not always accurate and more time is spent per patient using an interpreter compared with cases where there is no need for one.[30] In this study, patients reported that healthcare practitioners spoke in English and sometimes used medical jargon during the clinical encounter. It has been recommended that healthcare practitioners have at least a minimum understanding of their patients' languages and culture so as to facilitate effective communication.[31] The use of medical jargon with patients constitutes ineffective communication. Resource material is available in order to assist healthcare practitioners with using 'lay' language with patients.[32,33,34]

Healthcare practitioners need to discourage the perpetuation of patients' ideas about doctors being experts in their field who 'know it all', preventing patients from making enquiries about their clinical conditions. Patients need to be encouraged to ask questions since they are equal partners with healthcare practitioners in the management of their clinical conditions.[11] Patients should be encouraged to use the encounter with their healthcare practitioners to empower themselves. With the advent of the internet, the paradigm is changing[35] and healthcare practitioners need to prepare themselves to be engaged by patients regarding their clinical conditions.

Some patients expressed fear of inconveniencing their doctors – given their busy schedule – and were also reluctant to ask questions which they feared would be labelled as 'stupid'. The power gradient between a patient and the healthcare practitioner, where the latter is the dominant figure, has been challenged in recent years.[36,37] However, a minority of patients have still been found to perceive doctors as authoritarian (16% in South Africa, 17% in the United States and 20% in the United Kingdom).[38] The notion that the healthcare practitioner is an expert in the healthcare field has recently been counter-balanced by the realisation by healthcare practitioners that the patient is also an expert in the experience of his or her illness.[39] This has paved the way for a negotiated solution between the two 'experts', thus diminishing the power gradient. Medical schools need to promote this paradigm shift in their training programmes, to ensure that the future of healthcare practice is not characterised by the 'all-knowing healthcare practitioner' who has little to learn from his or her patients, but a future where the healthcare practitioner and patients collaborate and negotiate for better health outcomes.

Some patients indicated that they did not ask for clarity when healthcare practitioners indicated that they were uncertain with regard to the patient's condition. However, studies have shown that patients develop confidence in healthcare practitioners who are honest enough to admit that they are uncertain about certain aspects of patient care, prompting them to search for the information for their patients.[40] In our study, some patients had the notion that doctors 'know what they are doing', but others realised that the doctors 'appeared not to know' about their condition, whilst other inpatients became confused when there was 'conflicting information' from various doctors about their clinical conditions. Healthcare practitioners should avoid a situation where patients are confused by the conflicting information they receive from the healthcare practitioners in attendance. They need to share information amongst themselves about a given patient and endeavour to present a cohesive and comprehensive clinical picture to the patient.[41] Furthermore, it is a challenge for healthcare practitioners, not only those at DGMAH, to educate patients about the fact that there is frequently a need for healthcare practitioners to search for information relating to their patients' conditions and management, which is performed in the best interests of the patient.[42]

Regarding patient-related reasons for the inpatients not to seek clarity, it was of note that patients had a notion that healthcare practitioners held them in low esteem. That notion came as a result of their perception of how they were perceived by healthcare practitioners. They stated that healthcare practitioners 'did not regard (them) worth considering'. This could have been a combination of other factors already mentioned above, *inter alia*, the aloof stance toward patients that healthcare practitioners were seen to adopt, healthcare practitioners being too busy for patients and the negative attitude that they were perceived as having toward patients. Patients' perceptions of a negative attitude on the part of healthcare practitioners, especially for chronic diseases, has been documented.[43]

Those inpatients who had no reason for not asking for clarity on areas they did not understand presented a challenge to the healthcare practitioner to always invite questions following each healthcare practitioner–patient encounter.[12] Some inpatients indicated that they were not keen to seek clarity on their condition because they feared hearing bad news from the healthcare practitioners. Patients have been found to suffer from reactive depression following their hearing bad news, necessitating referral for psychosocial counselling.[44] However, withholding information from patients on the ground of their fear of bad news is not advised. Healthcare practitioners should therefore address their patients' fears and concerns during the breaking of bad news so as to help patients overcome this particular barrier.

Some patients indicated that they had already known about their clinical conditions before admission, hence they had seen no need to seek further clarity. It is highly unlikely that information received by a patient about their condition prior to admission was exhaustive. To this end, at the end of every communication with a patient, the healthcare practitioner should invite questions from the patient and make sure the patient indeed understands.[12]

Limitations of the study

The study did not specify the various cadres of the healthcare team (nurses, doctors, healthcare science personnel, etc.) to whom patients were referring in their responses. This lack of specificity makes it difficult to direct specific feedback to the relevant healthcare teams. There were no follow-up questions to establish a deeper understanding of the inpatients' responses. Errors could have been introduced during the translation of patients' responses from their mother tongue to English. This was minimised by the involvement of the expert in Linguistics in the translation.

The study was conducted in a tertiary institution, which limits its transferability to other settings. Nevertheless, tertiary hospitals as ultimate referral institutions should demonstrate a high standard of healthcare, including healthcare professional–patient relationships. Furthermore, revealing the socio-cultural and economical demographics of the participants could have helped the reader to judge the applicability of this research in other settings and could have helped with regard to the outlining of possible correlations and trends.

Practical implications and recommendations

Asking for clarification of information received by inpatients from healthcare practitioners is pivotal for an effective healthcare practitioner–patient encounter and will lead to greater understanding and therefore adherence to mutually-agreed therapies. The study has described, from the inpatient's perspectives, some of the factors that stand in the way of an effective two-directional communication between healthcare provider and patient. Healthcare professionals should make a conscious effort to develop attitudes and skills that motivate patient engagement through effective communication in plain language, which should include inviting the patients to ask questions after each healthcare professional–patient encounter as well as asking them to express their specific fears and concerns.

Conclusions

Reasons given by patients for not seeking clarity about their clinical conditions at DGMAH were based mainly on patients' perceptions of healthcare practitioners, their clinical conditions and perceptions of themselves. They perceived healthcare practitioners to be 'too busy', aloof, non-communicators and sometimes uncertain about patients' conditions. Although some had unquestioning trust in their healthcare practitioners others had experienced bad treatment from them. They had incapacitating clinical conditions, fear of bad news and an impression of adequate prior knowledge of their conditions. Some had the notion that healthcare practitioners held them in low esteem.

Future studies should investigate challenges faced by healthcare practitioners in a healthcare practitioner–patient encounter which are barriers in this encounter. Other future research could focus on factors that motivate patients to ask for clarification where they did not understand.

Acknowledgements

The authors would like to thank Nokulunga Mabuza, Phindile Ndimande, Frans Sekgwele, Kenny Mafala and Morongoe Mshoeng for their participation in data collection. We would also like to thank Nomkhosi Mabuza for her involvement in the extraction of data from the questionnaires.

Competing interests

The authors declare that they have no financial or personal relationship(s) that may have inappropriately influenced them in writing this article. This study was funded by the Medical Research Council (MRC) of South Africa (Grant number: M027, University of Limpopo [Medunsa Campus]).

Authors' contributions

LHM (University of Limpopo, Medunsa Campus) conceptualised the research idea and was the project leader. LHM, OBO (University of the Witwatersrand), IG (University of Limpopo, Medunsa Campus) and JVN (University of Limpopo, Medunsa Campus) were involved in the thematic data analysis and collaborative write-up. All authors were involved in the revision and approval of the final manuscript.

References

1. Mater Health Services. Patient charter – China. A guide for patients, carers and families. [document on Internet]. c2013 [cited 2013 Mar 21]. Available from http://www.mater.org.au/Files/Documents/Corporate/Patient-charter/MHS-106-04720-Mater-Patient-Charter-Chinese.PDF
2. Government of Western Australia, Department of Health. The Western Australian public patients' hospital charter. [document on Internet]. c2011 [cited 2013 Mar 21]. Available from https://www.health.wa.gov.au/services/downloads/Hospital_Charter_booklet.pdf
3. Health Professions Council of South Africa. Guidelines for good practice in the health care professions. National patients' rights charter – Booklet 3. [document on Internet]. c2008 [cited 2013 Mar 21]. Available from http://www.hpcsa.co.za/downloads/conduct_ethics/rules/generic_ethical_rules/booklet_3_patients_rights_charter.pdf
4. Medico-legal Practice Committee of the Law Society of Kenya. Draft of the national patients' right charter, 2012. [document on Internet]. c2012 [cited 2013 Mar 21]. Available from http://www.consumersinternational.org/media/1032556/kenya%20national%20patients'%20health%20charter.pdf
5. Munro SA, Lewin SA, Smith HJ, et al. Patient adherence to tuberculosis treatment: a systematic review of qualitative research. PLoS Med. 2007;4(7):e238. http://dx.doi.org/10.1371/journal.pmed.0040238
6. Mawela MP, de Villiers FP. The effect of admission on oral rehydration-related knowledge. Ann Trop Paediatr. 1999;19(1):75–81. http://dx.doi.org/10.1080/02724939992680
7. Zolnierek KB, DiMatteo MR. Physician communication and patient adherence to treatment: a meta-analysis. Med Care. 2009;47(8):826–834. http://dx.doi.org/10.1097/MLR.0b013e31819a5acc, PMid:19584762, PMCid:PMC2728700
8. Street RL Jr. Information-giving in medical consultations: The influence of patients' communicative styles and personal characteristics. Soc Sci Med. 1991;32(5):541–548. http://dx.doi.org/10.1016/0277-9536(91)90288-N
9. Stewart MA. Effective physician–patient communication and health outcomes: a review. CMAJ 1995;152(9):1423–1433. PMid:7728691, PMCid:PMC1337906
10. Cegala DJ, Marinelli T, Post D. The effects of communication skills training on compliance. Arch Fam Med. 2000;9(1):57–64. http://dx.doi.org/10.1001/archfami.9.1.57, PMid:10664643
11. Katz MG, Jacobson TA, Veledar E, et al. Patient literacy and question-asking behavior during the medical encounter: a mixed-methods analysis. J General Intern Med. 2007;22(6):782–786. http://dx.doi.org/10.1007/s11606-007-0184-6, PMid:17431697, PMCid:PMC2583801
12. Street RL Jr, Gordon HS, Ward MM, et al. Patient participation in medical consultations: why some patients are more involved than others. Med Care. 2005;43(10):960–969. http://dx.doi.org/10.1097/01.mlr.0000178172.40344.70
13. Chavunduka D, Dzimwasha M, Madondo F, et al. Drug information for inpatients in the community. World Health Forum. 1991;12(1):29–33. PMid:1859594
14. Creative Research Systems. Sample size calculator. [document on Internet]. c2013 [cited 2013 Oct 26]. Available from http://www.surveysystem.com/sscalc.htm
15. Darbyshire P, MacDougall C, Schiller W. Multiple methods in qualitative research with children: more insight or just more? Qualitative Research. 2005;5(4):417–436. http://dx.doi.org/10.1177/1468794105056921
16. Srivastava P, Hopwood N. A practical iterative framework for qualitative data analysis. Int J Qual Meth. 2009;8(1):76–84.
17. Lincoln YS, Guba EG. Naturalistic inquiry. Newbury Park, CA: Sage Publications; 1985.
18. Riessman CK. Narrative methods for the human sciences. Thousand Oaks, CA: Sage; 2008.
19. Anfara VA Jr, Brown KM, Mangione TL. Qualitative analysis on stage: making the research process more public. Educ Res. 2002;31(7):28–38.
20. Guba EG. Criteria for assessing the trustworthiness of naturalistic inquiries. ECTJ. 1981;29(2):75–91.
21. Slade L, Hoppmann CA. Time-sampling research in health psychology: potential contributions and new trends. The European Health Psychologist. 2011;13(4):65–69.
22. Faulkner M. Empowerment, disempowerment and the care of older people. Nurs Older People. 2001;13(5):18–20. http://dx.doi.org/10.7748/nop2001.07.13.5.18.c2183, PMid:12008615
23. Bruhn JG. Equal partners: doctors and patients explore the limits of autonomy. J Okla State Med Assoc. 2001;94(2):46–54. PMid:11288462
24. Westbrook JI, Duffield C, Li L, et al. How much time do nurses have for patients? A longitudinal study quantifying hospital nurses' patterns of task time distribution and interactions with health professionals. BMC Health Serv Res. 2011;11:319. http://dx.doi.org/10.1186/1472-6963-11-319
25. Hendrickson G, Doddato TM, Kovner CT. How do nurses use their time? J Nurs Adm. 1990;20(3):31–37. http://dx.doi.org/10.1097/00005110-199003000-00008, PMid:2313373
26. Wildschut A, Mqolozana T. Shortage of nurses in South Africa: relative or absolute? [document on Internet]. c2008 [cited 2013 Apr 01]. Available from https://www.labour.gov.za/downloads/documents/research-documents/nursesshortage.pdf

27. Department of Public Service and Administration. Batho Pele – putting people first. [page on Internet]. c2007 [cited 2013 Jan 24]. Available from http://www.info.gov.za/aboutgovt/publicadmin/bathopele.htm

28. Hurley AC, Volicer BJ, Hanrahan PA, et al. Assessment of discomfort in advanced Alzheimer patients. Res Nurs Health. 1992;15(5):369–377. http://dx.doi.org/10.1002/nur.4770150506, PMid:1529121

29. Drennan G, Swartz L. The paradoxical use of interpreting in psychiatry. Soc Sci Med. 2002;54(12):1853–1866. http://dx.doi.org/10.1016/S0277-9536(01)00153-8

30. Hampers LC, McNulty JE. Professional interpreters and bilingual physicians in a pediatric emergency department: effect on resource utilization. Arch Pediatr Adolesc Med. 2002;156(11):1108–1113. http://dx.doi.org/10.1001/archpedi.156.11.1108

31. Tang G, Lanza O, Rodriguez FM, et al. The Kaiser Permanente Clinician Cultural and Linguistic Assessment Initiative: research and development in patient–provider language concordance. Am J Public Health. 2011;101(2):205–208. http://dx.doi.org/10.2105/AJPH.2009.177055, PMid:21228282, PMCid:PMC3020187

32. Fagerlin A, Zikmund-Fisher BJ, Ubel PA. Helping patients decide: ten steps to better risk communication. J Natl Cancer Inst. 2011;103(19):1436–1443. http://dx.doi.org/10.1093/jnci/djr318, PMid:21931068, PMCid:PMC3218625

33. Centers for Disease Control and Prevention. Health Literacy. [page on Internet]. no date [cited 2010 Oct 25]. Available from http://www.cdc.gov/healthmarketing/healthliteracy/

34. Plain Language Association InterNational. Web sites for writers. [page on Internet]. c2009 [cited 2009 Jul 28]. Available from http://www.plainlanguagenetwork.org/Resources/websites.html

35. Kassirer JP. Patients, physicians, and the Internet. Health Aff. 2000;19(6):115–123. http://dx.doi.org/10.1377/hlthaff.19.6.115

36. Cahill J. Patient participation: a concept analysis. J Adv Nurs. 1996;24(3):561–571. http://dx.doi.org/10.1046/j.1365-2648.1996.22517.x, PMid:8876417

37. Coulter A. Partnerships with patients: the pros and cons of shared clinical decision-making. J Health Serv Res Policy. 1997;2(2):112–121. PMid:10180362

38. Pincock S. Patients put their relationship with their doctors as second only to that with their families. BMJ. 2003;327(7415):581. http://dx.doi.org/10.1136/bmj.327.7415.581-c, PMid:12969915, PMCid:PMC194117

39. Balint M. The doctor, his patient and the illness. London, UK: Pitman Books Ltd; 1964.

40. Haugli L, Strand E, Finset A. How do patients with rheumatic disease experience their relationship with their doctors? A qualitative study of experiences of stress and support in the doctor–patient relationship. Patient Educ Couns. 2004;52(2):169–174. http://dx.doi.org/10.1016/S0738-3991(03)00023-5

41. Davies C. Getting health professionals to work together: there's more to collaboration than simply working side by side. BMJ. 2000;320(7241):1021–1022. http://dx.doi.org/10.1136/bmj.320.7241.1021, PMid:10764344, PMCid:PMC1117928

42. Pellegrino ED, Thomasma DC. For the patient's good: the restoration of beneficence in health care. New York, NY: Oxford University Press; 1988. PMCid:PMC338480

43. Smit R. HIV/AIDS and the workplace: perceptions of nurses in a public hospital in South Africa. J Adv Nurs. 2005;51(1):22–29. PMid:15941457

44. Keller M, Sommerfeldt S, Fischer C, et al. Recognition of distress and psychiatric morbidity in cancer patients: a multi-method approach. Ann Oncol. 2004;15(8): 1243–1249. http://dx.doi.org/10.1093/annonc/mdh318, PMid:15277265

2

Improving the quality of care for patients with hypertension in Moshupa District, Botswana: Quality improvement cycle

Authors:
Cathy Kande[1]
Robert Mash[1]

Affiliations:
[1]Division of Family Medicine and Primary Care, Stellenbosch University, South Africa

Correspondence to:
Robert Mash

Email:
rm@sun.ac.za

Postal address:
Box 19063, Tygerberg, 7505, South Africa

Background: Although there are no prevalence studies on hypertension in Botswana, this condition is thought to be common and the quality of care to be poor.

Aim: The aim of this project was to assess and improve the quality of primary care for hypertension.

Setting: Moshupa clinic and catchment area, Botswana.

Methods: Quality improvement cycle.

Results: Two hundred participants were included in the audit. Sixty-eight per cent were women with a mean age of 55 years. In the baseline audit none of the target standards were met. During the re-audit six months later, six out of nine structural target standards, five out of 11 process target standards and one out of two outcome target standards were achieved. Statistically-significant improvement in performance ($p < 0.05$) was shown in 10 criteria although the target standard was not always met. In the re-audit, the target of achieving blood pressure control (< 140/90) in 70% of patients was achieved.

Conclusion: The quality of care for hypertension was suboptimal in our setting. Simple interventions were designed and implemented to improve the quality of care. These interventions led to significant improvement in structural and process criteria. A corresponding significant improvement in the control of blood pressure was also seen.

Améliorer la qualité de la prise en charge des patients souffrant d'hypertension dans le district de Moshupa, au Botswana: le cycle d'amélioration de la qualité

Présentation: Bien qu'il n'existe aucune étude portant sur la prévalence de l'hypertension au Botswana, il s'agit d'un problème de santé considéré comme courant, et la qualité de sa prise en charge est médiocre.

Objectif: L'objectif de ce projet était d'évaluer et d'améliorer la qualité des soins de santé primaire liés à l'hypertension.

Cadre: Centre médical et bassin de Moshupa, Botswana.

Méthodes: Cycle d'amélioration de la qualité.

Résultats: Deux cent personnes ont participé à l'étude. Soixante-huit pour cent d'entre elles étaient des femmes et l'âge moyen était de 55 ans. Au cours de l'étude subséquente menée six mois plus tard, six des neuf normes structurelles, cinq des 11 normes visées par le processus et une des deux normes visées par le résultat étaient effectives. Une amélioration statistiquement significative de la performance ($p < 0.5$) était observée pour 10 critères, bien que la norme visée n'ait pas été systématiquement atteinte. Au cours de l'étude subséquente, l'objectif consistant à procéder au contrôle de la tension artérielle (< 140/90) chez 70% des patients était réalisé.

Conclusion: La qualité de la prise en charge de l'hypertension était inférieure à la norme dans notre cadre. Des interventions simples ont été élaborées et mises en œuvres afin d'améliorer la qualité de cette prise en charge. Ces interventions ont conduit à une amélioration conséquente dans les critères structurels et relatifs aux processus. Une amélioration significative correspondante a également été observée dans le contrôle de la tension artérielle.

Introduction

Although there are no prevalence studies on hypertension in Botswana, hypertension is thought to be very common.[1] This condition is commonly asymptomatic, readily detectable by blood pressure measurement and can lead to complications if untreated.[2] The extrapolated statistics for Botswana suggest that there may be at least 800 000 individuals with raised blood pressure, which represents approximately 41% of the total population.[3] A cross-sectional study in Gaborone city council clinics in Botswana showed an even higher prevalence (61%) amongst the diabetic patients.[4] Hypertension is the most common reason for outpatient medical review.[4,5]

Hypertension has significant morbidity and mortality and is associated with adverse outcomes such as coronary artery disease, congestive cardiac failure, stroke and renal disease. This imposes more financial constraints on the health system, which is already burdened by the HIV pandemic. Based on the available evidence, the current US guidelines, published in the Seventh report of the Joint National Committee on prevention, detection, evaluation and treatment of high blood pressure (JNC 7), recommend maintaining blood pressure at less than 140/90 mmHg for most patients and less than 130/85 mmHg for patients with diabetes mellitus and renal disease.[5] However, the Society for Endocrinology, Metabolism and Diabetes of South Africa recommend a target of 130/80 mmHg for type 2 diabetes.[6]

There is evidence that treatment to specific targets can reduce morbidity and mortality.[5,7] A reduction of 5–6 mmHg in diastolic blood pressure (DBP) has been shown to reduce the incidence of stroke by 40%, coronary events by 15% and heart failure by 50%.[5] Non-pharmacological measures as well as medication can contribute to blood pressure reduction. For example, the Dietary Approaches to Stop Hypertension (DASH) low sodium diet reduces the systolic blood pressure (SBP) by 2–8 mmHg and weight reduction of 10 kg can contribute to a reduction of 5–20 mmHg.[5]

Despite this evidence, treatment in many settings is not very successful at achieving blood pressure control and meeting these targets. Control may remain poor as a result of limited resources, poor adherence to medication as well as inappropriate choice of medication. The National Health and Nutrition Examination Survey (NHANES III), conducted in the United States of America (USA) from 1988 to 1991, showed that 76% of known hypertensive patients had blood pressure measurements of 140/90 mmHg or higher.[5] A study conducted on veterans in the USA from 1990 to 1995 showed that more than 65% had blood pressure measurements of 140/90 mmHg or higher and 40% had measurements of 160/90 mmHg or higher.[5] Only 24% had their blood pressure controlled to less than 140/90 mmHg in a study conducted at five Department of Veterans Affairs sites in the USA.[8]

It is likely that the control of blood pressure and quality of care in Botswana is also problematic, although few studies exist to verify this. One study performed in Gaborone demonstrated that health workers frequently measure the patients' blood pressure incorrectly.[4]

There are guidelines that have been developed locally to improve the care of hypertensive patients. The South African Hypertension Society guideline was published in 2011 and a Botswana guideline in 2007.[7,9] Both guidelines address the processes of care for hypertensive patients.

Aim and objectives

The aim of this study was to improve the quality of care for hypertension at Moshupa clinic in Botswana. The specific objectives were to assess the current quality of care for hypertension; to plan and implement changes to improve the quality of care; to assess whether these changes were associated with a measurable improvement in the quality of care; and to make recommendations to the local Department of Health on how to improve the quality of care in primary care clinics.

Research methods and design

Ethical considerations

Ethical approval for the study was obtained from Stellenbosch University, reference N11/06/188.

Study design

This project was a quality improvement cycle comprising the following steps:

- Establishing an audit team.
- Setting up of criteria and target standards.
- Data collection.
- Data analysis.
- Data interpretation.
- Planning of changes in the facility and the implementation of the changes.
- Re-audit to detect changes in the quality of care.[10]

The setting

Moshupa district is situated in the southern part of Botswana. It has an estimated population of 22 811 which is served by 26 health facilities (eight clinics and 18 health posts).[11] There is no hospital in Moshupa and the district relies on a mission hospital in Kanye for referral. Laboratory, radiograph facilities and ECG machines are non-existent in the district and all health facilities refer to the mission hospital for these investigations.

Clinics are staffed with an average of six health workers whilst health posts have an average of three health workers. Moshupa clinic (the main clinic in Moshupa) offers 24-hour services. It is staffed with 10 nurses working in shifts, a lay counsellor, one health auxiliary, two cleaners and two ambulance drivers.

There are six doctors in the district. They are involved in consultation of adults and children in primary care, maternity and emergency care. Each doctor is allocated a number of health facilities that they visit on a monthly basis, but they visit clinics more regularly than health posts.

A dedicated hypertension clinic does not exist in the district and hypertensive patients are seen daily, together with other general patients, by doctors and nurses with different levels of expertise. Antihypertensive drugs are refilled monthly at the local clinics. The following antihypertensive classes are available: thiazide diuretics, loop diuretics (furosemide), calcium-channel blockers (nifedipine), beta blockers (propranolol, atenolol), angiotensin-converting enzyme inhibitors (captopril, enalapril). Health education is organised in each health facility in the morning and covers a variety of topics, with talks delivered by the health workers. At times, patients are also asked to deliver a health talk under the supervision of a nurse or health education assistant.

The present study focused on the Moshupa council clinic and the three health posts that were in its catchment area: Lothlakane West health post, Moshupa health post and Ralekgetho health post.

The audit team

The audit team was headed by the main researcher and included two doctors, one health auxiliary and four nurses. The team members felt motivated to participate in the quality improvement cycle as this would serve as a basis to audit other health programmes in which they had any active involvement. Prior to the audit, members had training on blood pressure measurement, which was not assessed in the study.

Setting of criteria and target standards

The audit team opted to use the South African Society of Hypertension guidelines,[7] which are the latest regional guideline based on internationally-accepted evidence. These guidelines also address the process of care in more detail and stratify the cardiovascular risk. The performance levels were set to be achievable targets and were based on the opinion of the audit team.

The South African Hypertension Society has established steps to follow to control BP. The first step is to evaluate the hypertensive patients with the following three objectives:[7]

(1) to assess lifestyle and identify other cardiovascular risk factors or concomitant disorders that may affect prognosis and guide treatment
(2) to reveal identifiable causes of high blood pressure
(3) to assess the presence or absence of target organ damage and cardiovascular disease (CVD).

In a nutshell, lifestyle modifications reduce blood pressure, prevent or delay the incidence of hypertension, enhance antihypertensive drug efficacy and decrease cardiovascular risk.[5] Further decisions with regard to the introduction of antihypertensive medications depend on the current blood pressure and the level of risk as described by the first step of evaluation of all hypertensive patients.

The choice of antihypertensive medications is also influenced by the presence of other co-morbid conditions, such as ischaemic heart disease, gout or asthma. In patients without such co-morbid conditions, the first antihypertensive medications are usually the thiazide or thiazide-like diuretics.

The guidelines classify hypertension as follows:

- Normal:
  - SBP 120–129 mmHg or DBP 80–84 mmHg
- High normal:
  - SBP 130–139 mmHg or DBP 85–89 mmHg
- Stage 1 (mild hypertension):
  - SBP 140–159 mmHg or DBP 90–99 mmHg
- Stage 2 (moderate hypertension):
  - SBP 160–179 mmHg or DBP 100–109 mmHg
- Stage3 (severe hypertension):
  - SBP >180 mmHg or DBP >110 mmHg

Furthermore, the guidelines recommend the following routine investigations:

- Body weight at every visit.
- Height at first visit.
- Body mass index at every visit.
- Abdominal obesity (waist circumference or waist-to-hip ratio) at every visit.
- Urinalysis at first visit and then yearly if normal. Repeated at the next visit if abnormal. If 2+ protein or 1+ haematuria, refer for or perform further investigations.
- Blood tests for creatinine, potassium, total cholesterol and fasting blood glucose should be done yearly.
- ECG should be done yearly.

Additional investigations are to be performed if secondary causes are suspected at the first visit or if refractory hypertension exists.

Treatment of hypertension should aim to achieve a target blood pressure of ≤140/90 mmHg for most patients; and a target blood pressure of ≤130/80 mmHg for patients with diabetes mellitus or chronic kidney disease.

The criteria were discussed during a meeting with the members of the audit team that agreed upon the performance levels. Performance levels were set for the structures relevant to hypertension management, the process of managing hypertensive patients and the outcome of the management of hypertension.

Structure

One would expect certain items to be available at each facility. A score of two was assigned for full compliance, a score of one for partial compliance and zero for non-compliance. Partial compliance meant that items were present, but not in good working condition or in insufficient quantities or expired. Target standards for the structure were the presence of:

- one functional anaeroid sphygmomanometer (blood pressure machine) at each facility
- a small, medium and large blood pressure cuff at each facility
- one functional weighing scale at each facility
- one functional height scale at each facility
- the hypertension guidelines (2011 Southern African Hypertension Society) at each facility

- investigation request forms (laboratory and ECG) at each facility
- specimen tubes for blood tests at each facility
- an ECG machine at each facility
- specimen bottles for urine at each facility.

Process

Target standards for the process were the following:

- 90% of records have the height recorded once
- 90% of records contain a weight measurement at each visit in the last year
- 90% of records have a classification of hypertension control in last year
- 70% of records demonstrate appropriate drug management as per the guidelines at each visit
- 60% of records have a serum creatinine recorded once yearly
- 60% of records have a fasting blood glucose recorded once yearly
- 60% of records have a record of urinalysis for protein, blood and glucose once yearly
- 90% of records have a random total cholesterol recorded once yearly
- 60% of records have an ECG recorded once yearly
- 80% of records have health education documented (either smoking, physical activity, diet or alcohol consumption) at each visit
- 90% of records have a body mass index recorded at each visit.

Outcome

Target standards for outcomes were:

- 70% of records have a blood pressure < 140/90 mmHg
- 70% of records have a blood pressure < 130/80 mmHg for high risk patients.

Study population

Our study population included all adult hypertensive patients aged 18 years and above, who visited the facilities with a documented diagnosis of hypertension over at least a six-month period. A sample-size calculation based on an 80% ability to detect a before–after difference with a *p* value of 0.05 recommended that 233 participants be included in the audit. Exclusion criteria were defined as pregnant women, patients from outside the Moshupa clinic catchment area and hypertensive patients aged less than 18 years.

Data collection

Clients were selected systematically by taking every second patient with hypertension who walked into the consulting room for their usual review during November 2011. The folders were then put aside and retrospective data collected from the patient's file using a data collection tool in order to measure the defined criteria. This was done by the doctors and nurses in charge at each of the selected sites. The structural criteria were evaluated by an inspection of the facility by the audit team.

Data analysis

Data were captured using a Microsoft Excel spread sheet and analysed by the Centre for Statistical Consultation at Stellenbosch University. Data analysis included frequency tables and comparison for significant change between the baseline audit and re-audit. Data were categorical in nature and a Chi-square test was used to detect significant differences ($p < 0.05$).

Data interpretation

The results of the actual performance were presented to the audit team for discussion and comparison with the target standards.

The planning and implementation of change

Plans for change in clinical practice were devised by the audit team to improve the quality of care of our hypertensive patients. The team had the mandate from the main researcher to ensure implementation and monitoring of any planned changes. A draft of the plan was submitted to every sister in charge and the management of the district.

The re-audit

Data collection, data analysis and interpretation were repeated six months after the initial audit in June 2012. This period allowed time for the changes to be implemented. Further recommendations were formulated so as to improve the quality of care to an optimal level. The same hypertension tools and same standards were used during the re-audit.

Results

Patient characteristics

There were 200 participants recruited from the four different sites: Moshupa clinic (n = 108; 54.0%), Moshupa health post (n = 56; 28%), Lotlhakane health post (n = 20; 10%) and Ralekgetho health post (n = 16; 8%). Moshupa had a larger population and the facilities there were busier than the smaller health posts. The participants' mean age was 55 years and their age distribution is shown in Figure 1. Out of this sample, 68% were women and 32% were men.

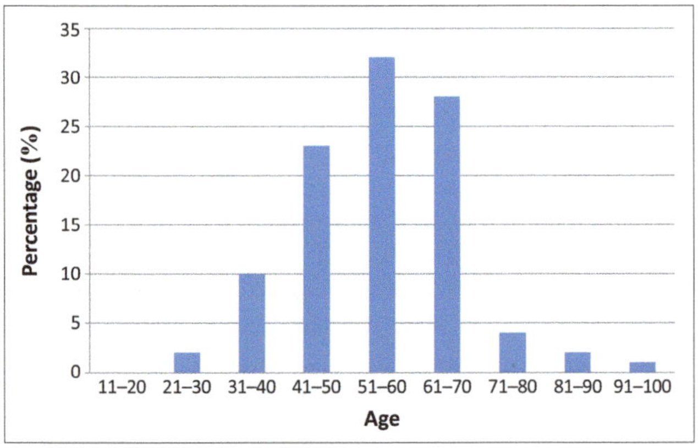

FIGURE 1: Age distribution of the sample.

Structural standards

The performance levels for structural criteria in both audits are compared in Table 1. There were four clinics and a maximum score of eight for compliance with the structural standards. Table 1 shows that six standards were achieved at baseline and nine standards in the re-audit.

Process standards

The performance level for process criteria are compared in Table 2 for both the baseline audit and the re-audit. Table 2 shows that none of the standards were achieved at baseline, but five out of 11 standards were achieved in the re-audit. There was a statistically-significant improvement during the re-audit for all the process criteria.

Outcome standards

Table 3 shows that control of blood pressure improved significantly and that the target of 70% controlled with blood pressure below 140/90 mmHg was achieved, albeit narrowly, in the re-audit.

Changes and implementation of changes

Recommendations were formulated by the audit team to address the poor performance seen in the baseline audit. Implementation of changes involved doctors, nurses and the pharmacist. The changes are summarised in Tables 4 and 5.

Discussion

Key findings and comparison with literature

The baseline audit demonstrated a poor quality of care for patients with hypertension and achieved none of the target standards. During the re-audit the structural criteria were the most improved, with six targets out of nine achieved. The process criteria showed five targets were achieved out of 11 and the outcome criteria met one target out of two. Significant improvement in performance was shown in 10 criteria although the target standard was not always met. Significant improvement in performance was the more important finding as the levels set were somewhat arbitrary and may have been too high and ambitious in many cases. It was possible to implement changes with simple interventions designed by the audit team and with regular follow up.

Improving the use of investigations was limited by the performance of the hospital-based laboratory, which often lacked reagents or had broken equipment. At the clinic level, the use of incorrect specimen bottles and forms resulted in some specimens being rejected.

TABLE 1: Results for structural target standards.

Structure standards	Baseline audit (Maximum score = 8)		Re-audit (Maximum score = 8)	
	Score (%)	Standard achieved	Score (%)	Standard achieved
There is at least a weighing scale in each facility	8 (100)	Yes	8 (100)	Yes
There is at least a height scale in each facility	0 (0)	No	8 (100)	Yes
There are laboratory request forms in each facility	5 (63)	No	8 (100)	Yes
There are specimen bottles for blood collection in each facility	4 (50)	No	6 (75)	No
There are hypertension guidelines available in each facility	2 (25)	No	8 (100)	Yes
There are functional blood pressure machines in each facility	8 (100)	Yes	8 (100)	Yes
There is a small, medium, large cuff in each facility	8 (100)	Yes	8 (100)	Yes
There are specimen bottles for urine collection in each facility	4 (50)	No	6 (75)	No
There is a functional ECG machine in each facility	0 (0)	No	0 (0)	No

TABLE 2: Results for the process standards (N = 200).

Process standard	Baseline audit		Re-audit		
	n (%)	Standard achieved	n (%)	Standard achieved	p-value
90% of patients have control of hypertension classified	48 (24)	No	112 (56)	No	< 0.001
90% of patients have height measured	31 (15)	No	157 (79)	No	< 0.001
90% of patients have weight measured	144 (72)	No	167 (84)	No	0.002
90% of patients have BMI calculated at each visit	25 (12)	No	156 (78)	No	< 0.001
60% of patients have total cholesterol checked annually	51 (26)	No	137 (69)	Yes	< 0.001
60% of patients have fasting blood glucose checked annually	22 (11)	No	120 (60)	Yes	< 0.001
60% of patients have urine checked for protein, glucose and blood annually	19 (10)	No	120 (60)	Yes	< 0.001
60% of patients have ECG performed	44 (22)	No	122 (61)	Yes	< 0.001
60% of patients have creatinine checked once annually	44 (22)	No	117 (58)	No	< 0.001
80% of patients have health education documented at each visit	71 (35.5)	No	144 (72)	No	< 0.001
70% of patients have appropriate drug management at each visit	108 (54)	No	152 (76)	Yes	< 0.001

TABLE 3: Results for outcome standards.

Outcome standards	Baseline audit (N = 200)		Re- audit (N = 200)		
	n(%)	Standard achieved	n(%)	Standard achieved	p-value
70% of records with BP < 140/90	97 (49)	No	139 (70)	Yes	< 0.001
70% of record with BP < 130/80 for high risk patients	32 (16)	No	53 (27)	No	< 0.001

TABLE 4: Changes in clinical practice for structural standards.

Structure standards	Recommendation of audit team	Action taken
There is at least a weighing scale in each facility	Weighing scales should be ordered by the nurse in charge of the facility.	Audit meeting were held every Thursday. The nurse in charge at each facility checked daily to ensure that patients' weight was taken at each visit.
There is at least a height measure in each facility	Height measure should be ordered by the nurse in charge.	Audit meeting were held every Thursday. Nurse in charge checked daily to ensure that height was measured at least once.
There are specimen bottles for blood and urine collection	Each nurse in charge should order enough specimen bottles for his/her facility.	A physical count was made on a daily basis. An order was made to the central medical store monthly or to the hospital for supply.
There are functional BP machines in each facility	Each nurse in charge should order BP machine for her/his facility.	An order of blood pressure machines was placed by the district pharmacist at the central medical store as part of her action plan.
There are hypertension guidelines in each facility in the consulting room	Doctors should photocopy guidelines and make them available in each consulting room.	Guidelines were available in the consulting room for easy and quick reference. The guidelines were made available at each facility by the audit team.
There are request forms for investigations	Nurse in charge should order or photocopy enough request forms for his/her facility. Soft copies should be available on the main clinic computer.	Request forms were printed from the computer on a daily basis and distributed to facilities where the audit was conducted. Forms were also ordered from central medical stores.

TABLE 5: Recommendations and actual changes for process standards.

Process standards	Recommendation of audit team	Action taken
90% of patients have their hypertension control assessed	Doctors and nurses to ensure that hypertension control is assessed for every patient.	An in-service training on hypertension guideline was held in clinics attended by nurses and doctors. Guidelines were distributed to participants. Meetings were held every Thursday afternoon. This needed to be reinforced by audit team.
90% of patients have their height measured	Doctors and nurses to ensure that height is measured at first visit.	The health auxiliary officer at the screening point measured height for each patient height scale was checked every morning.
90% of patients have weight measured	Doctors and nurses to ensure that weight is measured at each visit.	The health auxiliary measured weight for each patient and checked the weight scale every morning.
90% of patients have BMI calculated	Doctors and nurses to ensure that BMI is calculated at each visit.	BMI calculation was taught during training. Calculation was done at screening point or in the consultation room.
60% of patients have cholesterol checked and interpreted	Doctors and nurses to ensure that cholesterol is checked yearly.	Samples were collected from Monday to Thursday and transported to the hospital laboratory for analysis. The nurse in charge ensured specimens were transported in time. During our Thursday meeting emphasis was laid on the importance and interpretation of investigations in managing hypertensive patients.
60% of patients have fasting blood glucose checked and interpreted	Doctors and nurses to ensure fasting blood glucose checked yearly.	Samples were collected and sent to hospital for analysis. An order for glucometers has been placed. Thursday meeting discussed interpretation of results.
60% of patients have urine checked for protein, glucose and blood	Doctors and nurses to ensure urine checked yearly if normal and repeated at next visit if abnormal.	Samples were transported to the hospital from Monday to Thursday. Thursday meeting discussed urinalysis results.
60% of patients have ECG done and interpreted	Doctors to order ECG yearly.	There was a need to have an ECG machine locally. Clinics relied on the ECG machine at the hospital. Meetings were held to teach basic ECG interpretation. The audit team has advocated for purchase of at least one ECG machine in the district.
60% of patients have creatinine checked and interpreted	Doctors and nurses to order creatinine yearly.	There was need to have laboratory facility in Moshupa. Meeting were held on Thursdays to review shortfalls identified by the audit.
80% of patients have health education done and documented	Doctors and nurses to ensure ongoing health education.	Needs to be reinforced. Counselling on life style modification – diet, exercise, smoking and alcohol consumption in the management plan. The points discussed were to be documented on the patient's card. Patients were issued with a written plan documented in the medical record and tailored to individual patients. Health educators assisted with morning health talks.
70% of patients have appropriate drug management	Doctors and nurses to ensure appropriate medication is prescribed.	Hypertension guidelines were made available in the consulting room. In service training assisted with adherence to the guidelines.

BMI, body mass index.

Our study showed improved blood pressure control with 70% of records recording a blood pressure of less than 140/80 mmHg in the re-audit. These results are supported by a number of other studies where improving the technical quality of care was an effective strategy for improving blood pressure control and was achieved by relatively simple interventions within quality improvement cycles.[12,13,14,15]

Furthermore, JNC7 suggests that healthcare providers give insufficient attention to health education.[5] This study demonstrated that the frequency of health education improved, although the audit cannot assess the content or quality of the counselling.

Routine laboratory tests recommended in the South African guidelines included a 12-lead ECG, urinalysis, blood glucose, creatinine and total cholesterol. These laboratory tests were seldom carried out in the baseline audit, although this improved following the planning and implementation of change to clinical practice. This shows a lack of adherence on the part of the healthcare providers as suggested by the JNC 7 report.[5] Primary care in Botswana has not been organised for the adequate management of non-communicable diseases, such as hypertension, and yet this audit shows that significant improvement can easily be made when attention is given to the requirements. At the end of the study, however, none of the clinics had easy access to an ECG machine.

Limitations

Thirty-three patients were lost to follow up and the sample size with paired data was reduced to 200. The sample, however, appeared to be powered adequately to detect significant differences in the re-audit. Poor record keeping meant that not all activities were recorded in the notes and some patients kept their own records, which could not be traced at subsequent visits, resulting in missing data. The anaeroid sphygmomanometers were not calibrated regularly and thus the blood pressure measurements used in the audit were not taken under ideal conditions. The adherence of staff to the rules for blood pressure measurement was also not observed or assessed, although training on this was given prior to the audit.

Recommendations and implications

Improvement in performance should be seen as an ongoing process so that improvements are maintained and further improvements targeted. Such a commitment must involve the local facility staff and the district management. Realistic performance targets should be set from the baseline findings and the audit extended to other facilities and health programmes run in the district.

The process criteria need additional interventions with regards to access to investigations and essential equipment. ECG machines, glucometers and urine dipsticks need to be procured. The district still relies on the mission hospital for most of the investigations. The audit team advocated for procurement of basic equipment for the main clinic as well as a laboratory facility for the district.

Conclusions

The quality of care for hypertension was suboptimal in our setting as highlighted by the baseline audit. Simple interventions were designed and implemented to improve the quality of care of hypertensive patients. These interventions led to significant improvement in structural and process criteria. A corresponding significant improvement in the control of blood pressure was also seen. It is recommended that the quality improvement process be continued, expanded to other clinics and to other chronic conditions.

Acknowledgements

I would like to acknowledge my gratitude to the audit team and the clinic staff for their support. Thanks to Prof Daan G. Nel at the Centre for Statistical Consultation for help with the analysis.

Competing interests

The authors declare that they have no financial or personal relationship(s) which may have inappropriately influenced them in writing this article.

Authors' contributions

C.K. (University of Stellenbosch) performed the study as part of her MMed degree and was supervised by R.M. (University of Stellenbosch). The dissertation was adapted for publication jointly by C.K. and R.M.

References

1. Steyn K, Bradshaw D, Norman R, et al. Determinants and treatment of hypertension in South Africans: the first Demographic and Health survey. S Afr Med J. 2008; 98(5):376–380. PMid:18637309
2. Pinkney-Atkinson VJ. Hypertension treatment algorithm. PNT. 2008;12(1):37–41.
3. World Health Organization. Botswana Country Profile. [document on Internet]. [c2010] [cited 2013 Nov. 29]. Available from http://www.who.int/nmh/countries/bwa_en.pdf
4. Mengesha AY. Hypertension and related risks factors in type 2 diabetes mellitus (DM) patients in Gaborone City Council clinics, Gaborone, Botswana. Afr Health Sci. 2007;7(4):244–245. PMid:21499491, PMCid:PMC3074377
5. US Department of Health and Human Services. Complete report. The seventh report of the joint national committee on prevention, detection, evaluation, and treatment of high blood pressure. [document on Internet]. [c2004] [cited 2011 May 11]. Available from www.nhlbi.nih.gov/guidelines/hypertension/jnc7full.pdf
6. Amod A, Motala A, Levitt N, Berg J, Young M, Grobler N et al. The 2012 SEMDSA guideline for the management of type 2 diabetes (revised). JEMDSA. 2012;17(2 Suppl 1):S1–S95.
7. Seedat YK, Rayner BL. South African hypertension guidelines 2011. S Afr Med J. 2012;102(1):57–84.
8. Steyn K, Fourie J, Temple N (editors). Chronic diseases of lifestyle in South Africa: 1995–2005. Cape Town: Medical Research Council; 2006.
9. Ministry of Health. Botswana treatment guide 2007. Gaborone: Ministry of Health; 2007.
10. Mash B. How to audit or improve the quality of your service. In B Mash B, J Blitz-Lindeque (editors). South African Family Practice Manual. Cape Town: Van Schaik, 2006; p. 402–403.
11. Central Statistics Office. Population of towns, villages and associated localities. Gaborone: Central Statistics Office; 2002.
12. Cleveland Clinic Medicine Institute. Best practices in hypertension: the hypertension improvement project. [document on Internet]. [c2008] [cited 2013 Jul 24]. Available from http://www.amga.org/research/research/Hypertension/Compendiums/cleveland.pdf
13. De Vries E. Conference presentation. Auditing chronic disease care: does it make a difference. Presented at 15th National Family Practitioners Conference 11-12th May 2012. [page on Internet]. [c2012] [cited 2013 Nov. 29]. Available from http://saafp.org/conferences/index.php/ANFPC/2012/paper/view/257
14. Slingers N, De Villiers PJT. Evaluation of the effect of the introduction of a hypertension club on the management of hypertension at community health centre in the Cape Town Metropole. SA Fam Pract. 2009;51(2):143–147.
15. Onwukwe SC, Omole OB. Drug therapy, lifestyle modification and blood pressure control in a primary care facility, south of Johannesburg, South Africa: an audit of hypertension management. SA Fam Pract. 2012;54(2):156–161.

3

African Primary Care Research: Choosing a topic and developing a proposal

Author:
Bob Mash[1]

Affiliation:
[1]Division of Family Medicine and Primary Care, Stellenbosch University, South Africa

Correspondence to:
Bob Mash

Email:
rm@sun.ac.za

Postal address:
Box 19063, Tygerberg 7505, South Africa

This is the first in a series of articles on primary care research in the African context. The aim of the series is to help build capacity for primary care research amongst the emerging departments of family medicine and primary care on the continent. Many of the departments are developing Masters of Medicine programmes in Family Medicine and their students will all be required to complete research studies as part of their degree. This series is being written with this audience in particular in mind – both the students who must conceptualise and implement a research project as well as their supervisors who must assist them.

This article gives an overview of the African primary care context, followed by a typology of primary care research. The article then goes on to assist the reader with choosing a topic and defining their research question. Finally the article addresses the structure and contents of a research proposal and the ethical issues that should be considered.

Recherche africaine en soins de santé primaires: choisir un sujet et développer une proposition. Voici le premier article d'une série sur la recherche en soins de santé primaire dans le contexte africain. L'objectif de cette série est de renforcer les capacités de recherche en soins de santé primaire parmi les départements émergents de médecine familiale et de soins de santé primaire sur le continent. Beaucoup de départements développent actuellement des programmes de Masters de Médecine en Médecine familiale, et leurs étudiants devront effectuer des recherche dans le cadre de leur diplôme. Cette série est rédigée en ayant ce type de lecteurs particulier à l'esprit: les étudiants qui doivent conceptualiser et mettre en place un projet de recherche, ainsi que leurs superviseurs qui doivent les aider.

Cet article donne un aperçu du contexte africain de soins de santé primaire, suivi d'une typologie de recherche en soins de santé primaires. La suite de l'article aide le lecteur à choisir un sujet et à définir sa question de recherche. L'article s'achève en traitant de la structure et des contenus d'une proposition de recherche et des questions éthiques qui doivent être prises en compte.

Introduction

This is the first in a series of articles on primary care research in the African context. The aim of the series is to help build capacity for primary care research amongst the emerging departments of family medicine and primary care on the continent. Many of the departments are developing Masters of Medicine programmes in Family Medicine and their students will all be required to complete research studies as part of their degree. This series is being written with this audience in particular in mind – both the students who must conceptualise and implement a research project as well as their supervisors who must assist them. The emergence of a group of doctors, all of whom are required to perform primary care research, is also a major opportunity for the strengthening of primary healthcare.

The African context

Leading causes of the burden of disease in the African region include HIV, lower respiratory tract infection, diarrhoeal disease, malaria, neonatal infections, birth asphyxia, prematurity, tuberculosis, road traffic accidents and malnutrition.[1] Some countries, such as South Africa, also have a high burden of disease from violence and non-communicable chronic diseases.[1,2] Africa has the lowest life expectancy of all the world's regions.[1]

The African region has the lowest numbers of doctors, nurses and midwives per capita and primary healthcare systems are particularly underdeveloped.[1] The World Health Assembly has called for a multidisciplinary team approach to primary healthcare that would include community health workers, nurses, midwives, family physicians and allied health professionals.[3] The World Health Organization has called for a re-commitment to primary healthcare and has emphasised the need for four reforms: universal coverage to improve equity, service delivery reforms to make health systems more people centred, leadership reforms to make health authorities more reliable and public policy reforms to promote and protect the health of communities.[4] It is clear that the challenges facing primary care providers are immense, both in terms of the burden of disease in the people they care for and the organisational issues in the health systems they work within. The need for primary care research to assist in overcoming these challenges is also clear.

It is, however, difficult to generalise about Africa because of its vast geographic size and its huge variety of cultures, health systems and health needs. The intention of this article is not to suggest a list of research priorities or topics, but to present a conceptual framework for thinking about primary care research in our context. I will also outline the practical process of deciding on a topic and writing your research proposal.

Primary care research

Primary care research can be characterised as research that is not only about primary healthcare, but also conducted within and even by primary care providers. In the African context, one might also speak of research conducted in the health district as family physicians may also work as generalists in the district hospital.

One of the limitations of evidence-based medicine applied to the primary healthcare context is that much of the evidence is derived from hospital-based settings and populations and is difficult to generalise to primary care. Primary care has many differences from the hospital context, for example the range of conditions seen is different, the probability of severe disease in any encounter is far lower and providers are often managing multiple problems simultaneously. There is therefore a need for research to be conducted in primary care and to produce a more relevant evidence base. When thinking about primary care research, one can categorise it into the following types.[5]

Basic

Basic research has been defined as studies that 'help develop the research tools for primary care'.[5] The International Classification of Primary Care is one such tool that allows for the systematic coding of reasons for encounter, diagnoses and episodes of care.[6] More modest examples include the development of a 360-degree evaluation tool for assessing the impact of family physicians on the local health system or adaptation of the Primary Care Assessment Tool to local primary care systems.[7]

Clinical

Clinical research focuses on the burden of disease and the clinical processes involved. This may include the natural history, epidemiology, diagnosis and management of common clinical problems. Studies at a Masters level often focus on improving the quality of care or implementing guidelines for specific conditions or on understanding more about the patient's experience of care or perspective on their health. Large-scale clinical trials and observational studies are not usually feasible at a Masters level unless several students are co-opted as research assistants to contribute parts toward a larger study. Translational research may focus on whether an intervention is feasible in low-resource settings and whether the resultant benefits are worth the cost. Sometimes a systematic review may address a relevant specific clinical question.

Health services

Health services research focuses on the way primary care is organised and the processes involved. Key attributes of primary care, which cut across multiple clinical conditions, may be looked at, for example:[8]

- Access to primary care services: Availability of services, geographic accessibility, how care is organised in order to make it more accessible, affordability, acceptability of services to patients, actual utilisation and equality of access for different groups.
- Continuity of primary care: How well does the health service care for a patient over time and multiple illness episodes, what is the nature and quality of the relationship with the healthcare providers and how is the incremental information organised and accessed in the medical record?
- Coordination of primary care: How well does the health service coordinate a patient's care within and between levels of care? For example, between community-based and facility-based services, or between primary care and district hospitals, or with secondary care. How is care coordinated within the primary care team or facility?
- Comprehensiveness of care: Is the full range of services available to meet all the patient's health care needs?

Health systems

Health systems research is more at a policy level and may look at the relationship of health policies to other political, social or economic systems. It may also look at how policy is implemented and the impact on services, equity and health outcomes. For example, many of the human resource challenges for primary care are health systems issues, including the roles and responsibilities of the family physician in that system.

Educational

Research in this area focuses on the development of educational programmes for family medicine and primary care and continuing professional development. For example, research may look at the clinical skills that should be taught, the learning outcomes required or the use of learning portfolios. Research may also look at recruitment and retention of professionals, as well as career pathways.

Choosing a topic

Having outlined a broad typology of the different kinds of primary care research that are possible, the postgraduate student must eventually decide on a single topic for their research project. This section discusses some of the key considerations in choosing a topic.

One of the easiest routes for a postgraduate student is to become involved in a larger study that an established researcher has already designed. The advantage for the student is that they do not have to conceptualise the project from scratch, the researcher may already have obtained funding for the work and the work may have a higher impact. The advantage for the researcher is that they can expand the scope of their work through the use of multiple research assistants, build research capacity and produce a more significant piece of work.

Even if such a large-scale project is not available it can be helpful for key stakeholders and established researchers to suggest priorities to the students. At a local level the family physician trainer, facility or district manager and the student may discuss how best to use the opportunity for a research project to take things forward. The university and the department of health may also have documents outlining research priorities and key focus areas.

Often a student will generate potential research questions from reflection on their own challenges and experience in service delivery. Sometimes reading the scientific literature may prompt questions, seeing as most original research articles discuss the need for further research and unanswered questions. At an individual level, the student can judge the value of pursuing any research question by considering the following issues:

- How passionate or interested am I in this topic?
- What is the social value of this topic – how relevant or important is it to health needs in my context? Will answering this question make a difference?
- What is the scientific value of this topic – do I already know the answer to this question? What is the original contribution of this study to new knowledge? Sometimes the contribution to new knowledge is within the African context, even though the question may have been addressed elsewhere. It may be necessary to explore the literature before answering this question. Exploring the literature often leads to a new focus or more original question within the same area of interest.
- How feasible is it for me to answer – can I answer this question given my time, expertise and available resources? Students are often overly optimistic about the type of study design that is feasible. Clinical trials are often suggested, but in reality most Masters students do not have the time, financial resources or expertise to be a principal investigator of such a trial.

It can be helpful to actually rate your answers to the questions above to compare multiple possible research questions. It is usually helpful to discuss your ideas with your supervisor or a more experienced researcher. All comments and suggestions are worth considering seriously although you should not abandon your own viewpoint too easily.

Writing your research proposal

The following structure is widely accepted as being suitable for a research proposal.[9]

Project title

Your title should make clear the purpose of the research and sometimes the study design as well. It is likely that it will change as your research proposal evolves. Ensure that the final title is not too lengthy or obscure.

Cover page

Provide your name, student number, registered course, supervisors, collaborators, affiliations and contact details, that is, address, telephone, fax and email address.

Summary

You may well find this easier to write at the end, once you are clear about the project. It should summarise the project succinctly and stimulate interest in the topic. The summary is important because this may be the only part that key people look at, for example members of the ethics committee other than the designated reviewers or facility managers who must give permission for the research. The summary should also be structured into, for example, background, aim and objectives, methods and ethical considerations. It should not be longer than one to two pages.

Introduction

The introduction section to your proposal should convince the reader of the social and scientific value of your study. It would be unethical to conduct research that has no social or scientific value. You must construct a logical argument that utilises your review of the literature to support your argument for the social and scientific value of the research. In some studies it will also be important to present the theoretical basis and conceptual framework for the study. How to search, obtain and appraise the literature for this purpose, as well as how to construct this argument, are discussed in another article in this series. Note that no separate section for a literature review is proposed; instead, the literature is aligned with a specific purpose in the introduction.

Aim and objectives

You should define the main research question that you intend to answer and any hypothesis that will be tested. Your aim is often the same as your research question, but expressed as a statement rather than a question. You can then break down the broad aim into a number of secondary components or objectives. Be very careful that your choice of words here is an accurate reflection of what you intend to do (i.e. explore, measure, compare, evaluate). Your objectives are really aspects of the research question that the study will answer and should not be a description of the methodological steps. In the conclusion to your thesis you will conclude in terms of your findings for each of these objectives. Table 1 gives some examples of research questions, aims and objectives. If your research question is clearly formulated, the correct study design will be much easier to identify. However, if the research question is unclear, it is almost impossible to choose a correct design.

Methods

In this section, you need to consider the following aspects:

Study design

What type of design is appropriate to achieve your aim and answer your research question? The methods section will vary according to the type of study design and whether it is within an empirical-analytical paradigm (usually involving quantitative techniques such as randomised controlled trials, diagnostic studies, case-control studies, cohort studies or cross-sectional surveys), an interpretive-hermeneutic paradigm (usually qualitative techniques such as in-depth interviews or focus group interviews) or an emancipatory-critical paradigm (participatory action research). Many universities will also accept quality improvement cycles and project evaluations at a Masters level. It should be a clear and well-structured account of what you are going to do, of how you will establish the quality of what you plan to do and of any anticipated problems or limitations. Other articles in this series will discuss in detail the common study designs used by postgraduate family medicine students.

Setting

Describe the setting of the research study and study population. These could include, for example, the characteristics of the community involved as well as the facilities, staff and services available in the health system where the study is located.

Study population and sampling strategy

This refers to the manner in which you select people for the study or assign them to control or intervention groups. The study population should be defined in terms of who they are, where they are and any time periods. Define any inclusion or exclusion criteria. The size of the sample from this study population that you want to include in the study should be defined and justified. In quantitative studies, this requires a full explanation of the assumptions used in the calculation and usually needs the help of a statistician or at least advice from your supervisor. For simple sample-size calculations you can use an online statistical calculator or free software (for example, http://wwwn.cdc.gov/epiinfo/html/downloads.htm). The statistical issues vary depending on whether it is a representative sample, as in a survey, or whether a comparison of groups is involved. In qualitative studies, this relates to issues of saturation, whereby no new themes are being generated from further sampling. Once the sample size is clear then the process of obtaining this sample must be described. For example, will selection be random, systematic (every nth person) or purposeful and based on pre-defined criteria? How, in practical terms, will selection be done – by whom, where and how?

Interventions

In the case of an experimental-type design, describe the interventions that you will make on different groups.

Data collection

Describe the types of measurements or data collection methods that you will use. The validity of tools, such as questionnaires, needs to be established or you must describe how you will address this. It is usually better to use or adapt tools that have been developed and validated previously. The data collection tools such as interview guides or questionnaires are usually included as an appendix. This

TABLE 1: Examples of research questions, aims and objectives.

Examples	Research question	Aim	Objectives	Study design
Example 1	What do health-promotion officers think and feel about their implementation of a group diabetes education programme?	To explore what health-promotion officers think and feel about their implementation of a group diabetes education programme.	To explore their experience of the training they will receive on how to deliver and facilitate the education programme. To explore their views on the group diabetes education programme: the design of the programme, the resource materials provided, the information on diabetes, the facilitation style, the response of patients and any other issues.	Qualitative focus group interviews.
Example 2	What is the prevalence of substance abuse and its risk factors amongst adolescents attending high schools in the Example area?	To determine the prevalence of substance abuse and its risk factors amongst adolescents attending high schools in the Example area.	To determine the prevalence of tobacco smoking and use of alcohol, methamphetamine, cannabis, heroin, cocaine and any other illicit substances amongst adolescent high school students in the Example area. To evaluate the relationships between tobacco smoking, alcohol, cannabis and other illicit drug abuse. To evaluate the importance in this context of known factors associated with substance abuse. To evaluate any gender differences relevant to substance abuse.	Cross-sectional survey.
Example 3	How to improve the quality of care for congestive cardiac failure at Example Community Health Centre?	To assess and improve the quality of care for congestive cardiac failure at Example Community Health Centre.	To assess the current quality of care for congestive cardiac failure. To plan and implement changes to improve the quality of care. To assess if these changes are associated with a measurable improvement in the quality of care.	Quality improvement cycle.

section must also describe in practical terms the process of data collection – who will be involved, where this will happen, how they will do it and how language barriers will be addressed. Future articles in this series will focus on the use of questionnaires and qualitative interviews.

Data analysis

Describe how you will capture and store your data. Describe how you will check and clean your data prior to analysis. Describe the way in which you will analyse this data. Describe any software that you will use. You may need to consult a statistician for help to determine the appropriate statistical tests to use. Describe the steps in qualitative data analysis. Future articles in this series will focus on quantitative and qualitative data analysis.

Ethical considerations

Before embarking on any research study it is necessary to consider the ethical challenges. There are many examples in Africa of vulnerable communities being abused by researchers and of research findings being misrepresented. The following seven-point checklist has been developed specifically for health research in developing country settings:[10]

Social and scientific value

- Is the research question relevant?
- Is the research that is going to be reported been done previously? Sometimes, even if it has not been done in the researcher's own setting, it can still have scientific value.

Scientific validity

- Is the design and methodology of the study sound?
- Has the analysis process been considered?
- Is the sample size justified?

Fair selection of study population

- Has the study population been chosen fairly?
- Have any groups been excluded that could benefit from the research, because of non-scientific reasons, such as non-English or non-French speakers?
- Is the study population vulnerable in any way?

Favourable risk–benefit ratio

- Have the risks and benefits been assessed as accurately as possible?
- Is the risk–benefit ratio favourable?
- Are risks minimised?
- Are benefits maximised?

Independent review

- Where will the research be submitted for independent ethical review? Each university usually has an ethics committee responsible for this.
- Permission needed? Often the department of health or health facility has a process for giving permission to conduct the research.

Informed consent

- Has sufficient information been disclosed in a culturally- and linguistically-sensitive manner? The informed consent form should be written in simple, non-technical language and addressed directly to the person concerned.
- Waivers of informed consent? In some cases, such as the use of data obtained retrospectively from medical records for audit purposes, it may be impossible and unreasonable to find each patient in order to obtain informed consent. In situations such as this, a waiver of informed consent can be requested from the ethics committee.
- Children? Teenagers? Most countries have a legally-defined age at which children can consent to research. Below this age, informed consent must be obtained from the child's parent or legal guardian. Assent must still be obtained from the child. When your study population includes children, this can impose additional burdens on the research process in order to obtain consent.

Respect for participants and study communities

- Do the participants know they can withdraw from the study at any time?
- Have issues of confidentiality and privacy been addressed adequately? Participant names and personal details, such as telephone numbers, should not be sent to the statistician in the spreadsheet for analysis. Transcripts and quotations should not identify individuals. It may be necessary to protect confidentiality in data collection tools by the use of study codes rather than personal identifiers. Audiotapes of interviews should be stored securely and destroyed at a time specified in the proposal.

Timetable

Write a simple timetable of how long it will take to complete each part of the research from start to finish. A Gantt bar chart is another useful way of presenting the timetable.[11] This will include planning and gaining approval, data collection, data analysis and writing up. Be aware that planning and writing up often take longer than you anticipate. Think about how you will set aside time on a regular basis so as to complete the research project. The whole process can take two to three years, even for a relatively simple research project, thus students should plan their time accordingly. For example, you may need to schedule leave for data collection or writing up of your final thesis. Failure to complete the research assignment on time is a frequent reason for delay in graduating from the MMed programme.

Funding and budget

Present a budget of the financial support that you need in order to complete the research and describe the potential sources of funding. Consider whether you should submit formal funding proposals to bodies such as the Medical Research Council. Most Masters level research does not require large-scale funding and funds can be provided by the researcher themselves or the university.

References

List references to citations given in your proposal in an approved style, such as the Vancouver style, which is used in many journals.[12] It is important to be very careful about following the exact formatting and content requirements for the style and for each type of reference you use, such as a book, journal article or internet source. In Vancouver style, the citation is a number in square brackets or in superscript that is inserted after the full stop at the end of the sentence. References are listed in numerical sequence, in the order in which they are first used in the text. It is recommended, if you have access, that you use a reference manager software, which can automatically create citations and reference lists in different styles. Look carefully at the reference list at the end of this article for examples of how to format a journal article, book chapter or internet source.

Conclusion

This article introduces the series on primary care research and argues for the importance of building research capacity in the African context. The article presents an overview of the different types of primary care research and then focuses on the practical steps of choosing a research topic and writing the proposal. Future articles in the series will focus on different types of study design, data collection methods and data analysis. The final article will outline the writing of the thesis, research assignment or journal article.

Acknowledgements

This series is funded by the Stellenbosch University Rural Medical Education Partnership Initiative (SURMEPI).

Competing interests

The author declares that he has no financial or personal relationship(s) which may have inappropriately influenced him in writing this article.

References

1. Economist Intelligence Unit. The future of healthcare in Africa. [document on Internet]. c2012 [cited 2013 Aug. 12]. Available from: http://www.hst.org.za/publications/future-healthcare-africa
2. Bradshaw D, Norman R, Schneider M. A clarion call for action based on refined DALY estimates for South Africa. S Afr Med J. 2007;97(6):438, 440.
3. 62nd World Health Assembly. Primary health care, including health systems: Resolution 62.12. 18–22 May. Geneva: World Health Assembly. [document on Internet]. c2009 [cited 2013 Sep. 26]. Available from: http://www.15by15.org/wp-content/uploads/2009/05/primary_health_care_resolution_wha.pdf
4. World Health Organization. World Health Report – Primary Health Care: Now more than ever. Geneva: World Health Organization. [page on Internet]. c2008 [cited 2013 Sep. 26]. Available from: http://www.who.int/whr/2008/en/
5. Beasley JW, Starfield B, van Weel C, et al. Global health and primary care research. J Am Board Fam Med. 2007;20(6):518–526. http://dx.doi.org/10.3122/jabfm.2007.06.070172, PMid:17954858
6. WONCA International Classification Committee. International Classification of Primary Care (ICPC-2). 2nd ed. Oxford: Oxford University Press; 1998.
7. Bresick G. Assessing primary care performance – essential for revitalising district health services. 15th National Family Practitioners Conference. 11–12 May. Cape Town: SA Academy of Family Physicians; 2012.
8. Kringos DS, Boerma WGW, Hutchinson A, et al. The breadth of primary care: a systematic literature review of its core dimensions. BMC Health Serv Res. 2010;10:65. http://dx.doi.org/10.1186/1472-6963-10-65, PMid:20226084, PMCid:PMC2848652
9. Mash B, Blitz-Lindeque J, editors. South African Family Practice Manual. 2nd ed. Pretoria: Van Schaik; 2006.
10. Emanuel EJ, Wendler D, Killen J, et al. What makes clinical research in developing countries ethical? The benchmarks of ethical research. J Infect Dis. 2004;189(5):930–937. http://dx.doi.org/10.1086/381709, PMid:14976611
11. Wikipedia. Gantt Chart. [page on Internet]. No date [cited 2013 Sep. 03]. Available from: http://en.wikipedia.org/wiki/Gantt_chart
12. Van Dyk T, Coetzee M. Make sense of referencing: The Harvard, APA and Vancouver methods and the footnote system (3rd ed). Stellenbosch: Stellenbosch University Language Centre. [document on intranet]. c2010 [cited 2013 Sep. 26]. Available from: http://wiki.lib.sun.ac.za/images/a/a8/LanguageCentre_Reference_Techniques2010.pdf

Factors that influence contraceptive use amongst women in Vanga health district, Democratic Republic of Congo

Authors:
Kangale Izale[1]
Indiran Govender[2]
Jean-Pierre L. Fina[1]
John Tumbo[2]

Affiliations:
[1]Department of Family Medicine, Protestant University of Congo, Democratic Republic of Congo

[2]Department of Family Medicine and Primary Health Care, University of the Limpopo, Medunsa Campus, South Africa

Correspondence to:
Indiran Govender

Email:
indiran.govender@gmail.com

Postal address:
PO Box 222, Medunsa, 0204

Background: Contraception is often necessary in order to plan for children and without it there is a risk of unplanned pregnancies. In the Democratic Republic of Congo, this often results in abortions by untrained persons with resultant morbidity and mortality.

Aim: To investigate the factors that influence contraceptive use amongst women of childbearing age in the Vanga health zone.

Methods: Cross-sectional survey using interviewer-administered questionnaires.

Results: Of the 384 women recruited, a majority (46.1%) were in the 31–40 year age group; 52% had reached primary school and 88% did not have formal employment. One hundred and forty of the participants reported current use of contraception, with 60% of them using modern methods of contraception; 36.1% of them had begun using contraception before the age of 20; and the most common methods were oral contraceptive pills and injection, each accounting for 22.9%. There was variation in the duration of contraceptive use and the main reason for using contraception was to space children. Of the participants, 20.7% had been using contraception for more than two years. Seventy-seven (31.5%) of the women reported they did not use contraception because of a fear of side effects. Forty-four (18%) reported that they are unable to afford contraception, 38 (15.6%) had husbands who disapproved of contraceptive usage, 26 (10.6%) had a fear of infertility, 18 (7.4%) practised a religion that did not allow them to use contraception and 12 of the women (4.9%) did not use contraception because it was unavailable to them.

Conclusion: Barriers to contraception in our study were fears of side effects and infertility, cost, male partner's objection, unavailability of contraception and religious beliefs.

Les facteurs qui influencent l'utilisation des contraceptifs par les femmes dans le district de santé de Vanga, en République Démocratique du Congo.

Contexte: La contraception est souvent nécessaire pour la planification familiale, et sans elle on risque des grossesses non planifiées. En République Démocratique du Congo cela donne souvent lieu à des avortements par des personnes non qualifiées conduisant à la morbidité et mortalité.

Objectif: Etudier les facteurs qui influencent l'utilisation des contraceptifs chez les femmes en âge d'avoir des enfants dans la zone de santé de Vanga.

Méthodes: Etude transversale utilisant des questionnaires remplis par l'enquêteur.

Résultats: Des 384 femmes recrutées, la majorité (46.1%) appartenait au groupe d'âge de 31 à 40 ans; 52% avaient été à l'école primaire et 88% n'avaient pas d'emploi dans le secteur structuré. Cent quarante des participantes ont déclaré qu'elles utilisaient des contraceptifs, dont 60% utilisaient des méthodes modernes de contraception; 36.1% avaient commencé à utiliser la contraception avant l'âge de 20 ans; les méthodes les plus courantes étaient les pilules contraceptives orales et les injections, comptant chacune pour 22.9%. Il y avait une différence dans la durée d'utilisation des contraceptifs et la raison principale pour leur utilisation qui était l'espacement des naissances. Parmi les participantes, 20.7% utilisaient la contraception depuis plus de deux ans. Soixante-dix-sept femmes (31.5%) ont déclaré qu'elles n'utilisaient pas la contraception par crainte des effets secondaires. Quarante quatre (18%) ont déclaré qu'elles n'avaient pas les moyens d'utiliser la contraception, 38 (15.6%) avaient des maris qui étaient contre la contraception, 26 (10.6%) avaient peur de l'infertilité, 18 (7.4%) pratiquaient une religion qui ne leur permettait pas d'utiliser la contraception et 12 femmes (4.9%) n'utilisaient pas la contraception parce qu'elle n'était pas disponible pour elles.

Conclusion: Dans notre étude les barrières à la contraception étaient la crainte des effets secondaires et de l'infertilité, le coût, l'objection du partenaire mâle, la non disponibilité de la contraception et les croyances religieuses.

Introduction

Women worldwide are exposed to the risk of unwanted and unintended pregnancies as a result of ineffective or non-use of contraception. Women who are able to use known contraceptive methods are able to decide if and when they want children, as well as how many children they want.[1,2] Contraceptive practices entail contraceptive use or non-use, discontinuation of contraception and/or failure to use any of the contraceptive methods according to a specified set of guidelines.[3]

In the developing world, almost 137 million women who want to avoid pregnancy do not use any method of family planning.[4,5] Of the 210 million pregnancies that occur each year, almost 80 million are unplanned. Each year, approximately 42 million pregnant women seek termination of their unplanned pregnancy. Of the 20 million women who undergo unsafe abortions by untrained staff, 67 000 die annually. Almost all of these deaths (99%) occur in underdeveloped countries.[6]

Two nationally-representative surveys in Britain and Germany revealed that 67% of British and 96% of German women used contraception,[4] although contraceptive use patterns differed between East Germany, West Germany and Great Britain. Oral contraceptive use declined with age in both countries. Intrauterine device use and sterilisation increased with age. In Britain, oral contraceptive use was greater in urban areas than in rural areas. Intrauterine contraceptive device use and sterilisation rates were higher and oral contraceptive use rates were lower amongst married women as compared with never-married women. Increased church attendance was associated with a higher rate of condom usage. In Europe, there was no clear association between employment status and contraceptive practices.[4]

In South Africa, where contraceptives are provided free of charge, 30% to 50% of women present with unwanted and unplanned pregnancies and then seek termination of pregnancy.[3] In a 2009 report on Nigerian women, 31.5% believed that having sex once with a man would not result in pregnancy, although 90.0% knew about the benefits of family planning. Consideration of personal health and husband's approval were major determinants regarding the respondents' use of contraceptives. The authors concluded that there was a need for continuous education about contraception.[7]

From the literature, it is seen that contraceptive practices vary in Europe, South Africa and Nigeria and are influenced by the region in which the women live. In addition, whether they live in developing or developed countries also influences their practices, although these vary even in countries with similar economic statuses and amongst women of different age groups, education, social factors, marital status and religion.[4,5,7]

Sub-Saharan Africa has the highest fertility rate in the world, namely, 5.5 births per woman. Singh reports that one in every three births is involuntary.[5] The 1998 South African Demographics and Health Survey (SADHS) reported that 96% of women knew about contraception, although the rate of use of contraception was approximately 50%.[8] The conclusion of the study was that the low rate of condom use could be a result of lack of knowledge regarding how to use a condom, where to get condoms and the benefits of condom use. The SADHS study reported a decline in the level of knowledge of contraceptive methods from 1998 to 2008. When looking at married women, more than half (60%) used some method of contraception, with modern methods of contraception being used almost exclusively. Less than 0.1% of women relied on traditional methods and, of the modern methods, injectable contraception was the most widely used. Contraceptive use rose markedly as the education of the woman increased, as well as when the woman had at least three children.[9]

The traditional method of abstention is practised commonly in the Democratic Republic of Congo (DRC), resulting in a high rate of polygamy.[5] In the DRC, the contraception rate is estimated to be 8% for all methods and 2% for modern methods.[10] No study investigating factors influencing contraceptive use in the Vanga district was found.

Vanga health zone is one of the 515 health zones in the DRC, with the total population in the area being estimated at 244 839. In Vanga health zone, a programme of family planning was introduced in 1970 by Santé Rurale (SANRU), a USAID-funded programme for sustainable primary healthcare. However, contraception is not always available and women do not make regular use of these services. In Vanga hospital (the referral hospital), it is common to encounter diseases related to unsafe abortions, ranging from anaemia to sepsis and death. We sought to investigate the factors that influence contraceptive use amongst women of childbearing age in the Vanga health zone.

Research methods and design

Study design

This was a cross-sectional survey using interviewer-administered questionnaires. The questionnaire was administered by 38 trained interviewers. The questionnaire was translated from English to Kituba, then independently back translated to English, to check for distortions in the meaning and correctness of the translations.

Study population and sampling strategy

The total number of women of childbearing age in the region (18 to 49 years) was estimated to be 51 416, as determined by census.

Using Epi-Info (version 6.3), a confidence interval of 95%, a standard error of 0.01 and power of 80%, the sample size was calculated to be 384. Pregnant women were excluded from the study.

Systematic random sampling was used in order to recruit participants.

Data collection

Three variables were studied. These included socio-demographic variables, contraceptive practices of the women and factors leading to non-use of contraception. In assessing the practice of contraception, questions were asked about previous contraceptive use; age at first use of contraception; methods of contraception; and duration of current contraceptive use. To determine the factors influencing non-use of contraception, options presented included fear; inefficiency; partner's influence; unavailability of contraception; contraindications to usage; or non-awareness regarding contraception. The study was conducted over four months during 2009 and all women who were approached consented to participate in the study.

Data analysis

All data were entered onto an Excel spreadsheet and another person verified the data entries. Frequencies were calculated for each variable of interest and inferential statistics was used to determine the relationship between the variables by using SPSS software version 17.0. The statistical significance level was set at $p < 0.05$

Ethical considerations

Ethical approval for this study was obtained from the University of Limpopo Medunsa Campus Ethics Committee, MREC number MREC/M/111/2009:PG. Written informed consent was obtained from all the participants. Anonymity and confidentiality were assured. Permission was obtained from the manager of Vanga Health Zone central office.

Results

Baseline characteristics of the participants

The largest group amongst the 384 women recruited into the study fell into the31–40 year age group (n = 177; 46.1%). Two hundred and one (52%) had reached a primary school level of education. Three hundred and thirty-nine participants (88%) did not have any formal employment.

Three hundred and thirty-three of the women (86.9%) were married, 287 (74.7%) had experienced more than three pregnancies and 277 (72%) had more than three living children. The common religions were Protestant (n = 154; 51.6%) and Catholic (n = 198; 40.1 %), as is shown in Table 1.

One hundred and forty participants (36.5%) reported the current use of contraception, with 60% (n = 230) of those using modern methods of contraception; 61 (36.1%) of them had begun using contraception before the age of 20 (Table 2); and the most common methods of contraception were the oral contraceptive pill and injection, both 22.9% (n = 32).

TABLE 1: Baseline characteristics of the participants.

Baseline characteristics	Number	Percentage
Age group in years		
18–20	12	3.1
21–30	145	37.7
31–40	177	46.1
41–49	50	13.1
Occupation/Training		
Tailor	17	4.4
Nurse	60	15.6
Saleslady	26	6.7
Teacher	281	73.3
Educational level		
Primary school	201	52.3
High school	161	41.9
University	18	4.7
No education	4	1.0
Religion		
Catholic	154	40.1
Protestant	198	51.6
Muslim	2	0.5
Other religion	30	7.8
Marital status		
Married	333	86.9
Unmarried	51	13.1
Number of previous pregnancies		
0	12	3.1
1–2	95	22.1
≥ 3	287	74.7
Number of live children		
0	12	3.1
1–2	85	24.7
≥ 3	277	72.1
Tribe		
Mbala	186	48.4
Yansi	84	21.9
Muhungana	38	9.9
Songo	61	15.9
Other	15	3.9
Currently employed in the formal sector		
Yes	45	12

TABLE 2: Contraception use amongst women of reproductive age.

Descriptor	Number	Percentage
Age at the first use of contraception		
18–20	61	36.1
21–30	46	27.2
31–40	47	27.8
41–49	15	8.9
Contraceptive methods currently used		
Combined contraceptive oral pills	10	7.1
Male condom	32	22.9
Female condom	3	2.1
Tubal ligation	7	5.0
Coitus interruptus	35	25.0
Calendar method	20	14.3
Injectable hormonal method	32	22.9
Number of women using contraception according to age (n = 157)		
18–20	50	31.9
21–30	30	19.1
31–40	41	26.1
41–49	36	22.9
Women using contraception according to educational level (n = 140)		
Primary school	71	50.7
High school	63	45
University	4	2.9
No formal education	2	1.4

Characteristics of women taking contraception

One third of the current users of contraception (*n* = 31.9%) were younger than 20 and the largest group (*n* = 30; 21.4%) had been using contraception for anything from 13 months to two years. There was a wide variation in the duration of contraceptive use. The main reason for using contraception was for the spacing of children.

Seventy-seven (31.5%) of the women reported that they did not use contraception because of a fear of side effects (Table 3).

TABLE 3: Characteristics of women taking contraception.

Variable	Number	Percentage
Proportion of women using contraception according to marital status		
Married (*n*= 333)	123	37
Single (*n* = 51)	16	32
Use of contraception and number of children (*n* = 140)		
0	4	2.9
1–2	27	19.3
≥ 3	109	77.8
Contraception use and Tribe (*n* = 133)		
Mbala	69	52
Yansi	26	19.5
Muhungana	12	9
Songo	26	19.5
Duration of contraception use (*n* = 140)		
≤ 3 months	18	12.9
4–6 months	14	10
7–9 months	20	14.3
10–12 months	15	10.7
13 months–2 yrs	30	21.4
25 months–4 yrs	20	14.3
≥ 4 yrs	23	16.4
Reason for contraceptive use		
Does not want more children	38	27.1
Normal vaginal delivery is contraindicated	7	5
Pregnancy makes the woman very sick	15	10.7
Family spacing	63	45
Other reason	17	12.1
Reasons for not using contraception		
Fear of side effects	77	31.5
Fear of infertility	26	10.6
Distrust contraception	8	3.3
Husband's disapproval	38	15.6
Unavailability of the desired contraception	12	4.9
Complete absence of contraceptive methods.	17	7.0
Has contraindications to contraceptive use	4	1.6
Too expensive	44	18.0
Her religion disapproves use	18	7.4

Injectable contraception was used only by women who had children (Table 4).

Correlation analysis

Statistical analysis showed strong statistically-significant relationships between past use of contraception with age ($p = 0.000$) and number of children ($p = 0.000$). The comparison between non-use of contraceptives with age ($p = 0.005$) and the number of children ($p = 0.002$) were also of statistical significance (Table 5).

Discussion

This study sought to understand contraceptive use amongst women of childbearing age in the Vanga province of the DRC. This is very relevant in the DRC as well as Africa, in general, given the HIV epidemic and the high rate of unplanned pregnancy.

Many of the participants were in the 31 to 40 year age group (46.1%). Women aged 15 to 20 were more likely to use contraception (50%).

A demographic and health survey conducted in the DRC during 2007 showed that amongst sexually-active women, contraception use was as follows: 20% for women younger than 20, 39% for those aged 20–29, 24% for those aged 30–39 and 17% for those aged 40–49.[11] This differed from our findings since younger women in the Vanga region are now more aware of HIV and the benefits of contraception than five years ago, when the survey was conducted.

Slightly more than half (52.3%) of the 384 participants had primary school education, whereas four of the participants had no formal education. Of the women who had only a primary school education, 35% were using contraception, whilst only 22% of the women with University level education used contraception. In our survey, we had very few respondents who had University level education, however the proportion of these participants using contraception is low. It would thus seem that higher education is not a predictor for contraceptive use amongst these participants.

Most of our participants (88%) were without formal employment. This is consistent with most rural settings in

TABLE 4: Types and contraception used by women.

Variable	Oral contraception (%)	Male condom (%)	Female condom (%)	Tubal ligation (%)	*Coitus interruptus* (%)	Calendar method (%)	Injectable methods (%)
Tribe & type of contraception used							
Mbala	4	22	1	3	17	10	13
Yansi	3	3	1	0	10	4	8
Muhungana	1	1	0	3	4	3	3
Songo	3	7	0	1	5	3	8
Number of live children & type of contraception used							
0	0	1	0	0	2	1	0
1 or 2	1	10	0	0	8	7	2
≥ 3	9	21	2	7	25	13	30
Religion							
Protestant	5	20	3	8	26	14	21
Catholic	11	24	0	2	28	15	23

TABLE 5: Correlations analysis.

Variable	Pearson's correlation coefficient	*p*-value
Past use of contraception		
Age	-0.203	0.000*
Number of children	-0.213	0.000*
Number of live children	-0.173	0.001*
No practice of contraception		
Age	0.143	0.005*
Number of children	0.161	0.002*
Number of live children	0.139	0.006*

*, Statistically significant.

sub-Saharan Africa. During the demographic and health survey in the DRC in 2007, it was noted that the percentage of women who worked increased with age, where 81% of the 40–49 year age group were employed, whilst only 35% of those in the 15–19 year age group were employed.[11] The survey in 2007 found that 25% of all employment was in the sales and services sector,[11] which is consistent with our findings.

Christians made up the majority (92%) of the participants, with the most common denominations being Protestant (51.6%) and Catholic (40.1%). Our findings were consistent with results from the national survey, where 93% of women surveyed were Christian.[11] Natural contraceptive methods such as abstinence and the rhythm method are permissible for Catholics. Amongst Protestants, it is common for adherents to use birth control after the family is complete. Family planning was used for birth spacing rather than to restrict the overall size of families.[7]

In our study, 86% of the women were married. In the DRC as a whole, about 58% of all women are married.[11] This difference may be because early age marriages are common in Vanga. We found that contraceptive use was higher amongst married participants, whereas according to the national survey, contraception was used more by single women (69%) and male condoms were used most often.[11]

There was no significant difference between married and single participants regarding preference in terms of contraceptive methods. Dibaba reported that only 13% of married women in Asia used contraception.[12]

Of the women surveyed, 74.5% had experienced more than three child births and, of these, 72% had more than three children who were still alive. Tehrani, Farahani and Hashemi found that 50% of the women had one living child, 36.4% had two children and 11.7% had three. In the DRC, however, large families are common.[13]

Most participants were from the Mbala tribe (48.4%). This is the largest tribe in this region and members of the tribe use all forms of contraception, indicating that belonging to this tribe does not seem to prevent women from using any particular form of contraception.

One hundred and sixty-eight (43.7%) of the participants reported having used contraception in the past and 36.3 % of them had started using contraception before they were 20 years old. The national study found that about half of the participants (49%) had used at least one contraceptive method at some time in their lives.[11] In the study conducted by Bhatti in1995,[14] 5% had initiated contraceptive use at ages 15–19 years; 22% at ages 20–24 years; and 58% at ages 25–34 years. Our findings are thus similar to the national study in the DRC, in that slightly less than half of the women surveyed had ever used contraception.

In our survey, 36.4% of the women reported they were currently using contraception. Other research found that contraceptive use is similar in Kinshasa (42%) and Bas-Congo (40%).[11]

Sixty percent of the women in our study used modern contraceptive methods such as male condoms and injectable contraceptives (22.9% each). Tehrani, Farahani and Hashemi reported that natural methods (withdrawal and rhythm) were the most commonly-used contraceptive methods (61.0%), whilst the use of oral contraceptives, intra-uterine devices and condoms were at 22.9%, 10.1% and 6.0%, respectively.[11] From the demographic and health survey, the male condom (15%), oral contraceptive pill (4%) and injection (1%) were the most commonly-used modern contraceptive methods. Periodic abstinence (38%) was the most frequently-used traditional method, followed by withdrawal (23%).[11] It would thus seem that more women in the Vanga district use injectable hormones and male condoms as contraceptives as compared with the rest of the DRC. This may relate to the fact that SANRU has made these methods available to women in the Vanga district. A study by Masoda and Govender found that contraception price was a factor restricting its use in the DRC.[15]

We found that injectable contraceptive methods were the first choice amongst the women who had more than three children, followed by the male condom; whilst male condoms were the most common amongst women with one to two children and interrupted coitus was most common in the group without any children. The male condom was the most commonly-used method amongst the group of Mbala participants, whilst interrupted coitus was the most common method amongst Yansi and Muhungana participants. In the group of Songo participants, the most common method used was injectable contraception.

The intra-uterine device was the preferred method amongst women of childbearing age in Pakistan, followed by injectable contraceptives, oral contraceptive pills and male condoms. Only a minority (4%) of women preferred the use of the non-medical (traditional) methods of calendar and *coitus interuptus*.[14] In the United States, the most common methods used were the male condom (used at least once by 94% of study participants) and the pill (used at least once by 61%).[16] According to Berer, condoms are the mainstay of dual protection and will remain so until such time as other equally safe and effective methods are developed.[17]

Most participants (21.4%) have been using contraceptives for a short period of time (one to two years). This may be because of the increased involvement of non-governmental organisations, (NGOs) such as Santé Rurale (SANRU), over the past three years. Most of these NGOs are religion based and their activity has increased as the war in the DRC is stabilising. Many of the participants (45%) used contraception for spacing of their children.

The main reasons for not using contraceptives were a fear of side effects (31%), followed by disapproval of the husband (15%). The demographic and health survey found that women do not use contraceptives because of side effects (6%), medical contraindications (3%), refusal of the husband/ partner (5%) and religious restrictions (6%).[11] In our study, 7% said they did not use contraception because it was not allowed by their religion. Roman Catholics are forbidden to use medical or physical contraceptive methods.

Implications and recommendations

Women have been the primary subject of contraceptive and family planning research because most modern contraceptive methods were designed for use by women and because most programmes assume that women are primarily responsible for family planning.[18] However, a large proportion of women (15.6%) do not use contraception in the Vanga district because it is not permitted by their male partners, husbands in most instances. Cost of contraception is also a barrier to many women using contraception as it is free only at the non-governmental clinic (SANRU) and is sometimes out of stock, even at these clinics. This has also been found as a barrier in another study in the DRC.[15]

The participants' age and number of children impacts on their contraceptive use. The more children and the older a woman is, the more likely she is to use contraception. One of the contributing factors for this could be exposure to health education at ante-natal clinics and facilities located at the community level. The demographic and health survey also found that women with more children were more likely to use contraception.[8] The use of contraception was very low amongst woman with no children.[11] Tehrani, Farahani and Hashemi found in Tehran that age, women's level of education, their husbands' level of education and previous familiarity with contraceptive methods were the most important factors influencing contraceptive use.[11] A review conducted by Bongaarts and Bruce showed that socio-economic, behavioural and cultural factors influenced contraceptive use.[19]

Increasing the education of women regarding contraception and the various methods available could help to increase the use of family planning as we have found education to be an important predictor of contraception use. The other barriers to the use of contraception were religion and the objection of a woman's partner to contraceptive use. Male partners need to be involved actively in the choice and use of contraception and should be present during the consultation. It would be informative to carry out a similar study amongst the men in order to discover their views regarding contraceptive use. In this way, education which is designed to empower women may have a twofold effect. Firstly, women will become more aware of contraception and the choices available and, secondly, women will be empowered economically so they can be seen as equals in the Vanga district.

Limitations

Systematic sampling may have reduced the validity of the results. Using interviewers to assist in the completion of the questionnaires may have distorted the validity of responses as some participants may not have felt comfortable, thus giving responses that they thought were acceptable. We tried to reduce this by training the interviewers and asking them to maintain self-awareness and to demonstrate 'neutrality' during the interviews.

Conclusion

The main reason for women in this district to use contraception was for family spacing and women who had used contraception in the past were more likely to use it again. The fear of side effects was a major barrier to contraceptive use. Contraception methods and education regarding their use should be made easily accessible throughout the Vanga Health Zone.

Acknowledgements

The authors wish to thank the Department of Family Medicine staff who reviewed the original paper following a research writing retreat in the North West Province.

Competing interests

The authors declare that they have no financial or personal relationship(s) which may have inappropriately influenced them in writing this article.

Authors' contributions

K.I. (Protestant University of Congo) initiated the research, wrote up the first protocol and was involved in data collection. I.G. (University of the Limpopo) was involved in the writing of the protocol, analysis of the data and writing up of the research report. J.F. (Protestant University of Congo) was involved in the writing of the protocol, collection of the data and editing of the final research paper. J.T. (University of the Limpopo) assisted with analysis of the data and writing up of the research paper.

References

1. Maja TMM, Ehlers VJ. Contraceptive practices of women in Northern Tshwane, Gauteng Province. Health SA Gesondheid. 2004;9(4):42–52.
2. Centers for Disease Control and Prevention. Contraception [page on the Internet]. No date [cited 2012 Dec 05]. Available from: http://www.cdc.gov/reproductivehealth/unintendedpregnancy/contraception.htm

3. Department of Health, South Africa. National contraception policy guidelines [document on the Internet]. [2002] [cited 2012 Dec 15]. Available from: www.kznhealth.gov.za/contraception.pdf
4. Oddens BJ, Lehert P. Determinants of contraceptive use among women of reproductive age in Great Britain and Germany. I: Demographic factors. J Biosoc Sci. 1997;29(4):415–435. http://dx.doi.org/10.1017/S002193209700415X
5. Singh, S, Darroch JE, Vlassof, M & Nadeau, J. Adding it up: the costs and benefits of family planning and maternal and newborn health. New York: Guttmacher Institute and United Nations Population Fund; 2009.
6. World Health Organization. Unsafe abortion: global and regional estimates of incidence of unsafe abortion and associated mortality in 2003. 5th ed. Geneva: WHO; 2007.
7. Moronkola OA, Ojediran MM, Amosu A. Reproductive health knowledge, beliefs and determinants of contraceptives use among women attending family clinics in Ibadan, Nigeria. Afr Health Sci. 2006;6(3):155–159.
8. Moshia KM (2002) Contraceptive use and knowledge in South Africa: Evidence from the 1998 South African Demographic and Health Survey (SADHS). The XIV International AIDS Conference, Barcelona. July 7–12; 14: abstract no Mopec3350. Available from: http://ww1.aegis.org/conferences/iac/2002/MoPeC3350.html
9. Department of Health/UNDP. Millenium development goals. Goal 5: improve maternal health [document on the Internet]. 2010 [cited 2014 Mar 06]. Available from: http://www.statssa.gov.za/nss/Goal_Reports/GOAL%205-IMPROVE%20MATERNAL%20HEALTH.pdf
10. Ministère de la Santé Publique. Politique nationale de la santé [National health policy] [document on the Internet]. 2001 [cited 2014 Mar 05]. Available from: http://www.minisanterdc.cd/Articles/Reformesanitaire/D%82claration%20Politique%20nationale%20de%20la%20sant%82.pdf
11. Ministère du Plan et Macro International. Enquête Démographique et de Santé, République Démocratique du Congo 2007 [Demographic and Health Survey, the Republic of Congo 2007]. Calverton, Maryland, U.S.A; 2008.
12. Dibaba Y. Factors influencing women's intention to limit child bearing in Oromia, Ethiopia. Ethiop J Health Dev. 2009;23(1):28–33. http://dx.doi.org/10.4314/ejhd.v23i1.44834
13. Tehrani FR, Farahani FK, Hashemi M. Factors influencing contraceptive use in Tehran. Fam Pract. 2001;18(2):204–208. http://dx.doi.org/10.1093/fampra/18.2.204
14. Bhatti MH. Correlates of choice of contraceptive methods in Pakistan. Pak Dev Rev. 1995;34(4 Pt. III):889–898.
15. Masoda M, Govender I. Knowledge and attitudes about and practices of condom use for reducing HIV infection among Goma University students in the Democratic Republic of Congo. South Afr J Epidemiol Infect. 2013;28(1):61–68.
16. Abma JC, Martinez GM, Mosher WD, et al. Teenagers in the United States: sexual activity, contraceptive use, and childbearing, 2002. Vital Health Stat. 2004;23(24):1–48.
17. Berer M. Dual protection: more needed than practised or understood. Reprod Health Matters. 2006;14(28):162–170. http://dx.doi.org/10.1016/S0968-8080(06)28262-4
18. Hardee K, Ulin P, Pfannenschmidt, et al. The impact of family planning and reproductive health on women's lives: a conceptual framework. Geneva: Family Health International; 1996.
19. Bongaarts J, Bruce J. The causes of unmet need for contraception and the social content of services. Stud Fam Plann. 1995;26(2):57–75. http://dx.doi.org/10.2307/2137932

5

African Primary Care Research: Performing surveys using questionnaires

Authors:
Indiran Govender[1]
Langalibalele H. Mabuza[1]
Gboyega A. Ogunbanjo[1]
Bob Mash[2]

Affiliations:
[1]Department of Family Medicine, University of Limpopo, Medunsa Campus, South Africa

[2]Division of Family Medicine and Primary Care, Stellenbosch University, South Africa

Correspondence to:
Indiran Govender

Email:
indiran.govender@gmail.com

Postal address:
PO Box 222, Medunsa 0204, South Africa

The aim of this article is to provide practical guidance on conducting surveys and the use of questionnaires for postgraduate students at a Masters level who are undertaking primary care research. The article is intended to assist with writing the methods section of the research proposal and thinking through the relevant issues that apply to sample size calculation, sampling strategy, design of a questionnaire and administration of a questionnaire. The article is part of a larger series on primary care research, with other articles in the series focusing on the structure of the research proposal and the literature review, as well as quantitative data analysis.

La recherche sur les soins de santé primaire en Afrique: réaliser des sondages à l'aide de questionnaires. L'objectif de cet article est de fournir des directives pratiques pour la réalisation de sondages et l'utilisation de questionnaires, directives destinées aux étudiants de troisième cycle en année de Master qui mènent des recherches sur les soins de santé primaire. L'article est destiné à les aider à rédiger la section méthodologique de leur proposition de recherche et à réfléchir aux questions pertinentes relatives au calcul de la dimension de l'échantillon, à la stratégie d'échantillonnage, à l'élaboration d'un questionnaire et à son administration. L'article fait partie d'une série dédiée à la recherche sur les soins de santé primaire, et, comme d'autres articles composant cette série, traite essentiellement de la structure de la proposition de recherche, de l'étude bibliographique, et de l'analyse quantitative des données.

Introduction

This article is part of a series on African primary care research. In this article the authors address the use of surveys and questionnaires. This is a very common study design in primary care research and the article is intended to guide primary care researchers and postgraduate students at a Masters level with regard to the development of their research proposal. Other articles in the series focus on related issues such as the structure of the research proposal and the literature review, as well as quantitative data analysis.

Study design

The type of survey to be used should be described in the section on study design in your research proposal. For example, you may describe the design as a descriptive survey or an observational cross-sectional analytical study.

Surveys are used to obtain information on or to measure the distribution of selected characteristic(s) in a group or population of interest.[1,2] In simple terms, a survey encompasses any measurement procedure that involves administering a questionnaire to respondents. Questionnaires offer an objective means of collecting information about people's knowledge, beliefs, attitudes and behaviour. They can be used as the sole research instrument (such as in a cross-sectional survey) or within clinical trials and other epidemiological studies.[3,4]

Surveys are often descriptive in nature and help to quantify the frequency with which the variables of interest occur in a population. A cross-sectional survey can be used as a type of observational study, which goes beyond simple description to analyse and compare variables in the population. For example, a cross-sectional survey may divide the population into those who are adherent and non-adherent to antiretroviral treatment and then analyses the other variables collected in order to see if any are associated significantly with this outcome. In this type of observational study a hypothesis that certain variables may be associated with a particular outcome is tested.[2]

Before committing to a survey as your study design, consider if a questionnaire is the most appropriate tool. Sometimes, a questionnaire will be appropriate within a mixed methodology study – for example, to quantify the qualitative findings of an initial exploratory phase.

Study population

It is important to define your study population clearly before considering how you will sample from this population. Some researchers will also define a target population, which is the broadest population to which they would like to generalise their findings and then their study population, which is the population to which they actually have access. Often it is not possible to collect data from the entire study population and a representative sample must be selected, from whom data will be collected. The study population should be described in terms of people (who is included?), place (where are these people?) and, sometimes, time (over what time period?).

Sample size calculation

If collecting quantitative data with a view to testing a hypothesis or assessing the prevalence of a disease or problem, a minimum sample size should be calculated.[5] It is important to note that the formula for calculating sample size is different depending on whether the study is a descriptive survey or an observational cross-sectional study with analysis of comparison groups.

If you are planning a purely descriptive survey then your only concern is to estimate the variables you are interested in with sufficient precision so that you obtain a reasonably accurate picture of the situation in the larger target population. The calculation will tell you the size of the sample required to do this. If the main variable you are interested in measuring is a continuous variable, such as birth weight, then you will want a sufficient sample size in order to measure its mean value. If, however, the main variable you are interested in is a categorical variable, such as smokers and non-smokers, then you will want a sufficient sample size to measure the proportion of people with this variable. Your sample size will enable you to measure the point estimate of the variable within a certain confidence interval. A 95% confidence interval is usually chosen and, clearly, the larger the sample size the smaller the width of the 95% confidence interval and the more accurate the measurement.

To calculate sample size (N) for a mean you will need to decide how small you want the confidence interval (d) to be and you will also need to know the standard deviation (SD) of the variable that you are interested in. The formula to use will then be: $N = (1.96^2 \times SD^2)/d^2$. As an example, if you want to estimate the mean birth weight with a 95% CI of ± 50 g and the SD of birth weight is 500 g then $N = (1.96^2 \times 500^2)/50^2 = 384$. If the SD is not known then you should obtain it from published literature or subject experts and, if this is not possible, consider a pilot study to estimate it.

To calculate sample size (N) for a proportion, the same formula can be used but the SD for a proportion (p) is SD $= p \times (1-p)$. This implies (somewhat bizarrely) that you need to estimate the likely proportion in the population before you do your survey in order to calculate your sample size. For example, if you think the percentage of smokers is likely to be about 30% in your population then the SD = 0.3 x 0.7. If you also decide that you want the width of the 95% confidence interval to be 5% then the calculation will be $N = (1.96^2 \times 0.3 \times 0.7)/0.05^2 = 323$. If you have no idea of what the likely proportion will be then you can assume 50% for the sample size calculation.

If, however, your survey is intended to compare two groups for a particular outcome then it is no longer simply descriptive and the above sample size calculations no longer apply. In this situation you will need to consider the power of your sample size. Power is the ability to detect a difference that is actually present; it is related to the sample size, the difference that you want to detect, the variability in the data and the type of outcome variable you are dealing with (e.g. continuous or categorical). When you consult the statistician to make this calculation you will need to know what you consider to be the minimum clinically important difference between the groups and how large a risk you are willing to take that your inference will be wrong. Your inference may be wrong if you declare there is a difference, when in fact there is none (also called a type 1 or alpha error). The risk of this error is usually set at 5% or $p = 0.05$. Your inference may also be wrong if you declare there is no difference but in fact there is one (also called a type 2 or beta error). The risk of this error is often set between 10% – 20% or, conversely, a power of 80% – 90%.

Ultimately, your sample size calculation may also depend on practical issues such as your time and the feasibility of recruiting patients. Often, a compromise between accuracy or power and practicality must be reached. It is also good practice to involve a statistician in helping you with the sample size calculation. In your research proposal, you should list all of the assumptions that you have made in your calculation as described above.

Sampling

Sampling is selecting a group from a much larger population (study population) that is similar in its trait distribution (e.g. gender, ethnicity, age, income, etc.) to the larger population. Findings made from studying the group can then be generalised to the larger population. The required *size* of the sample has been calculated above, but sampling deals with the *actual selection* of the group.[6]

Without careful planning and choosing an appropriate method for sampling it is very easy to obtain a biased sample that does not represent the population. When this happens, it is difficult to extend the findings to the larger population and the validity of the research decreases. Therefore, in order to produce meaningful results, researchers must ensure that they have chosen an appropriate sampling method to select a representative sample of participants.[6]

The main threat to representativeness is bias. A biased sample (selection or participation bias) is one which contains characteristics that are different from those of the population. This bias may happen by chance, but is usually attributable to selection bias. Selection bias is present when participants are selected systematically in a way that increases the probability of their being different from the desired study population. For example, if a researcher recruits participants from a gym, they are more likely to be healthier and fitter than the rest of the general public; or, if the larger population is made up of 51% women and 49% men, a sample (regardless of size) that is made up of 38% women and 62% men is not representative. Participation bias is any influence that affects who participated during the study, such as those people who dropped out or refused to participate.[2,5,6]

Various sampling techniques can be used depending on the type of research to be conducted. The two major types of techniques are probability sampling and non-probability sampling.[6] In selecting a representative sample for a survey it is important to ensure that participants from the desired study population have an equal probability of being selected. Probability sampling is any sampling procedure that specifies the probability that each member of a population has of being selected. Probability sampling techniques include:[6,7]

Simple random sampling

This is when a list containing all of the population is created and used to select participants randomly. Random numbers can be generated, for example in an Excel spread sheet, to decide which people in the list to select. This random selection guarantees that each individual has an independent and equal chance of being selected. This method is very fair, unbiased and easy to carry out; it is the most common and highly-recommended technique. However, with simple random sampling there is no assurance of complete representativeness of the sample as those with rare features or conditions may be missed.[6,7]

Systematic sampling

This is a procedure of selection based on some simple, systematic rule such as every second or third person available or patients with odd numbers as the last digits of their medical files. The danger of this type of sampling is that there may be a hidden bias attached to the rule used to select people. For example if all male patients have a medical file ending in an odd number then only male patients will be selected in the example above. This can, however, be a practical approach to selecting people in a busy clinic where people present in no particular order.[6,7]

Stratified random sampling

A group selected from a population that reflects accurately certain segments of a population. In this type of sample, certain segments or traits are identified as being important to the research and the sample selected is controlled in order to ensure that those traits are accurately represented.[6,7] For example, in a survey of high school students you may stratify the sample by school or grade to ensure that equal numbers of students are selected from each. The students may still be selected in a random or systematic way within these strata.

Cluster sampling

This is when the sample is gained by the random selection of clusters from a list containing all of the possible clusters within a population. This method is easy for obtaining a large and relatively random selection of participants; however, the selections lack independence. For example, a study may select community health centres randomly out of the total number of such centres available and then recruit a group of patients from the selected centres. These patients form a cluster and may share similar characteristics that are different to clusters of patients from other centres. The effect of such clustering will need to be taken into account when considering the sample size, representativeness of the sample or when making comparisons between patients in the analysis.[6,7]

Non-probability sampling is any sampling procedure that cannot specify the probability that each member of a population has of being selected. This type of sampling is used when probability sampling is not feasible, but is generally not an acceptable approach to designing surveys. It is often used in qualitative research as described in the article on qualitative interviewing. Non-probability sampling techniques include convenience samples (including whoever happens to be available), quota sampling (a convenience sample of different subgroups such as men and women), purposive sampling (people selected on the basis of predefined criteria) and snowball sampling (people interviewed identify other people with the desired characteristics).[6,7]

It is important to know that it is better to collect fewer questionnaires with good quality responses than high numbers of questionnaires from participants which are inaccurate or incomplete. One way of reducing the amount of inaccurate or incomplete data is to set strict exclusion criteria at the start of the research. For example, many studies exclude participants who are unable to read or write in the language of the questionnaire and those with certain physical and mental disabilities that might interfere with their ability to give informed consent or to understand the questions asked. However, research that systematically excludes hard-to-reach groups is increasingly seen as unethical and additional strategies and resources may need to be built into the study protocol at the outset. Research participants must be able to give meaningful answers (with help from a professional interviewer if necessary).[2,3] The inclusion and exclusion criteria for sampling must be described clearly in the proposal.

Data collection (the questionnaire)

The data collection tool or questionnaire should be described in the research proposal and provided in full as an appendix. How the tool was obtained, adapted or developed should be described. The validity and reliability of the questionnaire should also be addressed in the proposal.

Using standardised and validated questionnaires

Just because a questionnaire has been piloted on a few colleagues, used in previous studies, or published in a peer-reviewed journal does not mean it is either valid or reliable. Development of a valid and reliable questionnaire is necessary in order to reduce measurement error. Measurement error is the discrepancy between respondents' attributes and their survey responses.

A valid questionnaire measures what it claims to measure. In reality, many questionnaires may not be valid. For example, a questionnaire that seeks to measure people's sexual behaviour may be less valid because it measures what they say they do, not what they actually do. Similarly, responses on questionnaires that ask health professionals how they manage particular diseases may differ significantly from actual clinical practice. An instrument developed in a different time, country, or cultural context may not be a valid measure in the group you are studying. If a valid questionnaire exists it should not be altered significantly as this affects the validity and reliability of the tool.[1,2,3] Minor adaptation to the language is, however, often needed in order to make it understandable to the local culture or context.

Reliable questionnaires yield consistent results from repeated samples and different researchers over time. Differences in results come from differences between participants, not from inconsistencies in how the items are understood or how different observers interpret the responses. A standardised questionnaire is one that is written and administered so all participants are asked precisely the same questions in an identical format and responses are recorded in a uniform manner.

Standardising a measure increases its reliability.[1,3,5] Three common types of reliability are inter-rater reliability (similarity between different raters using the same tool), test-retest reliability (similarity between repeated measurements on the same person) and internal consistency. Internal consistency is important for questionnaires and may be tested for by using the Cronbach's alpha statistical test, which measures how well items that are meant to measure a particular concept actually fit together in a questionnaire. For example, if the questionnaire has five questions that attempt to score how well a family physician teaches students then this test will quantify how well these questions work together to actually measure this attribute. A result of > 0.7 is considered 'good'. Standardised questionnaires can also report on their sensitivity (how good a test is at detecting who has the condition/disease) and specificity (how good a test is at detecting who does not have the condition/disease). Screening questionnaires should have a high sensitivity.[1,2,3]

Before designing your own questionnaire, consider using a standardised and validated existing questionnaire. A previously-validated and published questionnaire will save time and resources; results can be compared with other studies, you need only give outline details of the instrument when writing up the work and it may be easier to get the research published. However, be careful when translating an existing questionnaire.[3,4] It is also possible to perform your research study on the validation of a questionnaire itself, in preparation for its actual use in the future.

Increasingly, research on health services uses standardised questionnaires designed for producing data that can be compared across studies. For example, clinical trials routinely include measures of patients' knowledge and practice about a disease or condition, or satisfaction with health services. The validity of this approach depends on whether the type and range of closed responses reflects the full range of perceptions and feelings that people in all the different potential sampling frames might hold. Importantly, health status and quality of life instruments lose their validity when used beyond the context in which they were developed. Using one or more standard instruments alongside a short questionnaire could prevent the need to develop and validate a long list of new items.[3,8]

Designing your own questionnaire

It is not easy to construct your own questionnaire. With a computer it is possible to write one in a single evening provided the aim and objectives of the study are stated clearly. However developing a questionnaire that yields valid data to answer the research objectives is harder than one might think.[3,4] Inappropriate questions and lack of rigour inevitably lead to poor-quality data and misleading conclusions and recommendations. Using questionnaires can appear to provide quick answers to a research question, but may be inappropriately used, resulting in methodological errors.[3]

Structure of the questionnaire

The design depends on well-defined objectives for the research to which the content of the questionnaire can be aligned.[1,2] Avoid questions that do not address your study objectives directly, however interesting the questions might appear. It is unethical to ask about issues not covered in your objectives and irrelevant questions make the questionnaire longer and the data will most likely not be included in your analysis. Keep the questionnaire as short and as simple as possible in order to encourage a good response rate. A typical design for a questionnaire will have the following elements:[1]

- A clear and concise title.
- An introduction that explains the aim of the research and purpose of the questionnaire.
- Clear instructions on how to complete the questionnaire.
- Questions organised into appropriate sections. Typically, the questionnaire starts with relevant demographic data (e.g. age, sex) that is neutral rather than more sensitive topics. However, the most important issues should ideally be covered early on in case the respondent fails to complete all the questions.

Questionnaires should be in a language the participant understands and, when translating a questionnaire into another language, another translator should back translate it to verify that the original meaning has not been lost.

Types of questions

There are five types of questions that can be used: binary questions (e.g. yes/no or male/female), specific questions that do not specify options (e.g. How old are you?), multiple choice questions (in which the options should be mutually exclusive and exhaustive of all possible answers), multiple responses (where the respondent can select more than one of the options) and scaling questions (e.g. Likert or visual analogue-type scales).[9]

Wording of the questions

Begin with a few non-threatening and engaging items. Use simple and direct language. Place the most important items strategically in the first half of the questionnaire.[1,3] Two words that are often used inappropriately in question stems are 'frequently' and 'regularly'. A poorly-designed item might read, 'I frequently engage in exercise', and offer a Likert scale giving responses from 'strongly agree' through to 'strongly disagree'. However, 'frequently' implies frequency, so a frequency-based rating scale (with options such as 'at least once a day', 'twice a week', and so on) would be more appropriate. 'Regularly', on the other hand, implies a pattern. One person can regularly engage in exercise once a month whereas another person can regularly do so four times a week. Other words to avoid in question stems include commonly, usually, many, some and hardly ever.[3,10]

Avoid abbreviations and undefined terms that respondents may not be aware of, such as:

- Which type of diabetes do you have? ☐ T2DM ☐ T1DM
- What was your income last year?___________________

Last year may mean 12 months ending today, the previous financial year or calendar year. Income could be before or after tax.

Other pitfalls in question design include too long, ambiguous, double or triple questions in one sentence, unreasonable recall period, double negatives, response choices that are not mutually exclusive, response options that are not exhaustive or questions based on unstated assumptions.[3,10] In multiple response questions it may be useful to require an answer to every option (e.g. yes, no, don't know) as otherwise you may not know if the option was actually considered by the respondent.

Closed-ended questions enable researchers to collect aggregated data quickly, but the range of possible answers is set by the researchers, not the respondents, and the richness of potential responses is lower. Closed-ended items often cause frustration, usually because researchers have not considered all potential responses.[3,9] Ticking a particular box, or even saying 'yes', 'no' or 'maybe' can make respondents want to explain their answer; and such free text annotations may add richly to the quantitative data. A free text box may be inserted at the end of the questionnaire (or even after particular items or sections). Note that participants need instructions (perhaps with examples) on how to complete free text items in the same way as they do for closed questions.

If open-ended questions are used or free text comments are invited, the researcher(s) must plan in advance how this qualitative data will be analysed. The use of structured questionnaires, which have a few open-ended questions for comments or clarification is not qualitative research.[3,10] Usually, these qualitative responses are brief and can also be categorised and quantified. Rarely, if there are more in-depth responses, they can be transcribed and analysed as in qualitative research.[11] Adequate time, skills and resources for this analysis must be built into the study design; otherwise this will be a waste of participants' and researchers' time.[1,3,10]

Some respondents tend to agree with statements rather than disagree. For this reason, do not present items so that strongly agree always links to the same broad attitude. For example, on a patient satisfaction scale, if one question is 'my GP generally tries to help me out', another question should be phrased in the negative, such as 'the receptionists are usually impolite'.[1,3,10]

Empirical studies have repeatedly shown that low response rates are often because participants are unable to read or follow the questionnaire. In general, questions should be short and to the point (around 12 words or less), but for issues of a sensitive and personal nature, short questions can be perceived as abrupt and threatening and longer sentences are preferred.[1,3,10]

Analytical considerations

When designing your questions you should also think about the type of data that will be created and how this will be analysed. It is always better to collect continuous data whenever possible rather than categorical data as this allows you more flexibility and power in the final analysis. For example, collecting the actual age rather than asking people to tick an age category is preferred. In multiple choice questions it is preferable to not have too many categories as this will complicate the analysis, for example, when all categories must be compared in a contingency table. Please see the article on quantitative data analysis in this series.

Piloting of questionnaires

Questionnaires may fail because participants don't understand them, can't complete them, or get offended by them. Whether the researcher has constructed his own questionnaire or is using an existing instrument, they always pilot it on participants who are representative of the study population.[1,3] Approval from an ethics committee is necessary for this phase.[4,12]

Consider:

- How long do people take to complete it?
- Do any questions need to be repeated or explained?
- How do participants indicate that they have arrived at an answer?
- Do they show confusion or surprise at a particular response – if so, why?
- Short, abrupt questions may provoke short, abrupt answers.

Piloting will provide feedback to enable rephrasing of questions and will ensure a more valid and complete response. The piloting phase should include planning and testing the strategy for getting the questionnaire out and back, as well as when a reminder letter is needed. If researcher assistants are employed, they will require training.[1,3]

Data collection (procedures)

The way in which you will administer the questionnaire to collect your data needs to be fully described in the research proposal. You should also discuss any anticipated challenges in collecting data and how you plan to overcome them.

Survey questionnaires can be administered by personal interview (interviewer-administered), by self-administration (where the participant completes the questionnaire unassisted), or by telephone, mail (post), e-mail, cellphones or internet-based tools (such as a monkey puzzle).[1,2]

Mail surveys using questionnaires are a cheap method of gathering information, but often suffer from a low response rate. They are ideal for large sample sizes and/or when the sample comes from a wide geographic area. These take at least eight to 12 weeks to complete. There is no possibility of interviewer bias; however, respondents cannot be probed for more information.[3,10]

E-mail and internet surveys are very cost-effective and are the fastest method of distributing a survey. The internet user, however, does not represent the general population, although more are gaining access to the internet via their cellphones. Before undertaking an internet based surveys, consider this limitation.[1,2]

Factors that increase the response rates:[1,3,4,8,10]

- The questionnaire is clearly designed and has a simple layout with items grouped into logical and coherent sections.
- It offers participants incentives in return for completion.
- It has been thoroughly piloted and tested.
- Participants are notified about the study in advance with a personalised invitation.
- The aim of study and means of completing the questionnaire are explained clearly.
- A researcher is available to answer questions and to collect the completed questionnaire.
- If using a postal questionnaire, a stamped addressed envelope is included.
- The participants feel they are a stakeholder in the study.
- Questions are phrased in a way that holds the participant's attention.
- The questionnaire has clear focus and purpose and is kept concise.
- The questionnaire is appealing to look at.
- The questionnaire is delivered electronically (if appropriate).
- The researchers use reminders such as phone calls or other follow-up methods.

Advantages of written questionnaires[1,3,10]

- Questionnaires are very cost effective, especially when they involve large samples and many research questions.
- Questionnaires are familiar to most people and usually do not make people apprehensive.
- They reduce bias, with a uniform question presentation and no interpretation from another person.
- They are less intrusive than face-to-face or telephone interviews. Mailed questionnaires can be completed by the respondent in his own time.

Disadvantages of written questionnaires[1,3,10]

- Possible low response rate especially with postal surveys. This can lower confidence in the results. Response rates may vary from 10% to 90%.
- Inability to probe responses as they allow little flexibility in the response format. This can be overcome in part by allowing space for open questions and comments.
- The lack of personal contact results in the loss of visual cues, especially when dealing with sensitive issues.
- With postal questionnaires, the intended respondent may not be the person who actually completes the questionnaire.
- Not ideal for some respondents such as illiterate people, people who have reading problems and blind people.

Taking account of psychological and social influences

Survey research can never be completely objective. Researchers and participants are all human beings with psychological, emotional and social needs. A questionnaire means something different to participants and researchers. Researchers want data (with a view to publications, promotion, academic recognition and further income). This may lead to critical errors in piloting (e.g. piloting on friends rather than the target group), sampling (e.g. drifting toward convenience rather than random samples) and in the distribution, collection and coding of questionnaires. Staff employed to assist with a questionnaire study may not be familiar with all the tasks required to make it a success and may be unaware that covering up their ignorance or skill deficits will make the entire study unsound.[1,5,11]

Conclusion

This article has covered the methodological issues involved in planning a survey and using a questionnaire, which should be described in the research proposal. The sample size calculation, sampling strategy, questionnaire design and data collection strategy have all been discussed. Designing a survey with a questionnaire that produces usable data is not as easy as it might seem. Awareness of the pitfalls is essential when planning research.

Acknowledgements

The authors wish to thank Dr John Tumbo for proof reading and for providing valuable guidance for the writing of this article. The authors gratefully acknowledge funding received from the U.S. President's Emergency Plan for AIDS Relief (PEPFAR), through HRSA under the terms of T84HA21652., and via the Stellenbosch University Rural Medical Education Partnership Initiative (SURMEPI).

Competing interests

The authors declare that they have no financial or personal relationship(s) which may have inappropriately influenced them in writing this article.

Authors' contributions

All authors contributed to the initial manuscript and approved the final version. Further revisions were made by I.G. (University of Limpopo Medunsa Campus) and B.M. (Stellenbosch University).

References

1. StatPac. Research methods. [page on internet]. c2013 [cited 2013 Jul 9]. Available from: www.statpac.com/surveys/research-methods.htm
2. Davies B, Logan J. Research reading: a user-friendly guide for health professionals. 5th ed. Mosby: Canada; 2011.
3. Boynton PM, Greenhalgh T. Hands-on guide to questionnaire research. Selecting, designing, and developing your questionnaire. BMJ. 2004;328(7451):1312–1315. http://dx.doi.org/10.1136/bmj.328.7451.1312
4. Gillham B. Developing a questionnaire (real world research). London: Continuum; 2000.
5. Boynton PM. Hands-on guide to questionnaire research. Administering, analysing, and reporting your questionnaire. BMJ. 2004;328(7452):1372–1375. http://dx.doi.org/10.1136/bmj.328.7452.1372
6. Picciano A. Review of statistics – sampling procedures. [page on internet]. n.d. [cited 2013 Sep 2]. Available from: http://www.anthonypicciano.com/Sampling.html
7. Ogunbanjo GA. Making sense of statistics for the family practitioner: obtaining the "sample". SA Fam Pract. 2003;26(1):25.
8. Aaronson N, Alonso J, Burnam A. Assessing health status and quality-of-life instruments: attributes and review criteria. Qual Life Res 2002;11(3):193–205. http://dx.doi.org/10.1023/A:1015291021312
9. Leung WC. How to design a questionnaire. Student BMJ. 2001;09:171–216.
10. Presser S, Rothgeb JM, Couper MP, et al. Methods for testing and evaluating survey questionnaires. Hoboken, NJ: John Wiley & Sons; 2004. http://dx.doi.org/10.1002/0471654728
11. Mabuza L, Govender I, Ogunbanjo G, et al. African primary care research: qualitative data analysis and writing results. Afr J Prm Health Care Fam Med. 2014; In Press.
12. Babbie ER. Survey research methods. Belmont, CA: Wadsworth Publishing Co; 1973.

6

Price, availability and affordability of medicines

Authors:
Brenda S. Mhlanga[1]
Fatima Suleman[1]

Affiliations:
[1]Discipline of Pharmaceutical Sciences, School of Health Sciences, University of KwaZulu-Natal, South Africa

Correspondence to:
Fatima Suleman

Email:
sulemanf@ukzn.ac.za

Postal address:
Discipline of Pharmaceutical Sciences, School of Health Sciences, Westville Campus - University of KwaZulu-Natal, Private Bag X54001, Durban 4000, South Africa

Background: Medicines play an important role in healthcare, but prices can be a barrier to patient care. Few studies have looked at the prices of essential medicines in low- and middle-income countries in terms of patient affordability.

Aim: To determine the prices, availability and affordability of medicines along the supply chain in Swaziland.

Setting: Private- and public-sector facilities in Manzini, Swaziland.

Methods: The standardised methodology designed by the World Health Organization and Health Action International was used to survey 16 chronic disease medicines. Data were collected in one administrative area in 10 private retail pharmacies and 10 public health facilities. Originator brand (OB) and lowest-priced generic equivalent (LPG) medicines were monitored and these prices were then compared with international reference prices (IRPs). Affordability was calculated in terms of the daily wage of the lowest-paid unskilled government worker.

Results: Mean availability was 68% in the public sector. Private sector OB medicines were priced 32.4 times higher than IRPs, whilst LPGs were 7.32 times higher. OBs cost 473% more than LPGs. The total cumulative mark-ups for individual medicines range from 190.99% – 440.27%. The largest contributor to add-on cost was the retail mark-up (31% – 53%). Standard treatment with originator brands cost more than a day's wage.

Conclusion: Various policy measures such as introducing price capping at all levels of the medicine supply chain, may increase the availability, whilst at the same time reducing the prices of essential medicines for the low income population.

Le prix, la disponibilité et l'accessibilité financière des médicaments.

Contexte: Les médicaments jouent un rôle important dans les soins médicaux, mais les prix peuvent être un obstacle aux soins prodigués au patient. Peu d'études se sont penchées sur le prix des médicaments essentiels dans les pays à revenu faible et intermédiaire pour ce qui est des prix abordables pour le patient.

Objectif: Déterminer les prix, la disponibilité et l'accessibilité financière des médicaments sur le réseau de distribution au Swaziland.

Location: Les établissements privés et du secteur public à Manzini, au Swaziland.

Méthodes: On a utilisé la méthodologie standardisée conçue par l'Organisation Mondiale de la Santé et l'Action Internationale de la Santé pour étudier 16 médicaments pour maladies chroniques. Les données ont été collectées dans une région administrative, dans 10 pharmacies de détail privées et dans 10 établissements de santé publique. Les médicaments de marque originale (OB) et les équivalents génériques les moins chers (LPG) ont été contrôlés et ces prix ont été comparés aux prix internationaux de référence (IRP). Les prix abordables ont été calculés en fonction du salaire minimum journalier d'un fonctionnaire peu qualifié.

Résultats: La disponibilité était de 68% dans le secteur public. Les médicaments de marque originale (OB) du secteur privé coûtaient 32.4 fois plus cher que les IRP, alors que les LPG coûtaient 7.32 fois plus cher. Les OB coûtaient 473% plus cher que les LPG. Les majorations cumulatives totales des médicaments individuels vont de 190.99% à 440.27%. Le facteur majeur du coût additionnel était la majoration de détail (31% – 53%). Le traitement normal avec un médicament de marque originale coûte plus qu'une journée de salaire.

Conclusion: Différentes mesures telles que l'introduction d'un plafonnement des prix à tous les niveaux de la chaîne de ravitaillement des médicaments pourraient augmenter la disponibilité, tout en réduisant le prix des médicaments essentiels pour la population à faibles revenus.

Introduction

Access to medicines is influenced by many factors such as affordability, rational use, sustainable financing and reliable supply systems. One of the elements restricting access to medicines is high medicine prices.[1] This can have a detrimental effect on patients' health as well as the healthcare system in terms of lack of patient compliance with treatment and subsequent hospitalisation for serious complications. To increase access to medicines, one would thus need to ensure that medicines are affordable in order to counteract any existing barriers that might hinder medicine access. The stated goal of the 2011 Swaziland National Pharmaceutical Policy (SNPP) was to:

> ...[c]ontribute to improving the health of the Swaziland population by ensuring equitable access to and rational use of efficacious, good quality essential medicines and medical supplies and devices at affordable cost, particularly for vulnerable populations.[2]

One way of measuring affordability is to adjust prices by average income per person. This aids in understanding the value of a medicine with respect to the amount of income the average person has available to spend on pharmaceuticals. The SNPP has as objectives the development of pricing policies for medicines and encouraging generic prescribing and dispensing as well as generic substitution. These are meant to be part of future regulatory interventions.

Swaziland has a gross domestic product (GDP) per capita income of USD3073 and is classified as a lower middle-income country.[3] About 63% of the population are living below the upper poverty line of USD8.21 per capita per month.[3] The country's revenue has been affected severely by the global downturn. Southern African Customs Union (SACU) receipts were approximately 60% of government revenue in 2008. They were estimated at 9.3% in 2010. The 2006–2007 Demographic Health Survey (DHS) indicated that Swaziland was off track with regard to meeting its Millennium Development Goal (MDG) with health outcomes worsening as a result of high levels of HIV, AIDS and tuberculosis and limited progress with maternal, neo-natal and child health.[4]

The government, private sector, non-governmental organisations (NGOs) and faith-based organisations are all involved in the provision of health services.[5] There are primary, secondary and tertiary levels in the country. According to the SNPP, there are:

> ...1,018 449 inhabitants in Swaziland with about 78.9% residing in rural areas. 52% of the population is under the age of 20 years. The capital is Mbabane (population 69 000) and the largest city is Manzini (population 75 000). The Government, private sector, non-governmental organizations (NGOs), faith based organisations and traditional healers are involved in the provision of health services. There are 8 government hospitals, 2 mission hospitals, 1 industry supported hospital, 8 public health units, 5 health centres, and 218 clinics (type A+ B). In addition there are 73 mission health facilities (health centres, clinics and outreach sites), 62 private clinics and 22 industry-supported health centres and clinics.[2,5]

Swaziland has no established domestic pharmaceutical manufacturers. All medicines and medical supplies are imported. In the public sector, procurement is through an open tendering system. Procurement is restricted to items on the Swaziland National Essential Medicines List. Currently, there is no regulation for medicine pricing and thus no regulated dispensing fees. Medicine registration is not done in the country because the Pharmacy Act of 1929 does not have a process for registering and scheduling medicines, or licensing of sites for different types of pharmacies or inspections of such premises.[6] A new Pharmacy Bill and a Medicines and Related Substances Control Bill have been developed which provides for the establishment of a Pharmacy Council and a Medicines Regulatory Authority.[7]

Medicines are free at the point of delivery in the public sector, with a nominal user fee of USD1.16 charged for consultation in hospitals, USD0.58 for radiology and USD0.35 for laboratory tests (1USD = SZL8.6570 according to the exchange rate as at 12 December, 2012, the Central Bank of Swaziland). These may stand as a barrier regarding access to services for those with low or no income capacity. The weekly income for the lowest-paid government worker in Swaziland is USD44.46.[8]

Chronic shortages of medicines in public health facilities have been observed,[5] meaning that consumers are then forced to buy medicines in the private sector. Reliable evidence is required in order to understand what the specific problems are for one to come up with the best way to improve the situation, as well as whether governmental controls are necessary so as to ensure that essential medicines are available at the least cost to the consumer.

The aim of this study was to determine medicine prices, price structure, availability and affordability in the public health and private retail pharmacies in Swaziland. The objectives were to determine availability of medicines in both sectors, the differences between originator brand and generic medicine pricing, affordability of selected medicines and a comparison of prices in Swaziland against international reference prices. In addition, this study sought to identify the major cost drivers of medicine prices in Swaziland by examining the price components of selected medicines.

Research methods and design

Study design

A quantitative cross-sectional descriptive study design was employed.

Setting

The study was conducted in one administrative area (Manzini region) of Swaziland. Manzini City, which is within the Manzini region, is the largest city in Swaziland, with a population of 75 000.[9] The city is situated in the centre of the country and is considered to be the industrial capital, with various textile industries. There are three public hospitals and a public health unit located within the city. Manzini region has the largest number of licensed private retail pharmacies as compared with the other regions. More than 70% of the retail pharmacies in this region are located in Manzini City.

Study population and sampling strategy

Both the public and private sectors were examined. Ten private sector outlets were selected at random from an updated list of 14 registered pharmacies within Manzini. The public sector sample of 10 outlets included two national referral hospitals and two regional hospitals. The remaining six outlets were selected at random from the list of clinics and public health units providing treatment and care for non-communicable diseases.[8]

A total of 16 chronic disease medicines were included in the survey, of which four form part of the World Health Organization – Health Action International (WHO–HAI) list of global medicines, one is regional and 11 are supplementary. The sample selection was based on the disease burden of the country and only medicines found in the essential medicines list were selected. According to the Health Management Information System report of 2009, diabetes was reportedly amongst the top 10 leading causes of inpatient admissions.[8] Others that have added to the burden include cardiovascular diseases and cancers.[10] The selected medicines all have an International Reference Price (IRP). The 2011 Management Sciences for Health (MSH) reference prices were used.[11]

Data collection

Data collection took place between 12 December 2012 and 25 January 2013. The standardised methodology developed by WHO–HAI was used to conduct the survey.[1] As medicines in the public sector are free to all,[8] only data on medicine availability was collected from the public health facilities. Public-sector procurement prices were extracted from the procurement unit at the Ministry of Health. Private-sector patient prices and availability data were collected from the private retail pharmacies. To assess affordability, three common diseases namely asthma, hypertension and diabetes were selected and affordability of treatment was calculated using the daily wage of the lowest-paid unskilled government worker. A monthly treatment course was derived by multiplying the daily dose by 30. Price components data were collected in order to determine the various components that contributed to the final price of medicines.

Data were collected for two products, namely the originator brand (OB) and the lowest-priced generic equivalent (LPG) for each medicine found at each facility. Price data were not entered for products that were temporarily out of stock. Percentage availability was checked before leaving the facility to determine whether a back-up facility would have to be visited in order to conduct the survey again for those facilities with less than 50% of the survey medicines. To ensure data quality, data collection forms were reviewed every day after completion of the field work. Completeness of the forms, accuracy of unit prices and OB and LPG prices were double checked. Validation was undertaken for 20% of the facilities. These were selected randomly.

Five medicines were chosen for the price components study: Enalapril tablets, Atenolol tablets, Glibenclamide tablets, Metformin tablets and the Salbutamol inhaler. Key informants in the Ministry of Health, Ministry of Commerce and Trade and the Swaziland Revenue Authority were interviewed. Individual medicine prices were tracked from the time they are procured from manufacturers until they reach the patient. Information was obtained by interviewing both wholesalers and retailers.

Data analysis

Data were entered into a pre-programmed Microsoft Excel workbook (Part I).[12] Data entry was verified using the double entry and data-checker functions of the workbook. Summary tables and analyses such as median price ratios (MPRs) for all medicines, median MPRs, and percentage availability were generated automatically. The MPR is the ratio of the median price for each medicine across facilities divided by an IRP converted into local currency and is calculated when data are available from at least four facilities.

The availability of individual medicines was determined as being the percentage of facilities in which the medicine was found on the day of data collection. Mean availability was reported for the overall availability of the basket of medicines. Difference in percentage availability for OBs and LPGs of individual medicines and difference in average percentage availability for all OBs and LPGs would determine if the availability varies significantly between OBs and LPGs. Price components data were entered into a pre-programmed workbook (Part II).[13]

Ethical considerations

The study and the tools received ethical clearance from the Humanities and Social Sciences Research Ethics Committee, University of KwaZulu-Natal (HSS/1188/012M). For access to the Manzini healthcare premises and data, permission and ethical clearance was granted by the Ministry of Health, Swaziland.

Results

Availability

Mean availability of LPG medicines in the private sector was 77.50% ± 27.7% compared with 68.00% ± 22.3% in the public sector. Mean availability of OB medicines was higher in the public sector (80%) versus the private sector (40%). Medicines that had a particularly low availability in the public sector include aminophylline (30%) and propranolol (40%). Amlodipine, captopril and glibenclamide were found in over 90% of the outlets visited in the public sector. In the private sector, the LPGs for aminophylline and irbesartan had very low availability

(10% and 20% respectively), whilst atenolol, enalapril, glibenclamide, metformin and nifedipine were found in all the outlets.

Public-sector procurement prices

Only one price data point was found for any of the OB products since the government purchased medicines by generic names. Based on the MPRs' results for all 16 survey medicines, the public sector is procuring medicines at a slightly lower price than their IRPs (median MPR = 0.96). Half of the lowest-priced generic medicines were priced at 0.79 (25th percentile) to 1.72 (75th percentile) times their IRP. Medicines that were purchased at significantly less than IRPs include atenolol (0.65), captopril (0.72), irbesartan (0.25) and metformin (0.63). Examples of medicines for which the government was paying several times their IRPs include amlodipine (6.96), enalapril (3.86), phenytoin (7.56) and propranolol (2.97).

Private-sector patient prices

When private-sector medicine prices were compared with IRPs, the OB products were found to be priced at 32.4 times the IRPs. Within the basket this varied from 3.56 for irbesartan to 196.51 for glibenclamide. The median price of the lowest-priced generic equivalent was 7.32 times the IRP price. However, within the basket this varied from 1.50 for a salbutamol inhaler to 61.89 for amlodipine. To facilitate comparison of prices between the two product types, only those medicines where both the OB and LPG were available were included in the analysis. The results indicate that in the private sector, OBs cost 473% more, on average, than their generic equivalents. The median MPR for OB products in the private sector was 41.06 (range of 4.25–168.75) whilst for LPGs it was 8.67 (range 1.68–53.66). MPRs for the medicines are summarised in Table 1.

TABLE 1: Median price ratios for selected medicines, originator brand and generic equivalents in the private sector.

Medicine	Originator	Generic
Amlodipine 10 mg cap/tab	104.74	53.66
Atenolol 50 mg cap/tab	100.53	8.67
Carbamazepine 200 mg cap/tab	23.83	6.07
Enalapril 20 mg cap/tab	20.62	12.31
Glibenclamide 5 mg cap/tab	168.75	11.02
Metformin 500 mg cap/tab	5.54	3.29
Nifedipine Retard 20 mg cap/tab	44.93	5.19
Phenytoin 100 mg cap/tab	41.06	8.69
Salbutamol inhaler 100 mcg/dose	4.25	1.68

mg, milligrams per dosage form; cap/tab, capsules or tablets as a dosage form; mcg/dose, micrograms per dose of medicine.

Affordability of standard regimens

Affordability was measured only for medicines purchased from the private sector, since the government supplies medicines for free. The affordability of the LPGs, with the exception of enalapril, was less than one, with standard treatment costing slightly above a day's wage (1.2). Standard treatment with OBs cost more than a day's wage, except for metformin (0.9). Treating diabetes with glibenclamide required 6.7 days' wages and treating hypertension with atenolol needed 4.8 days' wages.

Price components

Price components for imported products were measured to investigate the differences in mark-ups and to determine the impact of tariffs, taxes and mark-ups on the price the patient pays. The country has no price-control regulation for medicines. No maximum mark-ups are set for the wholesaler or retailer. Over-the-counter medicines are charged 14% value added tax (VAT). Public-sector procurement is by open tender method, but it is limited to the Essential Medicines List. The tender price is Delivery Duty Paid. The price of the medicine is fixed for the duration of the tender contract period. The public sector has a generic medicine policy which does not apply to the private sector.

The mark-ups identified from the survey displayed wide variations for different medicines within the sector (Table 2). Retail mark-up contribution to the final price was the highest mark-up observed and ranged from 31% to 53%, the lowest being enalapril for both the originator and generic product. Metformin had the largest retail mark-up contribution to final price, with wholesale mark-up contribution being between 20% and 29%. The Cost, Insurance and Freight (CIF) contributed 18% to 34%. The landed price component (that is the price of the medicine after it arrives in a country and has passed all custom and import requirements and is transported to its first destination in the country) contributed from 4% to 8% of the final price.

The total cumulative mark-up was greater than 200% for all of the medicines with the exception of a generic salbutamol inhaler which had the lowest cumulative mark-up (190.99%). Metformin OB had the highest cumulative mark-up (440.27%), whilst glibenclamide and atenolol LPGs had a higher cumulative mark-up than the OBs (430.04% and 305.63% respectively). However, the patient still paid much less when buying these generics because their CIF price was low. Price components for enalapril were similar for the generic and

TABLE 2: Percent contribution of price components to final medicine price, originator vs. generic brands for selected medicines.

Medicine	Cost, insurance and freight	Landed price	Wholesale	Retail/dispensed price	Total percentage
Metformin 500 mg (OB)	18	4	27	51	100
Metformin 500 mg (LPG)	22	5	20	53	100
Salbutamol 100 mcg/dose (OB)	27	6	22	45	100
Salbutamol 100 mcg/dose (LPG)	34	8	26	32	100
Atenolol 50 mg (OB)	26	5	22	47	100
Atenolol 50 mg (LPG)	25	5	22	48	100

OB, originator brand; LPG, lowest-priced generic equivalent; mcg/dose, microgram per dose of medication.

originator products. It was also observed that the CIF price for the generic type was 94.8% that of the originator.

Discussion

In the public sector, only one of the survey medicines was found in the form of the OB product. This shows effective generic policy implementation in the public sector. In the private pharmacies, both the originator brands and generic equivalents were found, although generics were more widely available. Procurement prices in the public sector were very competitive, with medians below the IRPs. However, certain medicines such as phenytoin (MPR = 7.55) and amlodipine (MPR = 6.96) were priced considerably higher than their IRPs. The final patient prices for both LPGs and OBs were high in the private sector in terms of international pricing. LPGs were priced at nearly eight times their IRP, whilst OB medicines were priced at nearly 33 times their IRP. These disparities suggest substantial variation in price mark-ups between medicines.

The affordability of LPGs was generally good for all medicines, with standard treatment costing about a day's wage or less than the daily wage of the lowest-paid government worker in the private sector. However, the lowest-paid government worker is paid much more than the majority of the population. All the survey medicines were exempt from VAT as they are prescription medicines. The largest contributor to add-on costs was the retail mark-up. Generally, high mark-ups at different points in the supply chain can drastically increase prices and make medicines less affordable. Therefore, prices of medicines can be lowered substantially by reducing or regulating the mark-ups. Generics are more affordable than OBs and they would be more so if mark-ups were regulated.

About 63% of the population in Swaziland is living below the upper poverty line of USD8.21 per capita per month and, therefore, treatments which have been calculated to be affordable may still be too costly.[3] In addition, these costs do not include the other costs such as consultation and diagnostic tests. Finally, families generally require medicines for more than one member and may be confronted with unaffordable drug costs. Patients who cannot afford the private-sector costs may do without medicines completely. These findings are in line with other studies of affordability of chronic medicines which indicate that these medicines are unaffordable for many populations.[14,15,16,17]

Strengths and limitations

A major strength of this study is the use of the WHO–HAI medicine prices. The survey has allowed for the measurement of medicine prices and affordability in a reliable and standardised way that enables valid international comparisons to be made.

A limitation of the study is that availability is determined only for the list of survey medicines and therefore does not account for the availability of alternate forms, or of therapeutic alternatives for these medicines. Another limitation is that the MSH reference price is a median of recent procurement prices offered by for-profit and non-profit suppliers to international non-profit agencies for mostly generic products. This means that the MSH reference price is dependent on the number of supplier prices used which also determines the reliability of the MPRs. In cases where very few or no supplier prices are available and the buyer price is used as a proxy, MPR results can be skewed by a particularly high or low IRP. The quality of the products surveyed is another limitation of the study. The medicines are not yet registered in Swaziland and quality control testing was not performed. Assumption is made that they were of acceptable quality.

Recommendations

The findings of this study support the objectives of the SNPP, namely, to implement pricing policies to make medicines more affordable and available and to encourage generic prescription and dispensing as well as generic substitution. There is a need to uphold the generic policy implementation in the procurement of medicines in the public sector. Awareness creation and promotion of generic acceptance in the community and amongst healthcare professionals should be done. The use of IRPs as a benchmark should be encouraged in order to ensure lower procurement prices in the public sector.

A more comprehensive WHO–HAI based medicines price survey should be carried out to include more sectors and other essential medicines. There is clearly a need for a pricing policy to improve the availability of affordable generics. It should contain aspects of price control and incentives in order to reduce prices.

Conclusions

About one-third of the global population lacks reliable access to needed medicines, with this proportion being as high as 50% in some of the poorest countries of Africa and Asia.[18] One of the factors contributing to this lack of access is the price of medicines in countries. Whereas high-income industrialised countries often have health insurance systems, so that out-of-pocket payments for medicines are only required by 20% of the population, a lack of social insurance systems in developing nations contributes to the fact that up to 90% of people buy medicines through out-of-pocket payment.[19] The study has provided some insight into current issues related to price, availability and affordability of key medicines for the treatment of common chronic disease conditions in Swaziland. It has supported the need for policy development in terms of pricing policies and regulation of mark-ups that are required to increase availability, reduce prices, and improve affordability, which is the goal of the SNPP.

Acknowledgements

The authors wish to thank Ms Margaret Ewen (HAI-Europe) for her valuable comments.

Competing interests

The authors declare that they have no financial or personal relationship(s) that may have inappropriately influenced them in writing this article.

Authors' contributions

FS (University of KwaZulu-Natal) and BM (University of KwaZulu-Natal) conceptualised and designed the study. BM undertook the data collection and FS undertook data validation. Both authors were responsible for the final draft of the article.

References

1. World Health Organization, Health Action International. Measuring medicine prices, availability, affordability and price components. 2nd ed. Geneva: World Health Organization; 2008.
2. Kingdom of Swaziland. National pharmaceutical policy. 2nd ed. Swaziland: Ministry of Health [document on the Internet]. [2011] [cited 2014 Mar 02]. Available from: http://apps.who.int/medicinedocs/documents/s19028en/s19028en.pdf
3. The World Bank. Indicators [page on the Internet]. [2010] [cited 2013 Oct 07]. Available from: http://data.worldbank.org/indicator/
4. Central Statistical Office. Swaziland Demographic Health Survey 2006–2007. Swaziland: Ministry of Health; 2008.
5. World Health Organization Regional Office for Africa. Service Availability Mapping Report, 2010. World Health Organization, Regional Office for Africa; 2010.
6. Strengthening Pharmaceutical Systems (SPS)/USAID. Pharmaceuticals and the public interest: the importance of good governance [document on the Internet]. 2011 [cited 2014 Mar 07]. Available from: http://www.msh.org/sites/msh.org/files/sps_governance_pub_final_2011_0.pdf
7. Fakudze F. Harmonization initiative for the SADC region. Presentation at international conference on harmonisation of technical requirements for registration of pharmaceuticals for human use. [document on the Internet]. 2011 [cited 2014 Mar 02]. Available from: http://www.ich.org/fileadmin/Public_Web_Site/Meetings/C-GCG_Reports/June_2011_Cincinnati/SADC_Harmonization_Initiative_14_June_2011.pdf
8. Ministry of Public Service and Information. Establishment circular number 4 of 2010: Cost of living adjustment for 2010/11. Mbabane: MOPSI, 2010 Central Statistics Office. Swaziland Population and Housing Census, Mbabane, Swaziland; 2010.
9. Swaziland Ministry of Health. Essential health care package for Swaziland, 2010[document on the Internet]. 2010 [cited 2014 Mar 07]. Available from: http://www.gov.sz/images/stories/Health/essential%20health%20care%20package%20for%20swaziland.doc
10. Management Sciences for Health. International drug price indicator guide [password-protected database on the Internet]. [2011] [updated 2012; cited 2013 Oct 07]. Available from: http://erc.msh.org/dmpguide
11. World Health Organization/Health Action International. International medicines price workbook – Part I [file on the Internet]. [2011] [updated May 2008; cited 2013 Oct 07]. Available from: http://www.haiweb.org/medicineprices/manual/documents.html
12. World Health Organization/Health Action International. International medicines price workbook – Part II [file on the Internet]. [2011] [updated May 2008; cited 2013 Oct 07]. Available from: http://www.haiweb.org/medicineprices/manual/documents.html
13. Mendis S, Fukino K, Cameron A, et al. The availability and affordability of selected essential medicines for chronic diseases in six low- and middle-income countries. Bull World Health Organ. 2007;85(4):279–288. http://dx.doi.org/10.2471/BLT.06.033647
14. van Mourik MSM, Cameron A, Ewen M, et al. Availability, price and affordability of cardiovascular medicines: a comparison across 36 countries using WHO/HAI data. BMC Cardiovasc Disord. 2010;10:25. http://dx.doi.org/10.1186/1471-2261-10-25
15. Cameron A, Ewen M, Ross-Degnan D, et al. Medicine prices, availability, and affordability in 36 developing and middle-income countries: a secondary analysis. Lancet. 2009;373(9659):240–249. http://dx.doi.org/10.1016/S0140-6736(08)61762-6
16. Niëns LM, Cameron A, Van de Poel E, et al. Quantifying the impoverishing effects of purchasing medicines: a cross-country comparison of the affordability of medicines in the developing world. PLoS Med. 2010;7(8):e1000333. http://dx.doi.org/10.1371/journal.pmed.1000333
17. World Health Organization. Who Pays for Health Systems? In The World Health Report 2000. Geneva: World Health Organization, 2000; p.94–115.
18. WHO/WTO [World Health Organization/World Trade Organization Secretariats]. Report of the workshop on differential pricing and financing of essential drugs. Global Health Council. 8–11 April 2001; Høsbjør, Norway: Norwegian Foreign Affairs Ministry; 2001
19. Gelders S, Ewen M, Noguchi N, et al. Price, availability and affordability. An international comparison of chronic disease medicines. Background report prepared for the WHO planning meeting on the Global Initiative of Treatment of Chronic Diseases, Cairo, December 2005. World Health Organization [document on the Internet]. 2006 [cited 2014 Mar 02]. Available from: http://apps.who.int/medicinedocs/index/assoc/s14135e/s14135e.pdf

7

Ethical considerations of mobile phone use by patients in KwaZulu-Natal: Obstacles for mHealth?

Authors:
Caron L. Jack[1]
Maurice Mars[1]

Affiliations:
[1]Department of TeleHealth, Nelson R Mandela School of Medicine, University of KwaZulu-Natal, South Africa

Correspondence to:
Caron Jack

Email:
jackc1@ukzn.ac.za

Postal address:
Private Bag 07, Congella 4013, South Africa

Background: mHealth has the potential to facilitate telemedicine services, particularly in the developing world. Concern has been expressed about the confidentiality of health information that is relayed by mobile phone.

Aim: We examined the habits and practices of mobile phone use by patients in KwaZulu-Natal, South Africa.

Methods: We conducted a descriptive survey of two patient populations: 137 urban patients attending private practitioners and 139 patients in remote rural areas attending outpatient departments in Government-funded hospitals. The questionnaire covered several domains: demographics, mobile phone use, privacy and confidentiality and future use for health-related matters.

Results: Two hundred and seventy-six patients completed the questionnaire. We found that a third of our participants shared their mobile phone with others, 24% lent their phone to others and more than half received health-related messages for other people. Mobile phone theft was common, as was number changing. Thirty-eight percent of the people were not able to afford airtime for more than a week in the past year and 22% of rural patients were unable to keep their phone charged. Mobile phone signal coverage was significantly worse in the rural areas than in urban areas.

Conclusion: This study highlights the legal and ethical ramifications that these practices and findings will have on mHealth programmes in our setting. Healthcare providers and regulators will need to consider how patients use and manage their mobile phones when developing services and regulations.

Considérations d'ordre éthique sur l'usage des portables par les patients au KwaZulu-Natal: obstacles pour la santé mobile?

Contexte: La santé par téléphone portable peut faciliter les services de télémédecine, en particulier dans les pays en voie de développement. Certains craignent le manque de confidentialité des informations de santé transmises par téléphone portable.

Objectif: Nous examinons les habitudes et pratiques d'utilisation des portables par les patients au KwaZulu-Natal, en Afrique du Sud.

Méthodes: Nous avons mené une enquête descriptive sur deux groupes de patients: 137 patients urbains consultant des médecins privés et 139 patients dans les régions rurales éloignées en consultation externe dans les hôpitaux gouvernementaux. Le questionnaire couvrait plusieurs domaines: la démographie, l'utilisation des portables, la privauté et confidentialité, et l'utilisation future pour les questions liées à la santé.

Résultats: Deux cent soixante seize patients ont rempli le questionnaire. Nous avons trouvé qu'un tiers de nos participants partageaient leur portable avec d'autres personnes, que 24% le prêtaient à d'autres et que plus de la moitié recevaient des messages liés à la santé pour d'autres personnes. Les vols de portables étaient courrants ainsi que le changement de numéro. Trente-huit pour cent des gens n'avaient pas les moyens d'acheter du temps d'appel pour plus d'une semaine au cours de l'année passée et 22% des patients ruraux ne pouvaient pas garder leur portable chargé. La réception des portables était plus mauvaise dans les régions rurales qu'en ville.

Conclusion: Cette étude souligne les ramifications légales et morales que ces pratiques et résultats auront sur les programmes de santé mobile dans notre situation. Les prestataires de soins de santé et les autorités devront examiner comment les patients utilisent et gèrent leur téléphone portable dans le développement des services et règlements.

Introduction

Telemedicine, the practice of medicine over distance using information and communication technologies, has much to offer Africa with its high burden of disease and extreme shortage of health professionals,[1] but uptake has been disappointing.[2] This is, in part, because of a lack of connectivity in rural areas and high telecommunication costs.[3] Cellular or mobile phones have become a part of everyday life for many. With widespread signal coverage, they are seen as a means of facilitating telemedicine in Africa and the rest of the developing world.[4] mHealth is the term used to describe the broad use of mobile telecommunication and multimedia technologies for the delivery of healthcare.[5] mHealth is not another form of telemedicine, but is rather a means of data transmission using ubiquitous technology such as mobile phones and tablet computers. mHealth has, along with telemedicine, been identified as a practical solution with regard to reaching the health-related goals set out in the Millennium Development Goals (MDG) for health.[6] These are: improving maternal health; combating HIV, malaria and other diseases; and reducing child mortality. In alignment with these MDGs, South Africa's health priorities are maternal and child health and HIV.[7]

Mobile phone penetration has grown rapidly in Africa, albeit off a very low base, to 64%.[3] This does not mean that two-thirds of the population in Africa have mobile phones but that the number of active subscriber identity module (SIM) cards in circulation equates to two-thirds of the population. With an international average of 1.8 SIM cards per person, the proportion of people in Africa who own mobile phones was estimated to be 33% in 2012.[3] There are also indications that mobile phone penetration in Africa is increasing at a slower rate than the rest of the developing world and may be reaching saturation.[8] The median age in sub-Saharan Africa is 19 years and, with 43% of people living on less than USD1 per day (purchasing power parity), the cost of ownership of a mobile phone is out of reach of many people.[9] South Africa ranks third in Africa with regard to mobile phone penetration and therefore provides a robust platform for mHealth projects.[6]

A number of studies have shown the potential benefit that mobile phone use can have for healthcare in Africa.[10,11] Short message service (SMS) systems have been used to remind patients of appointments[12] and to take their medication,[11] for health education,[13,14] clinical care[15] and acquisition of data for disease surveillance,[16] all of which have improved patient outcomes.[17,18]

Concerns over patient confidentiality, privacy, autonomy and the security of personal and clinical data have been raised in all areas of telemedicine and medical informatics.[19] The concepts of confidentiality and privacy are culture dependent and the importance and impact of this on mHealth solutions in Africa need further study. In the WelTel Kenyan HIV medication adherence trial, HIV-positive patients were reminded by SMS to take their medication.[20] Patient eligibility was not dependent on owning a mobile phone but rather on having access to one or, for the illiterate, having a literate person available to take and convey the message. Confidentiality and the fear of stigma did not appear to be an issue, as a secondary analysis of the data from this trial revealed that the researchers overcame issues of confidentiality and stigma by sending a weekly check-in text message of 'Mambo-How are you?', requiring an active response from the participants stating that they were well or they had a problem, rather than using direct questions.[21] In a study in Botswana on patients' views regarding participating in a mobile phone-based dermatology service, only two of 75 people were concerned about privacy issues, but 43 people did not feel that photographs of the face were acceptable.[22]

Little has been published on confidentiality and privacy of data when using mobile phones for general clinical healthcare beyond the research arena, especially in the developing world. In thinking about the utility of mobile devices with regard to supporting patient-provider communication it is important to consider the following: (1) mobile device and network access (handset availability, capacity to keep battery charged, network availability, SIM card registration, airtime); (2) communication standards (voice or text, regulations or best practice for provider-initiated communications, availability of audit trail); and (3) sustainability (changing contact information, cost).

The aim of this study was to determine the access, availability and use of mobile devices amongst patients in KwaZulu-Natal, South Africa and thereby identify any ethical issues relating to patient–provider communication.

Research methods and design

Study design and setting

A descriptive, survey of two patient populations was undertaken in KwaZulu-Natal: urban patients consulting private, fee-for-service medical practitioners in Durban, a large city; and patients attending government-subsidised outpatient services in remote rural hospitals.

Sampling strategy

The estimated sample size was 264 participants, based on the survey formula of $n = z^2(p(1\text{-}p))/c^2$, with the following parameters: 95% confidence level (z = 1.96), margin for error (c = 6%) and a worst-case percentage for picking a choice for the variables of interest (p = 50%). A convenience sample representing different socio-economic groups was selected.

Data collection

Data were collected over a period of three months. A questionnaire covering four domains, namely, patient demographics, mobile phone use, privacy and confidentiality and mobile phone use for health-related matters, was designed by the authors. The questionnaire used may be found in the Appendix. The questionnaire was piloted with several participants for validation and to check for ambiguities. Privacy and confidentiality were addressed by determining whether the respondent was the sole user of the mobile phone, whether the phone or SIM card was shared with others and if others used their SIM cards in the respondent's phone. The questionnaire also looked at mobile phone theft. Mobile phone use included issues such as financing of mobile phone calls, availability of airtime, ability to keep a mobile phone charged, sophistication of the mobile phone used, number changing and the reliability of the network signal. Health-related use addressed mobile phone use for contacting hospitals or doctors and for taking health-related messages for others. In order to maximise response rates the questionnaire was administered to the study participants by the author, with the assistance of an interpreter where necessary.

Data analysis

The Chi Square test was used for analysis of categorical data with alpha set at 5%. Missing data were not included in the percentage and *p*-value calculations.

Ethical considerations

The study was undertaken with the approval of the Biomedical Research Ethics Committee of the University of KwaZulu-Natal (reference number BE063/09) and verbal informed consent was obtained from the participants. All participants were over the age of 18 and no personal or identifying information was obtained.

Results

A total of 276 people agreed to complete the questionnaire (137 urban and 139 rural patients). Thirteen of the rural responders (9.3%) did not own a mobile phone and were excluded from further analysis, leaving a total of 263 respondents, 137 urban (52%) and 126 rural (47.9%). Whilst it was envisioned that there would be two groups in the study, a third group emerged from the rural group, namely, those who work in urban areas, but reside in rural areas. The number of people in each of the three groups was as follows: urban (n = 137; 52.1%), rural (n = 83; 31.6%) and both areas (n = 43; 16.4%). Seventy percent of the respondents were women.

A third of all participants (n = 97; 36.9%) shared use of their mobile phone with others. Over half of the people (n = 131; 53.6%) took messages for others and 22.2% (n = 55) lent their phone to others. Rural respondents were significantly more likely to share SIM cards with other people and significantly more likely to be contacted by hospitals trying to contact other people (Table1).

Responses to questions related to connectivity, airtime and sophistication of mobile phone are shown in Table 2. Few people have mobile phone contracts and rural patients are significantly less likely to have a contract than urban patients (n = 3; p < 0001). In the past year, over a third of people (n = 95; 38.7%) went without airtime for more than a week, a quarter (n = 62; 25%) changed their mobile phone number and 23% (n = 58) had their mobile phone stolen. Significantly fewer rural respondents were able to keep their phones charged, with 22% reporting this as a problem (n = 19; p < 0004). Mobile phone signal coverage was significantly worse in rural areas. The rural cohort appeared to have older or simpler phones without a camera (n = 43; 57.3%).

Mobile phone use is shown in Table 3. Rural patients were significantly less likely to use their phones to contact their doctor (n= 31; p < 0001) or use the SMS feature (n = 60; p < 0001).

Discussion

The study adopted a 'bottom up' approach to identify how patients use and manage their mobile phones and whether

TABLE 1: Habits and practices of how people use their mobile phones.

Habit/Practice	Urban %	Rural %	Both %	*p*
I am the only user of the phone	88/131 (67.0)	52/75 (70.7)	26/41(63.4)	-
I lend my phone to other people	26/132 (19.7)	18/75 (30.7)	11/41(26.8)	-
I share SIM cards with other people	5/132 (3.8)	10/75 (13.3)	3/41 (7.3)	0.04
Other people put their SIM card in my phone	24/125 (19.2)	18/71(25.4)	7/38 (18.4)	-
I put my SIM card in other people's phones	28/129 (21.7)	16/71 (22.5)	10/41(24.4)	-
The hospital contacts other people through my mobile phone	14/126 (11.1)	33/74 (44.6)	5/38 (13.2)	< 0.001
I take messages on my phone for other people	54/130 (41.5)	58/74 (78.4)	19/40 (47.5)	< 0.001

SIM, subscriber identity module.
p, significant at < 0.05

TABLE 2: Connectivity and network issues.

Variable	Urban %	Rural %	Both %	*p* %
I buy airtime on contract	37/133 (27.8)	3/75 (4.0)	7/43 (16.3)	< 0.0001
I have been without airtime for more than a week in the last year	44/129 (34.1)	36/75 (48.0)	15/41 (36.6)	-
My number has changed in the past year	28/131 (21.4)	22/75 (29.3)	12/41 (29.3)	-
I am able to keep my battery charged	129/131 (98.5)	66/85 (78.0)	40/43 (93.0)	0.0004
I get a good phone signal at home	120/127 (94.5)	60/74 (81.1)	38/42 (90.5)	0.01
My phone has a camera	119/131 (90.8)	43/75 (57.3)	38/43 (88.7)	< 0.0001
I have had a mobile phone stolen	31/131 (23.7)	14/75 (18.7)	13/43 (30.2)	-

p, significant at < 0.05

TABLE 3: How patients use their mobile phones.

I use my mobile phone to	Urban %	Rural %	Both %	*p*
Contact the hospital	97/130 (74.6)	49/75 (65.3)	29/41 (70.7)	N/S
Contact my doctor	108/130 (83.1)	31/75 (41.3)	33/41 (80.5)	< 0.001
SMS	125/130 (96.2)	60/75 (80.0)	39/41 (95.1)	< 0.001

p, significant at < 0.05

this would have implications on mHealth interventions within our setting. The key findings were that people in KwaZulu-Natal share mobile phones and SIM cards and take health-related messages for other people. In addition, it was found that mobile phone theft is a problem. This raises issues of possible breaches of confidentiality and privacy of patient information that could have legal and ethical implications for mHealth programmes, patients and healthcare providers if not taken into consideration.

Respect for privacy and confidentiality are seen as being fundamental human rights and are cornerstones of medical ethics, protected by law in most countries; but privacy and confidentiality are culturally-dependent concepts. Differences in the importance of privacy have been noted between Western and Japanese subjects[23] and there have been recent changes in the understanding of privacy in China following changes in its economic policy.[24] In most African cultures, where collective family decision-making is the norm, confidentiality is viewed in a different light.[25] The word for confidentiality in isiZulu, the indigenous language of KwaZulu-Natal, was understood by only 30% of isiZulu-speaking people attending an outpatient clinic.[26] In the Botswanian study on the perceptions of HIV-positive patients regarding the provision of a mobile phone-based dermatology service, few were concerned about privacy as this was guaranteed by the researchers.[22] Kenyan HIV-positive patients received messages on shared phones and illiterate patients allowed others to receive SMS messages on their behalf which reminded them to take their medication.[20] In South Africa, where a stigma is attached to being HIV positive, a woman was killed by her community when her HIV status became known, showing that privacy and confidentiality are of major importance.[27] Sharing of SIM cards can allow text messages and information to be saved from a phone to the SIM card in some instances or vice versa.

Many healthcare providers (HCPs) and patients are now communicating with each other via SMS within a clinical setting.[28] In the United Kingdom, the Medical Protection Society (MPS) has published recommendations for communicating with patients by SMS and notes that the SMS now forms part of a legal medical record. They recommend that HCPs take informed consent from patients if they are going to communicate via SMS and say that this should be noted in the patient's medical file.[29] The recommendation does not, however, address patient-initiated SMSs. Consent is seen as a protective measure for both the HCP and the patient, providing some proof that both parties were agreeable to this form of communication and understand the risks involved.

With over a quarter of respondents in this study having changed their mobile phone number or having had their phone stolen within the past year, patient contact details would need to be verified and updated at each clinic visit. Programmes providing other SMS or mobile phone services would have to be informed of every change of number or theft. This would not, however, prevent breaches of confidentiality when messages are sent after the theft or number change but before the next clinic appointment.

Sharing of mobile phones amongst patients has also been documented in Kenya, where 41% of people were reported to share phones. Education, income, literacy, geographic location, gender and lack of electricity were cited as the primary reasons for not owning a phone.[30] Illiteracy has been shown to have an impact on the use of SMS amongst rural South Africans, which would limit the use of SMS services to convey health information. In one rural community, the ratio of outgoing calls to SMS was 17:1.[18] Eighty percent of rural patients in the current study use the SMS facility on their phones and 86% of rural patients want to receive medical reminders via SMS.

In rural areas, approximately 20% of people cannot keep their phones charged and do not have good signal reception. Very few have airtime contracts, with rural people being less likely to have one. Airtime is purchased on a 'pay-as-you-go' basis, with the most common voucher being the lowest denomination of R5.00 (± $0.50), which buys approximately four minutes of call time. Rural patients, whilst saying that they can contact the hospital using their mobile phone, indicated that they would only do so in an emergency situation requiring an ambulance as they perceive calling the hospital to be expensive. Half the rural patients were without airtime for more than a week during the past year, as were a third of the urban patients. If mHealth is to be integrated fully into the South African healthcare system, financial support or viable solutions, such as a substantial lowering of the cost of airtime for health programmes, will be needed for sustainability and cognisance will have to be taken of the fact that phones may be off the network at various times.

Over 40% of rural patients' phones did not have a camera, suggesting that these were older, entry-level phones and the difference between the groups was significant ($p < 0.001$). It is expected that this will change as more people upgrade their current phone and their old phones filter into the rural areas. To benefit rural populations, providers of mHealth services need to offer solutions that work across a spectrum of phones, including older technologies.

In South Africa, the Health Professions Council of South Africa (HPCSA), which is the statutory body that regulates all medical practitioners and medical practice, has drafted guidelines for the practice of telemedicine. They define telemedicine as:

> [*t*]he exchange of information amongst healthcare professionals at a distance for the purpose of facilitating, improving and enhancing clinical, educational and scientific healthcare and research, particularly to the under serviced areas in the Republic of South Africa.[31]

Significantly, this definition fails to mention the use of information and communication technologies, of which the mobile phone is one. The draft guidelines propose that a telemedicine consultation should only take place where there is an established patient–practitioner relationship, unless in an emergency, that all telemedicine activities require written informed consent and that written records be kept at both the send and receive site for each encounter. These requirements are problematic for mHealth services such as call centres, SMS services for general healthcare advice, education and medication reminders and telephonic consultation for a primary or second opinion. An attempt to implement a telephone-based clinical service was condemned as unethical by the HPCSA, which then also deemed telemedicine unethical because of concerns over confidentiality and privacy, amongst others.[32] Landline telephones, however, are used routinely in clinical practice and have been since at least 1879,[33] without the need for written informed consent and/or the requirement of written records. Regulatory consistency is thus required.

Limitation

The use of convenience sampling may be considered to be a limitation of the study as the results may not be representative of the total population of mobile phone users in KwaZulu-Natal.

Conclusion

It would be both prudent and ethically wise to obtain informed consent from patients in our setting prior to using mobile phones for health-related activities, as the findings of this study has identified potential breaches in maintaining the confidentiality of patient information. Consent would not, however, prevent breaches of confidentiality when phones and SIM cards are shared or when health messages are taken for other people. Obtaining consent in this instance would inform and alert the patient to these risks.

Further studies are needed in other African countries in order to determine if mobile phone use practices found in this study are common, connectivity specific, or driven by expediency or culture.

Acknowledgements

We wish to acknowledge and thank Mr Bhekhani Hlombe and Mr Cunden Chetty from the Department of TeleHealth for their kind assistance in data collection and in arranging visits to the outlying rural hospitals.

Competing interests

The authors declare that they have no financial or personal relationship(s) which may have inappropriately influenced them in writing this article.

Authors' contributions

CLJ (Nelson R Mandela School of Medicine) conducted and designed the study, performed the primary analysis, drafted the manuscript and collected the data. MM (Nelson R Mandela School of Medicine) was involved in conceptualisation of the study, contributed to the interpretation of the data and drafted the manuscript. Both authors read and approved the manuscript prior to submission.

References

1. World Health Organization. The World Health Report 2006 – working together for health [page on the internet]. 2006 [cited 2013 Aug 19]. Available from: http://www.who.int/whr/2006/en/
2. Mars M. Telemedicine in KwaZulu-Natal: from failure to cautious optimism. J Telemed Telecare. 2007;13(Suppl. 3):57–59. http://dx.doi.org/10.1258/135763307783247310
3. International Telecommunication Union. Measuring the information society [document on the Internet]. 2012 [cited 2013 Aug 22]. Available from: http://www.itu.int/en/ITU-D/Statistics/Documents/publications/mis2012/MIS2012_without_Annex_4.pdf
4. Aker JC, Mbiti IM. Mobile phones and economic development in Africa. J Econ Persp. 2010;24(3):207–232. http://dx.doi.org/10.1257/jep.24.3.207
5. World Health Organization. [homepage on the internet]. Towards the development of an mHealth strategy: A literature review. WHO Press, Geneva,2008 [cited 2013 Dec 29]. Available from: http://www.who.int/goe/mobile_health/mHealthReview_Aug09.pdf
6. GSMA. GSMA announces new global research that highlights significant growth opportunity for the mobile industry [homepage on the internet]. 2012 [cited 2013 Aug 22]. Available from: http://www.gsma.com/newsroom/gsma-announces-new-global-research-that-highlights-significant-growth-opportunity-for-the-mobile-industry
7. Department of Health. eHealth Strategy South Africa 2012–2016 [document on the internet]. 2012 [cited 2013 Dec 29]. Available from: http://www.hst.org.za/publications/e-health-strategy-south-africa-2012-2016
8. Mars M. The digital divide: still a reality. Global Telemedicine and eHealth Updates. 2013;6:277–280.
9. Global Health Observatory. World health statistics 2013 [homepage on the internet]. 2013 [cited 2013 Aug 19]. Available from: http://www.who.int/gho/publications/world_health_statistics/2013/en/
10. Free C, Phillips G, Felix L, et al. The effectiveness of M-health technologies for improving health and health services: a systematic review protocol. BMC Research Notes. 2010;6(3):250. http://dx.doi.org/10.1186/1756-0500-3-250, PMID: 20925916.
11. Mahmud N, Rodriguez J, Nesbit J. A text message-based intervention to bridge the healthcare communication gap in the rural developing world. Technol Health Care. 2010;18(2):137–144. doi: 10.3233/THC-2010-0576, PMID:20495253
12. Hasvold PE, Wootton R. Use of telephone and SMS reminders to improve attendance at hospital appointments: a systematic review. J Telemed Telecare. 2011;17(7):358–364. http://dx.doi.org/10.1258/jtt.2011.110707, PMID: 21933898
13. Gold J, Lim MSC, Hellard ME, et al. What's in a message? Delivering sexual health promotion to young people in Australia via text messaging. BMC Public Health. 2010;10:792. http://dx.doi.org/10.1186/1471-2458-10-792, PMID: 21190584
14. Gisore P, Shipala E, Otieno K, et al. Community based weighing of newborns and use of mobile phones by village elders in rural settings in Kenya: a decentralised approach to health care provision. BMC Pregnancy and Childbirth. 2012;12:15. http://dx.doi.org/10.1186/1471-2393-12-15, PMID: 22429731
15. Gilbert JW. Telemedicine by cell phone technology. Pediatr Neurosurg. 2010;46(5):408. http://dx.doi.org/10.1159/000318749, PMID: 21412030
16. Thinyane H, Hansen S, Foster G, et al. Using mobile phones for rapid reporting of zoonotic diseases in rural South Africa. Stud Health Technol Inform. 2010;161:179–189. PMID: 21191171
17. Noordam C, Kuepper BM, Stekelenburg J, et al. Improvement of maternal health services through the use of mobile phones. Tropical Med Int Health. 2011;16(5):622–626. http://dx.doi.org/10.1111/j.1365-3156.2011.02747.x, PMID: 21342374

18. Kaplan WA. Can the ubiquitous power of mobile phones be used to improve health outcomes in developing countries? Global Health. 2006;2:9. http://dx.doi.org/10.1186/1744-8603-2-9, PMID: 16719925

19. Kaplan B, Litewka S. Ethical challenges of telemedicine and telehealth. Camb Quart Healthc Ethics 2008;17(4):401–416. http://dx.doi.org/10.1017/S0963180108080535, PMID: 18724880

20. Lester RT, Ritvo P, Mills EJ, et al. Effects of a mobile phone short message service on antiretroviral treatment adherence in Kenya (WelTel Kenya1): a randomised trial. Lancet. 2010;376(9755):1838–1845. http://dx.doi.org/10.1016/S0140-6736(10)61997-6, PMID: 21071074

21. Van der Kop ML, Karanja S, Thabane L, et al. In-depth analysis of patient–clinician cell phone communication during the WelTel Kenya1 antiretroviral adherence trial. PLoS ONE. 2012;7(9):e46033. http://dx.doi.org/10.1371/journal.pone.0046033

22. Azfar RS, Weinberg JL, Cavric G, et al. HIV positive patients in Botswana state that mobile teledermatology is an acceptable method for receiving dermatology care. J Telemed Telecare. 2011;17(6):338–340. http://dx.doi.org/10.1258/jtt.2011.110115, PMID: 2184417

23. Adams AA, Murata K, Orito Y, et al. Emerging social norms in the UK and Japan on privacy and revelation in SNS. Int Review Inform Ethics. 2011;16(12):18–26.

24. Fan L, Buchanan W, Lo O, et al. SPoC: protecting patient privacy for e-health services in the cloud. In: eTELEMED 2012. 2012; p.99–104.

25. Ndebele P, Mfutso-Bengo J, Masiye F. HIV/AIDS reduces the relevance of the principle of individual medical confidentiality among the Bantu people of Southern Africa. Theor Med Bioethics. 2008;29(5):331–340. http://dx.doi.org/10.1007/s11017-008-9084-y, PMID: 19048391

26. Jack C, Singh Y, Hlombe B, et al. Language, cultural brokerage and informed consent: will technological terms impede telemedicine use? Pan-African Ethics, Human Rights and Medical Law Conference. Johannesburg, South Africa, May 6–8, 2013.

27. Cullinan K. AIDS martyr's killers may face justice. City Press [article on the Internet]. 2001 [cited 2014 Mar 10]. Available from: http://www.health-e.org.za/1999/11/17/aids-martyrs-killers-may-face-justice/

28. Hyodo K, Chihara K, Yasumuro Y, et al. Doctor-to-patient communication by 2.5G mobile phone; preliminary study. Internat Congress Series. 2005;1281:196–199. http://dx.doi.org/10.1016/j.ics.2005.03.239

29. Medical Protection Society. Communicating with patients by text message [homepage on the internet]. 2013 [cited 2013 Aug 22]. Available from: http://www.medicalprotection.org/uk/england-factsheets/communicating-with-patients-by-text-message

30. Wesolowski A, Eagle N, Noor AM, et al. Heterogeneous mobile phone ownership and usage patterns in Kenya. PLoS ONE. 2012;**7**(4):e35319. http://dx.doi.org/10.1371/journal.pone.0035319, PMID: 2255814

31. Kekana M, Noe P, Mkhize B. The practice of telemedicine and challenges to the regulatory authorities. S Afr J Bioethics Law 2010;3(1):33–37.

32. Bateman C. Cutting- edge telemedicine venture freezes as official bodies frown. S Afr Med J. 2011;101(6):368, 372. PMID: 21920090

33. Aronson SH. The Lancet on the telephone 1876–1975. Med Hist. 1977;21(1):69–87. http://dx.doi.org/10.1017/S0025727300037182, PMID: 320411

Appendix starts on the next page →

APPENDIX: Questionnaire

Mobile Telephone Usage Questionnaire

Please circle or tick answer

Q1: Demographics:

Male	Female

Age	

Q2: Area:

Town	Farm	Both

Q3: Do you own and use a mobile phone?

Yes	No

a. If you answered 'yes' please complete the following:

Current age	
Owns mobile phone	
Contract	
Pay as you go	
Number for life	

Q4: Does anyone in your household use a cellular phone?

Yes	No

a. If you answered 'yes' please complete the following:

Family member	
Current age	
Owns mobile phone	
Contract	
Pay as you go	
Number for life	

Q5: Are you the only user of the mobile phone?

Yes	No

Q6: Do you lend your mobile phone to other people?

Yes	No

Q7: Has your mobile phone number changed in the past year?

Yes	No

Q8: Do you share SIM cards with other people?

Yes	No

Q9: Do other people put their SIM cards into your mobile phone?

Yes	No

Q10: Do you put your SIM card in anyone else's mobile phone?

Yes	No

Q11: Does the hospital contact other people using your mobile phone number?

Yes	No	N/A

Q12: Do you receive messages for other people on your mobile phone?

Yes	No	N/A

Q13: Do you use your mobile phone to contact the hospital?

Yes	No

Q14: Are you able to contact your doctor via mobile phone?

Yes	No

Q15: Do you use the SMS/MMS service on your mobile phone?

Yes	No

Q16: Does your mobile phone have a camera?

Yes	No

Q17: Do you get good mobile phone signal from your home?

Yes	No

Q18: Has your mobile phone ever been stolen?

Yes	No

Q19: Do you want to receive medical advice or medical reminders via SMS on your phone?

Yes	No

Q20: Do you ever have a time when you do not have any airtime for more than a week?

Yes	No

Q21: Are you able to keep your mobile phone battery charged?

Yes	No

Q22: When you visit the farm are you able to use your mobile phone?

Yes	No

8

Prevention of mother-to-child transmission in HIV audit in Xhosa clinic, Mahalapye, Botswana

Authors:
Stephane Tshitenge[1]
Andre Citeya[2]
Adewale Ganiyu[1]

Affiliations:
[1]School of Medicine, University of Botswana, Botswana

[2]Mahalapye District Health Management Team, Botswana

Correspondence to:
Stephane Tshitenge

Email:
stephane.tshitenge@mopipi.ub.bw

Postal address:
PO Box 49, Mahalapye, Botswana

Background: The Mahalapye district health management team (DHMT) conducts regular audits to evaluate the standard of services delivered to patients, one of which is the prevention of mother-to-child-transmission (PMTCT) programme. Xhosa clinic is one of the facilities in Mahalapye which provides a PMTCT programme.

Aim: This audit aimed to identify gaps between the current PMTCT clinical practice in Xhosa clinic and the Botswana PMTCT national guidelines.

Setting: This audit took place in Xhosa clinic in the urban village of Mahalapye, in the Central District of Botswana.

Methods: This was a retrospective audit using PMTCT Xhosa clinic records of pregnant mothers and HIV-exposed babies seen from January 2013 to June 2013.

Results: One hundred and thirty-three pregnant women registered for antenatal care. Twenty-five (19%) knew their HIV-positive status as they had been tested before their pregnancy or had tested HIV positive at their first antenatal clinic visit. More than two-thirds of the 115 pregnant women (69%) were seen at a gestational age of between 14 and 28 weeks. About two-thirds of the pregnant women (67%) took antiretroviral drugs. Of the 44 HIV-exposed infants, 39 (89%) were HIV DNA PCR negative at 6 weeks. Thirty-two (73%) children were given cotrimoxazole prophylaxis between 6 and 8 weeks.

Conclusion: The PMTCT programme service delivery was still suboptimal and could potentially increase the mother-to-child transmission of HIV. Daily monitoring mechanism to track those eligible could help to close the gap.

Le contrôle de prévention de la transmission du VIH (PTME) de la mère à l'enfant à la clinique Xhosa de Mahalapye au Botswana.

Contexte: L'équipe de gestion sanitaire du district de Mahalapye (DHMT) procède à des contrôles réguliers pour évaluer le niveau des services donnés aux patients, tels que le programme de prévention de la transmission du VIH de la mère à l'enfant (PTME). La clinique Xhosa est l'un des établissements à Mahalapye qui offre un programme PTME.

Objectif: Cette évaluation avait pour but d'identifier l'écart entre les pratiques cliniques PTME actuelles à la clinique Xhosa et les directives nationales du PTME du Botswana.

Lieu: Cette évaluation a eu lieu à la clinique Xhosa dans le village de Mahalapye, dans le District central du Botswana.

Méthodes: Il s'agissait d'une rétrospective basées sur les rapports du PTME de la clinique Xhosa des mères enceintes et des bébés exposés au virus VIH examinés de janvier à juin 2013.

Résultats: Sur les cent tente-trois femmes enceintes inscrites pour les soins prénataux, vingt-cinq (19%) savaient leur état séropositif car elles avaient été testées avant leur grossesse ou avaient été testées séropositives lors de leur première visite prénatale à la clinique. Plus des deux-tiers des 115 femmes enceintes (69%) avaient été examinées pendant la gestation entre 14 et 28 semaines. Environ les deux-tiers des femmes enceintes (67%) prenaient des médicaments antirétroviraux. Parmi les 44 enfants exposés au VIH, 39 (89%) étaient séronégatifs par test d'ADN-PCR à six semaines. Trente-deux enfants (73%) avaient reçu un traitement prophylactique au cotrimoxazole entre 6 et 8 semaines.

Conclusion: Le service du PTME était encore sous-optimal et pourrait augmenter la transmission du VIH de la mère à l'enfant. Un mécanisme de contrôle quotidien et de dépistage des personnes concernées pourrait permettre de réduire l'écart.

Introduction

Background

Botswana's high HIV burden is an immediate threat to child survival as children born with HIV are vulnerable to both disease and death.[1] The introduction of the Prevention of Mother-to-Child Transmission (PMTCT) programme has resulted in a significant reduction in the number of children born with HIV.

It has been a decade since the PMTCT programme was launched in the country. In this time, the spread of HIV from mother-to-child has decreased from about 40% to 4%.[2] The Botswana government aims to reduce mother-to-child transmission to less than 1% by 2016.[3] The Botswana PMTCT guidelines state that: (1) all HIV-positive pregnant women with a CD4+ cell count above 350 cells/mm^3 should be initiated on triple antiretroviral prophylaxis (TAP) at 14 weeks; (2) all HIV-positive pregnant women with a CD4+ cell count below 350 cells/mm^3 or who are at the World Health Organization (WHO) clinical stage 3–4 should be initiated on highly-active antiretroviral therapy (HAART), regardless of their gestational age; (3) all HIV-exposed infants should be initiated on cotrimoxazole (CTX) prophylaxis at six to eight weeks.[1]

The PMTCT programme is run in all health facilities across the country and has been integrated into antenatal care (ANC) as well as maternity and post-natal care. The Mahalapye district health management team (DHMT) conducts regular audits to evaluate the standard of services (such as PMTCT) that are delivered to patients. Xhosa clinic is one of the facilities in Mahalapye DHMT that provide the PMTCT programme.

Aim and objectives

This audit aimed to identify gaps between the current PMTCT clinical practice in Xhosa clinic and the Botswana PMTCT national guidelines. The objectives were:

1. to determine the HIV status of pregnant women at their first ANC visit
2. to determine the proportion of pregnant women who booked early (before 28 weeks) for ANC appointments
3. to establish whether HIV-positive pregnant women with a CD4+ cell count above 350 cells/mm^3 were initiated on TAP at 14 weeks
4. to establish whether HIV-positive pregnant women with a CD4+ cell count below 350 cells/mm^3 or in WHO clinical stage 3–4 were initiated on HAART, regardless of their gestational age
5. to determine the HIV results of HIV-exposed infants at 6–8 weeks
6. to establish whether all HIV-exposed infants were initiated on CTX prophylaxis at 6–8 weeks.

Research method and design

Setting

Xhosa clinic is one of the 45 health facilities in Mahalapye, an urban village in the Central District of Botswana. The clinic provides only outpatient services and is one of the main antiretroviral (ARV) therapy service providers in the Mahalapye health district.

Audit design

This was a retrospective audit using PMTCT Xhosa clinic registers, namely the ANC register and the Baby PCR (polymerase chain reaction) testing register.

Sample

All pregnant women enrolled on PMTCT services and all HIV-exposed infants aged 6–8 weeks seen at Xhosa clinic between January 2013 to June 2013 were included in the study.

Data collection and analysis

All ANC records of pregnant mothers and all records of Baby PCR tests of HIV-exposed babies from 01 January to 30 June 2013 were included. The following data were collected: gestational age, pregnant mother's HIV test at the first visit, CD4+ results, ARV treatment and HIV-exposed infants on CTX. All data collected from records of HIV-exposed babies were included. The standard of PMTCT patient management was adopted from the Botswana PMTCT and the Botswana Safe Motherhood Initiative guidelines.[1,3] Data were fed into a spreadsheet for analysis. Descriptive statistics such as frequencies were used to analyse the pooled data and the results were presented in graphics (bar charts) and tables. The audit team reported their findings to the Mahalapye DHMT.

Ethical considerations

The clinical audit was approved by the Mahalapye DHMT (reference PBRS/2014). No patient identifier information (e.g. name, clinic number, address) was used. Access to the records was restricted to the audit team and information collected was stored securely in an electronic file with password. The electronic file was destroyed after completion of the audit. Information gathered during the audit process were only used for purposes of the audit. Only the summarised data to allow future comparison with any re-audit were kept. The audit in no way intended to victimise any particular person.

Results

One hundred and thirty-three pregnant women registered for ANC from January 2013 to June 2013. Twenty-five (19%) knew their HIV-positive status as they had been tested before their pregnancy or had tested HIV-positive at their first ANC visit (Figure 1). The majority of the women either did not know their HIV status (n = 55; 41%) or tested HIV negative (n = 53; 40 %) at their first ANC visit.

Eighteen of the 133 pregnant women did not have their gestational age recorded in the register, but the gestational age of the majority of the remaining 115 women (n = 102; 89%) was before 28 weeks at their first antenatal visit (Figure 2). More than two-thirds of the 115 pregnant women (n = 79; 69%) were seen at a gestational age of between 14 and 28 weeks; whilst only 23 (20%) were seen at a gestational age of below 14 weeks. Only 13 of the pregnant women (11%) booked their first ANC visit after 28 weeks of gestation.

About two-thirds of the pregnant women (n = 45; 67%) took ARV drugs as TAP or HAART; whilst 33% (n = 22) of the pregnant women were eligible, but were not initiated on ARV drugs (Figure 3). The majority of those on ARV drugs took HAART (n = 52; 78%).

The Xhosa clinic Baby PCR testing register indicated that 44 HIV-exposed infants were reviewed at ages 6 and 8 weeks during the study period. Out of the 44 HIV-exposed infants, 39 (87%) were HIV DNA (proviral HIV) PCR negative at six weeks, one (2.3%) was HIV DNA PCR positive, three (6.8%) results were still pending and one (2.3%) sample had been lost (Figure 4). Thirty-two (73%) children were given CTX prophylaxis between 6 and 8 weeks; whilst 12 (27%) of the HIV-exposed infants were not initiated on CTX prophylaxis (Figure 5).

Discussion

This audit was part of the routine monitoring of the service delivery to our patients. In our audit, the proportion of the HIV-positive pregnant women (19%) was far from the HIV prevalence of 32% amongst ANC clinic attendees in Botswana.[1,4,5] Close to half of pregnant women (41%) did not know their HIV status at the first visit. One may argue that the lower proportion of HIV-positive pregnant women from our audit, compared with the national one, did not reflect the true picture as a significant number of pregnant women with unknown HIV status contributed to the total.

The majority of pregnant women (87%) booked for their first ANC visit either before 14 weeks or between 14 and 28

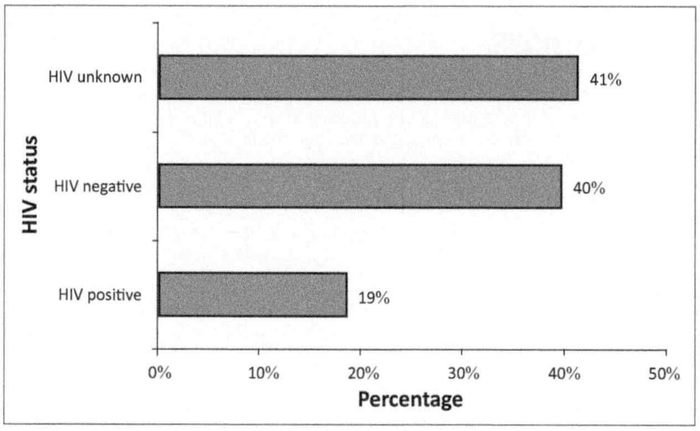

FIGURE 1: Bar chart demonstrating proportion of HIV status in women at their first antenatal care visit, Xhosa clinic, January 2013 to June 2013.

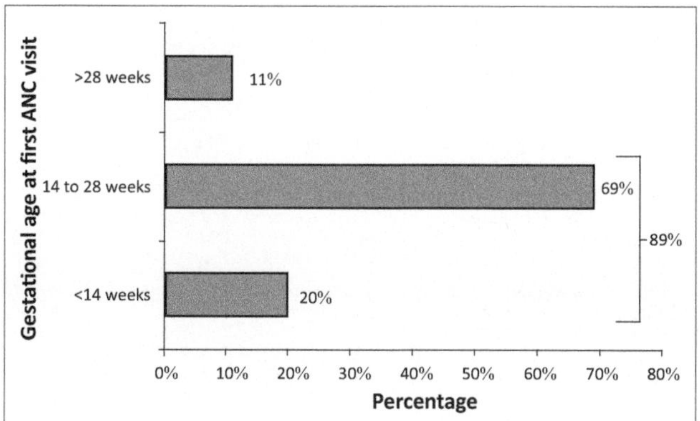

ANC, antenatal care.

FIGURE 2: Bar chart demonstrating gestational age of pregnant women at first antenatal care visit, Xhosa clinic, January 2013 to June 2013.

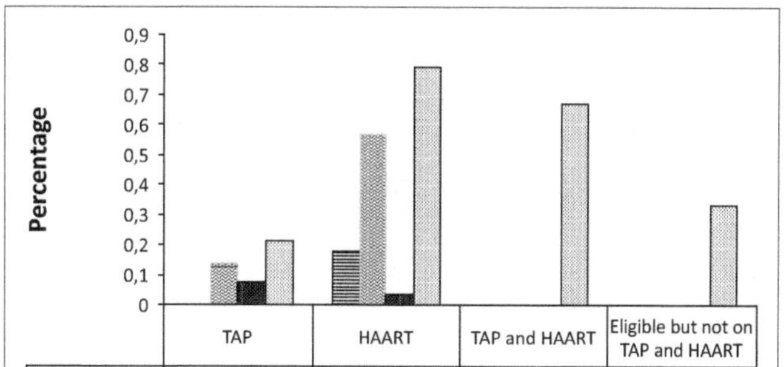

	TAP	HAART	TAP and HAART	Eligible but not on TAP and HAART
< 14 weeks		18%		
14-28 weeks	14%	57%		
> 28 weeks	7.3%	3.5%		
Total	21%	18%	67%	33%

TAP, triple antiretroviral therapy; HAART, highly-active antiretroviral therapy.

FIGURE 3: Bar chart demonstrating eligible patients on triple antiretroviral therapy or highly-active antiretroviral therapy versus eligible patients not initiated on treatment.

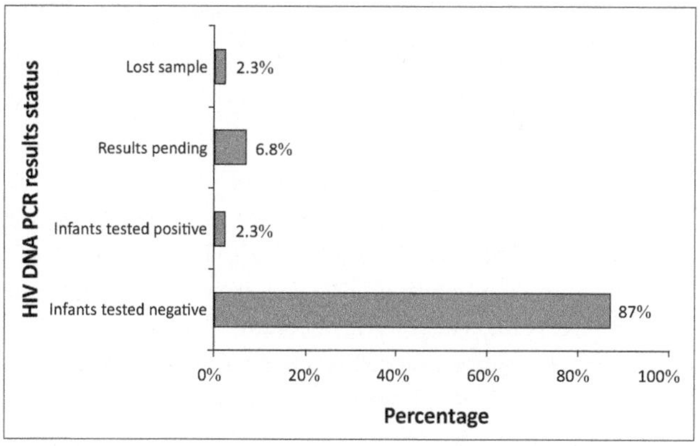

DNA PCR, deoxyribonucleic acid polymerase chain reaction.

FIGURE 4: Bar chart demonstrating results of HIV DNA PCR at 6–8 weeks of HIV-exposed infants, Xhosa clinic, January 2013 to June 2013.

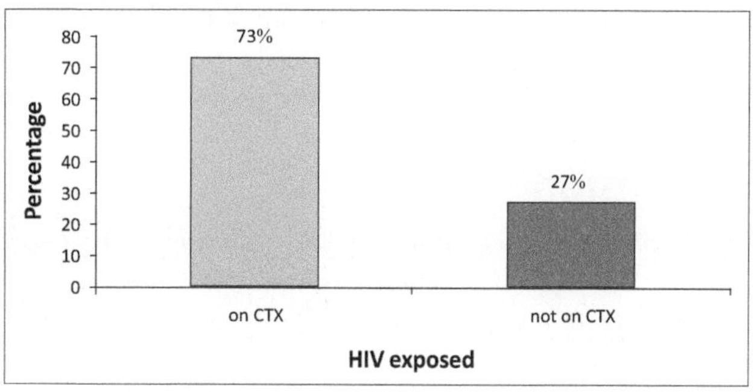

CTX, cotrimoxazole prophylaxis.

FIGURE 5: Bar chart demonstrating HIV-exposed infants given cotrimoxazole prophylaxis from 6–8 weeks, Xhosa clinic, January 2013 to June 2013.

weeks, which implied that the majority of these clients came on time to seek appropriate care.

The majority of pregnant women (67%) on ARV drugs were on a HAART regimen. The criteria for initiation of HAART are when the patient's CD4+ count is below 350 cells/mm^3 and/or when the patient is classified as being at WHO clinical stage 3 or 4.[1,6,7] The high proportion of pregnant women on HAART could suggest that there was good collaboration between the infectious disease centre clinic (IDCC) and the ANC clinic.

The proportion of HIV-positive pregnant women who were eligible for TAP or HAART, but not yet initiated on this regimen, was significant (33%). The PMTCT guidelines recommend that all eligible pregnant women should be given appropriate service. Poor documentation and inadequate monitoring could contribute to this inadequate service delivery. The transmission of HIV from mother to newborn increases in the absence of in utero PMTCT intervention.[8,9] It was estimated that during the period where PMTCT intervention in utero was absent in Botswana, the transmission estimates each year ranged from 684 to 1367.[1]

The majority of HIV-exposed infants (89%) tested negative. Only one (2.3%) HIV DNA PCR result was positive. This proportion was below the national proportion of 4% and the global target of 5% by 2015,[1,2,10] but only a small number of children were tested. About three-quarters of the HIV-exposed infants (73%) were given prophylaxis between six and eight weeks. More effort should be put into covering the 27% of infants who did not receive appropriate services.

Recommendations

The Mahalapye DHMT healthcare providers in Xhosa clinic should encourage the general public and patients to test for HIV in order to reduce the proportion of people who do not know their HIV status. Mahalapye DHMT should conduct health facility and community talks in order to educate mothers regarding early ANC booking. Daily monitoring to track those eligible for TAP, HAART and CTX should be implemented in the Xhosa clinic in order to reduce the proportion of eligible women and HIV-exposed children who are not on appropriate drugs. The effort to improve the current clinical practice with regard to PMTCT intervention during pregnancy and care of exposed babies could include more home care visits. More emphasis should be put to record keeping. We also recommended regular audits of clinical practice in order to measure the services provided to clients.

Conclusion

The findings of this audit showed that there are gaps between the clinical practice in Xhosa clinic with regard to its PMTCT programme and the standard set by Botswana PMTCT guidelines. The PMTCT programme service delivery was still suboptimal with regard to the administration of ARV to HIV-positive pregnant women and in the provision of CTX prophylaxis to HIV-exposed infants. The audit was conducted in one institution in Mahalapye DHMT, so the findings cannot be generalised to the whole region.

Acknowledgements

The audit team acknowledges the valuable contributions of Xhosa clinic staff with regard to making the registers available, as well as their willingness to help.

Competing interests

The audit team declares that there were no financial or personal relationship(s) that may have inappropriately influenced them in writing this article.

Authors' contributions

S.T. (University of Botswana) was responsible for the conceptualisation of the study, data analysis, write up of the report and compilation of this manuscript. A.C. (Mahalapye District Management Health Team) was responsible for the conceptualisation of the study and data collection. A.G. (University of Botswana) was responsible for editing.

References

1. Botswana Ministry of Health. Botswana prevention of mother-to-child (PMTCT) transmission of HIV: pocket guide. [document on the Internet] 2011 [cited 2014 May 01]. Available from: http://www.hiv.gov.bw/sites/default/files/documents/BTP%20-%20PMTCT-Pocket%20Guide.pdf
2. Government of Botswana. Botswana millennium development goals: status report 2010. [document on the Internet] 2010 [cited 2014 May 01]. Available from: http://www.undp.org/content/dam/undp/library/MDG/english/MDG%20Country%20Reports/Botswana/botswana_2010.pdf
3. Botswana Ministry of Health. The Safe Motherhood Initiative (SMI). National guidelines for antenatal care and the management of obstetric emergencies and prevention of mother-to-child transmission of HIV in Botswana. Gaborone: Botswana; 2005.
4. World Health Organization. Summary country profile for HIV/AIDS treatment scale-up. [document on the Internet] 2004 [cited 2014 May 01]. Available from: http://www.who.int/3by5/en/Botswana.pdf
5. Botswana Ministry of Health. 2009 Botswana second generation HIV antenatal sentinel surveillance technical report. Gaborone: Botswana; 2009.
6. Botswana Ministry of Health. 2012 Botswana national HIV & AIDS treatment guidelines. Gaborone: Botswana; 2012.
7. World Health Organization. Antiretroviral drugs for treating pregnant women and preventing HIV infection in infants. Geneva: WHO; 2010.
8. Torpey K, Kasonde P, Kabaso M, et al. Reducing pediatric HIV infection: Estimating mother-to-child transmission rates in a program setting in Zambia. J Acquir Immune Defic Syndr. 2010;54(4):415–422. http://dx.doi.org/10.1097/QAI.0b013e3181e36616
9. Cooper ER, Charurat M, Mofenson L, et al. Combination antiretroviral strategies for the treatment of pregnant HIV-1-infected women and prevention of perinatal HIV-1 transmission. J Acquir Immune Defic Syndr. 2002;29(5):484–494. http://dx.doi.org/10.1097/00126334-200204150-00009
10. UNAIDS. Countdown to zero – global plan towards the elimination of new HIV infections among children by 2015 and keeping their mothers alive: 2011–2015. Geneva: UNAIDS; 2011.

The diabetic foot risks profile in Selebi Phikwe Government Hospital, Botswana

Authors:
Stephane Tshitenge[1]
Adewale Ganiyu[1]
Deogratias Mbuka[1]
Joseph M. Shama[2]

Affiliations:
[1]Family physicians and lecturers, Department of family medicine, School of Medicine, University of Botswana, Botswana

[2]Hospital superintendent, Selebi Phikwe Government Hospital, Botswana

Correspondence to:
Stephane Tshitenge

Email:
stephotshitenge@yahoo.com

Postal address:
PO Box 49, Mahalapye, Botswana

Aim: The present study aimed: (1) to evaluate the proportion of each diabetic foot (DF) risk category, according to the International Working Group on the Diabetic Foot (IWGDF) consensus, in patients attending the diabetic clinic in Selebi Phikwe Government Hospital (SPGH) and (2) to examine some of the factors that may be associated with the progression to higher risk categories such as anthropometric measurements, blood pressure, glycosylated haemoglobin (HbA1c) and lipid profile.

Methods: A retrospective, cross sectional chart review of patients who had attended the diabetic clinic in SPGH from January 2013 to December 2013 was performed. Patients were included if they had undergone a foot examination. Patients with amputation due to accident were excluded. The DF risk category was assessed by determining the proportion of patients in each of four risk categories, as described by the IWGDF consensus.

Results: The study encompassed 144 records from patients reviewed for foot examination from January to December 2013. Patients' ages were between 16 and 85 years, 46 (40%) were male and 98 (60%) were female. The majority (122, [85%]) of patients were in DF risk category 0, whilst a limited number of patients were classified in risk category 1 (10, [6.9%]), risk category 2 (7, [4.9%]) and risk category 3 (5, [3.5%]). Most of the patients had the type 2 diabetes mellitus (139, [97%; 95% CI 92% – 99%]). Patients' ages were associated with the progressively higher DF risk categories. The adjusted odd ratio was 1.1 (95% CI 1.03–1.14; $p = 0.004$).

Conclusion: The present study revealed that about 15% of patients attending the SPGH diabetic clinic were categorised in higher risk groups for diabetic foot; patients' ages were linked to the higher DF risk categories.

Le profil des risques du pied diabétique à l'Hôpital gouvernemental de Selebi Phikwe, au Botswana.

Objectif: Cette étude a pour but: (1) d'évaluer la proportion de catégorie de risques du pied diabétique (DF), selon le Groupe de Travail International sur le document de consensus sur le pied diabétique (IWGDF), chez les patients fréquentant la clinique pour diabétiques de l'Hôpital gouvernemental de Selebi Phikwe (SPGH) et (2) d'examiner les facteurs associés à la progression vers des catégories de risques plus élevés tels que les mesures anthropométriques, la tension sanguine, l'hémoglobine glycosylée (HbA1c) et le taux de lipides.

Méthodes: On a effectué une révision rétrospective et transversale des graphiques des patients qui avaient fréquenté la clinique pour diabétiques du SPGH de janvier 2013 à décembre 2013. Les patients qui avaient subi un examen du pied ont été acceptés. Les patients ayant subi une amputation à la suite d'un accident ont étés exclus. La catégorie à risque du pied diabétique a été évaluée par la détermination de la proportion de patients dans chacune des quatre catégories à risque, comme il est décrit dans le document de consensus IWGDF.

Résultats: L'étude comprend 144 dossiers de patients évalués pour l'examen du pied de janvier à décembre 2013. Les patients avaient de 16 à 85 ans, 46 (40%) étaient des hommes et 98 (60%) des femmes. La majorité (122, [85%]) des patients étaient dans la catégorie à risque de pied diabétique 0, alors qu'un nombre limité de patients étaient classés dans la catégorie à risque 1 (10, [6.9%]), la catégorie à risque 2 (7, [4.9%]) et la catégorie à risque 3 (5, [3.5%]). La majorité des patients avaient le type 2 de diabète mellitus (139, [97%; 95% CI 92% – 99%]). L'âge des patients correspondait à des catégories à risque progressivement plus élevé de diabète du pied. Le rapport de risques ajusté était de 1.1 (95% CI 1.03–1.14; $p = 0.004$).

Conclusion: Cette étude a révélé qu'environ 15% des patients fréquentant la clinique pour diabétiques de SPGH étaient classés dans des groupes à risque plus élevé de pied diabétique; l'âge des patients était lié aux catégories de risques plus élevé de pied diabétique.

Introduction

Lower limb problems such as foot ulceration, infection and amputation are common in people with diabetes.[1,2,3,4,5] Recent reports have highlighted the significance of prompt recognition of the high-risk foot and the standardised provision of preventive measures,[6,7] as they can help to avoid the development of foot lesions, minimise morbidity and costs resulting from those complications. Strategies such as patient and staff education, multi-disciplinary management of foot ulcers, and close monitoring can lessen the amputation rate.[8, 9,10,11]

High risk of foot complications is associated with: a history of prior ulcer or amputation, Charcot foot, poor glycaemic control, trauma, peripheral neuropathy and/or peripheral vascular diseases, infections, foot structure deformity, impaired vision, old age, male gender, and ethnicity (black people and Hispanic people).[4, 12, 13, 14]

Several risk-stratification schemes have been suggested; none of these classification systems has been universally adopted to foretell complications. The International Working Group on the Diabetic Foot (IWGDF) system seems to be the most endorsed and simplified risk-stratification system used.[15] This system classifies patients into four risk categories. In risk category 0, patients are considered to have protective sensation or there is no foot deformity. In risk category 1, patients are considered to have an impending risk, as they have a loss of protective sensation (LOPS). In risk category 2, patients have high risk, as they have LOPS in their feet with evidence of the high-pressure zone (callus/deformity) or poor circulation. In risk category 3, patients have a history of plantar ulceration or neuropathic fracture (Charcot foot).[4, 12, 15] Risk stratification also serves as a guide to schedule patient review; risk category 0, 1, 2 and 3 patients are reviewed annually, semi-annually, quarterly and monthly to quarterly, respectively.[4]

The aim of the present study was: (1) to evaluate the proportion of each diabetic foot (DF) risk category, according to IWGDF consensus,[4] in patients attending a diabetic clinic in Selebi Phikwe Government Hospital (SPGH), a district primary care facility in Botswana; and (2) to examine some of the factors that may be associated with the progression to higher risk categories such as anthropometric measurements, blood pressure, glycosylated haemoglobin (HbA1c) and lipid profile.

Contribution to field

There is a paucity of data available from Sub-Saharan Africa on DF risk categories and the predisposing factors. The majority of available data are from studies conducted in secondary and tertiary settings. Therefore, it was deemed necessary to conduct such a study in a primary care setting. It is hoped that the public will benefit from this study, as it attempts to document the prevalence of DF risk categories in primary healthcare in Selebi Phikwe, Botswana and the Sub-Saharan region.

Ethical considerations

Ethical clearance for the study was obtained from the University of Botswana (URB/IRB/1406) and the Ministry of Health [PPME 13/18/1 VIII (79)]. Permission for data collection at SPGH was also obtained from the hospital management. A waiver of patient consent was obtained from the Institutional Review Board (University of Botswana) since the study required only examination of routinely maintained medical records.

Research methods and design

Study design

A retrospective, cross sectional chart review was performed of patients who had attended the diabetic clinic in SPGH from January 2013 to December 2013.

Context and sampling of the study

The present study involved reviewing all diabetes mellitus (DM) patients' records: both type 1 and type 2 diabetes mellitus. Patients were booked for foot assessment as they arrived at the clinic and they were reviewed as per IWGDF recommendations.[4]

The SPGH is situated in the Central District of Botswana. It provides primary healthcare in outpatient clinics such as the diabetic clinic. The clinic has been operational since October 2010; in 2011, one nurse had formal training on diabetic care.

Data collection and procedure

Records of patients booked for foot review during the study period were selected. Those from patients with amputation due to accident were excluded.

Data were collected from a checklist form used routinely in the clinic, which captures information such as: demographics (gender, age); type of DM; history of hypertension; and anthropometric measurements (weight, height, body mass index, waist circumference). Laboratory data (blood sugar, HbA1c, kidney function, lipid profile) and clinical variables such as a DF risk category were collected as well. The laboratory results (HbA1c, lipid profile) obtained within the previous six months were used for the study.

Data analysis

Data distribution was checked, then summarised by calculating the mean ± standard deviation (s.d.) for normally distributed variables, and the frequency in percentages for binomial and the median ± interquartile range (IQR), if skewed. A Kruskal-Wallis rank test was performed to measure the differences between the medians of factor DF risk category with regards to independent variables such as: age, hypertension, systolic and diastolic blood pressure, body mass index (BMI), blood sugar level, HbA1c, LDL-C, HDL-C, total cholesterol and triglyceride. The Tukey's quick test was used as a *post hoc* test to find where these differences between median DF risk categories lied. To control for possible confounding variables, variables were selected with a significant level of association ($p \leq 0.2$), their normality, linearity and homoscedasticity were checked and they were fitted into the ordinal regression model. Results were expressed as a coefficient, adjusted odds ratio (OR) and 95% confidence interval (CI). All statistical analyses were carried out using an R software version 3.0.0 with R commander package version 1.9-6. The level of significance was set at $p < 0.05$.

Results

In 2013, the SPGH clinic registered 402 patients. Of these, 149 patients were included in the present study because they were reviewed for foot examination from January to December 2013. Five records were discarded, as they had missing data on most sections. There were no patients reviewed with an amputation during the study period.

Demographic characteristics of the study population

Out of the 144 records included in the present study, 46 (40%) were male and 98 (60%) were female. Patients were aged between 16 and 85 years; their mean age was 55 years old (95% CI 53–57 years old).

Diabetic foot risk category

The majority (122, [85.0%]) of patients in the present study were in the DF risk category 0; whilst fewer were classified in risk category 1 (10, [6.9%]), risk category 2 (7, [4.9%]) and risk category 3 (5, [3.5%]). Overall, the proportion of patients with LOPS, high-pressure zone (callus and/or deformity), poor circulation, history of plantar ulceration or neuropathic fracture deformity was 15.0%.

Clinical and laboratory profile of the study population

As shown in Table 1, most of the patients in the study had type 2 DM (139 [97%; 95% CI 92% – 99%]). About three-quarters (74%; 95% CI 64% – 82%) of patients were diagnosed with hypertension. The average systolic blood pressure was 140 mm Hg (95% CI 135 mmHg – 144 mmHg). The majority (62/105, [59%]) had uncontrolled blood sugar (HbA1c above 7.0%), the mean HbA1c was 8.1% (95% CI 7.7% – 8.7%). The mean low-density lipoprotein cholesterol was 3.6 mmol/L (95% CI 2.9 mmol/L – 4.3 mmol/L). More than half of the patients had a BMI above 28 kg/m^2 (95% CI 26 kg/m^2 – 40 kg/m^2).

Association between diabetic foot risk category with demographic and clinical variables

The only demographic variable that was significantly different between risk categories was age (p = 0.005, as shown in Table 2). Subsequent analysis (depicted in Figure 1) shows that median age is significantly different only between categories 0 and 1 (p < 0.001). The results of the ordinal logistic regression analysis are shown in Table 3. Patients' ages were associated with the progressively higher DF risk categories. The adjusted odd ratio was 1.1 (95% CI 1.03 – 1.14; p = 0.004).

The study did not detect any significant differences between the median of DF risk categories in other variables, as their p values were above 0.05.

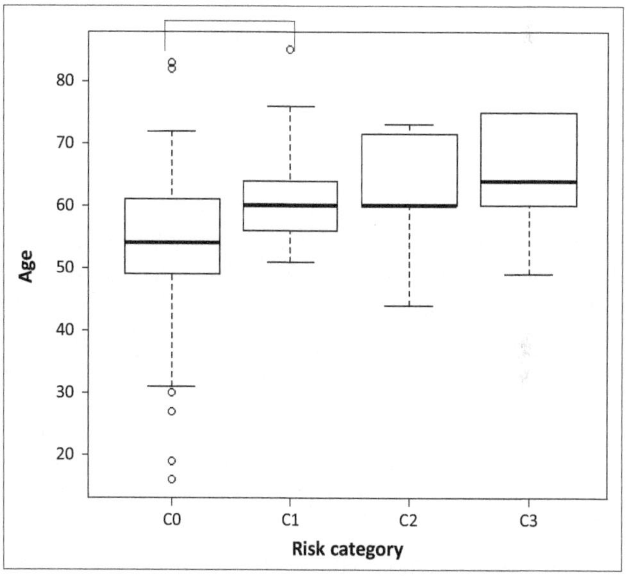

C0, DF risk category 0; C1, DF risk category 1; C2, DF risk category 2; C3, DF risk category 3.

FIGURE 1: Boxplots of the age for each of the DF risk category in patients reviewed for foot examination at the diabetic clinic, January to December 2013.

TABLE 1: Clinical and biological profile of patients reviewed for foot examination at the diabetic clinic, January to December 2013.

Profile	Variables						95% CI
	%	*n*	mean	s.d.	median	IQR	
Type 2 diabetes mellitus	97	139	-	-	-	-	96–98
Hypertension number	70	101	-	-	-	-	65–75
Systolic blood pressure (mmHg)	-	-	140	27	-	-	135–144
Diastolic blood pressure (mmHg)	-	-	77	11	-	-	75–78
Body mass index (kg/m^2)	-	-	-	-	28	8.2	26–40
Waist circumference (cm)	-	-	106	13	-	-	102–111
Fasting blood sugar (mmol/L)	-	-	8.0	3.5	-	-	7.4–8.5
Haemoglobin A1c (%)	-	-	8.1	2.3	-	-	7.7–8.7
High density lipoprotein cholesterol (mmol/L)	-	-	1.2	0.4	-	-	1.1–1.3
Low-density lipoprotein cholesterol (mmol/L)	-	-	3.6	0.9	-	-	2.9–4.3
Triglyceride (mmol/L)	-	-	-	-	1.6	1.0	1.4 -1.8
Total cholesterol (mmol/L)	-	-	5.1	1.1	-	-	4.9–5.3

SPGH, Selebi Phikwe Government Hospital; s.d., standard deviation; IQR, interquartile range; mmol/L, millimol per litre.

TABLE 2: Kruskal-Wallis test, association between diabetic foot risk category and variables in patients reviewed for foot examination at the diabetic clinic, January to December 2013.

Variables	Diabetic foot risk category				Kruskal-Wallis *p*-value
	0	1	2	3	
Age, mean (s.d.), year	54.0 ± 9.9	60.0 ± 8.6	60.0 ± 1.4	64.0 ± 7.7	0.005
Systolic blood pressure, mean (s.d.), mmHg	134.0 ± 25.2	137.0 ± 33.1	138.0 ± 20.5	167.0 ± 20.1	0.13
Diastolic blood pressure, mean (s.d.), mmHg	76.0 ± 11.5	76.0 ± 9.4	79.0 ± 1.4	79.0 ± 4.7	0.72
Body mass index, median (IQR), kg/m^2	30	27	27	24	0.25
Waist circumference mean (s.d.), cm	104.0 ± 13.0	108.0 ± 15.0	108.0	97.0	0.36
Fasting blood sugar, mean (s.d.), mmol/L	7.3 ± 3.6	7.9 ± 2.1	7.3 ± 0.6	7.3 ± 2.4	0.8
Haemoglobin A1c, mean (s.d.), g%	7.7 ± 2.3	6.9 ± 3.8	6.7	7.7 ± 0.96	0.84
High density lipoprotein cholesterol, mean (s.d.), mmol/L	1.1 ± 0.4	1.1 ± 0.3	1.2	1.0 ± 0.25	0.5
Low density lipoprotein cholesterol, median (IQR), mmol/L	3.4 ± 0.99	3.3 ± 0.4	3.2	3.3	0.98
Triglyceride, median (IQR), mmol/L	1.6 ± 1.04	1.9 ± 0.8	1.4	1.5 ± 1.1	0.37
Total cholesterol, median (SD), mmol/L	5.2 ± 1.2	5.1 ± 0.8	5.0	4.8 ± 0.6	0.48

SPGH, Selebi Phikwe Government Hospital; s.d., standard deviation; IQR, interquartile range; mmol/L, millimol per litre; kg/m^2, kilogram per meter square.
$p < 0.001$

Discussion

The present study revealed that amongst the patients reviewed for foot examination in the SPGH diabetic clinic, the majority (85%) were in DF risk category 0, whilst 15% were categorised in higher risk groups. A total of 6.9% of patients were classified in risk category 1, 4.9% in risk category 2 and 3.5% in risk category 3. One primary care setting study produced comparable results of prevalence with 8.4% for risk category 1, and 4.5% for risk category 2; but the prevalence of risk category 3 was higher (13.0%).[16] In another study from a tertiary care setting, a higher prevalence of 17% for risk category 1, 11% for risk category 2 and 7% for category 3 was reported.[17] The present study's patients were in lower-risk categories than from the previous studies. It can be speculated that there was misclassification of the patients' DF to a lower-risk group in the present study; this could be due to only one nurse having had formal training for diabetic foot care. On the other hand, the present study's findings may reflect the true prevalence; if so, there would be a need to elucidate with further study factors that contributed to the lower DF risk classification of the present study's population.

In the present study, the majority of patients had hypertension, were overweight or obese (70%); 59% had uncontrolled blood sugar for at least the past three months (mean HbA1c = 8.1%) and showed elevated levels of LDL-C (mean LDL-C = 3.6 mmol/L). The partnership between hypertension and obesity is a common finding in type 2 diabetes. Biologic parameters such as HbA1c and LDL-C are not desirable for diabetic patients [18,19,20]; thus, they did not show an association with higher DF risk categories. These findings showed similarity with a recent study.[17] The patients in the present study had a mean age of 55 years, and it is known that type 2 diabetes patients over the age of 50 years struggle to regulate their blood sugar.[21]

The present study's findings revealed that patient's ages showed significant differences in the medians between the DF risk categories; this was trivial only between DF risk categories 0 and 1 ($p < 0.001$). These findings were comparable with previous reports.[22] The present study's

TABLE 3: Ordinal logistic regression with the DF risk category as the dependent variable and both age and SBP as independent variables, in patients reviewed for foot examination at the diabetic clinic, January to December 2013.

Risk factors	Regression coefficient	Two tailed *p*-value	Adjusted odd ratio	95% CI
Age	0.08	0.004	1.1	1.03-1.14
SBP	0.02	0.1	1.0	0.99-1.04

SPGH, Selebi Phikwe Government Hospital; DF, diabetic foot; SBP, systolic blood pressure.

findings showed dissimilarity with a central Saudi Arabian study, as it failed to establish a positive association between increased SBP with the progressively higher DF risk categories. [23] It was not part of the present study to assess the length of time that a patient had diabetes and its influence to the progression to higher DF risk categories.

There is little known about DF risk-category prevalence in primary healthcare settings in Sub-Sahara Africa. The importance of screening and sorting DF risk categories has the merit of being able to recognise patients in danger of lower extremity events and to implement time-appropriate care, more especially amongst older patients.

The limitations of the present study were: its retrospective and cross-sectional design, which consequently meant that the causal relationships between DF risk categories and variables, such as age, could not be recognised. Further investigations with a different design are recommended in order to clarify the influence of misclassification of DF risk categorisation.

Recommendations

It is recommend that foot examination and risk categorisation should become part of the routine management of diabetic patients in primary care in Botswana and Sub-Saharan Africa. More healthcare providers should be empowered with these skills. A more rigorous, prospective and multi-centre study is required to shed more light on the magnitude of the DF risk in Botswana.

Conclusion

The present study revealed that about 15% of patients attending the SPGH diabetic clinic were categorised in the high-risk groups for diabetic foot; patients' ages were linked to the higher DF risk category. The present study provides additional data on the prevalence of DF risk categories in primary care settings in Botswana and the Sub-Saharan African region. Further prospective, large and multi-centre investigations are required to endorse these findings.

Acknowledgements

The authors acknowledge the valuable contributions of the SPGH staff in the availing of registers and their willingness to help.

Competing interests

The authors declare that they have no financial or personal relationship(s) that may have inappropriately influenced them in writing this article.

Authors' contributions

S.T. (University of Botswana) was responsible for the conceptualisation of the study, data analysis, write up of the report and compilation of this manuscript. D.M. (University of Botswana), J.M.S. (Selebi Phikwe Government Hospital) and A.G. (University of Botswana) were responsible for editing.

References

1. Hall V, Thomsen RW, Henriksen O, Lohse N. Diabetes in Sub-Saharan Africa 1999–2011: Epidemiology and public health implications. A systematic review. BMC Public Health. 2011;11:564. http://dx.doi.org/10.1186/1471-2458-11-564
2. Levitt NS. Diabetes in Africa: Epidemiology, management and healthcare challenges. Heart. 2008;94(11):1376–82. http://dx.doi.org/10.1136/hrt.2008.147306
3. Maher D, Waswa L, Baisley K, Karabarinde A, Unwin N, Grosskurth H. Distribution of hyperglycaemia and related cardiovascular disease risk factors in low-income countries: A cross-sectional population-based survey in rural Uganda. Int J Epidemiol. 2011;40(1):160–71. http://dx.doi.org/10.1093/ije/dyq156
4. Frykberg RG, Zgonis T, Armstrong DG, et al. Diabetic foot disorders: A clinical practice guideline. The journal of foot and ankle surgery. 2006. http://dx.doi.org/10.1016/S1067-2516(07)60001-5
5. Christensen DL, Faurholt-Jensen D, Faerch K, et al. Prevalence of glucose intolerance and associated risk factors in rural and urban populations of different ethnic groups in Kenya. Diabetes Res Clin Pract. 2009; 84(3):303–10. http://dx.doi.org/10.1016/j.diabres.2009.03.007
6. Singh N, Armstrong DG, Lipsky BA. Preventing foot ulcers in patients with diabetes. JAMA. 2005;293:217–28. http://dx.doi.org/10.1001/jama.293.2.217
7. Morbach S. Structures of diabetic foot care. European endocrine disease. 2006.
8. Farber JS. Diabetes management office-based screening, prevention, and management of diabetic foot disorders. Primary Care: Clinics in Office Practice. 2007; Volume 34, Issue 4, 873-885. http://dx.doi.org/10.1016/j.pop.2007.07.001
9. Helfand AE. Assessing and preventing foot problems in older patients who have diabetes mellitus. Clin Podiatr Med Surg. 2003;20:573–82. http://dx.doi.org/10.1016/S0891-8422(03)00040-5
10. Nyamu PN, Otieno CF, Amayo EO, McLigeyo SO. Risk factors and prevalence of diabetic foot ulcers at Kenyatta National Hospital. East African Medical Journal. 2003;80(1).
11. Jbour AS, Jarrah NS, Radaideh AM, et al. Prevalence and predictors of diabetic foot syndrome in type 2 diabetes mellitus in Jordan. Saudi Med J 2003; 24:761–764.
12. Shojaiefard A, Khorgami Z, Larijani B. Independent risk factors for amputation in diabetic foot. Int J Diabetes Dev Ctries. 2008;28:32–37. http://dx.doi.org/10.4103/0973-3930.43096
13. Kozek E, Górska A, Fross K, Marcinowska A, Citkowska A, Sieradzki J. Chronic complications and risk factors in patients with type 1 diabetes mellitus--retrospective analysis. Przegl Lek. 2003; 60:773–777.
14. Rheeder P. The diabetic foot. JEMDSA. 2004;9(3).
15. Apelqvist J, Bakker K, Van Houtum WH, Schaper NC. Practical guidelines on the management and prevention of the diabetic foot based upon the International Consensus on the Diabetic Foot (2007). Diabetes/ metabolism research and reviews guidelines. Diabetes Metab Res Rev. 2008;24(Suppl 1):S181–S187. http://dx.doi.org/10.1002/dmrr.848
16. Stephen J, Najarian R, Stolusky T, et al. Identifying Diabetic Patients at High Risk for Lower-Extremity Amputation in a Primary Healthcare Setting. Diabetes care. 1992;15(10).
17. Shahbazian H, Yazdanpanah L, Latifi SM. Risk assessment of patients with diabetes for foot ulcers according to risk classification consensus of international working group on diabetic foot. Pak J Med Sci. 2013;29(3):730–734. http://dx.doi.org/10.12669/pjms.293.3473
18. Seedat YK, Rayner BL. South African Hypertension Guideline 2011. SAMJ. 2012;102(1).
19. Klug EQ, Raal FJ, Marais AD, et al. South African Dyslipidaemia Guideline Consensus Statement. S Afr Med J. 2012;102:177–188.
20. Amod A, Ascott-Evans BH, Berg GI, et al. The 2012 SEMDSA Guideline for the Management of Type 2 Diabetes. JEMDSA. 2012;17(2):S1–S95.
21. Kibachio JM, Omolo J, Muriuki Z, Juma R, Karugu L, Ng'ang'a Z. Risk factors for diabetic foot ulcers in type 2 diabetes: A case control study, Nyeri, Kenya. African Journal of Diabetes Medicine. 2013;21(1):n.p.
22. Abolfotouh MA, Alfaifi SA, Al-Gannas AS. Risk factors of diabetic foot in central Saudi Arabia. Saudi Med J. 2011;32(7):n.p.

10

Body adiposity indices are associated with hypertension in a black, urban Free State community

Authors:
Ronette Lategan[1]
Violet L. van den Berg[1]
Corinna M. Walsh[1]

Affiliations:
[1]Faculty of Health Sciences, University of the Free State, South Africa

Correspondence to:
Ronette Lategan

Email:
nutrition@ufs.ac.za

Postal address:
PO Box 339 (G24), Bloemfontein, 9300, South Africa

Background: Non-communicable diseases, including hypertension, are increasing rapidly in resource-poor, developing countries amongst populations transitioning from traditional to westernised lifestyles; and are associated with excess weight.

Aim: To investigate the relationship between hypertension and various indices of body adiposity in a transitioning, urban, black population.

Setting: Three hundred and thirty-nine adults (25–64 years) from a larger cross-sectional study (Assuring Health for All in the Free State) conducted in Mangaung, South Africa, were included.

Methods: Standard techniques were used to determine blood pressure, HIV status, body mass index (BMI), waist-to-height ratio (WHtR) and body adiposity index (BAI).

Results: Approximately 40% of the sample was HIV-positive and 63.4% hypertensive, with the greatest risk of hypertension being amongst older men. Based on BMI, 23.0% were overweight and 32.1% obese. Waist-to-height ratio showed that 58.6% had increased cardiovascular risk. Mean BAI was 34.1%, whilst 76.3% had a body fat percentage in the overweight/obese category. Waist circumference representing increased cardiovascular risk was found in 44.3% of women and 3.9% of men. Significant positive correlations between mean arterial blood pressure and BMI ($r = 0.261$; $p < 0.001$), WHtR ($r = 0.357$; $p < 0.001$) and BAI ($r = 0.245$; $p < 0.001$) were found. WHtR was a stronger predictor of mean arterial pressure than BMI or BAI. HIV status showed an inverse correlation with all adiposity indices ($p < 0.001$).

Conclusion: Our findings promote WHtR as a practical screening tool for increased hypertension risk in populations undergoing westernisation, and support weight loss as a first-line intervention for the prevention and management of hypertension.

Les indices d'adiposité corporelle sont associés à l'hypertension dans une communauté africaine et urbaine de la province de l'Etat libre.

Présentation: Les maladies non transmissibles, notamment l'hypertension, connaissent une augmentation rapide dans les pays aux ressources limitées et en voie de développement parmi les populations en transition entre un style de vie traditionnel et un style de vie occidentalisé; elles sont également associées à un excédent de poids.

Objectif: Etudier la relation entre l'hypertension et différents indices d'adiposité corporelle dans une population africaine, en transition et urbaine.

Cadre: Trois cent trente-neuf adultes (âgés de 25 à 63 ans) sélectionnés à partir d'une étude transversale de plus grande envergure (Assurer la Santé pour Tous dans l'Etat Libre) réalisée à Mangaung, en Afrique du Sud, ont été inclus.

Méthodes: Des techniques standards ont été utilisées afin de déterminer la tension artérielle, la séropositivité, l'indice de masse corporelle (IMC), le rapport taille-hanche (RTH) et l'indice d'adiposité corporelle (IAC).

Résultats: Environ 40% de l'échantillon étaient séropositifs et 63.4% étaient hypertensifs, le risque d'hypertension le plus élevé étant observé chez les hommes âgés. Sur la base de l'IMC, 23% étaient en surpoids, et 32.1 étaient obèses. Le RTH indiquait que 58.6% présentaient un risque cardiovasculaire accru. L'IAC moyen était de 34.1%, et 76.3% des participants à l'étude avaient un pourcentage de graisse corporelle entrant dans la catégorie surpoids/obèse. La circonférence de la taille représentant un risque cardiovasculaire accru a été mesurée à 44.3% chez les femmes et à 3.9% chez les hommes. Des corrélations significatives entre la tension artérielle moyenne et l'IMC ($r = 0.261$; $p < 0.001$), le RTH ($r = 0.357$; $p < 0.001$) et l'IAC ($r = 0.245$; $p < 0.001$) ont été observées. Le RTH était une variable causale plus importante de la tension artérielle moyenne que l'IMC ou l'IAC. La séropositivité présentait une corrélation inverse avec tous les indices d'adiposité ($p < 0.001$).

Conclusion: Nos conclusions indiquent que le RTH devrait être utilisé comme outil de dépistage pratique du risque d'hypertension accru chez les populations en transition, et que la perte de poids devrait être recommandée comme intervention de première ligne pour la prévention et la gestion de l'hypertension.

Introduction

Hypertension is a leading cause of morbidity in middle-income countries. It is gaining significance in low-income countries, contributing to an increasing global disease burden.[1,2] Underdiagnosis and/or inadequate treatment of hypertension may cause organ damage and premature death,[1,3] affecting the economy of a country and making prevention and early intervention important objectives for health authorities worldwide.

It has been estimated that hypertension accounted for 9% of deaths in South Africa in 2000, making it the second-highest cause of mortality after sexually-transmitted diseases.[2] South Africa has been undergoing a transition from traditional diets and more active lifestyles to typically Western diets and more sedentary practices. These trends are associated with the high prevalence of obesity amongst black South Africans, particularly women in urban areas.[3]

A strong relationship exists between body weight and blood pressure, with the risk of developing hypertension being two to six times higher in overweight than in normal weight individuals.[1] Overweight and general adiposity are associated independently with an increased risk for heart failure.[4] A strong relationship also exists between the degree of obesity as measured by body mass index (BMI) and waist circumference (WC), and the prevalence of ischaemic stroke, regardless of gender or race.[5] Weight loss as a first-line treatment for lowering blood pressure is therefore generally recommended.[1,3,6,7] It has been found that 5.1 kg of weight loss caused a reduction of 4.44 mmHg and 3.57 mmHg in systolic and diastolic pressure, respectively, translating to a reduction of 1.05 mmHg in systolic and 0.92 mmHg in diastolic pressure per kilogram of weight lost.[7] Markers of general obesity and indicators of abdominal obesity are good predictors of cardiovascular risk. Waist circumference (WC), waist-to-height ratio (WHtR), BMI and visceral fat percentage are strong predictors of arterial stiffness in morbidly obese female patients.[8]

The World Health Organization (WHO) recognises two thresholds for abdominal obesity as measured by WC, depicting different levels of risk for metabolic (including cardiovascular) complications. Increased risk is at a WC of > 80 cm in women and > 94 cm in men, with substantially increased risk at a WC of > 88 cm for women and > 102 cm for men.[9] Even a WC within the higher parameters of normal cut-off points is associated with a high prevalence of hypertension in older adults, independent of BMI and other hypertension risk factors.[10]

The risk for metabolic complications occurs at different levels of adiposity (indicated by BMI) and central obesity (indicated by WC) in different populations. It has been recommended that the current BMI cut-off points should be retained as international classification, but that more detail be added for reporting purposes (18.5 kg/m^2 – 23 kg/m^2 increasing but acceptable risk; 23 kg/m^2 – 27.5 kg/m^2 increased risk; and ≥ 27.5 kg/m^2 high risk) to facilitate international comparison.[11] Different ethnicity-specific cut-off points have also been suggested for WC.[12]

As no ethnicity-specific WC recommendations exist for South Africans, the recommendations for sub-Saharan Africa[13,14] (80 cm for women; 94 cm for men) can be considered, which are approximately 10% lower than the recommendation for North Americans.[12]

WHtR is regarded as a better and more sensitive obesity marker than BMI for predicting hypertension and as an early marker of metabolic health risks.[15,16] An advantage of WHtR is that the same cut-off point (0.5) can be used for both men and women of different ethnic groups.[15]

Body adiposity index (BAI), a direct estimate of percentage body fat calculated from hip circumference and height, is an easily-obtained measure to predict the risk for obesity-related diseases.[17]

Despite strong evidence that supports the association between body weight and hypertension, Schutte et al.[18] failed to show a strong relationship between obesity markers (BMI and fat percentage) and blood pressure amongst black South African women.

The high prevalence of HIV infection in South Africa should be considered. Hypertension is equally common amongst both HIV-infected and -uninfected individuals. Although multivariate models link increasing age, higher BMI, longer duration of infection and diabetes to hypertension in HIV-infected populations, the prevalence of hypertension is apparently not influenced by HIV status or the use of highly active antiretroviral therapy (HAART).[19,20,21,22,23]

The Assuring Health for All in the Free State (AHA-FS) study investigated the double burden of infectious diseases and undernutrition, on the one hand, and obesity and its comorbidities on the other, in a low-income, black, urban community in central South Africa. Hypertension occurred in 56.9% (n = 415) of the study population and mean systolic and diastolic blood pressure measurements were 135.5 ± 23.9 mmHg and 89.8 ± 17.4 mmHg, respectively.[24] The high prevalence of hypertension in this population was the motivation for investigating its primary causes. The objective of this substudy, therefore, was to invesitgate to investigate the relationship between blood pressure and various indices of body adiposity (BMI, WC, WHtR and BAI) in a transitioning urban black population, whilst taking into account the influence of HIV.

Research methods and design

Approval to conduct the study was obtained from the Ethics Committee of the Faculty of Health Sciences, University of the Free State in Bloemfontein, South Africa.

For this cross-sectional study, data from the urban AHA-FS study[24] were used. Data were collected over a period of two weeks in March 2009 from six areas in Mangaung, South Africa, namely Freedom Square, Turflaagte, Namibia, Kagisanong, Chris Hani and Rocklands. Households were selected by proportional cluster sampling, stratified by area and formal plot/squatter households in open areas. Using randomly selected X- and Y-coordinates, 100 starting points were selected. Trained field workers approached five adjacent households from each starting point in order to obtain written informed consent from eligible adults (25–64 years). In the AHA-FS study, a variety of measurements, including body weight, height, waist and hip circumferences were taken, blood pressure was measured and blood samples were drawn for various biochemical tests. A subsample, with complete data sets for age, gender, blood pressure, body weight, height and HIV status, was included in this study.

Blood pressure was measured by a registered medical practitioner according to recognised guidelines.[25,26] Hypertension was defined as systolic blood pressure of ≥ 140 mmHg and/or diastolic blood pressure ≥ 90 mmHg.[1] Participants using prescription medication for the management of hypertension at the time of the interview were also classified as hypertensive.[25,26]

HIV status was determined from fasting venous blood samples. Primary screening for HIV was performed using the Enzygnost HIV Integral II Ag/Ab test (Dade Behring, Marburg, Germany) and results were confirmed by the Vironostika HIV Uni-Form II Ag/Ab test (bioMérieux, Marcy l'Etoile, France).

Anthropometric measurements were taken by trained final-year Dietetics students, under supervision of the researchers. Body weight was determined using WHO guidelines[27] on a floor-type Seca 770 digital scale (Medical Scales and Measuring Systems Seca kk., Japan) with accuracy to 100 g and a maximum capacity of 200 kg. Height was measured[27] with a Seca stadiometer (Medical Scales and Measuring Systems Seca kk., Japan) accurate to the nearest 5 mm. BMI (kg/m^2) was calculated and interpreted according to WHO guidelines.[27,28] Waist circumference was measured with a non-stretch measuring tape, midway between the top of the superior iliac crest and the lowest rib in the mid-axillary line.[9]

Waist circumference was interpreted according to WHO guidelines[9] as increased risk of metabolic complications at > 80 cm in women and > 94 cm in men; and as a substantially-increased risk of metabolic complications at a WC > 88 cm in women and > 102 cm in men. WHtR was determined by dividing WC (cm) by height (cm). A WHtR of ≥ 0.5 indicates an increased risk for non-communicable diseases (NCDs) in both genders.[15]

Hip circumference was measured at the widest portion of the buttocks parallel to the floor, accurate to the nearest 5 mm.[27]

Hip circumference and height were used to calculate BAI (see formula below),[17] which provides an accurate estimate of body fat percentage when compared to dual-energy X-ray absorptiometry (DXA).[17]

BAI (% body fat) = hip circumference (cm) ÷ height $(m)^{1.5}$ – 18. BAI results were interpreted according to the classification proposed by Ricciardi et al.[29] namely:

- low body fat: 10% – 15% (men); 14% – 20% (women)
- average body fat: 16% – 18% (men); 21% – 25% (women)
- above average body fat: 19% – 20% (men); 26% – 29% (women)
- overweight body fat: 21% – 25% (men); 30% – 35% (women)
- obese body fat: ≥ 26% (men); ≥ 36% (women).

Statistical analysis

Analysis of data was performed with PASW (Predictive Analytics SoftWare) statistics software by SPSS version 18 (Chicago, SPSS Inc.). Frequencies and percentages were used to express categorical data. Means and standard deviations, or percentiles, as appropriate, were used to express quantitative variables. Comparisons of means were performed using *t*-tests. Chi-square tests, two-tailed Pearson correlations, point bi-serial correlations and multivariate logistic regression models were used to describe and test associations between variables; and relative risk of incidence was calculated.

Ethical considerations

Ethical clearance was granted by the Ethics Committee, Faculty of Health Sciences, University of the Free State, Bloemfontein, South Africa (ETOVS number 21/07).

Results

Age, blood pressure, anthropometry and HIV status

A total of 339 adults (76 men [22.4%]; 263 women [77.6%]) with a mean age of 44.3 years (range 25–64 years) were included in the study. Table 1 summarises the participants' information in terms of age, blood pressure (systolic, diastolic and mean arterial pressure) and anthropometry.

More than a third (39.8%; n = 135) of the sample was HIV-infected and the mean BMI was significantly lower ($p < 0.001$) in HIV-infected participants (24.9 ± 7.4 kg/m^2), compared with HIV-uninfected participants (29.6 ± 9.2 kg/m^2). In 41.6% (n = 141) of individuals, systolic blood pressure was ≥ 140 mmHg, whilst 46.6% (n = 158) had a diastolic blood pressure of ≥ 90 mmHg, indicating hypertension. Approximately one quarter (25.4%; n = 86) of participants used antihypertensive medication at the time of the study. Consequently, 63.4% (57.9% [n = 44] men and 65.0% [n = 171] women) of the participants were classified as hypertensive.

Distribution of body fat indices

The distribution of body fat indices of the participants is summarised in Table 2 A, B, C and D.

Based on BMI, 18.4% (n = 14) of the men and 65.8% (n = 173) of the women were overweight/obese. With regard to WC, using cut-off points for sub-Saharan populations, 6.5% (n = 5) of the men (WC > 94 cm) and 66.8% (n = 175) of the women (WC > 80 cm) showed increased health risk.

An overweight/obese BMI was associated significantly (χ^2 = 144.533; $p < 0.001$) with high-risk WC (> 88 cm in women; > 102 cm in men). Based on a WHtR of ≥ 0.5, 19.7% (n = 15) of the men and 69.8% (n = 183) of the women were at risk. When taking BAI into consideration, 73.7% (n = 56) of the men and 77.1% (n = 202) of the women had body fat percentages in the overweight/obese category.

TABLE 1: Age, blood pressure and anthropometric measurements of participants (N = 339, unless indicated otherwise).

Variable	Mean	Standard deviation (SD)	Range
Age			
Years	44.3	± 10.6	25–64
Blood pressure (mmHg)			
Systolic pressure			
Total group	135.5	± 23.7	72–203
Men (n = 76)	134.8	± 22.8	87–188
Women (n = 263)	135.7	± 24.0	72–203
Diastolic pressure			
Total group	89.8	± 17.6	46–188
Men (n = 76)	86.6	± 15.2	54–119
Women (n = 263)	90.7	± 18.1	46–188
Mean arterial pressure			
Total group	105.0	± 18.0	59–191
Men (n= 76)	102.7	± 15.6	68–133
Women (n = 263)	105.7	± 18.5	59–191
Height (cm)	159.4	± 7.9	139.8–180
Weight (kg)	70.1	± 21.4	31.9–140
Body mass index (BMI; kg/m²)			
Total group	27.8	± 8.8	13.3–55.7
Men (n = 76)	21.4	± 5.6	14.5–49.9
Women (n = 263)	29.6	± 8.7	13.3–55.7
Waist circumference (WC; cm)			
Men (n = 76)	78.1	± 13.9	47–134
Women (n = 262)	88.9	± 17.1	59–143
Waist-height ratio (WHtR) (N = 338)	0.55	± 0.11	0.27–0.91
Hip circumference (cm) (N = 338)	104.5	± 18.2	73.5–165
Body adiposity index (BAI; %)			
Men (n = 76)	24.1	± 5.2	16.8–50.7
Women (n = 262)	37.1	± 9.5	19.2–66.1

Occurrence of hypertension in relation to age, gender and body fat indices

A major risk factor for increased arterial blood pressure is age. To assess the effect of age, participants were stratified according to mean age into two age groups, namely > 44 years (n = 172) and ≤44 years (n = 167). Hypertension was significantly more prevalent in the older group (χ^2 = 45.526; $p < 0.0001$). A relative risk for hypertension of 1.78 (95% confidence interval [CI] 1.48; 2.13) was calculated, indicating that the older group had a 78% higher risk of being hypertensive than the younger group. When genders were compared, controlling for age, the relative risk for hypertension was 2.4 (95% CI 1.47; 3.91) for men and 1.66 (95% CI 1.37; 2.01) for women. The occurrence of hypertension in relation to BMI categories is shown in Table 3.

When stratified into low to normal BMI (< 25 kg/m²; low risk) and overweight/obese BMI (≥ 25 kg/m²; high risk), 76.5% (n = 143) of the overweight/obese group had hypertension, which was a significant finding (χ^2 = 30.611; $p < 0.0001$) in this group. After controlling for age, participants > 44 years with an overweight/obese BMI had a relative risk of 1.25 (95% CI 1.06; 1.46) of being hypertensive, compared with a normal/underweight BMI. In the ≤44 years group, the relative risk of being hypertensive was 2.69 (95% CI 1.75; 4.15) when being overweight/obese versus being normal/underweight.

When applying a multivariate logistic regression model (mean arterial pressure as independent variable and age and BMI as dependent variables), BMI and age accounted for 14.8% of the change in arterial pressure. For every one year increase in age, or every 1 kg/m² increase in BMI, a 0.48 mmHg increase in mean arterial pressure could be expected ($p < 0.001$).

TABLE 2 A: Body mass index (BMI) according to the categories recommended by the WHO for international classification.[11]

BMI kg/m²	Classification	Men (n = 76)		Women (n = 263)	
		n	%	n	%
< 18.5	Underweight	19	25.0	21	8.0
18.5–24.9	Normal	43	56.6	69	26.2
25.0–29.9	Overweight	11	14.5	67	25.5
30.0–34.9	Obese Class I	0	0	39	14.8
35.0–39.9	Obese Class 2	2	2.6	32	12.2
≥ 40.0	Obese Class 3	1	1.3	35	13.3

TABLE 2B: Waist circumference (WC) according to the categories recommended by the WHO.[9]

Level of risk	Gender-specific cut-offs		Men (n = 76)		Women (n = 262)	
			n	%	n	%
Low risk	Men: Women:	< 94 cm < 80 cm	71	93.4	87	33.2
Increased risk	Men: Women:	94–102 cm 80–88 cm	2	2.6	59	22.5
High risk (central obesity)	Men: Women:	> 102 cm > 88 cm	3	3.9	116	44.3

TABLE 2C: Waist-to-height ratio (WHtR).[16]

Level of risk	Universal cut-offs	Men (n = 76)		Women (n = 262)	
		n	%	n	%
Low risk	< 0.5	61	80.3	79	30.2
At risk	≥ 0.5	15	19.7	183	69.8

TABLE 2D: Body adiposity index (BAI) according to body fat % categories.[29]

Body fat (%)	Gender-specific cut-offs	Men (n=76)		Women (n=263)	
		n	%	*n*	%
Low	Men: 10–15% Women: 14–20%	0	0	2	0.8
Average	Men: 16–18% Women: 21–25%	4	5.3	30	11.5
Above average	Men: 19–20% Women: 26–29%	16	21.1	28	10.7
Overweight	Men: 21–25% Women: 30–35%	39	51.3	72	27.4
Obese	Men: ≥ 26% Women: ≥ 36%	17	22.4	130	49.6

TABLE 3: Distribution of normotensive and hypertensive participants across BMI categories.

Body mass index (BMI)	Normotensive (n = 124)		Hypertensive (n = 215)	
	n	%	*n*	%
Weight				
Underweight (< 18.5 kg/m²)	23	18.5	17	7.9
Normal weight (18.5–24.9 kg/m²)	57	46.0	55	25.6
Overweight (25.0–29.9 kg/m²)	23	18.5	55	25.6
Obese				
Class I (30.0–34.9 kg/m²)	5	4.0	34	15.8
Class II (35.0–39.9 kg/m²)	6	4.8	28	13.0
Class III (≥ 40 kg/m²)	10	8.1	26	12.1

TABLE 4: Waist circumference in relation to the prevalence of hypertension.

Waist circumference category	Men (n = 76)				Women (n = 262)			
	Normotensive (n =3 2)		Hypertensive (n = 44)		Normotensive (n = 92)		Hypertensive (n = 169)	
	n	%	*n*	%	*n*	%	*n*	%
Lower risk (n = 159) (Women: ≤ 88 cm; Men: ≤ 102 cm)	32	42.1	39	51.3	52	19.8	35	13.4
Increased risk (n = 61) (Women: 80–88 cm; Men: 94–102 cm)	0	0	2	2.6	21	8.0	38	14.5
Central obesity (n = 118) (Women: > 88 cm; Men: > 102 cm)	0	0	3	3.9	19	7.3	97	37.0

In Table 4, the prevalence of hypertension according to WC categories is summarised, indicating an increased prevalence of hypertension with increasing WC for women ($\chi^2 = 32.062$; $p < 0.0001$). An independent samples *t*-test confirmed that WC in the hypertensive group was significantly higher than the normotensive group and correlations showed that mean arterial blood pressure correlated significantly with WC in both men ($r = 0.262$; $p < 0.05$) and women ($r = 0.382$; $p < 0.001$).

When female participants were stratified according to WC as > 88 cm and ≤ 88 cm and controlled for age (< 44 years and ≥ 44 years), older women with high-risk WC had a relative risk of 1.29 (95% CI 1.08; 1.53) of being hypertensive; whilst younger women with high-risk WC had a relative risk of 2.22 (95% CI 1.56; 3.14) of being hypertensive.

Both WHtR ($r = 0.357$; $p < 0.001$) and BAI ($r = 0.245$; $p < 0.001$) correlated significantly with mean arterial blood pressure. A significant relation was found between a WHtR of ≥ 0.5 (increased risk) and the prevalence of hypertension ($\chi^2 = 43.057$; $p < 0.001$). WHtR ($r = 0.357$) showed a stronger correlation with mean arterial pressure than BMI ($r = 0.261$) or BAI ($r = 0.245$).

HIV status and blood pressure

Mean arterial pressure was correlated inversely to HIV status ($r = -0.217$; $p < 0.001$). However, partial correlation indicated that this inverse association resulted from the effect of age and adiposity levels on blood pressure. When using a point bi-serial correlation, HIV status showed an inverse correlation with BMI ($r = -0.262$; $p < 0.001$), WC ($r = -0.364$; $p < 0.001$), WHtR ($r = -0.299$; $p < 0.001$), and BAI ($r = -0.226$; $p < 0.001$) in women.

Discussion

The prevalence of hypertension, which affected 63.4% of the total group in this low-income, urban, black population, compares with 61.8% reported for an African-American population older than 40 years.[30] The high prevalence of hypertension, especially amongst a population that included younger participants, raises concern.

More than half (55.1%; $n = 187$) of the participants had BMIs above normal (23.0% overweight; 32.1% obese). This is higher than the WHO estimate of 45.1% for the prevalence of overweight/obesity in the general South African population[27] and the 48% reported for South Africans from 18 companies participating in a health-risk screening programme.[31] For men, the prevalence of overweight/obesity was lower (18.4%) than the prevalence described for Free State men in the South African National Health and Nutrition Examination Survey study (25.3%), but for women, the prevalence was higher (65.8% vs 63.7%).[32] The mean BMI for this study (27.8 kg/m²) was lower than the mean of 29.8 ± 0.2 kg/m² for Americans of combined races,[30] as well as the mean of 30.1 kg/m² in African-Americans as reported previously.[33]

With regard to above-normal BMIs, 14.5% (n = 11) and 3.9% (n = 3) of men (mean BMI 21.4 kg/m²) and 25.5% (n = 67) and 40.3% (n = 106) of women (mean BMI 29.6 kg/m²) were overweight and obese, respectively. This finding corresponds with data from the South African Demographic and Health Survey,[34] reporting 18.7% of urban black men as overweight and 8.1% as obese (mean BMI 23.1 kg/m²) and 27.1% of urban black women as overweight and 33.8% as obese (mean BMI 28.1 kg/m²). Our findings confirmed the trend that black South African women have substantially higher BMIs than their male counterparts, as reported previously. Charlton et al.[35] reported a mean BMI of 28 kg/m² in black South African men (37.7% obese) and 33.5 kg/m² in black South African women (67.9% obese) in Cape Town. The Transition and Health During Urbanisation of South Africans (THUSA) study[36] reported that 28.6% of black South African female participants were obese and 53.8% had a BMI > 25 kg/m². Contrary to the higher BMIs found amongst women in South Africa, a mean BMI of 26.4 kg/m² for American men and 26.2 kg/m² for women have been reported.[37]

The high prevalence of overweight/obesity in this population, linked to the prevalence of hypertension, agrees with the International Study of Salt and Blood Pressure (INTERSALT),[38] reporting a strong, significant, independent association of BMI with blood pressure.

BMI in this study was related significantly ($p < 0.001$) to to WC. Black South African women had a similar mean WC (88.9 cm) than American women (88.5 cm).[37] In contrast, black South African men in our study had a lower mean WC (78.1 cm) than American men (95.6 cm). The incidence of high-risk WC was higher than the national data for urban black South Africans[34] (3.9% versus 3.1% for men; and 44.3% versus 39.1% for women). Charlton et al.[35] also described a higher mean WC in a black population, namely 92.6 cm in men and 92.4 cm in women.

Mashele et al.[39] found that, similar to our findings, urbanised hypertensive black South African men and women were typically older, more obese and had a larger WC compared with their normotensive counterparts.

Based on WHtR and BAI as obesity indices, a high percentage of participants in the current study were at increased risk for NCD. WHtR was increased in 58.6% (n = 198) of participants, whilst 76.3% (n = 258) of all participants had a BAI in the overweight/obese category. We found a slightly stronger association of hypertension with WHtR than with BMI and BAI, although all three indices were associated significantly with mean arterial blood pressure. These findings concur with a meta-analysis[40] reporting that measures of abdominal obesity were better predictors of cardiovascular disease risk than BMI. More importantly, however, WHtR could be seen as a simple tool to screen for hypertension in this particular community. At a primary healthcare level, the community could be taught to use a piece of string equal to their height; if the string cannot go around the waist at least twice, the risk for hypertension and other non-communicable diseases is reflected.

Almost 40% (n = 135) of participants in our study were infected with HIV. Although the prevalence of hypertension showed an inverse association with HIV status, this association was found to result from the lower body adiposity as represented by lower BMI, WHtR, BAI and WC, which are associated with HIV infection. A similar lack of significant associations between hypertension and HIV status has been reported previously.[19,20,21,22,23]

A degree of bias is acknowledged. More women may have participated because the research was conducted during a week day, resulting in less men attending because of being formally employed. More ill people may have participated due to free medical examinations being conducted during the study.

Conclusion

Obesity, hypertension and HIV occurred commonly amongst participants in this study. The prevalence of hypertension was not influenced significantly by HIV status when adiposity was taken into account. WHtR was related significantly to mean arterial pressure and seemed to be a stronger predictor of mean arterial pressure than BMI or BAI. Obesity was more prevalent in women than men; and, in women, hypertension was related significantly to WC and BMI. These results support weight loss as the first line of intervention for the treatment and prevention of hypertension with its accompanying disease burden. We propose that WHtR may be an easy and practical way of screening for hypertension and motivating communities to decrease their waist circumference. Future research to assess the impact of a simple nutrition message, 'Stay healthy by keeping your waist circumference less than half of your height', is recommended.

Acknowledgements

The researchers acknowledge the Department of Biostatistics, Faculty of Health Sciences, University of the Free State, for providing assistance with the analysis and interpretation of data. The Fulbright program (USA) is acknowledged for research assistance during writing of the report. Dr. Daleen Struwig, medical writer, Faculty of Health Sciences, UFS, is acknowledged for technical and editorial preparation of the manuscript for publication.

The study received financial support from the South African National Research Foundation (NRF); grant number TTK2006050800013.

Competing interests

The authors declare that they have no financial or personal relationship(s) which may have influenced them inappropriately in writing this article.

Authors' contributions

R.L. (University of the Free State) planned the project, collected and interpreted data, performed part of the statistical analysis and wrote the article; V.L.vdB. (University of the Free State) was the study leader, made substantial scientific contributions and assisted in writing the article; and C.W. (University of the Free State) was the co-study leader, the principle investigator of the larger AHA-FS study, collected and interpreted data and assisted in writing the article. All the authors approved the final version of the manuscript.

References

1. Couch SC, Krummel DA. Medical nutrition therapy for hypertension. In: Mahan KL, Escott-Stump S, editors. Krause's food and nutrition therapy. 12th ed. Philadelphia: WB Saunders Company, 2008; p. 865–898.
2. Norman R, Gaziano T, Laubscher R, et al. Estimating the burden of disease attributable to high blood pressure in South Africa in 2000. S Afr Med J. 2007;97(8 Pt 2):692–698. PMID: 17952226
3. Steyn K. Hypertension in South Africa. In: Steyn K, Fourie J, Temple N, editors. Chronic diseases of lifestyle: 1995–2005. Technical report. Cape Town: South African Medical Research Council, 2006; p. 80–96.
4. Hu G, Jousilahti P, Antikainen R, et al. Joint effects of physical activity, body mass index, waist circumference, and waist-to-hip ratio on the risk of heart failure. Circulation. 2010;121:237–244. http://dx.doi.org/10.1161/CIRCULATIONAHA.109.887893, PMid: 20048205
5. Yatsuya H, Folsom AR, Yamagishi K, et al. Race- and sex-specific associations of obesity measures with ischemic stroke incidence in the Atherosclerosis Risk in Communities (ARIC) Study. Stroke 2010;41(3):417–425. http://dx.doi.org/10.1161/STROKEAHA.109.566299 , PMid: 20093637
6. Appel LJ. ASH position paper: dietary approaches to lower blood pressure. J Clin Hypertens. 2009;11(7):358–368. http://dx.doi.org/10.1111/j.1751-7176.2009.00136.x, PMid: 19583632
7. Neter JE, Stam BE, Kok FJ, et al. Influence of weight reduction on blood pressure: a meta-analysis of randomized controlled trials. Hypertension. 2003;42(5):878–884. http://dx.doi.org/10.1161/01.HYP.0000094221.86888.AE, PMid: 12975389
8. Nordstrand N, Gjevestad E, Dinh KN, et al. The relationship between various measures of obesity and arterial stiffness in morbidly obese patients. BMC Cardiovasc Disord. 2011;11:7. http://dx.doi.org/10.1186/1471-2261-11-7, PMid: 21284837
9. World Health Organization. Waist circumference and waist-hip ratio: report of a WHO expert consultation, Geneva, 8–11 December 2008 [document on the internet]. c2011 [cited 2011 Jun 7]. Available from: whqlibdoc.who.int/publications/2011/9789241501491_eng.pdf
10. Levine DA, Calhoun DA, Prineas RJ, et al. Moderate waist circumference and hypertension prevalence: the REGARDS study. Am J Hypertens. 2011;24(4):482–488. http://dx.doi.org/10.1038/ajh.2010.258, PMid: 21233800
11. WHO Expert Consultation. Appropriate body-mass index for Asian populations and its implications for policy and intervention strategies. Lancet. 2004;363(9403):157–163. http://dx.doi.org/10.1016/S0140-6736(03)15268-3, PMid: 14726171
12. Alberti KG, Eckel RH, Grundy SM, et al. Harmonizing the metabolic syndrome: a joint interim statement of the International Diabetes Federation Task Force on Epidemiology and Prevention; National Heart, Lung, and Blood Institute; American Heart Association; World Heart Federation; International Atherosclerosis Society; and International Association for the Study of Obesity. Circulation. 2009;120(16):1640–1645. http://dx.doi.org/10.1161/CIRCULATIONAHA.109.192644, PMid: 19805654
13. Eckel RH, Grundy SM, Zimmet PZ. The metabolic syndrome. Lancet. 2005;365(9468):1415–1428. http://dx.doi.org/10.1016/S0140-6736(05)66378-7, PMid: 15836891
14. Balkau B, Charles MA. Comment on the provisional report from the WHO consultation. European Group for the Study of Insulin Resistance (EGIR). Diabet Med. 1999;16(5):442–443. http://dx.doi.org/10.1046/j.1464-5491.1999.00059.x, PMid: 10342346
15. Ashwell M, Hsieh SD. Six reasons why the waist-to-height ratio is a rapid and effective global indicator for health risks of obesity and how its use could simplify the international public health message on obesity. Int J Food Sci Nutr. 2005;56(5):303–307. http://dx.doi.org/10.1080/09637480500195066, PMid: 16236591
16. Sayeed MA, Mahtab H, Latif ZA, et al. Waist-to-height ratio is a better obesity index than body mass index and waist-to-hip ratio for predicting diabetes, hypertension and lipidemia. Bangladesh Med Res Counc Bull. 2003;29(1):1–10. PMid: 14674615
17. Bergman RN, Stefanovski D, Buchanan TA, et al. A better index of body adiposity. Obesity. 2011;19(5):1083–1089. http://dx.doi.org/10.1038/oby.2011.38, PMid: 21372804
18. Schutte AE, Huisman HW, Van Rooyen JM, et al. Should obesity be blamed for the high prevalence rates of hypertension in black South African women? J Hum Hypertens. 2008;22(8):528–536. http://dx.doi.org/10.1038/jhh.2008.35, PMid: 18432254
19. Medina-Torne S, Ganesan A, Barahona I, et al. Hypertension is common among HIV-infected persons, but not associated with HAART. J Int Assoc Physicians AIDS Care. 2012;11(1):20–25. http://dx.doi.org/10.1177/1545109711418361, PMid: 21876213
20. Bloomfield GS, Hogan JW, Keter A, et al. Hypertension and obesity as cardiovascular risk factors among HIV seropositive patients in Western Kenya. PLoS ONE. 2011;6(7):e22288. http://dx.doi.org/10.1371/journal.pone.0022288, PMid: 21779407
21. Baekken M, Os I, Sandvik L, et al. Hypertension in an urban HIV-positive population compared with the general population: influence of combination antiretroviral therapy. J Hypertens. 2008;26(11):2126–2133. http://dx.doi.org/10.1097/HJH.0b013e32830ef5fb, PMid: 18854751
22. Jung O, Bickel M, Ditting T, et al. Hypertension in HIV-1-infected patients and its impact on renal and cardiovascular integrity. Nephrol Dial Transplant. 2004;19(9):2250–2258. http://dx.doi.org/10.1093/ndt/gfh393, PMid: 15238630
23. Bergersen BM, Sandvik L, Dunlop O, et al. Prevalence of hypertension in HIV-positive patients on highly active retroviral therapy (HAART) compared with HAART-naïve and HIV-negative controls: results from a Norwegian study of 721 patients. Eur J Clin Microbiol Infect Dis. 2003;22(12):731–736. http://dx.doi.org/10.1007/s10096-003-1034-z, PMid: 14610658
24. Van Zyl S, Van der Merwe LJ, Walsh CM, et al. Risk-factor profiles for chronic diseases of lifestyle and metabolic syndrome in an urban and rural setting in South Africa. Afr J Prim Health Care Fam Med. 2012;4(1), Art. #346, 10 pages. http://dx.doi.org/10.4102/phcfm.v4i1.346
25. Wallace C, Xue MZ, Caulfield M, et al. Genome scans in hypertension. In: Dominiczak AF, Connell JMC, editors. Handbook of hypertension, vol. 24. Genetics of hypertension. Edinburgh: Elsevier, 2007, p. 49–66.
26. National Institutes of Health; National Heart, Lung, and Blood Institute; National High Blood Pressure Education Program (NIH). The seventh report of the joint national committee on prevention, detection, evaluation, and treatment of high blood pressure [document on the internet]. c2004 [cited 2013 May 10]. Available from: http://www.nhlbi.nih.gov/guidelines/hypertension/jnc7full.pdf
27. World Health Organization. WHO STEPS surveillance: guide to physical measurements. Step 3: guide to physical measurements (step 2) [document on the internet]. c2008 [cited 2011 Jun 7]. Available from: www.who.int/chp/steps/Part3_Section3.pdf
28. World Health Organization. Global database on body mass index 2011 [homepage on the internet]. c2011 [cited 2011 Feb 21].Available from: http://apps.who.int/bmi/index.jsp?introPage=intro_3.html
29. Ricciardi R, Metter EJ, Cavanaugh EW, et al. Predicting cardiovascular risk using measures of regional and total body fat. Appl Nurs Res. 2009;22(1):2–9. http://dx.doi.org/10.1016/j.apnr.2007.01.011, PMID: 19171289
30. Reis JP, Michos ED, Von Mühlen D, et al. Differences in vitamin D status as a possible contributor to the racial disparity in peripheral arterial disease. Am J Clin Nutr. 2008;88(6):1469–1477. http://dx.doi.org/10.3945/ajcn.2008.26447, PMid: 19064505
31. Kolbe-Alexander TL, Buckmaster C, Nossel C, et al. Chronic disease risk factors, healthy days and medical claims in South African employees presenting for health risk screening. BMC Public Health 2008;8:228. http://dx.doi.org/10.1186/1471-2458-8-228, PMid: 18601718
32. Shisana O, Labadarios D, Rehle T, et al. The South African National Health and Nutrition Examination Survey (SANHANES-1). [document on the internet]. c2013 [cited 2013 Oct 30]. Available from: http://www.hsrc.ac.za/uploads/pageContent/3893/SANHANES-launch%20edition%20(online%20version).pdf
33. Ehret GB, Morrison AC, O'Connor AA, et al. Replication of the Wellcome Trust genome-wide association study of essential hypertension. Eur J Human Genet. 2008;16(12):1507–1511. http://dx.doi.org/10.1038/ejhg.2008.102, PMid: 18523456
34. Department of Health. South Africa Demographic and Health Survey 2003, full report. Pretoria: Department of Health; 2007. Available from: www.mrc.ac.za/bod/sadhs.htm
35. Charlton KE, Steyn K, Levitt NS, et al. Diet and blood pressure in South Africa: intake of foods containing sodium, potassium, calcium, and magnesium in three ethnic groups. Nutrition. 2005;21(1):39–50. http://dx.doi.org/10.1016/j.nut.2004.09.007, PMid: 15661477
36. Kruger HS, Venter CS, Vorster HH, et al. Physical inactivity is the major determinant of obesity in black women in the North West Province, South Africa: the THUSA study. Nutrition. 2002;18(5):422–427. http://dx.doi.org/10.1016/S0899-9007(01)00751-1, PMID: 11985949
37. Flegal KM, Graubard BI. Estimates of excess deaths associated with body mass index and other anthropometric variables. Am J Clin Nutr. 2009;89(4):1213–1219. http://dx.doi.org/10.3945/ajcn.2008.26698, PMid: 19190072
38. Intersalt Cooperative Research Group. Intersalt: an international study of electrolyte excretion and blood pressure. Results for 24 hour urinary sodium and potassium excretion. BMJ. 1988;297(6644):319–328. http://dx.doi.org/10.1136/bmj.297.6644.319, PMid: 3416162
39. Mashele N, Van Rooyen JM, Malan L, et al. Cardiovascular function and psychological distress in urbanised black South Africans: the SABPA study. Cardiovasc J Afr. 2010;21(4):206–211. PMid: 20838719
40. Lee CM, Huxley RR, Wildman RP, et al. Indices of abdominal obesity are better discriminators of cardiovascular risk factors than BMI: a meta-analysis. J Clin Epidemiol. 2008;61(7):646–653. http://dx.doi.org/10.1016/j.jclinepi.2007.08.012, PMid: 18359190

Integrating HIV care and treatment into primary healthcare: Are clinics equipped?

Authors:
Talitha Crowley[1]
Ethelwynn L. Stellenberg[1]

Affiliations:
[1]Division of Nursing, Faculty of Medicine and Health Sciences, Stellenbosch University, South Africa

Correspondence to:
Talitha Crowley

Email:
tcrowley@sun.ac.za

Postal address:
PO Box 19063, Francie van Zijl Drive, Tygerberg 7505, South Africa

Background: The demand for HIV care and treatment services is increasing rapidly and strategies to sustain long-term care should be employed. The decentralisation and integration of HIV care and treatment services into primary healthcare (PHC) is vitally important in order to ensure optimal access to life-saving antiretroviral therapy and ongoing chronic care. Conversely, the PHC system is fraught with the current burden of disease.

Setting: The study was conducted in PHC clinics in the uMgungundlovu district, Kwa-Zulu Natal.

Aim: The objectives of the study were to assess whether PHC clinics were equipped to deliver integrated HIV services and to evaluate the availability of resources as well as support systems for HIV care and treatment in PHC clinics.

Methods: A quantitative, cross-sectional descriptive study was undertaken in 20 randomly-selected, eligible clinics in the uMgungundlovu district, KwaZulu-Natal, South Africa. An evaluation instrument was completed through observations and review of the clinic data records. Criteria were based on the World Health Organization's guide to indicators for antiretroviral programmes as well as South African HIV standards for PHC facilities.

Results: None of the clinics were equipped adequately. Clinics with a higher patient load had poorer scores, whilst clinics providing antiretroviral therapy were better equipped in terms of human resources and infrastructure.

Conclusion: HIV services are an essential part of primary healthcare and clinics need to be equipped adequately in order to render this service. It is unlikely that the over-burdened health system would be able to cope with an increased number of patients on antiretroviral therapy in the long term, whilst maintaining quality of services, without support being given to PHC clinics.

L'intégration des soins et du traitement du VIH dans les services de santé primaire: les cliniques sont-elle équipées pour cela?

Contexte: La demande des services de soins et traitement du VIH augmente rapidement; aussi faudrait-il employer des stratégies pour maintenir les soins à long terme (devraient être employées). La décentralisation et l'intégration de ces services dans les soins de santé primaires (SSP) sont (est) importantes pour assurer un accès optimal au traitement de sauvetage et aux soins continus.

Objectifs: Evaluer si les cliniques de SSP étaient équipées pour offrir des services intégrés du VIH. Evaluer la disponibilité des ressources ainsi que des systèmes de soutien pour les soins et traitement du VIH.

Méthodes: Une étude descriptive quantitative, transversale a été menée dans 20 cliniques (aléatoirement) sélectionnées au hasard dans le district d'uMgungundlovu, au KwaZulu-Natal, en Afrique du Sud. Un instrument d'évaluation a été complété par observation et revue des données. Les critères étaient fondés sur les indicateurs de programmes antirétroviraux de l'Organisation Mondiale de la Santé, et sur les normes sud-africaines pour (sur) le VIH.

Résultats: Aucune des cliniques n'était correctement équipée. Les cliniques à (a) charge élevée de patients avaient les (plus pauvres) scores les plus bas; celles de thérapies antirétrovirales étaient mieux équipées en ressources humaines et infrastructures.

Conclusion: Les services du VIH sont une partie essentielle des soins de santé primaires ; les cliniques doivent être équipées pour rendre ce service. Il est peu probable que le système de santé surchargé sera (serait) en mesure de faire face à une augmentation du nombre de patients sous traitement antirétroviral à long terme, tout en maintenant la qualité des services, sans soutien apporté aux centres de SSP.

Introduction

Social value

There has been a significant expansion in the need for HIV care and treatment in Africa as well as in the world.[1] Such a scale-up of treatment brings unique challenges that warrant investigation. One of the critical challenges is the delivery of long-term care for the increasing population of clients on antiretroviral therapy within the context of overburdened health systems.[2]

The global incidence of HIV seems to have stabilised, but the number of people receiving antiretroviral therapy has increased, with 6.65 million people receiving antiretroviral therapy by the end of 2010.[1] With the introduction of the World Health Organization (WHO) Global Health Sector Strategy on HIV/AIDS, 2011–2015[3] and the UNAIDS 2011–2015 Strategy: Getting to Zero,[4] there is a renewed focus on sustainable models for the delivery of long-term HIV care and treatment. In order to promote accessible, equitable and sustainable HIV services within resource-constrained systems, HIV programmes need to be decentralised (brought closer to the people) and integrated with other health services.[2] A primary healthcare (PHC) approach is generally considered as being central to providing equitable healthcare.[5,6,7]

Scientific value

Current trends suggest increased support for the decentralisation of HIV treatment and care services, task shifting and the integration of these services within the PHC system.[2,8]

The decentralisation of care includes the provision of HIV care and treatment such as antiretroviral therapy, both in PHC clinics and within communities.[9] In general, task shifting is a characteristic of decentralisation. Tasks traditionally performed by higher cadres are shifted to lower cadres with less training such as non-physician clinicians, nurses, nurse-assistants, community healthcare workers and people living with HIV.[10]

'Integration' is described differently by various authors but, in broad terms, means services previously provided vertically which are now delivered as a package of care within mainstream health services.[6,8] The integration of HIV services into primary healthcare has the benefit of promoting coherent and holistic services. It increases access to care, allows more people to be treated, improves retention in care, saves costs and potentially leads to improved patient outcomes.[11,12,13] However, the evidence for the benefits of decentralisation and integration of HIV care and treatment is not definitive and a number of studies found no difference in health-related outcomes or access to antiretroviral therapy.[6,14,15]

It has been found that the integration of HIV care and treatment services in primary healthcare benefit the larger PHC system.[12] Nevertheless, ongoing challenges such as logistical and infrastructural constraints as well as adding tasks to overburdened staff are barriers to successful integration.[12,16,17]

It is apparent that the decentralisation and integration of HIV care and treatment into primary healthcare has potential benefit, yet there are few clear recommendations for effective integration of HIV care and treatment into primary healthcare.[15] This study describes the evaluation of PHC clinics within a health district in South Africa with a high HIV burden, to establish whether these clinics are equipped for integrated HIV care and treatment services.

Given the potential benefit of the integration of HIV care and treatment services to improve access to care and provide continuity of long-term care, it is crucial to identify available resources in PHC clinics that will enable quality HIV care and treatment services. Furthermore, quantifiable methods to assess whether clinics are equipped fully for integration of care could be beneficial with regard to measuring progress.

Conceptual framework

The conceptual framework for the study was based on Donabedian's model for healthcare quality evaluation,[18] which constitutes of structure, process and outcome indicators. For the purpose of this study, the structure and process indicators according to the Donabedian model were applied in order to evaluate the objectives as determined for the study. Several indicators, grouped in clusters such as recording and reporting, physical space, basic HIV services rendered and laboratory capacity, were used to evaluate whether clinics were equipped for integrated services (Figure 1).

Aim and objectives

The objectives of the study were to assess whether PHC clinics were equipped adequately for the delivery of integrated HIV services and to evaluate the availability of resources and support systems for HIV care and treatment in PHC clinics.

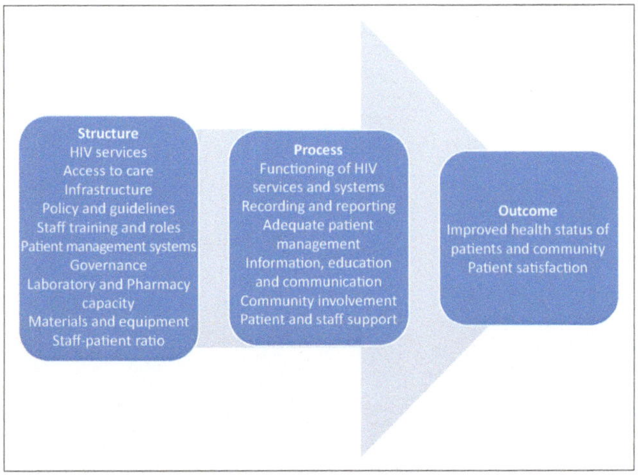

FIGURE 1: Conceptual framework indicating indicator clusters.

Research method and design

Study design

A quantitative cross-sectional descriptive design was used.

Setting

The study was conducted in PHC clinics in the uMgungundlovu district, Kwa-Zulu Natal. Kwa-Zulu Natal has the highest HIV prevalence in South Africa (39.5%).[19]

Study population and sampling strategy

The target population for the purpose of this study was provincial clinics and local government clinics of the uMgungundlovu District, KwaZulu-Natal. The eligibility criteria for choosing clinics were the following:

- Clinics were operational from a permanent location.
- Service delivery took place every week day for eight hours per day.
- A comprehensive PHC service was provided.

The target population for the purpose of this study was 47 clinics. A simple random sample of 20 (43%) of the clinics was drawn in order to ensure representation of the target population. The sample was selected by assigning numbers to the clinics on the list obtained from the district office. Numbers were selected randomly by a third party to ensure that each clinic had an equal chance of being selected.

Data collection

The researcher collected all data with the use of an instrument. A new instrument based on the literature, the WHO's guide to indicators for monitoring and evaluating national antiretroviral programmes[20] and HIV standards for PHC facilities in South Africa,[21] was developed by the researcher. The instrument was divided into Section A, which included demographical data about the clinic, and Section B, which contained indicator clusters such as: recording and reporting; physical space; basic HIV services rendered; laboratory capacity; and pharmacy capacity (Figure 1).

Pilot test

Pilot testing of the instrument was conducted in two clinics that were not part of the sample. It was identified during the pilot test that the instrument only allowed for dichotomous responses. During data collection, it was observed that many of the indicators should rather be measured categorically and the instrument was consequently adapted. Clinics were given a score out of '3' for each of the 136 indicators, where a score of '3' was allocated if all requirements were met; '2' for most requirements met; '1' for few requirements met; and '0' for no requirements met. A minimum acceptable score of 80% was decided upon, including meeting the critical criteria, for clinics to be equipped adequately to deliver integrated HIV care and treatment services. Critical criteria were indicators that were regarded as essential for effective functioning and their selection was based on the literature. These 87 critical points included indicators such as whether the clinic had 12 months of patient data available, the implementation of infection prevention and control procedures and the provision of basic HIV services, such as HIV testing and counselling. Data from the pilot test were not included in the main study.

Validity and reliability

The face and content validity of the instrument were strengthened by pilot testing the instrument and consultations with experts in HIV systems research, nursing research and a qualified statistician. Detailed field notes were taken of observations made and information from clinic data records so as to promote accurate scoring.

Main study

Data for the main study were collected from clinic data records and from observations made by the researcher from December 2008 to January 2009. Clinic managers were consulted when relevant data could not be found.

Data analysis

Data were entered into Microsoft Excel by the researcher and a statistical analysis program, STATISTICA (Release 8), was used to analyse the data. Comparisons between variables such as clinic demographical data, indicators and the overall clinic score were made by using appropriate techniques, such as Fisher exact, Mann-Whitney U and Spearman correlations. These techniques are all used on smaller sample sizes in order to ensure the accurate interpretation of results. A 5% significance level ($p < 0.05$) was used as a guideline to determine significant relationships.

Ethical considerations

Ethical approval for the study was obtained from the Health Research Ethics Committee at the Faculty of Medicine and Health Sciences, University of Stellenbosch (N08/09/237). Permission to conduct the research was obtained from the KwaZulu-Natal provincial research committee, the uMgungundlovu district manager and local municipality managers. Written informed consent was obtained from clinic managers before data collection. The interruption of clinic procedures was limited since the researcher obtained data from clinic data registers and observations. Clinic names were coded and data de-identified in order to protect anonymity.

Results

Clinic demographical data

The ratio between provincial and local government clinics was 3:2 (Table 1). Most clinics ($n = 13$; 65%) were open on all week days for eight hours per day, six clinics (30%) were open for 24 hours for seven days per week and one clinic (5%) was open on weekdays and on Saturdays. Non-governmental organisations (NGOs) employed staff for the antiretroviral therapy (ART) programme in eight (40%) clinics. Statistical analysis revealed that clinics that had NGO support for the HIV programme were more likely to provide ART as part of their HIV care and treatment services (Fisher exact $p < 0.01$).

Indicator clusters

Recording and reporting were assessed by evaluating whether clinics had a complete set of data available for the 12 months prior to the study. Only 11 clinics (55%) had complete data available for the primary healthcare head count, HIV counseling and testing (HCT) and TB monitoring.

Physical space comprised storage space for medical supplies as well as consultation rooms. Only six (30%) clinics had sufficient storage space for nutritional supplements and medication. In 10 (50%) of the clinics, the number of consultation rooms was not sufficient for the current purposes. Sharing of consultation rooms between healthcare workers was observed to be a common practice, posing concerns for patient privacy. Clinics that provided ART had more consultation and counseling rooms available than clinics where ART was not provided (Mann-Whitney U $p < 0.01$).

Adequate referral systems are central to the functioning of decentralised ART services. Reliable transport systems for patient referral were only available in eight (40%) clinics, whilst two (10%) clinics did not have a dedicated telephone or cellphone line in order to communicate with referral facilities. With regard to patient information, education and communication (IEC), HIV educational material in local languages was only available in seven (35%) of the clinics.

Basic HIV services included indicators such as the provision of family planning, sexually-transmitted infection management and HIV counseling and testing (HCT). All of the basic HIV services were available and utilised, with half (50%) of the clinics proving ART and 15 (75%) clinics preparing patients for ART initiation, including antiretroviral adherence preparation and baseline blood investigations. All of the clinics (100%) provided HCT and CD4 blood testing, although provider-initiated counseling and testing (PICT) was only practised in five (25%) clinics. At the time of the study, professional nurses did not initiate patients on ART and in 19 (95%) of the clinics, less than half of the staff members had received any HIV-related training. In two (10%) of the clinics, it was observed by the researcher that there were no dedicated professional nurses for managing patients on ART and patients collected medication from untrained staff, such as enrolled nurses. There was no significant difference between clinics that did and did not provide ART with regard to staff trained in HIV management (Mann-Whitney U $p = 0.47$).

TABLE 1: Demographical data of clinics (n = 20).

Variable	n	%
Local government (municipality)	8	40
Provincial government	12	60
Clinics with NGO support for HIV programme	8	40
Clinics with no NGO support for HIV programme	12	60
Clinics where ART was available	10	50
Clinics where ART was not available	10	50

n, number of clinics; NGO, non-governmental organisation; ART, antiretroviral therapy.

Adherence to the policies and national treatment guidelines or protocols is important for ensuring safe patient care. Updated policies and guidelines that were organised in a file could only be located in two (10%) of the clinics. The implementation of universal infection precautions were found to be challenging in three clinics (15%) since there were no handwashing basins or alcohol-based hand disinfectant and a lack of sharp containers and medical waste bins.

Patient support was found to be lacking as nine clinics (45%) did not have functional support groups for HIV-positive patients on-site and three (30%) clinics providing ART did not have a system in place for tracing clients that default on their treatment. However, clinics providing ART were more likely to have a functional support group for people living with HIV (Mann-Whitney U $p = 0.01$).

Community involvement, defined as being any evidence of interaction between the clinic and community-based organisations or the provision of community services, was absent in 18 (90%) of the clinics. Of the clinics that engaged with the community, one clinic (5%) interacted with traditional healers in the community to support patients on ART to adhere to therapy and one clinic (5%) had a record of community health workers (CHWs) who were active in the community for referral of patients for home-based or palliative care. None of the clinics had a social worker on-site and none of the clinics had a record of referring patients for home-based or palliative care.

Laboratory and pharmaceutical services are both essential components of the provision and monitoring of ART. Adequate laboratory services were available in more than half (n = 15; 75%) of the clinics. However, only eight (40%) of the clinics had a turn-around time of less than two weeks on certain blood results and two (10%) of the clinics experienced problems with the system for transport of specimens to the laboratory. The laboratory system could also not be accessed electronically in any of the clinics.

Dispensaries (dedicated medicine rooms) were used for storing medication in 19 (95%) of the clinics and one clinic (5%) used cupboards in the patient consultation rooms. Insufficient storage space for storing medication existed in half (50%) of the dispensaries. These clinics did not have sufficient shelf space for medication. There were no dedicated storage areas and boxes containing medication or medical supplies were stacked on the floors of consultation rooms and dispensaries. Adequate security for the dispensary was only available in 12 (60%) of the clinics. In four (20%) of the clinics, the room where the medication was kept was not air-conditioned as the air-conditioner was broken at the time. All the clinics had essential medicines available, although functional stock-outs of essential drugs were reported by clinic managers in 18 (80%) of the clinics.

With regard to governance and management, only three clinics (15%) were supervised every three months by the district HIV/AIDS coordinator. Provincial government clinics were significantly more likely to be visited every three months by the HIV/AIDS coordinator than local government clinics (Mann-Whitney U $p < 0.01$). The latter finding could suggest communication challenges between the HIV/AIDS coordinator and local government clinics.

In nine (45%) of the clinics, the clinic building was not adequately maintained. Problems observed by the researcher with regard to maintenance were numerous and included: walls requiring painting, leaking roofs, 'rotten' ceilings that were falling down, sewerage systems that were out of order, poor air-conditioning and leaking toilets. There was lack of electricity or water supply in some of the park homes outside the clinics that were utilised for HIV services. Basic equipment such as otoscopes, thermometers, blood pressure monitors and measuring jugs for mixing paediatric medication was missing or not functioning properly in two (10%) of the clinics.

Average monthly patient statistics were calculated where clinics had at least three months of data available (Table 2). There were large variations in the PHC monthly headcount, which could be attributed to the fact that some clinics rendered a 24-hour service and some only an eight-hour daily service. Some of the rural clinics did not have a very high patient headcount. Furthermore, there could be differences in how the clinics counted and documented their PHC headcount.

Clinics where ART was provided reflected a significantly higher PHC headcount than clinics that did not provide ART (Mann-Whitney U $p < 0.01$).

The average number of patients seen per staff member (Registered Nurse, Enrolled Nurse and Enrolled Nurse Assistant) per day was 22.77 (SD = 9.87), with a minimum of 9.76 and a maximum of 49.94.

Clinics with higher PHC headcounts had significantly more staff members than clinics with lower headcounts (Spearman $r = 0.87$, $p < 0.01$). Furthermore, clinics that provided ART had significantly more staff compared with clinics that did not provide ART (Mann-Whitney U $p < 0.01$). The provision of ART as part of HIV care and treatment services was therefore associated with increased PHC headcounts and the employment of more staff members.

Clinic score

Although five (25%) clinics obtained an average clinic score percentage of more than 80%, none of the clinics met all critical points. The high mean of 73.98 (SD = 6.93) for the total score signifies that PHC clinics have the potential to provide quality integrated HIV treatment and care services should they receive adequate support.

The clinic scores were affected significantly by the number of staff members as well as the patient load (number of patients seen by each nursing staff member per day) of the clinic. Clinics with more staff members were more likely to achieve a high score for the instrument than clinics with less staff members (Spearman $r = 0.71$, $p < 0.01$). Furthermore, the higher the average number of patients seen by each staff member per day (patient load), the lower the average score (Spearman $r = -0.63$, $p < 0.01$). This may denote the importance of sufficient human resources to ensure quality of services.

Clinics where an NGO was providing additional resources for the ART programme obtained a significantly higher score than clinics where there was no NGO involvement (Mann-Whitney U $p = 0.01$). NGO support for the ART programme in the form of human and other resources may therefore improve PHC capacity for HIV care and treatment services.

Discussion

Key findings

The results indicated that most basic HIV care and treatment services were provided in PHC clinics. However, PHC clinics were not equipped adequately to render integrated HIV care and treatment services. This was because of a lack of capacity on both a clinical and health system level. Although half of the clinics already provided ART, the provision of ART is not the primary indicator for determining whether clinics are equipped to render quality integrated services. Key elements such as recording and reporting, human resource constraints, physical space and support systems needed to be addressed.

Aspects of HIV care and treatment such as the availability of physical space, trained healthcare professionals, updated guidelines, essential drugs, nutritional support, support groups and tracing of defaulters were found to be lacking. These findings are consistent with studies conducted in other provinces in South Africa.[16,17]

Clinics that provided ART had more staff available. The average monthly ART patient headcount for these clinics

TABLE 2: Clinic statistics.

Average monthly statistic	*n*	Mean	Standard deviation	Minimum	Maximum
PHC headcount	20	3850.55	2397.33	959	9438
HCTs done	20	124.05	69.99	27	301
CD4 counts done	18	74.06	57.82	15	239
ART up-referrals	16	17.31	12.76	2	40
ART follow-ups	9	225.44	199.09	21	558
Patients on waiting list for ART	10	42.6	66.6	4	229

n, number of clinics; PHC, primary healthcare; HCT, HIV counseling and testing; CD4, cluster of differentiation 4; ART, antiretroviral therapy.

was 225.44 (SD = 199.09). The ART rollout would inevitably increase the patient load of clinics and this was confirmed in the results. If human and other resources do not increase, other initiatives for managing patients on ART in the long term need to be explored. Workload and capacity constraints as well as logistical and infrastructural challenges and a lack of supervision and support were ongoing challenges that were documented in other studies.[8,16,17,22]

Discussion of key findings

Integrating additional services into primary healthcare without providing the adequate human resources and ongoing support could compromise the quality of care provided to patients and have long-term repercussions for reaching strategic developmental and global health goals.

Essential HIV care and treatment services as well as managerial and infrastructural support are key components for ensuring quality services. The provision of ART at a PHC level should be supported with additional human resources, infrastructure and the implementation of comprehensive models for integration of care.

Strengths and limitations

Limitations included that the study was conducted in one district within the context of a high HIV burden of disease and the results may therefore not be generalised to other settings. The number of clinics that was used was limited because of the depth of assessment in each of the clinics. The instrument and the scoring system used needs further testing in order to assess the reliability. Scores could have been calculated for individual structure and process indicator clusters which may prove beneficial in identifying specific areas that need improvement.

Implications or recommendations

With the ongoing effort to promote nurse-led services, emphasis should be placed on evaluating individual clinics with regard to resources and management systems for integrating HIV care and treatment services. Certain organisational systems, protocols and resources should be in place in order to ensure quality of care and continuity of services. Districts and clinics may vary with regard to human resources and infrastructure, necessitating individualised interventions.

However, HIV resources have been found to rehabilitate the PHC infrastructure[12] and a follow-up study is therefore necessary in order to evaluate the impact of the escalated ART rollout since 2010 on PHC clinics in South Africa.

Conclusion

The shift from doctor-led hospital-based care to nurse-led primary healthcare necessitates careful consideration for patient safety and quality of care. The clinics evaluated in this study were not equipped adequately for integration of HIV care and treatment into PHC services. Integration of HIV care and treatment services into primary healthcare could have detrimental effects on the quality of long-term HIV care and treatment within the current overburdened PHC system.

With a renewed focus on the provision of primary healthcare and integration of HIV care and treatment in mainstream health services, additional resources and support should be allocated to PHC clinics in order to sustain long-term HIV care that is of a high quality and will not compromise other services. Such an approach will inevitably strengthen the larger PHC system in order to address the quadruple burden of disease in South Africa.

Acknowledgements

We would like to thank all the clinic managers at the participating clinics who accommodated the data collection.

Competing interests

The authors declare that they have no financial or personal relationship(s) which may have inappropriately influenced them in writing this article.

Authors contributions

T.C. (Stellenbosch University) conducted the research, analysed and interpreted the data and wrote the manuscript. E.L.S. (Stellenbosch University) supervised the research and reviewed and edited the manuscript.

References

1. WHO, UNAIDS, UNICEF. Global HIV/AIDS response: epidemic update and health sector progress towards Universal Access. Progress report 2011 [document on the Internet]. 2011 [cited 2014 Mar 09]. Available from: http://www.aidsdatahub.org/sites/default/files/documents/UNAIDS_Global_HIVAIDS_Response_Progress_Report_2011.pdf
2. Ross DA, South A, Weller I, et al. HIV treatment and care systems: the way forward. AIDS. 2012;26(Suppl 2):S147–S152. http://dx.doi.org/10.1097/QAD.0b013e32835bde37
3. World Health Organization. Global health sector strategy on HIV/AIDS 2011–2015 [document on the Internet]. 2011 [cited 2014 Mar 09]. Available from: http://www.who.int/hiv/pub/hiv_strategy/en/
4. UNAIDS. UNAIDS strategy 2011–2015 [page on the Internet]. 2010 [cited 2014 Mar 09]. Available from: http://www.unaids.org/en/aboutunaids/unaidsstrategygoalsby2015/
5. De Maeseneer J. Primary health care in Africa: Now more than ever! Afr J Prm Health Care Fam Med. 2009;1(1), Art. #112, 3 pages. http://dx.doi.org/10.4102/phcfm.v1i1.112
6. Dudley L, Garner P. Strategies for integrating primary health services in low- and middle-income countries at the point of delivery. Cochrane Database Syst Rev. 2011;7: CD003318. http://dx.doi.org/10.1002/14651858.CD003318.pub3
7. Munderi P, Grosskurth H, Droti B, et al. What are the essential components of HIV treatment and care services in low and middle-income countries: an overview by settings and levels of the health system? AIDS. 2012;26(Suppl 2):S97–S103. doi: 10.1097./QAD.0b013e32835bdde6
8. Uebel KE, Joubert G, Wouters E, et al. Integrating HIV care into primary care services: quantifying progress of an intervention in South Africa. PLoS One. 2013;8(1):e54266. http://dx.doi.org/10.1371/journal.pone.0054266
9. Kredo T, Ford N, Adeniyi FB, et al. Decentralising HIV treatment delivery in lower- and middle-income countries. Cochrane Database Syst Rev. 2013;6:CD009987. doi: 10.102/14651858.CD009987
10. World Health Organization. Task shifting: global recommendations and guidelines [document on the Internet]. 2008 [cited 2014 Mar 09]. Available from: http://www.who.int/healthsystems/TTR-TaskShifting.pdf
11. Fatti G, Grimwood A, Bock P. Better antiretroviral therapy outcomes at primary healthcare facilities: an evaluation of three tiers of ART services in four South African provinces. PLoS One. 2010;5(9):e12888. http://dx.doi.org/10.1371/journal.pone.0012888

12. Pfeiffer J, Montoya P, Baptista AJ, et al. Integration of HIV/AIDS services into African primary health care: lessons learned for health system strengthening in Mozambique – a case study. J Int AIDS Soc. 2010;13:3. http://dx.doi.org/10.1186/1758-2652-13-3

13. Long L, Brennan A, Fox MP, et al. Treatment outcomes and cost-effectiveness of shifting management of stable ART patients to nurses in South Africa: an observational cohort. PLoS Med. 2011;8(7):e1001055. doi: 10.1371./journal.pmed.1001055

14. Fairall L, Bachmann MO, Lombard C, et al. Task shifting of antiretroviral treatment from doctors to primary-care nurses in South Africa (STRETCH): a pragmatic, parallel, cluster-randomised trial. Lancet. 2012;380(9845):889–898. http://dx.doi.org/10.1016/S0140-6736(12)60730-2

15. Sweeney S, Obure CD, Maier CB, et al. Costs and efficiency of integrating HIV/AIDS services with other health services: a systematic review of evidence and experience. Sex Transm Infect. 2012;88(2):85–99. http://dx.doi.org/10.1136/sextrans-2011-050199

16. Cameron D, Gerber A, Mbatha M, et al. Nurse-initiation and maintenance of patients on antiretroviral therapy: are nurses in primary care clinics initiating ART after attending NIMART training? S Afr Med J. 2012;102(2):98–100.

17. Georgeu D, Colvin CJ, Lewin S, et al. Implementing nurse-initiated and managed antiretroviral treatment (NIMART) in South Africa: a qualitative process evaluation of the STRETCH trial. Implement Sci. 2012;7:66. http://dx.doi.org/10.1186/1748-5908-7-66

18. Donabedian A. Quality assessment and monitoring. Eval Health Prof. 1983;3(6):363–375. http://dx.doi.org/10.1177/016327878300600309

19. Republic of South Africa. Global AIDS response progress report 2012 [document on the Internet] 2012 [cited 2014 Mar 09]. Available from: http://www.unaids.org/en/dataanalysis/knowyourresponse/countryprogressreports/2012countries/ce_ZA_Narrative_Report.pdf

20. World Health Organization. National AIDS programmes: a guide to indicators for monitoring and evaluating national antiretroviral programmes [document on the Internet]. 2005 [cited 2014 Mar 09]. Available from: http://www.who.int/hiv/pub/me/naparv.pdf

21. Pleaner M, Moleko W, Sibanyoni M. HIV standards: a self-assessment tool to improve HIV services at primary health care facilities. Johannesburg, South Africa: RHRU; 2008.

22. Rashidian A, Shakibazadeh E, Karimi-Shahanjarini A, et al. Barriers and facilitators to the implementation of doctor-nurse substitution strategies in primary care : qualitative evidence synthesis. Cochrane Database Syst Rev. 2013;2:CD010412. http://dx.doi.org/10.1002/14651858.CD010412

12

Body mass index of 16-year olds in urban Maseru, Lesotho

Authors:
Violet L. van den Berg[1]
Lisemelo Seheri[1]
Jacques Raubenheimer[2]

Affiliations:
[1]Department of Nutrition and Dietetics, University of the Free State, South Africa

[2]Department of Biostatistics, University of the Free State, South Africa

Correspondence to:
Violet van den Berg

Email:
vdbergvl@ufs.ac.za

Postal address:
PO Box 339, Bloemfontein 9300, South Africa

Background: Overweight and/or obesity amongst children and adolescents is a global epidemic with health consequences that track into adulthood. No data are currently available regarding overweight/obesity amongst adolescents in Lesotho.

Aim and setting: To assess the prevalence of overweight and/or obesity and the associated risk factors amongst 16-year olds in urban Maseru, Lesotho.

Method: A cross-sectional descriptive study was conducted on a systematic sample of 16-year olds in grade four (N = 221; 56.6% girls) from randomly-selected schools in urban Maseru. Diet histories and data on lifestyle, physical activity and knowledge, attitudes and/or perceptions and practices regarding nutrition were obtained during structured interviews and body mass index (BMI) was determined.

Results: Amongst these 16-year olds, 27.2% girls and 8.3% boys were overweight and/or obese based on World Health Organization cut-offs for BMI; 39.8% were insufficiently active or inactive; 6.4% used alcohol regularly; and 11.7% used tobacco. Whilst 28.1% reported no television watching/electronic gaming/computer usage (combined screen time) outside school, 23.6% reported ≥ 4 hours of combined screen time outside school. Most (91.4%) consumed < 3 servings of vegetables/day; 86.4% consumed < 2 servings of fruits/day; and 95.5% consumed < 2 servings of dairy/day. The majority consumed maize porridge (56.1%), bread (63.8%) and margarine/oil/fat (82.3%) daily and added sugar to their food (74.2%). Fruits, vegetables, dairy, meat, pulses and traditional foods were only consumed weekly or less often. Most bought from tuck shops (18.6% daily; 54.3% weekly). Various gaps in knowledge, perceptions and practices were identified that may benefit from educational intervention.

Conclusions: The current study identifies westernised dietary and lifestyle changes, along with overweight and/or obesity, amongst 16-year old adolescents in Lesotho.

Indice de masse corporelle chez les adolescents de 16 ans dans l'agglomération de Maseru, au Lesotho.

Contexte: L'excès de poids/obésité chez les enfants et adolescents est une épidémie mondiale qui a des conséquences sur la santé qui se poursuivent à l'âge adulte. A l'heure actuelle il n'existe aucune donnée sur l'excès de poids/obésité chez les adolescents du Lesotho.

Objectif et lieu: Evaluer la prévalence d'excès de poids/obésité et les facteurs de risques qui lui sont associés chez les adolescents de 16 ans dans l'agglomération de Maseru, au Lesotho.

Méthode: On a effectué une étude descriptive transversale sur un échantillon systématique d'enfants de 16 ans de grade quatre (N = 221; 56.6% de filles) d'écoles sélectionnées au hasard dans l'agglomération de Maseru. Au cours d'entretiens structurés on a noté les antécédents alimentaires et les données sur le mode de vie, l'activité physique et les connaissances, attitudes/perceptions et pratiques relatives à la nutrition ainsi que l'indice de masse corporelle (BMI).

Résultats: Parmi ces adolescents de 16 ans, 27.2% des filles et 8.3% des garçons étaient en surpoids / obèses selon les seuils de l'OMS pour l'IMC; 39.8% n'étaient pas assez actifs/inactifs; 6.4% buvaient de l'alcool régulièrement; et 11.7% ont fait l'usage de tabac. Alors que 28.1% ne regardaient pas la télévision/ n'utilisaient pas les jeux électroniques/ l'ordinateur (temps passé devant un écran) en dehors de l'école, 23.6% passaient ≥ quatre heures devant un écran en dehors de l'école. La plupart (91.4%) consommaient moins de trois portions de légumes par jour; 86.4% consommaient moins de deux portions de fruits par jour; et 95.5% consommaient moins de deux portions de produits laitiers par jour. La majorité consommait de la bouillie de maïs (56.1%), du pain (63.8%) et de la margarine/ de l'huile/des corps gras (82.3%) chaque jour et ajoutait du sucre à leurs aliments (74.2%). Ils mangeaient des fruits, des légumes, des produits laitiers, de la viande, des légumes secs et de la nourriture traditionnelle chaque semaine ou moins souvent. La plupart d'entre eux achetait à manger au kiosque (18.6% chaque jour; 54.3% chaque semaine). On a identifié des lacunes dans leurs connaissances, perceptions et pratiques qui pourraient être améliorées par l'éducation.

Conclusions: Cette étude identifie les changements dus à l'influence occidentale dans le mode de vie et l'alimentation des adolescents de 16 ans du Lesotho, ainsi que le surpoids et l'obésité.

Introduction

The World Health Organization (WHO) recognises the epidemic of childhood overweight/obesity as being one of the most serious global public health challenges of the 21st century.[1] Obesity in childhood and adolescence has been identified as a key predictor for obesity in adulthood, as well as the early onset of insulin resistance, hypertension, dyslipidemia, and type 2 diabetes.[1,2,3] In addition, morbidity and mortality in the adult population are increased in individuals who were overweight as adolescents, even if they lose the extra weight during adulthood.[2,3]

In the United States, national representative data gathered for the period 2008–2009 indicated that 33.0% of boys and 30.4% of girls aged two to 19 are overweight and/or obese.[4] In the 25 countries constituting the European Union, the prevalence of overweight/obesity is currently 16% – 22% amongst seven- to 17-year olds.[5] The epidemic also affects developing countries,[1,6] with the recent prevalence of overweight/obesity amongst five- to 19-year olds at 41.8% in Mexico, 22.1% in Brazil, 22.0% in India and 19.3% in Argentina.[6] In addition, studies of secular trends indicate that the prevalence of overweight and/or obesity is escalating at an alarming rate, both in developed and in developing countries.[6]

In 2004, the International Obesity Task Force estimated that less than 1% of children aged five to 17 years were overweight and/or obese in the sub-Saharan African region.[6] However, the South African Health of the Nation Survey for 2001–2004 found that 13.3% of boys and 22.3% of girls aged six to 13 years, were overweight and/or obese;[7] whilst the 1st South African National Youth Risk Behaviour Survey (SAYRBS) for 2002 reported that 7% of boys and 25% of girls aged 13 to 19 years were overweight/obese.[8] When the SAYRBS was repeated in 2008, 11.2% of boys and 27.8% of girls adolescents (13 to 19 years old), were found to be overweight and/or obese.[9] More recently, the South African National Health And Nutrition Examination Survey (SANHANES-1) found that 10.2% of boys and 22.3% of girls aged 10 to 14 years fell into this classification.[10]

The development of childhood overweight and/or obesity is attributed to a complex interplay between genetics and environmental factors.[11] In developing countries, as a result of' aggressive advertising practices, relatively low cost of energy-dense foods and improved purchasing power',[6] children and adolescents are increasingly abandoning more prudent traditional diets 'in favour of foods high in saturated fat and refined carbohydrates, sweetened carbonated beverages and diets low in polyunsaturated fatty acids and fiber'.[6,11]

Simultaneously, because of increased indoor leisure activities and entertainment, unsafe neighbourhoods and lack of open spaces in communities, these children and adolescents are also becoming increasingly more sedentary.[6] Studies show that these specific patterns of nutrition and lifestyle transition are strongly associated with urbanisation and are highly conducive to the development of obesity, insulin resistance, cardiovascular diseases and type 2 diabetes.[6,12]

Moreover, in developing countries, intrauterine energy and nutrient deprivation are common amongst food-insecure mothers, also leading to metabolic adaptations in the foetuses which predispose them to future overweight and related metabolic disturbances, particularly when exposed during childhood to the above-mentioned transitional diet and lifestyle.[13]

The problem of overweight and obesity amongst children and adolescents in developing countries is further complicated by false traditional beliefs about and low knowledge of health and nutrition, as well as by specific socio-cultural perceptions regarding nutrition, gender roles and overweight and/or obesity amongst parents, caregivers and school children.[6] Whilst various studies have focused on urbanisation, nutrient and lifestyle transition and overweight/obesity and their related health risks in the South African pediatric and adolescent population,[12,14,15] few studies to date have investigated these problems in other sub-Saharan African countries.

The Kingdom of Lesotho is a small mountainous country of just over 30 300 km^2, completely encircled by the Republic of South Africa. The climate is semi-arid with unpredictable weather patterns frequently characterised by droughts, heavy rainfall and hailstorms in summer, followed by very cold winters with frost and snow in the higher areas.[16] The population of 1 936 181 (July 2013 estimate) consists of 99.7% Basotho.[17] In 2010, 27% of the population lived in urban areas and it was estimated that the urban population will increase annually by 3.5% from 2010 to 2015.[16] Around 35.0% of the population is aged below 15 years (2010 estimate).[16]

To date, however, no study has focused on overweight and/or obesity amongst children and adolescents in Lesotho. This study is therefore the first to report on overweight/obesity, the risk factors for weight gain, as well as knowledge, attitudes, perceptions and practices regarding overweight and/or obesity amongst adolescents (represented in this study by 16-year olds) in urban Lesotho. The study was restricted to one age group because the data were collected by a single researcher on a very limited budget. The age of 16 was chosen since national surveys often report overweight and obesity prevalence for adults in the population, namely, those over the age of 16 years. These data may serve to raise awareness of the emerging problem of overweight/obesity amongst the youth in Lesotho as a developing country where emphasis is placed on the prevention of undernutrition only; and to motivate future larger-scale surveys to assess the full extent of the problem amongst children and adolescents in the country. The results may also be used as baseline data to design intervention programmes to address the identified problems.

Research methods and design

Setting

The study was conducted amongst learners attending school in urban Maseru who were already 16 or had turned 16 in 2010. Maseru is the capital of Lesotho, located in the western low lands. It is by far the most populated city in the country

(220 000 in 2010).[17] In Lesotho, learners in urban areas start primary school at age 5 to 6 years. Primary education takes 7 years, followed by 3 years of junior secondary and 2 years of senior secondary education. In the Lesotho school system the majority of 16-year olds are in Form 4.

Study population and sampling strategy

There are 20 schools in urban Maseru, of which 2 are private and 3 are single-gender. The private and the single-gender schools were included non-randomly in the sample. A further 5 schools were selected randomly from the remaining 15 mixed-gender public schools, so that a total of 10 schools was included in the study. There were 2510 students enrolled in Form 4 over these 10 schools for the 2010 school year. As coverage of a tenth of the population in the sample was considered both representative and practically achievable, a sample of 251 learners was selected to participate in the study. From each school, a number of learners proportionate to the size of the Form 4 class of that school, were chosen systematically from the admissions lists obtained from the various schools. Adolescents were eligible to be included in the study if they were 15 (turning 16 in 2010) or 16 years old and were in Form four in 2010. Adolescents were excluded from the study if they were aged 16 years, but not in Form 4 in 2010. A meeting was conducted with the selected learners at each school in order to inform them about the study. During these contact sessions, letters explaining the purpose of the study were handed out to all selected learners to read and to take home to their parents or legal guardians. Learners who wanted to participate in the study were required to return signed letters of consent from their parents or legal guardians and were also required to also sign letters giving their assent regarding inclusion. Learners retained the written information sheets.

Data collection

Structured interviews were conducted in private with each participant in the participant's language of choice (English or Sesotho), in empty classrooms at the relevant schools. During the interview, weight and height were measured and questionnaires were used to collect data on socio-demography, dietary intakes, physical activity, screen watching habits, smoking habits and alcohol consumption, as well as knowledge, perceptions, attitudes and practices regarding nutrition. All data were collected by a single researcher who is a native of Maseru, Lesotho and is therefore familiar with the language and culture of the area; and who was trained in nutrition and the relevant research techniques at the University of the Free State in South Africa.

Anthropometry

During the interview, the researcher recorded the height and weight of each participant using standardised techniques[18] and calibrated equipment.

Lifestyle factors

During the structured interviews, participants were asked: whether or not they consume alcohol; to indicate the types of alcoholic beverages they usually drink (red wine, white wine, beer, liquor or others which they could specify); to report how often they usually consume alcohol over a period of a week; and to indicate the volume of consumption of these different types of alcoholic beverages during the 7 days prior to the interview. In addition, participants were asked whether or not they had ever tried to smoke cigarettes or had ever used snuff; and to indicate on how many days in the 30 days prior to the interview they had smoked cigarettes or used snuff. As these may be sensitive questions for adolescents to answer since they are legally not permitted to purchase alcohol or tobacco products and are advised not to use these substances, the participants were reassured about the confidentiality with which the information would be treated. Participants were also asked to report the number of hours that they spend per day watching television, playing electronic games, using a computer or accessing the internet (which was noted as combined screen time).

Physical activity information was obtained with questions adapted from the SAYRBS[8,9] which was in turn adapted specifically for South African adolescents from the International Physical Activity Questionnaire [IPAQ].[19]

Dietary intake and eating habits

In order to assess the overall balance of daily intake of foods from the basic food groups (starch; fruit; vegetable; milk and milk products; and meat and meat alternatives), as well as to quantify and evaluate daily intakes of energy and macronutrients, a 24-hour recall was administered during the structured interviews. Food photographs, packaging and local household utensils were used to assist participants in recalling portion sizes and food choices.

Food choices and dietary patterns were assessed by means of a non-quantified food frequency questionnaire (FFQ), which was administered during the same interview so as to determine how often particular foods within each food group were being consumed. The FFQ was adapted by the researcher to reflect foods from each of the food groups that are commonly used in Lesotho. Indigenous food choices such as wild fruits and traditional vegetable and traditional starch dishes were also included. An additional category included salty snacks, fast foods and beverages, as well as taking a packed lunch to school and buying from the school's tuck shop.

Knowledge, perceptions, attitudes and practices

Knowledge, perceptions, attitudes and practices regarding nutrition were recorded during the structured interviews by means of 49 questions adapted from the questionnaire used in the South African Food Consumption Survey Baseline for Food Fortification.[20] The current questionnaire included: 12 questions to assess knowledge regarding selection of food items, ways in which foods are handled and methods in which foods are prepared (providing the options 'true', 'false' or 'do not know'); 7 questions to assess attitude toward food and nutrition (providing the options 'agree, 'disagree or 'do not know'); 9 questions to assess nutrition practices (providing the options 'regularly, 'occasionally or 'never'); 10 questions to assess attitude toward obesity (providing the options 'true', 'false' or 'do not know'); 6 questions to assess perceptions regarding the causes of obesity (providing the options 'true', 'false' or 'do not know'); and 5 questions to assess knowledge regarding the relationship between obesity and health (providing the options 'true', 'false' or 'do not know').

Data analysis

Reliability interviews were conducted one month after the initial interview on every 10th participant. If more than 20% of the answers to the questions differed between the 2 interviews, these questions were regarded as unreliable and excluded from the analysis. No questions were excluded.

Statistical analysis was performed by the Department of Biostatistics of the Faculty of Health Science of the University of the Free State and was generated by SAS® software 9.3 (SAS Institute, Cary, NC 2014). Categorical data were presented as frequencies and percentages; and continuous data as medians and percentiles.

Body mass index (BMI) was interpreted according to the WHO Z-score expanded tables which classify BMI-for-age as overweight if greater than + 1 standard deviation (SD) of the mean (equivalent to BMI 25 kg/m^2 at 19 years) and as obese if greater than +2SD of the mean (equivalent to BMI 30 kg/m^2 at 19 years).[21] However, as these charts only became available in 2006, the CDC (US Centers for Disease Control and Prevention) data tables for BMI-for-age[22] and the International Obesity Task Force (IOTF) age-specific cut-off-points[23] for BMI at age 16 years were included so as to allow for comparison of the results with earlier studies in other countries. Pearson correlation analysis was used to evaluate associations between BMI and energy and macronutrient intakes ($p \leq 0.05$ was considered significant).

Physical activity data were analysed according to the guidelines of the IPAQ.[19] According to the IPAQ, 'vigorous physical exercise comprises participation in activities that would make the participant sweat and breathe hard for at least 20 minutes'.[19] For the purposes of the current study, participants were considered to have participated in sufficient vigorous physical activity if they reported having engaged in activities such as soccer, netball, rugby, basketball or running for at least 20 minutes on 3 or more days in the 7 days preceding the data collection. Moderate physical exercise comprises 'participation in activities that would not make the participant sweat or breathe hard for at least 30 minutes'.[19] In this study, participants were considered to have participated in sufficient moderate physical activity if they reported having engaged in activities such as walking, slow bicycling, skating, pushing a lawn mower, mopping, polishing or sweeping floors for at least 30 minutes on 5 or more days in the week preceding the data collection. Participants were considered to have been insufficiently active if they participated in some physical activity during the seven days preceding the data collection, but did not meet the above levels of activity. Participants were considered inactive if they did not report any participation in physical activity during the seven days preceding the data collection. For the purpose of this study, the frequencies were aggregated for participants who reported different combinations of both moderate and vigorous activity.

Usual daily food intakes were quantified from the record of usual daily intakes, using standard exchange lists compiled according to the recommendations of the American Dietetic Association[24] and specifically adapted for South African and Lesotho food by quantifying portion sizes from the SA Medical Research Council's (MRC) Food Composition Tables[25] and the SA MRC Food Quantity Tables.[26] Intakes were thus expressed as servings from the different food groups and evaluated according to the recommendations of the United States Agricultural Department's Food Guide Pyramid 1992 (USAD-FGP),[27] which quantifies the recommended daily number of portions to be consumed from each food group (6–11 from the starch group; 2–4 from the fruit group; 3–5 from the vegetable group; 2–3 from the milk and milk products group; and 2–3 from the meat and meat alternatives group). The exchange lists were also used to calculate the daily energy and macronutrient intakes, which were assessed compared to the estimated average requirements (EAR) for 16-year olds.[28]

The frequency with which a list of specific foods was included in the diet (recorded with the non-quantified FFQ) was expressed as the percentage of the participants that consume the individual food items on a daily, weekly, monthly or occasional basis, or never.

The answers to the questionnaire assessing knowledge, attitudes, perceptions and practices toward nutrition and obesity, were expressed as the percentage of the participants who chose the various answer options provided. The knowledge sections of the questionnaire were also scored according to the number of correct answers achieved.

Ethical considerations

The study protocol was approved by the Ethics Committee of the Faculty of Health Sciences, University of the Free State (ETOVS NR 162/09). Permission to carry out the research was obtained from the Chief Inspector in the Ministry of Education in Lesotho and from the heads of the schools involved in the study. Participation in the study involved no risk to the participants. In cases where health risks were identified in a subject during the study, participants received free dietetic advice and counseling. All information in the study was kept strictly confidential. During the reporting of the results the focus was strictly on group trends so that individual information remains confidential within the study.

TABLE 1a: Body weight status of 16-year-old students from schools in urban Maseru.

Body weight (N = 221)	Males (n = 96)				Females (n = 125)			
	Overweight		Obese		Overweight		Obese	
	n	%	n	%	n	%	n	%
WHO†	5	5.2	3	3.1	28	22.4	6	4.8
CDC†	3	3.1	3	3.1	20	16.0	6	4.8
IOTF†	9	9.4	0	0.0	25	20.0	4	3.2

Note: BMI classified according to the following growth standards for 16-year olds.
†, World Health Organization (WHO) percentile charts.
‡, US Centers for Disease Control and Prevention (CDC) 2000 percentile charts.
§, International Obesity Task Force (IOTF) age-specific cut-off points.

TABLE 1b: Physical activity levels of 16-year-old students from schools in urban Maseru.

Self-reported physical activity levels (N = 221)	n	%
Vigorously active: Participants who participated in at least 20 minutes of activity that would make them sweat and breathe harder than normal on at least 3 days during the 7 days preceding the interview.	81	36.7
Moderately active: Participants who participated in at least 30 minutes of activity that would make them sweat or breathe hard on at least 5 days the 7 days preceding the interview.	52	23.5
Insufficiently active: Participants who participated in some physical activity during the 7 days preceding the interview, but did not reach the above levels of activity	58	26.2
Inactive: Participants who did not report any participation in physical activity during the 7 days preceding the interview	30	13.6

TABLE 1c: Lifestyle habits of 16-year-old students from schools in urban Maseru.

Approximate number of self-reported hours spent watching television or using a computer outside school hours (N = 221	TV		Computer		Combined screen time	
	n	%	n	%	n	%
None (has no TV and/or computer or does not use it)	67	30.3	188	85.0	62	28.1
1 hour/day	36	16.3	12	5.4	35	15.8
2 hours/day	50	22.6	10	4.5	43	19.5
3 hours/day	34	15.4	4	1.8	29	13.1
4 hours/day	24	10.9	3	1.4	24	10.9
≥ 5 hours/day	10	4.5	4	1.9	28	12.7

TABLE 1d: Lifestyle habits related to self-reported alcohol usages of 16-year-old students from schools in urban Maseru.

Self-reported alcohol usage (N = 221)	n	%
Non-drinker: Males/females who never consume alcohol	206	93.2
Occasional drinker: Males/females who consume < 1 unit/week	1	0.5
Low drinker: Males who consume 1–10 units/week; females who consume 1–7 units/week	8	3.6
Moderate drinker: Males who consume 11–21 units/week; females who consume 8–14 units/week	3	1.4
Heavy drinker: Males who consume > 21 units/week; females who consume >14 units/week	3	1.4

TABLE 1e: Lifestyle habits related to self-reported tobacco usage of 16-year-old students from schools in urban Maseru.

Self-reported tobacco usage (N = 221)	n	%
Participants who have never smoked cigarettes, not used snuff	190	86.0
Participants who only used snuff	5	2.3
Participants who smoked cigarettes before, but not during the past month	14	6.3
Participants who smoked cigarettes on ≥ 1 days in the past month	10	4.5
Participants who smoked cigarette ≥ 20 days in the past month	2	0.9

Results

A total of 221 learners participated in the study, representing a response rate of 88.4% (7 participants did not bring consent from their parents or legal guardians; 15 were absent from school because of unpaid school fees at the time of the study; and eight withdrew from the study, citing busy schedules).

Socio-demographic status

The final sample of 221 participants consisted of slightly more girls (n = 125, 56.6%) than boys (n = 96, 43.4%). All were Basotho; and the majority attended mixed-gender schools (n = 139, 62.9% mixed-gender schools; n = 82, 37.1% single-gender schools) and lived at home (n = 198, 89.6% at home; n = 23, 10.4% in school hostels) during the school term.

Body weight status

Based on the WHO percentile charts for BMI, 8 (8.3%) of the boys and 34 (27.2%) of the girls were overweight and/or obese. More overweight and/or obese adolescents were identified by the WHO standards than with either the CDC percentile charts or the IOTF age-specific cut-off points (Table 1).

Lifestyle practices

The lifestyle practices of the participants are combined in Table 1. For the 7 days preceding the data collection, just more than a third (n = 81, 36.7%) of the participants reported sufficient vigorous activity, whilst almost a quarter (n = 52, 23.5%) reported sufficient moderate activity. More than one in 3 participants reported insufficient activity (n = 58, 26.2%) or being inactive (n = 30, 13.6%) in the week prior to the study. No significant correlations were found between BMI category and level of physical activity.

The majority (n = 188, 85%) of the participants reported that they did not play electronic games, use computers or access the internet outside school hours, with 67 (30.3%) also reporting that they did not watch television outside school hours. Almost a third (n = 62, 28.1%) reported no combined screen time (watching television, playing electronic games, using computers or accessing the internet outside school hours), whilst 23.6% (n = 52) reported 4 or more hours of combined screen time per day outside school hours.

Although 206 (93.2%) participants reported no alcohol drinking behaviour, 6.4% (n = 14) reported drinking at least one to 10 units per week (boys) or one to 7 units per week (girls). The most consumed types of alcohol were beer or cider. One in 10 (n = 26, 11.7%) reported that they had smoked tobacco (n = 12, 5.4%) on at least one day in the month prior to the interview and a minority (n = 5, 2.3%) used snuff.

Dietary intake

The mean (± SD) daily intakes for energy and macronutrient intakes, quantified from the records of usual daily food consumption, were slightly higher for boys than girls (Table 2). The mean energy intake of boys was only 53.9% of the recommended EAR, whilst that of the girls was 66.1% of the recommended EAR for this age group. The reported mean fat intake was at around 20% of total energy intake, whilst around two thirds of mean energy intake was contributed by carbohydrate.

In the whole group (N = 221), BMI had a significant and positive correlation with total daily energy intakes (R = 0.2; p = 0.01) and daily carbohydrate intakes (R = 0.3; $p < 0.01$); and showed a trend toward a positive correlation with daily protein intakes (R = 0.1; p = 0.09), but did not have a significant correlation with daily fat intakes (R = 0.1; p = 0.14).

Compared with the recommendations for healthy eating as depicted in the USDA FGP,[28] the majority of the participants (Table 3) did not meet the minimum daily requirements for vegetables (n = 202, 91.4%), fruit (n = 192, 86.7%) and milk and milk products (n = 201, 91.0%), whilst 37.6% (n = 83) did not meet the minimum daily intakes of meat and meat alternatives. Most (n = 165, 74.7%) had higher than recommended daily intakes of starchy foods which agree with the high percentage of energy derived from carbohydrates.

These trends were confirmed by the FFQ (Table 4), in which the majority of participants indicated that they consumed maize porridge (n = 124, 56.1%), bread (n = 141, 63.8%) and margarine/butter/oil (n = 182, 82.3%); and that they added sugar (n = 164, 74.2%) and salt (n = 191, 86.4%), respectively, to food and/or drinks on a daily basis. Fresh or frozen vegetables and fruits, milk, cheese and yoghurt

TABLE 2: Energy and macronutrient intakes of 16-year-old students from schools in urban Maseru.

Daily intakes (mean ± SD)	Males (n = 96)	EAR males 14-18 yrs*	Females (n = 125)	EAR females 14-18 yrs*
Energy (kJ)	7178.9 ± 2349.1	13 298	6576.5 ± 1006.5	9946
Carbohydrate (g) (Expressed as % of total energy intake)	276.8 ± 53.1 (65.3%)	130	260.6 ± 49.9 (67.3%)	130
Protein (g) (Expressed as % of total energy intake)	69.1 ± 14.9 (16.3%)	46	62.0 ± 12.3 (16.0%)	52
Fat (g) (Expressed as % of total energy intake)	36.1 ± 17.0 (19%)	-	35.0 ± 13.9 (20.3%)	-

*, EAR (Estimated average requirements) of 14–18 year old males and females.[28]

TABLE 3: Daily intakes from the basic food groups of 16-year-old students (N = 221) from schools in urban Maseru compared to the USDA Food Guide Pyramid recommendations†.

Intakes from the different food groups	Recommendations‡	n	%
Starchy foods			
Below recommendations	< 6 servings per day	2	0.9
Within recommendations	6–11 servings per day	54	24.4
High intakes	> 11 servings per day	165	74.7
Vegetables			
Below recommendations	< 3 servings per day	202	91.4
Within recommendations	3–5 servings per day	18	8.1
High intakes	> 5 servings per day	1	0.5
Fruits			
Below recommendations	< 2 servings per day	191	86.4
Within recommendations	2–4 servings per day	30	13.6
High intakes	> 4 servings per day	0	0.0
Milk and milk products			
Below recommendations	< 2 servings per day	211	95.5
Within recommendations	2–3 servings per day	10	4.5
High intakes	> 3 servings per day	0	0.0
Meat and meat alternatives			
Below recommendations	< 2 servings per day	83	37.6
Within recommendations	2–3 servings per day	45	20.4
High intakes	> 3 servings per day	93	42.1

USDA, U.S. Department of Agriculture; †, Evaluated according to the food groups and recommendations of the American Department of Agriculture's Food Guide Pyramid.[27]

TABLE 4: Frequency of food consumption of 16-year-old students from schools in urban Maseru (N = 221).

Food and food groups	Daily		Weekly		Monthly		Occasionally		Never	
	n	%	*n*	%	*n*	%	*n*	%	*n*	%
Breads, cereal, rice and pasta										
Maize meal (stiff porridge / pap)	124	56.1	93	42.1	1	0.5	1	0.5	3	1.4
Lesheleshele (soft sorghum porridge)	11	5.0	53	24.0	41	18.6	6	2.7	110	49.8
Motoho (fermented sorghum meal porridge)	3	1.4	21	9.5	73	33.0	23	10.4	101	45.7
Bread Brown/White	141	63.8	76	34.4	2	0.9	0	0.0	2	0.9
Cereal	23	10.4	45	20.4	37	16.7	1	0.5	65	29.4
Rice/mealie rice	2	0.9	177	80.1	21	9.5	0	0.0	21	9.5
Samp	2	0.9	106	48.0	66	29.9	4	1.8	43	19.5
Poone (mealies)	1	0.5	8	3.6	9	4.1	160	85.5	34	15.4
Pasta	1	0.5	84	38.0	52	23.5	2	0.9	82	37.1
Popcorn	4	1.8	80	36.2	59	26.7	1	0.5	77	34.8
Vegetables										
Fresh/frozen	66	29.9	130	58.8	9	4.1	16	7.2	0	0.0
Wild vegetables	0	0.0	15	6.8	10	4.5	29	13.1	138	62.4
Lepu (pumpkin leaves)	0	0.0	0	0.0	0	0.0	136	61.5	85	38.5
Fruit										
Fresh/frozen	56	25.3	118	53.4	35	15.8	12	5.4	0	0.0
Wild fruits	1	0.5	4	1.8	6	2.7	25	11.3	185	83.7
Fruit juice	19	8.6	104	47.1	95	43.0	3	1.4	0	0.0
Milk and milk products										
Fresh milk	35	19.0	111	50.2	42	15.8	0	0.0	33	14.9
Mafi (fermented milk)	0	0.0	75	33.9	62	28.0	4	1.8	80	36.2
Cheese	6	2.7	56	25.3	47	21.3	0	0.0	109	49.3
Yoghurt	6	2.7	69	31.2	74	33.5	2	0.9	70	31.7
Meat and meat alternatives										
Chicken	2	0.9	173	78.3	46	20.8	0	0.0	1	0.5
Red meat	2	0.9	144	65.2	60	27.1	1	0.5	14	6.3
Bacon/Polony/Vienna/Ham/Russian	38	17.1	108	48.9	32	14.5	1	0.5	14	6.3
Fish	0	0.0	95	43.0	71	32.1	1	0.5	54	24.4
Eggs	12	5.4	140	63.3	35	15.8	0	0.0	34	15.4
Peas/Beans/Lentils/Soy beans	1	0.5	139	62.9	54	24.4	0	0.0	27	12.2
Likahare (Tripe / Offal)	0	0.0	51	23.1	88	39.8	11	5.0	71	32.1
Peanuts/Nuts	6	2.7	72	32.6	67	30.3	2	0.9	74	33.5
Fats, oils and sugar										
Peanut butter	11	5.0	87	39.4	41	18.6	3	1.4	79	35.7
Salad dressing/Mayonnaise	8	3.6	126	57.0	47	21.3	2	0.9	38	17.2
Coffee creamer	18	8.1	45	20.4	24	10.9	8	3.6	126	57.0
Butter/Margarine/Oil	182	82.3	28	12.7	5	2.3	2	0.9	4	1.8
Sweets/Chocolates	57	25.8	102	46.2	23	10.4	0	0.0	39	17.6
Add sugar to food/drinks	164	74.2	40	18.1	4	1.8	5	2.3	8	3.6
Jam	8	3.6	60	27.1	44	19.9	7	3.2	102	46.2
Cordials	79	35.7	88	39.8	30	13.6	0	0.0	24	10.9
Fizzy drinks (soda)	12	5.4	93	42.1	71	32.1	79	35.7	26	11.7
Ice cream	0	0.0	36	16.3	31	14.0	82	37.1	72	35.6
Others										
Add salt to food	191	86.4	14	6.3	2	0.9	2	0.9	12	5.4
Dry packet chips (crisps)	45	20.4	134	60.6	21	9.5	1	0.5	20	9.0
Take a lunchbox to school	13	5.9	91	41.1	4	1.8	0	0.0	113	51.1
Tuck shop	41	18.6	120	54.3	22	10.0	1	0.5	37	16.7
Traditional dishes	0	0.0	9	4.1	31	14.0	14	6.3	167	75.6
Beer/Cider/Wine/Liqueur	0	0.0	18	8.1	17	7.7	15	6.8	171	77.4
Dietary supplements	9	4.1	5	2.3	2	0.9	5	2.3	200	90.5

were mostly consumed on a weekly basis, or less often. Most participants reported that they never consumed wild vegetables (n = 138, 62.4%) or wild fruits (n = 185, 83.7%). Similarly, traditional foods such as *lesheleshele* [soft porridge made from sorghum meal], *motoho* [fermented soft porridge made from sorghum meal], *lepu* [stewed pumpkin leaves] and *mafi* [fermented milk], as well as traditional dishes (*nyekoe, potele, lipolokoe, seqhaqhabola* and *tsóeu-koto*), were consumed infrequently. Whereas meat and meat alternatives such as chicken, red meat, fish, eggs and pulses were only consumed weekly or less often, most participants reported that they consume high-fat processed meats such as bacon, polony, viennas, ham and Russians daily (n = 38, 17.1%) or weekly (n = 108, 48.9%). One in 4 (n = 57, 25.8%) reported that they consume sweets/chocolates daily; one in 5 (n = 45, 20.4%) that they consume packet chips (crisps) daily; and more than a third (n = 79, 35.7%) that they drink cordials/cordials/fizzy drinks daily. More than half (n = 113, 51.1%) reported that they never take a packed lunch to school and only about 6% (n = 13) that they take lunch daily, whilst most reported that they would rather buy from the schools' tuck shops on a daily basis (n = 41, 18.6%) or weekly (n = 120, 54.3%). On the FFQ, almost a 10th (n = 18, 8.1%) of the participants reported using alcohol on a weekly basis, compared to the 6.4% (n = 14) that admitted to weekly intakes of alcohol on the lifestyle questionnaire. Most participants (n = 200, 90.5%) never used dietary supplements.

Knowledge, perceptions, attitudes and practices regarding nutrition

Although most participants had high scores on the part of the questionnaire related to nutrition knowledge (Table 5, Questions 1 to 12; mean score 75% correct answers), certain topics for nutrition education were identified. Only half (n = 122, 55.2%) knew that soya mince was a healthy alternative to meat (Table 5, Question 8); only half (n = 109; 49.3%) knew that sugar is not a source of vitamins and minerals (Table 5, Question 6); just over a third (n = 82, 37.1%) knew that high alcohol consumption can cause weight gain (Table 5, Question 10); and only 30.8% thought that one should eat a lot of sugar in order to have energy (Table 5, Question 5).

The participants mostly agreed with statements depicting positive attitudes toward good nutrition (Table 5, Questions 13 to 19). The participants' answers to questions regarding nutrition practices (Table 5, Questions 20 to 28) supported the results obtained from the records of usual daily intakes and the FFQ in portraying low intakes of vegetables and fruit (Question 20) and pulses (Question 21) and regular intakes of cold drinks/fizzy drinks (Question 23). Adding sugar and butter/margarine/oil to cooked vegetables did not seem to be a regular practice in this population.

Attitudes, perceptions and knowledge regarding obesity

The participants had mixed attitudes toward obesity, as well as toward efforts to lose weight or to be thin (Table 6, Questions 29 to 39). Almost 70% (n = 152) felt that 'fat people cannot work hard' (Table 6, Question 32) and 40% (n = 88) that 'fat people are unhappy' (Table 6, Question 34). Regarding the acceptability of obesity, only 25 (11.4%) agreed with the statements that 'fat people have more friends' (Table 6, Question 30); more than half (n = 123, 55.5%) felt that 'children do not like their mothers to be fat' (Table 6, Question 31); and about a 5th (n = 42, 18.9%) felt that 'men

TABLE 5a: Responses of 16-year-old students from schools in urban Maseru to questions related to knowledge regarding nutrition.

Knowledge of participants regarding nutrition (N = 221)	Options	n	%
1. Most nutrients are lost during the cooking.	True†	192	86.9
	False	20	9.0
	Do not know	9	4.1
2. Nutrient losses from fruits and vegetables can occur as a result of long storage.	True†	142	64.3
	False	49	22.2
	Do not know	30	13.6
3. Healthy foods help protect against illness.	True†	216	97.4
	False	5	2.3
	Do not know	0	0.0
4. Eating lots of different kinds of foods is healthier than eating a few kinds.	True†	170	76.9
	False	37	16.7
	Do not know	14	6.3
5. You should eat a lot of sugar to have energy.	True	68	30.8
	False†	137	62.0
	Do not know	16	7.2
6. Sugar contains vitamins and minerals.	True	66	29.9
	False†	109	49.3
	Do not know	39	20.8
7. Dry beans, peas, lentils are a healthy choice to eat in place of meat.	True†	180	81.4
	False	26	11.8
	Do not know	15	6.8
8. Soya mince is as healthy as meat.	True†	122	55.2
	False	57	25.8
	Do not know	42	19.0
9. It is not healthy for pregnant women to drink alcohol.	True†	204	92.3
	False	16	7.2
	Do not know	1	0.5
10. Drinking a lot of beer and wine can make you put on weight.	True†	82	37.1
	False	111	50.2
	Do not know	28	12.7
11. Eat at least three meals a day.	True†	213	96.4
	False	5	2.3
	Do not know	3	1.4
12. Eating breakfast every morning is healthy	True†	210	95.0
	False	7	3.2
	Do not know	4	1.8
Mean number (%) of correct answers for questions 1 to 12 (N = 221): 9.0/12 (75.0%)			

†, Correct answer.

TABLE 5b: Responses of 16-year-old students from schools in urban Maseru to questions related to attitudes regarding nutrition.

Attitudes of participants regarding nutrition (N = 221)	Options	n	%
13. I only buy food that is good for my body.	Agree Disagree Do not know	124 85 12	56.1 38.5 5.4
14. I eat what I like, and do not care if it is healthy or not.	Agree Disagree Do not know	95 124 2	43.0 56.1 0.9
15. I have a right to buy foods that are healthy for my body.	Agree Disagree Do not know	216 5 0	97.7 2.3 0.0
16. I believe that the food I eat now will affect my health in future	Agree Disagree Do not know	137 57 27	62.0 25.8 12.2
17. I do not need to care about eating healthy to keep my weight constant.	Agree Disagree Do not know	28 187 6	12.7 84.6 2.7
18. I just do not have the time to think about food and nutrition.	Agree Disagree Do not know	67 141 13	30.3 63.8 5.9
19. I do not have to care about food unless the doctor or nurse talks about it.	Agree Disagree Do not know	36 181 4	16.3 81.9 1.8

TABLE 5c: Responses of 16-year-old students from schools in urban Maseru to questions related to practices regarding nutrition.

Practices of participants regarding nutrition (N = 221)	Options	n	%
20. Do you eat five vegetables and fruits a day?	Regularly Occasionally Never	25 128 68	11.3 57.9 30.8
21. Do you eat dry beans, split peas, lentils, soya twice or more/ week?	Regularly Occasionally Never	72 109 40	32.6 49.3 18.1
22. Do you drink water in between meals?	Regularly Occasionally Never	156 44 21	70.6 19.9 9.5
23. Do you drink cold drinks / fizzy drinks every day?	Regularly Occasionally Never	41 130 50	18.6 58.8 22.6
24. Do you eat cake, pastries or biscuits in between meals every day?	Regularly Occasionally Never	17 101 103	7.7 45.7 46.6
25. Do you add salt to your food at table?	Regularly Occasionally Never	76 81 64	34.5 36.8 28.6
26. Do you like to add sugar to vegetables in the cooking process?	Regularly Occasionally Never	25 54 142	11.4 24.5 64.1
27. Do you like to add butter/margarine/oil to cooked vegetables?	Regularly Occasionally Never	12 43 166	5.5 19.5 75.0
28. Do you often buy take-away foods?	Regularly Occasionally Never	15 88 118	6.8 40.0 53.2

prefer fat women' (Table 6, Question 33). Regarding weight loss, just under half (n = 98, 44.5%) felt that 'it is difficult to lose weight' (Table 6, Question 38) and about a third (n = 74; 33.6%) that 'if one loses weight, one looks unattractive with loose skin' (Table 6, Question 39). Only 18.6% (n = 35) of participants felt that 'people who eat healthy foods are thin' (Table 6, Question 35). Regarding physical activity, 92.3% (n = 204) agreed that 'if one exercises daily (Table 6, Question 36), one feels healthy' and 188 (85%) agreed that they 'enjoy exercise' (Table 6, Question 37).

Asked about some of the causes of overweight/obesity (Table 6, Questions 39 to 44), about a third (n = 71, 32.3%) thought that weight gain ('getting fat') may be caused by using 'lots' of sugar in tea (Table 6, Questions 41), or eating late in the evening (Table 6, Question 39) (n = 71, 32.3%; and n = 60, 27.3%, respectively). About half (n = 107, 48.6%) thought that drinking a lot of water could help one to eat less (Table 6, Question 43). Although most (n = 174, 78.6%) thought that 'lots' of fat/oil in food could cause weight gain (Table 6, Question 42) and most (n = 130, 58.6%) thought that eating a 'lot' of fat in food does not make one feel comfortable (Table 6, Question 44), a third (n = 64; 29.1%) did not think that eating fat on meat could cause weight gain and 30 (13.6%) did not know (Table 6, Question 40).

The last part of the questionnaire tested the participants' knowledge and perceptions on the relationship between obesity and health (Questions 45 to 49). Not all participants related obesity to diabetes (n = 152, 68.6%) (Table 6, Question 45), hypertension (n = 178, 80.5%) (Table 6, Question 46) and infertility (n = 65, 29.4%) (Table 6, Question 49), whilst only half agreed that weight loss would be beneficial to people with diabetes (Table 6, Question 48). The mean knowledge score on this part of the questionnaire, calculated from the number of correct responses to questions 45 to 49, was 59.6%.

TABLE 6a: Responses of 16-year-old students from schools in urban Maseru to questions related to attitudes regarding obesity.

Attitude of participants towards obesity (N = 220*)	Options	n	%
29. Fat people have more friends.	True	25	11.4
	False	118	53.6
	Do not know	77	35.0
30. Children do not like their mothers to be fat.	True	122	55.5
	False	54	24.4
	Do not know	44	20.0
31. Fat people cannot work hard	True	152	69.1
	False	57	25.9
	Do not know	11	5.0
32. Men prefer fat women.	True	41	18.6
	False	117	53.2
	Do not know	62	28.2
33. Fat people feel unhappy.	True	88	40.0
	False	64	29.1
	Do not know	68	30.9
34. People who eat healthy food are thin.	True	41	18.6
	False	155	70.5
	Do not know	24	10.9
35. If one exercises daily, one feels healthy.	True	203	92.3
	False	9	4.1
	Do not know	9	3.6
36. I enjoy bodily exercise.	True	187	85.0
	False	29	13.2
	Do not know	4	1.8
37. It is difficult to lose weight.	True	98	44.5
	False	98	44.5
	Do not know	24	10.9
38. If one loses weight, one looks unattractive with loose skin.	True	74	33.6
	False	107	48.6
	Do not know	39	17.7

TABLE 6b: Responses of 16-year-old students from schools in urban Maseru to questions related to perceptions regarding obesity.

Perceptions of participants regarding the causes of obesity (N = 220*)	Options	n	%
39. If one eats late in the evening, one is likely to get fatter.	True	60	27.3
	False	116	52.7
	Do not know	44	20.0
40. Fat on meat does not make one fatter.	True	64	29.1
	False	126	57.3
	Do not know	30	13.6
41. Lots of sugar in tea makes one fatter.	True	71	32.3
	False	113	51.4
	Do not know	36	16.4
42. Lots of oil and fat in food make one fatter.	True	173	78.6
	False	36	16.4
	Do not know	11	5.0
43. When one drinks a lot of water, one eats less.	True	107	48.6
	False	81	36.8
	Do not know	32	14.5
44. When one eats a lot of fat in food, one feels comfortable.	True	58	26.4
	False	129	58.6
	Do not know	33	15.0

TABLE 6c: Responses of 16-year-old students from schools in urban Maseru to questions related to knowledge regarding obesity.

Knowledge of participants regarding the relationship between obesity and health (N = 220†)	Options	n	%
45. Thin people get more sugar diabetes than fat people.	True	21	9.5
	False‡	151	68.6
	Do not know	48	21.8
46. More fat people than thin people suffer from high blood pressure.	True‡	177	80.5
	False	21	9.5
	Do not know	22	10.0
47. Thin people get tired easier than fat people.	True	7	3.2
	False‡	205	93.2
	Do not know	8	3.6
48. Fat people with sugar diabetes become healthier when they lose weight.	True‡	110	50.0
	False	47	21.4
	Do not know	63	28.6
49. Thin women do not get pregnant easily.	True	16	7.3
	False‡	156	70.9
	Do not know	48	21.8
Mean number (%) of correct answers for questions 45 to 49 (N = 220): 3.6/6 (59.6%)			

†, One participant was unavailable to complete this part of the questionnaire during a structured interview.
‡, Correct answer.

Discussion

This study identifies overweight and/or obesity as an emerging health problem amongst Basotho adolescents in urban Lesotho, with 6% to 9% of 16-year-old boys and 21% to 27% of 16-year-old girls being overweight and/or obese, depending on the growth standards used. The study identified several known risk factors for adolescent overweight/obesity amongst these 16-year-old Basotho, including insufficient or no physical activity in almost 40%; more than 4 hours per day of combined screen time in almost a quarter (23.6%); regular alcohol consumption in 6.4%; and tobacco use in 14% of participants; as well as evidence of nutritional transition toward more unhealthy westernised eating habits. Some misperceptions regarding nutrition and obesity were also clear in a substantial proportion of the participants. This is significant as only a decade ago overweight/obesity was considered to be low in sub-Saharan countries compared with other developing countries.[6] This concurs with a recent report describing increasing trends of overweight/obesity amongst children < 5 years in African countries, which may eventually track into adolescence.[29] The majority of sub-Saharan countries, including Lesotho, however, have limited available representative data on overweight/obesity prevalence because public health and nutrition-related efforts have been focused mostly on undernutrition and food safety.[30]

In the current study, overweight and/or obesity was classified according to the WHO growth standards, the CDC growth standards and the IOTF age-specific cut-off points. The WHO growth standards,[21] released in 2006, were developed based on longitudinal data of children from six different cohorts representing different cultures and ethnic settings around the world. The WHO aimed to develop a single international growth standard that represents the best description of physiological growth in all children, as well as to establish the breastfed infant as the normative for growth and development.[21] The CDC cut-off points were developed based on five nationally-representative surveys of American children conducted between 1963 and 1994.[22] The IOTF cut-off points were based on children living in six countries (i.e., United States, Brazil, Great Britain, Hong Kong, Netherlands and Singapore) and were extrapolated to the widely-accepted definitions for adult overweight and obesity of BMI ≥ 25 and BMI ≥ 30, respectively.[23] Studies (none yet from Africa) comparing results using the three different standards report varying results.[31,32,33] In the current study, the WHO standards in comparison with the CDC standards identified more of the 16-year-old boys and girls as overweight, but similar numbers as obese. By contrast, the IOTF cut-off points identified fewer obese boys and girls, but more overweight boys than the other two standards (Table 1). These findings highlight the importance of considering the definitions used to classify BMI when studying and comparing prevalence data for overweight and/or obesity between studies and countries.

The prevalence of overweight and/or obesity found in the current study amongst 16-year-old Basotho in urban Maseru is slightly lower than that reported for adolescents in surrounding South Africa. Using the IOTF cut-offs, 9.4% of boys and 23.2% of girls in the current study were identified as overweight/obese (Table 1). According to the SAYRBS2008 (which compared BMI to the IOTF cut-offs), 12.1% of black males and 36.2% of black females between 13 and 19 years old were overweight and/or obese.[9] The prevalence of overweight and obesity amongst the Basotho adolescents was also lower than amongst American adolescents, particularly amongst boys. The USYRBS20114 (which compared BMI to the CDC growth standards) found that 30.5% of American black males and 38.2% of American black females in Grades 9 to 12, were overweight/obese, compared with 6.2% of the Basotho males and 20.8% of the Basotho females (when using CDC cut-offs and combining the overweight and obese categories; Table 1) in the current study. These results, therefore, point to emerging overweight/obesity amongst Basotho adolescents, represented in this study by 16-year olds in urban Maseru; a problem which to date has not been identified or targeted specifically in Lesotho.[30]

Lack of sufficient physical activity is one of the major risk factors for overweight and/or obesity in children and adolescents.[6,8,9] Apart from assisting in weight control, adequate physical activity also reduces the risk for non-communicable diseases independently of weight.[34] It has also been suggested that physically-active adolescents are more likely to adopt other healthy behaviour such as avoiding tobacco, alcohol and drug use, as well as demonstrating higher academic performance at school.[31] Surveys in the United States and South Africa[9] reported ethnic differences with regard to activity level. The current study found that combined insufficient and no physical activity (39.8%) was almost as common amongst these Basotho adolescents as amongst their South African counterparts (41.7% reported in the SAYRBS2008).[9] However, only 36.7% of the Basotho participants participated in significantly vigorous activity in the week preceding the data collection, compared with43.0% of black South African adolescents.[9] Comparison with the findings of the USYRBS2011,[4] as well as with many other studies, is difficult because different standards were used to classify physical activity levels. However, sedentary behaviour seems to affect a substantial proportion of Basotho adolescents.

Extended screen time per day is considered to be a risk for childhood and adolescent overweight and/or obesity as it constitutes a form of sedentary behaviour.[4,8,9] Compared with South African adolescents (29.3% nationally and 30% black South Africans),[9] fewer Basotho adolescents in this study (23.6%), reported spending 4 hours or more per day of combined screen time (watching television, playing electronic games, using a computer or the internet) outside school hours, whilst almost a third reported no screen time outside school hours. The Basotho adolescents watched considerably less television than American adolescents. According to the USYRBS 2011,[4] 32.4% of adolescents nationally and 54.6% of black adolescents watch more than 3 hours of television per day, compared with 15.4% of the

Basotho adolescents who reported watching 4 hours or more of television per day. Similarly in the United States, 31.1% of adolescents nationally and 38.1% of black adolescents used a computer outside school or played video games for more than 3 hours per day,[4] compared with only 3.3% of the Basotho adolescents who reported 4 or more hours of such activities outside school. A possible limitation of the current study (as well as in the USYRBS[4] and SAYRBS[8,9]) is that social interaction on cellphones was not included as a form of sedentary behaviour, since adolescents may spend hours engaged in these activities.

Evidence from cross-sectional and prospective studies indicate that 3 or more units of alcohol per day (≥ 21 units per week) may contribute to overweight and obesity.[35] Although only 1.4% of the Basotho adolescents reported drinking 14 to 21 units of alcohol per week (Table 1), excessive alcohol use independent of weight is also recognised as a major risk factor for non-communicable diseases.[34] Furthermore, studies indicate that alcohol exposure in adolescence predicts heavy alcohol use later in life.[36] Self-reported alcohol use amongst the Basotho adolescents in the current study was substantially lower than in the United States and surrounding South Africa. Of the Basotho adolescents, only 6.8% reported using any alcohol and 2.4% reported drinking more than a unit per week, compared to the United States where 38.7% of adolescents nationally (and 30.5% of black adolescents) reported consuming any alcohol in the month prior to the USYRBS2011,[4] as well as South Africa where nationally 34.9% adolescents and 31.8% of black adolescents, reported consuming any alcohol in the month prior to the SAYRBS2008.[9] However, the USYRBS[4] and SAYRBS[8,9] made use of anonymous self-reported questionnaires, whereas in the current study structured interviews were conducted with the participants, which may have resulted in under-reporting of their actual alcohol (and tobacco) use.

Tobacco use is the single largest cause of preventable death through non-communicable diseases in the world today.[34] Smokers on average weigh less than non-smokers, because nicotine increases energy expenditure and can reduce appetite (making smoking attractive to adolescent girls).[37] By contrast, however, heavy smokers tend to weigh more than light smokers or non-smokers, especially in persons of lower socio-economic status.[37] Smoking causes hormonal imbalances which contribute to insulin resistance and obesity-related non-communicable diseases; in addition, smokers also tend to be more inactive and have a poorer diet, than non-smokers, both of which are conducive to weight gain.[37] The majority of smokers start using tobacco before the age of 19 years.[9] In the current study, 11.7% of the Basotho participants reported that they had ever tried smoking cigarettes in their lifetime (5.9% on at least more than one day in the month prior to the interview) and 2.3% reported using snuff. In South Africa, the SAYRBS2008 survey[9] reported that nationally 29.5% of learners and 24.4% of black adolescents had ever smoked cigarettes in their lifetime (with 21.0% nationally and 24.5% on at least more than one day in the month prior to the interview). The USYRBS2011 survey[4] reported that 44.7% of adolescents nationally and 39.1% of black adolescents had ever tried smoking cigarettes (even a puff or two) in their lifetime (with 18.1% nationally and 10.5% on at least more than one day in the month prior to the interview). The current study may be identifying the emergence of alcohol use and cigarette smoking amongst Basotho adolescents, although the problem at this stage does not seem to be as outspoken as in surrounding South Africa or other developed countries. Under-reporting or failure to disclose drinking and smoking habits during a face-to-face interview in the current study, as opposed to anonymous questionnaires used in other surveys[4,8,9] could, however, have been a limitation.

Taken together, the lifestyle habits in the current study indicate that a transition toward a more sedentary lifestyle, as well as early onset of alcohol use and cigarette smoking, both of which are conducive to weight gain and likely to track into adulthood, may be emerging amongst Basotho adolescents, who are represented in this study by 16-year-old adolescents.

Similarly, analysis of the dietary habits shows a nutritional transition taking place amongst these adolescents. Traditional African diets described in the 1950s were associated with low risk for non-communicable diseases.[38] Amongst South Africans, the nutritional transition associated with rapid urbanisation, which has been taking place over the last few decades, is typically characterised by increased intake of total fat, animal protein, sugar and salt; and decreased intake of plant protein, dietary fiber and other complex carbohydrates.[38] The Basotho adolescents in this study reported that maize porridge and bread were still the staple foods which are consumed, almost to the exclusion of most other nutritious foods, by most adolescents on a daily basis (Tables 2, 3 and 4). Fruits and vegetable intakes were very low with only a 10th of the participants consuming at least two servings of fruit and three servings of vegetables per day (Table 2) and only a third reporting that they include vegetables and fruit in their diet on a daily basis (Table 3). Traditional wild vegetables and fruits were consumed only rarely. Vegetables and fruits are sources of vitamins, minerals, fiber and numerous phytochemicals which protect against non-communicable diseases;[39] adequate intake of fruits and vegetables has also been linked inversely to the risk of overweight and/or obesity in adults and children.[40]

Observational studies demonstrate a significant inverse association between dairy or calcium intake and body weight, body fat or BMI.[41] Mechanisms for this association may include stimulation of calcium influx into adipocytes, activation of lipogenesis and inhibition of lipolysis by increased calcium; as well as by reduction of fat absorption and increased faecal fat excretion, which are caused by calcium forming insoluble soaps with dietary fat.[42] Reaching an optimum peak bone density (at around the age of 30) is also considered the best way to counteract the early onset of osteoporosis. Consuming an adequate amount of milk or dairy products is considered the most practical, effective and relatively inexpensive and safe way (when compared with the cost of and risk reported for calcium supplement use) to acquire adequate calcium in order to optimise bone density.[42] Dairy intake was, however, very low in this population, with more than 90% of participants not consuming the required two to three servings per day. Furthermore, only one in five participants reported consuming dairy on a daily basis whilst 15% reported that they never consume dairy products. The high level of lactose intolerance amongst blacks people in sub-Saharan Africa[43] may prevent the use of fresh milk; but the intake of fermented milk, which forms part of traditional diets, was also low (Table 4).

The non-quantified FFQ (Table 3) also indicates frequent intake of fatty processed meats, sugary drinks and tuck-shop treats, with low intake of all traditional foods. These trends were not reflected clearly in the 24-hour recall data and in the relatively low total energy intakes calculated from the 24-hour recall data (Table 2). This may reflect what is referred to as the 'flat-slope syndrome' in which participants with high actual consumption often underestimate their intake of food and drink on recall.[18]

The adolescents showed good basic knowledge about nutrition (average knowledge score of 75%) and overall they portrayed a negative attitude toward overweight and/or obesity, as well as an appreciation for the important role that sound nutrition plays in a healthy lifestyle. Their knowledge regarding the role of overweight/obesity in health was, however, lower (average score of just under 60%). The most concerning finding was the substantial proportion of adolescents who have certain misperceptions regarding nutrition and obesity, as was clear from the responses (Table 5 and 6). These misperceptions highlight areas that need to be targeted through educational programmes in order to address the emerging problems of overweight/obesity amongst adolescents in Lesotho.

Implications and recommendations

The results of the current study amongst 16-year olds in urban Maseru raise awareness of the fact that Lesotho may be faced with an emerging health issue of adolescent overweight and/or obesity, a problem which is known to track into adulthood and which contributes significantly to morbidity and mortality in later life.[2,3] With public health and nutrition-related efforts in Lesotho to date having been focused largely on the prevention of undernutrition, these results highlight the need to intervene with educational programmes targeted at school children so as to increase nutritional knowledge and to prevent overweight/obesity. As the current study (for logistical reasons) only included 16-year-old adolescents attending school in Maseru, this survey needs to be repeated on a larger scale to represent all children below 18 years from all parts of Lesotho; and should be designed to compare urban and rural data regarding the prevalence of dietary and lifestyle risk factors of weight gain.

Conclusion

The current study, which is the only one as yet to perform an investigation specifically looking at overweight and/or obesity amongst adolescents in Lesotho, finds evidence of transition towards westernised dietary patterns characterised by high sugar and fast-food intakes and low fruit, vegetable and dairy consumption, as well as increased sedentary behaviour, amongst 16-year-old school goers in urban Maseru. Such a transition, if occurring amongst Basotho adolescents, puts them at risk for adult obesity and associated non-communicable diseases which will increase the healthcare burden on a low-income developing country with existing high levels of poverty. These data raise awareness of the emerging problem of overweight and/or obesity and the related risk factors amongst the youth in developing countries where emphasis is still placed only on the prevention of undernutrition.

Acknowledgements

The authors thank the head masters, teachers and learners of the various schools in urban Maseru for their cooperation and participation in this study. This study was not supported by outside funding.

Competing interests

The authors declare that they have no financial or personal relationship(s) that may have inappropriately influenced them in writing this article.

Author contributions

V.L.vd.B. (University of the Free State) was the study leader and made substantial interpretational contributions and wrote the article. L.S. (University of the Free State) planned the project and collected and interpreted the data to fulfil the requirements of the degree Magister in Nutrition at the University of the Free State. J.R. (University of the Free State) advised on the study design and sampling procedures and also performed the statistical analysis.

References

1. World Health Organization. Prioritizing areas for action in the field of population-based prevention of childhood obesity: A set of tools for Member States to determine and identify priority areas for action [document on the Internet]. c2012 [cited 2014 Oct 18]. Available from: http://www.who.int/dietphysicalactivity/childhood/tools/en/
2. Reilly JJ, Kelly J. Long-term impact of overweight and obesity in childhood and adolescence on morbidity and premature mortality in adulthood: Systematic review. Int J Obes (Lond). 2011;35(7):891–898.
3. Deckelbaum RJ, Williams CL. Childhood obesity: The health issue. Obes Res. 2001;9 Suppl 4:239S–243S.
4. Eaton JK, Kann L, Kinchen S, et al. Youth risk behavior surveillance – United States, 2011. Surveillance Summaries, 2012/61(SS04);1–162 [page on the Internet]. c2012 [cited 2013 Nov 02]. Available from: http://www.cdc.gov/mmwr/preview/mmwrhtml/ss6104a1.htm
5. European Association for the Study of Obesity. Facts &statistics [page on the Internet]. c2013 [cited 2014 Oct 18]. Available from: http://www.easo.org/task-forces/childhood-obesity-cotf/facts-statistics
6. Gupta N, Goel K, Shah P, et al. Childhood obesity in developing countries: Epidemiology, determinants, and prevention. Endocr Rev. 2012;33(1):48–70.
7. Armstrong ME, Lambert MI, Lambert EV. Secular trends in the prevalence of stunting, overweight and obesity among South African children (1994–2004). Eur J Clin Nutr. 2011;65(7):835–840.

8. Reddy SP, Panday S, Swart D, et al. Umthenthe Uhlaba Usamila: The 1st South African youth risk behaviour survey 2002 [document on the Internet]. c2003 [cited 2014 Oct 18]. Available from: http://www.mrc.ac.za/healthpromotion/YRBSpart1.pdf

9. Reddy SP, James S, Sewpaul R, et al. Umthente Uhlaba Usamila: the 2nd South African youth risk behaviour survey 2008 [document on the Internet]. c2010 [cited 2013 Nov 02]. Available from: http://www.mrc.ac.za/healthpromotion/yrbs_2008_final_report.pdf

10. Human Sciences Research Council. SANHANES-1 Media Release 6 August 2013. Media release No. 2: nutritional status of children [document on the Internet]. c2013 [cited 2013 Nov 07]. Available from: http://www.hsrc.ac.za/uploads/pageContent/3895/02%20NUTRITIONAL%20STATUS%20OF%20CHILDREN.pdf

11. Qi L, Cho YA. Gene-environment interaction and obesity. Nutr Rev. 2008;66(12):684–694.

12. Delisle H, Ntandou-Bouzitou G, Agueh V, et al. Urbanisation, nutrition transition and cardiometabolic risk: The Benin study. Br J Nutr. 2012;107(10):1534–1544.

13. Rolland-Cachera MF, Deheeger M, Maillot M, et al. Early adiposity rebound: Causes and consequences for obesity in children and adults. Int J Obes (Lond). 2006;30 Suppl 4:S11–S17.

14. Department of Health, Republic of South Africa. South African Demographic and Health Survey 2003. Full report [document on the Internet]. c2003 [cited 2013 Nov 06]. Available from: http://measuredhs.com/pubs/pdf/FR206/FR206.pdf

15. Steyn K, Fourie J, Temple N. Chronic diseases of lifestyle in South Africa: 1995–2005. Technical Report [document on the Internet]. c2006 [cited 2013 Nov 06]. Available from: www.mrc.ac.za/chronic/cdl1995-2005.pdf

16. About.com. Education: Geography: Lesotho [page on the Internet]. c2005 [cited 2014 Oct 22]. Available from: geography.about.com/library/cia/blclesotho.htm

17. Central Intelligence Agency. CIA World Factbook, Lesotho: people and society [page on the Internet]. n.d. [cited 2013 Nov 06]. Available from: https://www.cia.gov/library/publications/the-world-factbook/geos/lt.html

18. Lee RD, Nieman DC. Nutritional assessment. 4th ed. Boston: McGraw Hill; 2007.

19. Craig CL, Marshall AL, Sjöström M, et al. International physical activity questionnaire: 12-country reliability and validity. Med Sci Sports Exerc. 2003;35(8):1381–1395.

20. Labadarios D, Swart R, Maunder EMW, et al. Executive summary of the National Food Consumption Survey-Fortification Baseline (NFCS-FB-I): South Africa, 2005. S Afr J Clin Nutr. 2008;21(3)(Suppl 2):245–300.

21. World Health Organization Multicentre Growth Reference Study Group. WHO child growth standards: length/height-for-age, weight-for-age, weight-for-length, weight-for-height and body mass index-for-age: methods and development [document on the Internet]. c2006 [cited 2013 Nov 06]. Available from: http://www.who.int/childgrowth/standards/Technical_report.pdf

22. Kuczmarski RJ, Ogden CL, Guo SS, et al. 2000 CDC growth charts for the United States: methods and development [document on the Internet]. c2000 [cited 2013 Nov 06]. Available from: http://www.cdc.gov/growthcharts/2000growthchart-us.pdf

23. Cole TJ, Bellizi MC, Flegal KM, et al. Establishing a standard definition for child overweight and obesity worldwide: International survey. BMJ. 2000;320(7244):1240–1243.

24. Wheeler ML, Franz M, Barrier P, et al. Macronutrient and energy database for the 1995 Exchange Lists for Meal Planning: A rationale for clinical practice decisions. J Am Diet Assoc. 1996;96(11):1167–1171.

25. Wolmarans P, Danster N, Dalton A, et al. Condensed food composition tables for South Africa. Cape Town: Medical Research Council; 2010.

26. Langenhoven ML, Conradie PJ, Wolmarans P, et al. MRC food quantities manual. 2nd ed. Cape Town: Medical Research Council; 1991.

27. Shaw A, Fulton L, Davis C, et al. Using the food guide pyramid: A resource for nutrition educators [document on the Internet]. n.d. [cited 2014 Oct 18]. Available from: http://milk.procon.org/sourcefiles/usingthefoodguidepyramid.pdf

28. Institute of Medicine of the National Academies Food and Nutrition Board. Dietary reference intakes for energy, carbohydrates, fiber, fat, fatty acids, cholesterol, protein, and amino acids [document on the Internet]. c2005 [cited 2013 Nov 06]. Available from: http://www.nal.usda.gov/fnic/DRI/DRI_Energy/energy_full_report.pdf

29. De Onis M, Blössner M, Borghi E. Global prevalence and trends of overweight and obesity among preschool children. Am J Clin Nutr. 2010;92(5):1257–1264.

30. Lobstein T, Baur L, Uauy R. Obesity in children and young people: A crisis in public health. Obes Rev. 2004,5(Suppl 1):4–104.

31. Shields M, Tremblay MS. Canadian childhood obesity estimates based on WHO, IOTF and CDC cut-points. Int J Pediatr Obes. 2010;5(3):265–273.

32. Twells LK, Newhook LA. Obesity prevalence estimates in a Canadian regional population of preschool children using variant growth references. BMC Pediatr. 2011;11:21.

33. De Sousa Lopes HM. Diagnostic accuracy of CDC, IOTF and WHO criteria for obesity classification, in a Portuguese school-aged children population [document on the Internet]. c2012 [cited 2014 Oct 18]. Available from: http://repositorio-aberto.up.pt/bitstream/10216/62314/3/Hugo%20de%20Sousa%20LopesTeseDiagnostic%20accuracy%20of%20CDC%20IOTF%20and%20WHO%20criteria%20for%20obesity%20classification%20in%20a%20Portugues-e%20schoolaged%20children%20population%20Mestrado%20em%20Sade%20Pblica.pdf

34. World Health Organization. Global strategy on diet, physical activity and health: physical activity and young people [page on the Internet]. c2013 [cited 2013 Nov 07]. Available from: http://www.who.int/dietphysicalactivity/factsheet_young_people/en/index.html

35. Wannamethee SG. Alcohol, overweight and obesity. In: RR Watson, VR Preedy, S Zibadi, eds. Alcohol, Nutrition, and Health Consequences. New York: Humana Press, 2013; pp. 371–381.

36. Merline A, Jager J, Schulenberg JE. Adolescent risk factors for adult alcohol use and abuse: Stability and change of predictive value across early and middle adulthood. Addiction. 2008;103(Suppl 1):84–99.

37. Chiolero A, Faeh D, Paccaud F, et al. Consequences of smoking for body weight, body fat distribution, and insulin resistance. Am J Clin Nutr. 2008;87(4):801–809.

38. MacIntyre UE, Kruger HS, Venter CS, et al. Dietary intakes of an African population in different stages of transition in the North-West Province, South Africa: The THUSA study. Nutr Res. 2002;22(3):239–256.

39. Van Dokkum W, Frølich W, Saltmarsh M, et al. The health effects of bioactive plant components in food: Results and opinions of the EU COST 926 action. Nutr Bull. 2008;33(2):133–139.

40. Ledoux TA, Hingle MD, Baranowski T. Relationship of fruit and vegetable intake with adiposity: A systematic review. Obes Rev. 2011;12(5):e143-150.

41. Van Loan M. The role of dairy foods and dietary calcium in weight management. J Am Coll Nutr. 2009;28(Suppl 1):120S–129S.

42. Anderson JJB. Bone health. In: KL Mahan, SL Escott-Stump, eds. Krause's Food, Nutrition and Diet Therapy. 12th ed. Philadelphia: Elsevier, 2008; pp. 532–562.

43. Segal I, Gagjee PP, Essop AR, et al. Lactase deficiency in the South African black population. Am J Clin Nutr. 1983;38(6):901–905.

13

An examination of the factors fueling migration amongst Community Service practitioners

Authors:
Candice Reardon[1]
Gavin George[1]

Affiliations:
[1]Health Economics and HIV and AIDS Research Division (HEARD), University of KwaZulu-Natal, South Africa

Correspondence to:
Gavin George

Email:
georgeg@ukzn.ac.za

Postal address:
Health Economics and HIV and AIDS Research Division (HEARD), University of KwaZulu-Natal, 4th Floor J Block, Durban 4041, South Africa

Background: Research is needed in order to understand the potential influence of the Bilateral Agreement between South Africa and the United Kingdom (UK), as well as other more recent international and local policies restricting movement of South African health workers abroad; and to determine what effect they have on the migration intentions and plans of health professionals in South Africa.

Aim: The aims were to (1) explore the migration intentions and the factors that influence these intentions amongst Community Service (CS) nurses and doctors; (2) explore their views and opinions about the Bilateral Agreement between the UK and South Africa (SA) and other UK policies around the recruitment and employment of foreign health professionals; and (3) understand the impact of these policies on the migration plans of these CS doctors and nurses.

Method: Qualitative focus groups and interviews were conducted with 23 CS doctors and nurses. To supplement this, 6 interviews were conducted with nurses and a doctor who had worked in the UK.

Results: A higher disposition toward moving abroad was apparent amongst those who had experienced a challenging and frustrating CS year. Poor working conditions, including long work hours, high patient loads and inadequate resources and equipment, as well as low salaries and the perceived ambivalence of the government to the complaints of health practitioners, were influencing decisions to migrate abroad.

Conclusion: The findings suggest that government efforts to better manage, recognise and respect the work and contribution of health professionals to the country would go a long way toward retaining health professionals.

Un examen des facteurs d'incitation à la migration des professionnels de la santé et de leurs opinions sur la politique restreignant leurs déplacements.

Contexte: Un accord bilatéral et d'autres politiques existent aujourd'hui entre le Royaume-Uni et l'Afrique du Sud, visant à endiguer la migration des professionnels de la santé en Afrique du Sud vers le Royaume-Uni. Des recherches sont nécessaires pour comprendre l'influence potentielle de cet accord bilatéral, et d'autres politiques interdisant la circulation des travailleurs de la santé sud-africains à l'étranger, et l'effet qu'ils ont sur les intentions d'émigration et les plans des professionnels de la santé en Afrique du Sud.

Objectifs: Les objectifs étaient spécifiquement (1) d'explorer les intentions d'émigration des infirmières et des médecins des services communautaires, ainsi que les facteurs qui influent sur ces intentions, (2) d'explorer leurs points de vue et opinions à propos de l'accord bilatéral entre le Royaume-Uni et SA et à propos des autres politiques du Royaume-Uni sur le recrutement et l'emploi des professionnels de santé étrangers, et (3) de comprendre l'impact de ces politiques sur les plans d'émigration des médecins et des infirmières de services communautaires.

Méthodes: Des groupes de discussion et des entrevues qualitatives ont été organisés avec 23 médecins et infirmières de services communautaires. Nous avons eu six entretiens avec des infirmières et un médecin qui avaient travaillé au Royaume-Uni.

Résultats: Une plus grande disposition à se déplacer à l'étranger était évidente parmi ceux qui avaient connu une année de service communautaire difficile et frustrante. Les mauvaises conditions de travail, y compris de longues heures de travail, les charges élevées de patients et l'insuffisance des ressources et de l'équipement ainsi que les bas salaires et l'ambivalence apparente du gouvernement aux plaintes des praticiens de la santé ont influencé ces médecins à émigrer à l'étranger.

Conclusions: Les résultats suggèrent que les efforts du gouvernement pour améliorer la gestion, reconnaître et respecter le travail et la contribution des professionnels de la santé dans le pays contribuerait grandement à retenir les professionnels de la santé.

Introduction

The health workforce constitutes one of the 6 key building blocks for a well-functioning health system.[1] In 2006, the World Health Organization (WHO) estimated that 37% of trained doctors and 7% of trained nurses had migrated from South Africa (SA) to work abroad.[2] The emigration rate of nurses is calculated to be between 1% and 2% per year, which means that by 2008, between 2128 and 4256 nurses would have left the country.[3] By 2015, it has been estimated that SA will experience a critical 'gap' of 15 380 staff nurses, 22 121 professional nurses, 3930 doctors and 5677 medical specialists.[4]

Evidence suggests that health professionals are considering emigration as a result of the prospects of a better life in their destination country.[5] Crush, Pendleton and Tevera,[5] in their 2005 study, found that a substantial proportion of South African health professionals had already taken active steps to emigrate. Similarly, in 2007, Pendleton, Crush and Lefko-Everett[6] found that 13.9% of the registered South African health professionals in their study had applied for work permits, 5.5% were in the process of applying, 6.2% had applied for or were applying for a permanent residence permit in their destination country and roughly 30.2% had already applied for professional registration in their country of interest. South African health professionals showed a preference for destination countries such as Australia and New Zealand, the United Kingdom (UK), Europe, North America and Canada.[6]

Other studies amongst South African heath workers revealed that financial factors, better job opportunities for themselves and schooling opportunities for children abroad as well as the high crime rate in SA were significant factors encouraging these health workers to emigrate.[7] Another important pull factor attracting health professionals to countries overseas is the opportunity to gain international experience.[8] According to Oberoi and Lin,[9] however, push factors motivating health professionals to leave SA can exert a more powerful influence on their emigration decisions than the factors attracting them to their destination country. The major push factors that emerged most frequently in their interviews were poor remuneration, lack of job satisfaction, lack of future prospects for further education and career development, poor working conditions, HIV and poor quality of life.[9] In a South African study, medical and nursing students cited poor working conditions within the public health sector, including long work hours, high patient loads, inadequate resources and occupational hazards as being the primary push factors encouraging them to consider leaving the country.[10]

In SA, there have been various initiatives by the government specifically aimed at strengthening the rural healthcare system that has been weakened by internal migration to the private health sector and the migration of health workers to other countries. The development and implementation of the Occupation Specific Dispensation (OSD) was based on the recognition that improvement in the conditions of service and remuneration for health professionals constituted the most urgent priority. Dispensations for specific occupational categories include unique salary structures for each identified occupation in the public service, centrally-determined grades and job profiles, career-progression opportunities and other employment practices.[11]

The introduction of Community Service (CS) for all categories of health professionals was aimed at further alleviating staff shortages in rural and under-served areas. It has been argued that the introduction of CS has not stopped doctors from leaving to spend time overseas after their CS year. Reid[12] found that an increasing proportion of CS doctors between 1999 (34%) and 2001 (43%) intended to work overseas after their CS year. Of Reid's sample, 20% said they would consider working in rural or under-served areas in the future, which he argues is adequate reason for the government to implement an appropriate and systemic set of incentives that could encourage these health professionals to practise in rural areas, circumventing the requirement for young health professionals to endure their year of obligatory service.[12] Based on these findings it has been argued that CS defeats its own end because health professionals may assume they have fulfilled their duty and compensated society for the costs of their study.[12,13] Other opponents have thrown harsher criticism at the current policy around medical internships and CS, referring to it as 'cruel and degrading' with 'no other professional group in the country subjected to such levels of exploitation and discrimination by the state'.[13] A lack of supervision, compounded by extraordinary high levels of overtime, have been identified as two key problems of CS requiring urgent attention.[14,]

SA has entered into a number of bilateral agreements with foreign governments aimed at moderating the outflow of South African health professionals and alleviating health worker shortages in the country. In the 1990s, the South African government began placing pressure on the UK to refrain from recruiting South African doctors. In 1999, the former President of SA, Nelson Mandela, publicly accused the UK of poaching South Africa's health professionals.[15] This culminated in the endorsement of a Memorandum of Understanding (MOU)[16] between the UK and SA in 2002 as a response to the recruitment of health workers from developing countries. The MOU, although no longer in force today, took a dynamic flexible approach to encouraging ongoing dialogue between the UK and SA around human resources for health, healthcare capacity and development with regular assessment and adjustment by both countries.[17] The Bilateral Agreement covered a wide range of areas with a view to sharing and disseminating best practice between the two countries. It also offered the opportunity for nationals from both the UK and SA to benefit from time-limited placements in either country, thereby creating transcultural opportunities for both clinical personnel and healthcare managers.[8,15]

Around the same time as the Bilateral Agreement between SA and the UK was in existence, the UK *Code of Practice for the International Recruitment of Healthcare Professionals*,[18] developed in 2001, prohibited National Health Service organisations from recruiting health workers from certain countries, including SA, unless a government-to-government agreement existed with that country. Although this was respected widely by the public sector, private-sector organisations sustained their recruitment efforts, resulting in a net rise in foreign health workers in the UK in 2002.[19] Consequently, the UK Code of Practice was revised in 2004 to ensure that all healthcare organisations, including the private sector, adhered to its recruitment guidelines as well as to cover the recruitment of both temporary and permanent staff.[18]

Objective of the study

There is a paucity of empirical research studies that have examined the views and opinions of CS practitioners toward the Bilateral Agreement between the UK and SA[16] and other policies such as the UK Code of Practice,[18] which sought to curb the large outflow of South African health workers to the UK. One of the research objectives of this study was to understand how the increased difficulty faced by South African health professionals in gaining employment in the UK and other countries, may influence their future emigration plans and intentions. Moreover, this study sought to gain an understanding of the emigration considerations and intentions of CS doctors and nurses, including both the push and pull factors that influence their decisions to remain in or leave SA.

To provide a point of comparison with the data from the CS practitioners, interviews were conducted with South African nurses and doctors that had worked in the UK in order to establish the factors that fuelled their migration abroad. The attitudes and opinions of the returned health professionals toward the Bilateral Agreement and stricter UK policies were also sought in order to provide an important point of comparison between older health professionals who have worked abroad and younger nurses and doctors who have not.

Contribution to the field

Nurses and doctors coming to the end of their obligatory CS are at a critical stage in their careers. There is research to suggest that fewer CS practitioners are wanting to remain in the public service after their year of CS[12] and that the proportion wanting to go overseas after their year of obligatory service has increased.[20] In view of this, this research sought to explore the work experiences of health professionals during their CS year and any influence this may have on their intentions and plans to leave SA. Moreover, this study showcases the main factors fuelling their migration desires and intentions, as well as how these may influence their migration plans in view of stricter policies around immigration and employment in the UK.

Research method and design

Design

A qualitative approach was used for this study in order to provide rich and in-depth explorations and verbal descriptions which resulted in sufficient detail to describe the views and opinions of CS practitioners toward migration and foreign employment policies.

Sampling strategy

The researchers were granted access to 2 public hospitals in KwaZulu-Natal. In total, 29 participants took part in this study. This figure comprised 23 CS nurses and doctors (15 CS doctors and 8 CS nurses) and 6 health professionals (5 nurses and 1 doctor) who had worked in the UK. Twenty-one participants were women and 8 were men. Twenty participants were black South Africans, 7 were Indian and 2 were white South Africans. The focus groups and interviews were all conducted in early 2011.

In order to access CS nurses and doctors, two hospitals were approached for the study. Approval was sought from the medical managers at both hospitals to interview their CS nurses and doctors. The researcher was unable to contact the nursing manager in order to set up focus groups with the CS nurses at the Durban hospital. Altogether, two focus groups with CS nurses and two with CS doctors were conducted at a district hospital located in the Pietermaritzburg area and four focus groups with CS doctors were carried out at a regional-level hospital located in the greater Durban area. All CS doctors and nurses in the two hospitals were notified in writing about the study by their CS representative or their medical or nursing manager and a proposed schedule of focus group dates and times circulated to them. The researchers had originally intended to conduct eight focus groups because of the study's time constraints, thus only eight focus group sessions were planned for. The CS practitioners were under no obligation to attend the focus group sessions; those interested self-selected into the study.

To supplement this data, six interviews were conducted with nurses and doctors who had worked abroad in the UK. These individuals were sourced from the database of Africa Health Placements (AHP), a social profit organisation who had helped find them employment on their return from the UK. Two interviews with a doctor and nurse who had worked in the UK were conducted over the phone. The other four interviews were conducted in person with the nurses at their hospitals.

Materials

The focus group discussion questions were developed in alignment with the research objectives. The overarching categories of questions included: (1) their emigration considerations and reasons for emigrating or wanting to emigrate; (2) personal views and opinions about the Bilateral Agreement and other UK policies; and (3) the potential impact of these policies on their emigration plans and intentions. The interview schedule used with the nurses and doctor who had worked in the UK sought to solicit their views and opinions about the Bilateral Agreement between SA and the UK as well as other UK immigration and employment policies, their reasons for wanting to work abroad and their comparative experiences of working in the UK and SA.

Procedure

The focus groups and interviews were conducted at a time that was convenient for the nurses and doctors at their place of employment and lasted between 40 and 50 minutes. Two interviews with a doctor and nurse who had worked in the UK were conducted over the phone. The other four interviews were conducted in person with the nurses at their hospitals. The fieldwork was conducted by a female, junior researcher with no medical training. The focus groups and interviews were recorded and transcribed verbatim.

Analysis

As recommended by Bogdan and Biklen,[21] the transcripts were read twice by the researcher in order to familiarise herself with the data before coding began. The coding was data driven as themes were allowed to emerge from the text. Opler's terminology of 'expressions' and 'themes' was used in coding the data.[22] 'Expressions' denote the basic units of data or incidents in the text that develop into themes and subthemes through a process of synthesising and comparison across cases.

Descriptive codes were used to identify basic expressions that were found in individual transcripts. These were compared with expressions emerging from other interviews and, after being categorised into subthemes, were given more analytical coding labels. Ryan and Bernard's[22] techniques for identifying themes from basic expressions in the text were used. The process of analysing the data moved from descriptive to analytical coding as recommended by Gibbs.[23]

Ethical considerations

Ethical approval was gained from the University of KwaZulu-Natal (UKZN) Biomedical Research Ethics Committee (Ref: BE191/010) as well as from the KwaZulu-Natal Provincial Department of Health (Ref: HRKM146/10). All participants involved in the study were informed about the nature of the study and what their participation would entail. Ethical issues such as the voluntary and informed nature of participation, anonymity and confidentiality were addressed within the informed consent forms that were handed to the respondents. The focus groups and interviews were conducted in private rooms at the hospitals, at a time that was convenient for the participants. The interviews and focus groups were recorded with the respondents' permission. All identifying information has been taken off the transcripts so as to ensure confidentiality of the respondents' accounts. Every participant was provided with a copy of the final report after completion of the study, as prescribed by good ethical practice.[23] In the presentation of the findings, no identifying information of the participants or the hospitals is provided in order to ensure confidentiality of their accounts.

Results

Migration considerations

All but four doctors were considering the possibility of emigrating at some stage in their careers. The desire to work abroad for a temporary period of time before they decide on permanent settlement abroad was reported often. The doctors who were less inclined to want to leave the country were located in one hospital in the Pietermaritzburg area and reported having a positive CS year. In comparison, the group of doctors who voiced the strongest desire to leave the country were from the hospital situated in the greater Durban area; these doctors expressed many frustrations and complaints about their CS experience.

Most of the doctors considering emigration shared the same plans; they would specialise in SA and after that reassess the situation in the country and their job prospects, only emigrating if they thought it necessary.

In contrast, the majority of the nurses had not given much thought to leaving SA and did not have much knowledge or information about working and living abroad. Some nurses ($n = 4$) expressed an openness to the possibility of emigrating, although this was not articulated with any definite plans to do so. A number of significant deterrents to migrating abroad emerged from the nurses' group discussions that appeared to root them in the country for at least the near future. These included the contractual obligation they had with the provincial Department of Health, caring for their children and the lower-job grade that they would probably work at overseas. In particular, the nurses expressed dislike for the work that some expatriate nurses abroad had to endure in nursing homes, which included caring for the elderly and looking after their less 'medical' needs. The following quote from a community service nurse indicates that she regards the nature of the work done in care homes as degrading and undignified for themselves as professional nurses, which might dissuade her from working abroad:

> 'She was a sister when she was in here in SA and then when she went there she was making tea for the *gogos* there [*Gogos is a Zulu word commonly used in SA to refer to elderly women or grandmothers*]. Why you making tea for those? So there it's just bringing your dignity down.' (Community service nurse, Regional public hospital in Pietermaritzburg area)

Push and pull factors for working abroad

Push factors

It was agreed unanimously that push factors were stronger motivations weighing in on participants' emigration considerations than pull factors. The influence that push factors play in the nurses and doctors' desire to migrate abroad is reflected in the following quote by a doctor:

> 'There's no reason why we should want to leave ... Like I said, I love South Africa and I will always regard this as home ... However there are factors here that make me think twice about remaining. And it's definitely the push factors because even money-wise you can make a living in South Africa ... it's just there's too many push factors that force you out of here.' (CS doctor, Regional public hospital in greater Durban area)

These push factors included poor salaries, poor and frustrating working conditions, job uncertainty after CS, crime and the poor state of the healthcare system in SA. One doctor shared frustrations about not being able to afford his basic material needs even after qualifying as a doctor:

> 'I've been driving [*a*] Jetta 2 1990 model, after Medical School, after graduating … So frustrating … Go overseas, make quick bucks and come back, get the car and all those things. So we can't even buy – I'm talking about a car here … we can't even afford to buy a house, after years and years of graduating from Medical School. Those things are so frustrating and pushing you to go.' (CS doctor, Regional public hospital in greater Durban area)

The increase in salaries brought about by the OSD was viewed positively by some respondents from both hospitals, whilst others felt it would not have the desired effect of attracting and retaining health workers in the public healthcare system. One doctor from the Pietermaritzburg hospital believed that the OSD would obviate the problem of medical doctors having to work abroad after qualifying to pay off study loans. Another CS doctor, who had worked previously in the UK, recognised the salary benefit from the OSD and believed it was far more lucrative to work in the public rather than the private health sector. However, two doctors in the same focus group disagreed with this doctor's sentiments about the OSD. They believed that the salary increases from the OSD were not strong enough incentives to deter them and other doctors from going overseas. Their beliefs about the inadequacy of the OSD are reflected in the following quote:

> 'I mean it's quite dependent on your overtime … you should be able to get a salary, a decent salary where you were able to pay for your house and your car and educate your children and all of that, without having to do overtime. But if you look at it, we're not getting paid enough. I mean if you don't do overtime then it's quite a big chunk of your salary … It's not a good enough incentive, I think, to stay.' (CS doctor, Regional public hospital in greater Durban area)

Secondly, several doctors complained about experiencing very poor working conditions that were making them debate whether to remain in the country. Their primary complaints centred on a lack of proper medical equipment and a high burden of disease and patient mortality. Several doctors expressed sadness and frustration about not being able to do more for their patients because of the lack of resources and heavy patient loads, which they felt limited their ability to deliver good patient care.

Other factors related to the healthcare system, such as a lack of money being invested for improvements, the poor treatment of doctors and the severe health worker shortages, were also identified as being significant push factors. Severe staff shortages could leave doctors feeling as though they were constantly being forced to 'fill the gap'. Another doctor reported that the shortages in her hospital had made her stagnate in her medical training because of the lack of senior staff available for supervision and mentoring. She believed that the UK would offer her a better-resourced setting with better learning opportunities.

Finally, several doctors shared their anxieties and concerns about their job opportunities following their CS year. One doctor lamented that he was 'currently facing unemployment' as a result of the freezing of posts which he blamed on the government's frugal investment of money into the healthcare system. Although two doctors, both based in the Pietermaritzburg hospital, were against their fellow doctors leaving SA, they expressed understanding and sympathy for their fellow white South African doctors who, they believed, were inclined to pursue work opportunities abroad because of the lack of specialist training posts available to them. The issue of particular race groups being at a disadvantage in the selection for specialist posts was also articulated by three doctors in the Durban hospital who believed that they would receive fairer opportunities for enrolment in specialist training programmes in the UK or Canada. In the following quote, one doctor describes her experience of being turned down for a position in a specialist training programme in the province:

> 'I've applied for a registrar post and I got a very nice reply from the head of the department stating that the fact that 67% of the province of KZN is made up of black South Africans, therefore they have to give 67% of their posts to black South Africans; so therefore you have a better chance of applying to one of the other Med Schools in the country. So I feel lately I would stand a better chance there [*in the UK*], not being discriminated by the colour of your skin because I think I'm a good doctor and you should be given a fair opportunity.' (CS doctor, Hospital in greater Durban area)

Pull factors

The most common pull factors reported included the higher salaries and earning potential in foreign countries, better training and job opportunities, opportunities to travel and practise first-world medicine, as well as having a better quality of life. Several nurses, including those having worked in the UK, reported that higher salaries abroad, which would enable them to fulfill their children's educational and material needs, were a key motivator to migrate. In the following quote, a nurse articulates how the higher salary she received in the UK helped their family's financial situation:

> 'The only thing that pushed me out of the country was that my girls were all going to the University. Three of them, one after the other, so I couldn't finance them to that extent, so I had to leave the country just to try and make some money to pay for them.' (Nurse, District public hospital, Rural northern KZN)

Conversely, family relationships and commitments played an important role insofar as encouraging three doctors, all from the Pietermaritzburg hospital, to remain in the country to work. However, these doctors were referring to the importance of sustaining the relationships with their siblings and parents and did not have children to consider.

The improved quality of life abroad included perceptions of a safer environment for themselves and their family, reasonable working hours and patient loads as well as a higher standard of living. For one doctor, central to the better working environment overseas was the lower levels of stress he would endure and the increased resources that would reduce his 'suffering' at work:

> 'The two main benefits – basically financially [sic] and working in a stress free environment. You know, not suffering, calling the nurse for this and that and trying to find this, trying to find needles and you can't find them, you prescribe a drug for a patient and it's not there or unaffordable … and the workload … I mean people that have worked there say that it's just a stress-free environment.' (CS doctor, Regional public hospital in greater Durban area)

The ability to travel more easily if one were to be based in the UK or Canada was also appealing to many of the doctors. Several doctors also mentioned wanting to experience practising medicine in a first-world context, where there were fewer resource shortages and more manageable patient loads. It was also believed that working abroad would provide better opportunities to really help the patients they treated as well as to develop as a doctor.

Three of the nurses who had worked in the UK alluded to a curiosity that attracted them to working abroad. Coupled with their curiosity about working in a foreign country was their desire to gain experience working as a nurse or doctor in a foreign healthcare system that would provide them with valuable experience that they could re-invest into SA's healthcare system on their return. Fewer contractual constraints and the flexibility to work where you want and when you want, as opposed to the restrictions against moonlighting for health professionals in SA, were attractive features of work life abroad for a few of the CS nurses interviewed.

Views about stricter UK immigration and employment policies

The doctors who were reluctant to leave SA were more supportive of the Bilateral Agreement and the stricter policy changes in the UK. Three doctors believed that the impact of the stricter policies and the ban on active recruitment from developing nations such as SA would curb the huge outflow of South African doctors and improve the healthcare system. In the following quote, one doctor emphasises the overall benefit to the South African health system and the country as a whole that stricter migration policies can produce:

> 'I think it's maybe a good thing because it obviously keeps more doctors in the country; the hospitals become better staffed so the patient care gets better. So I think for the country it's actually a better thing. Probably for the doctors themselves it's not very helpful, but for the country, I think it's actually better.' (CS doctor, District public hospital in Pietermaritzburg area)

The stricter policies around the employment and emigration of South African doctors to the UK, as well as the difficulty this created for doctors wanting to leave, also garnered support from three doctors on the grounds that it would ensure that the doctors who are leaving are serious about going to work abroad. It was felt that the ban on active recruitment was a good thing because the ease of gaining access to the UK through an agency would encourage more doctors to go abroad, including those who were less committed and resolved in their motivation to work there. One doctor also felt that the introduction of the Professional and Linguistic Assessments Board (PLAB) exams for doctors wanting to work in the UK was a good policy change; firstly, because it would ensure that only high quality doctors from South Africa were entering the UK workforce and secondly, because the exams will help prepare South African doctors for the working environment in the UK. The PLAB exam is the main route by which International Medical Graduates demonstrate that they have the necessary skills and knowledge to practise medicine in the UK.

The majority of nurses seemed either indifferent to the policies or thought they were 'fair'. It is reasoned that the indifference expressed by some of the nurses occurred because many of them were not entertaining definite plans to go abroad and, thus, these policies were irrelevant for them in their prospective career path at the time of the study.

The majority of the doctors, however, shared negative views and frustrations relating to the stricter policies on immigration, employment and recruitment of South African doctors in the UK. In most instances, the South African government was the target of their frustration and complaints, rather than the UK government who had implemented the UK Code of Practice.[18] The negative views expressed by the doctors related to three subthemes: (1) the restriction to their freedom to emigrate; (2) being discriminated against because of their occupation; and (3) the South African government's unfair treatment of them.

Several doctors and two nurses argued that the stricter policies and the prohibition against recruiting South African doctors to the UK constituted a restriction to their freedom to migrate. There was a shared belief that health professionals should be free to decide which country they want to work in and for how long. Owing to the greater difficulty for doctors to enter the UK, five doctors described feeling 'forced' to remain in country, yet in earlier discussions many of these same doctors reported feeling 'pushed out' or 'forced to leave' the country because of their negative working conditions. This predicament – being pushed to go even though they did not want to, but forced to stay – is expressed by a doctor in the following statement:

> 'They've taken the short cut blocking the border saying "you can't get out". You have to stay whether you like it or not and the conditions are not going to improve, in fact they are going to get worse. After this they increase the internship from one year to two years and the CS … they know they've blocked the borders, we can't do anything. You have to stay you have to do all those things.' (CS doctor, Regional public hospital in greater Durban area)

Many doctors complained that the policies were unfair because they discriminated against them as health professionals. Furthermore, it was agreed widely that the South African government was unfair in its attempt to prohibit the active recruitment of South African health professionals by foreign governments. The perceived unfairness also related to their failure to address the poor working conditions causing the doctors to want to migrate and not treating them as well as health professionals are treated by foreign governments. The South African government was seen to be taking 'short cuts' and acting 'selfishly' and 'in their own interests'. Rather than working toward prohibiting active recruitment of health professionals, the doctors reported that the South African government should take action to encourage health professionals to remain in the country:

> 'You see, the government and the UK has [*sic*] a bilateral agreement – doctors are not involved. You see our department, they just make these laws and say "this is what you have to do", without coming to us and finding out the reasons why people are moving. Instead of looking at those reasons and trying to address them, they take short cuts in trying to prevent doctors going … that's why we say if we get the opportunity we're heading out.' (CS doctor, Regional public hospital in greater Durban area)

The relative ease with which UK doctors could come to SA without having to write the PLAB exam was a source of frustration and fuelled perception about unfair treatment by both governments. Two doctors, who intended to remain in SA, also felt that the UK doctors coming to SA should write a similar entrance exam to the PLAB exams in the UK to ensure that no preference was seen to be given to foreign doctors from developed nations.

Potential impact of the Bilateral Agreement and stricter policies on emigration

Participants were asked what kind of impact they felt the stricter UK policies and the prohibition of recruitment of South African doctors by the UK would have on doctors' emigration plans. The doctors believed that the policies could have three different levels of impact: (1) they would reduce the outflow of doctors to the UK; (2) they would encourage doctors migrate to other countries; or (3) they would not deter those health workers with strong motivations to migrate.

Only three doctors believed that the stricter policies would assist in reducing the number of doctors migrating abroad. Several doctors believed that South African doctors will simply try to work in another country to which they are able to gain easier entry. The ease with which South African doctors can gain entry into other first-world countries such as Canada would reportedly influence two of the doctors to emigrate to Canada rather than the UK, even though the UK was the preferred country destination. In the following statement, one doctor explains how difficulties in gaining entry into the UK will not deter her from leaving SA:

> 'I'm looking at emigration out of South Africa … If Ireland won't take me I will look for somewhere else who is willing to take me if the environment is better for my lifestyle, for my family, that type of thing. I'm not going to stay in South Africa just because they've restricted me from going to the UK.' (CS doctor, Regional public hospital in greater Durban area)

Several doctors considering migrating to the UK in the future said that the stricter policies and the difficulty in gaining access to the country would not deter them or other healthcare professionals from moving to the UK if they felt the long-term benefit to their lives and careers was worth the difficulty in getting there. Even doctors intending to remain in SA agreed that the stricter policies and difficult immigration processes would not deter those doctors who were fed up with enduring their frustrations in SA.

Discussion

The findings indicate that the overwhelming majority of doctors have a desire to work abroad after their CS year, with some intending to specialise in SA before they move abroad and others considering migration should they not find a medical officer post after their CS year. This concurs with other quantitative studies[5,6,10] which have found that a large proportion of medical and nursing students in SA are considering migrating abroad within a few years after their graduation.

Our findings also confirm those of Oberoi and Lin,[9] in that push factors appeared to exert a stronger influence on participants' desires and decisions to emigrate than pull factors. The most salient push factors articulated by the doctors and nurses included poor salaries, poor working conditions and resource shortages, heavy workloads, job uncertainty after their CS and the overall poor state and lack of investment in the healthcare system. Family relationships constituted either a push or pull factor, depending on the nature of the relationship; CS nurses with children were more inclined to see working abroad as an opportunity to provide better for their children, whilst CS doctors' relationships with their parents, siblings and extended families encouraged them to remain in the country.

The most predominant pull factors included higher salaries and earning potential in foreign countries, better training and job opportunities, opportunities to travel and practise first-world medicine, as well as the possibility of a better quality of life. The allure of better salaries abroad is a common finding in the literature.[9,10,19,24] Amongst nurses, better salary prospects abroad were highly sought after in the context of their children's educational and material needs, as were the perceived flexibility and autonomy of being able to work where and when they wanted as opposed to their current contractual constraints and the restrictions against moonlighting in other health facilities. Perceptions of an improved quality of life included a less stressful and frustrating work environment as well as prospects of a higher standard of living and a safer environment within which to live.

The nature of participants' views, whether favourable or unfavourable, about the stricter policies for recruitment and employment of foreign health professionals in the UK and the Bilateral Agreement, appeared to be associated with their migration desires and current level of job satisfaction. There were mixed views as to whether the introduction of the OSD has had or will have a potential impact on the exodus of healthcare professionals from SA; and again, these views seemed to be informed by participants' migration desires and intentions. In contrast to some doctors' disbelief that the OSD could curb emigration, research has shown that the OSD has made significant strides in closing the gap between the salaries earned abroad and those now earned in SA.[25]

Views supporting stricter policies restricting the migration of SA health workers abroad were premised on the perceived overall benefit that would accrue to the health system and the country should more doctors be available in the public sector. Furthermore, it was believed that stricter policies would ensure that only the most resolved health professionals would succeed. Most views and opinions expressed regarding the Bilateral Agreement and the stricter migration and recruitment policies tended to be negative, however, evoking frustration and anger amongst participants. Negative views were often directed at the South African government and were perceived as a restriction to their freedom, discrimination against them as health professionals and unfair treatment. The Melbourne Manifesto (A Code of Practice for the International Recruitment of Health Care Professionals),[26] adopted in 2002, places a degree of responsibility on countries who are experiencing substantial losses of health professionals to examine the reasons for these outflows, particularly with regard to addressing working conditions, incentives and educational opportunities, in order to encourage health professionals to remain in the country.[26]

The majority of participants, particularly those with a desire and intention to migrate, believed that the policies would not deter doctors, including themselves, from attempting to pursue work opportunities in the UK and would possibly even result in health professionals trying to enter other first-world countries in order to escape the frustrating and challenging work environment of the public health system in SA.

Limitations of the study

The groups of CS practitioners were not representative of the population of CS nurses and doctors in the province because of the way in which the participants were accessed. The focus groups had to be arranged at a time that was convenient for most of the doctors and nurses, which excluded several of the doctors and nurses as a result of their working schedules. Because of this, the CS nurses and doctors self-selected for the study, which could bring about differences between the sample selected for the study and the CS nurses and doctors who did not take part. Furthermore, the fact that the focus groups with the CS doctors were conducted in the last month of their CS year may have influenced their thoughts around migrating and their anxieties and concerns around the perceived job uncertainty for them in the following year.

Recommendations

The findings underscore the importance of ensuring that CS nurses and doctors experience a fulfilling and productive CS year in order to help retain them in the public sector (and the country) thereafter. The findings also underscore the need for the South African government to have a better engagement with and inform health professionals about policies and bilateral agreements that can directly affect their work experiences and migration plans. In view of the findings, it is believed that this would go a long way toward improving health professionals' perceptions of the government as their employer, as well as toward placating their frustrations regarding working in the public healthcare system. The government has acknowledged the importance of better management of its health workforce through garnering a deeper understanding of the key issues and challenges facing its workforce.[4] Our findings reinforce these efforts to strengthen Human Resource Management strategies, suggesting greater attention be paid to salient push factors identified by this study as well as to better engagement with regard to migration policies, bilateral agreements and even temporary migration opportunities available to health professionals.

If the South African government intends to embark on efforts to encourage the return of South African health professionals working abroad, it is then imperative that it begins to improve the working conditions and general state of the public healthcare system in South Africa which may have incited these health professionals to leave in the first place. This is in line with recommendations made by the Code of Practice for the International Recruitment of Health Care Professionals (Melbourne Manifesto).[26] Although salary increases have been achieved through the implementation of the OSD, the findings of this study suggest that increased salaries without improvements to working conditions and resources will not be sufficient to encourage health professionals to return to or remain in SA.

Conclusion

The majority of CS doctors in our study expressed desires and intentions to migrate abroad shortly after completion of their CS. The push factors, relating to the conditions in which they work, their salaries and the state of the healthcare system, had a strong influence on their decision to leave the country. During this critical early period in the careers of nurses and doctors, the findings show that it is of utmost importance that these practitioners be made to feel that they have been engaged with in an adequate fashion by the South African government with regard to their complaints about their working conditions, low salaries and heavy workloads. For many considering migrating, the knowledge that the government would attempt to or was in the process of improving their working conditions would make them reconsider leaving. In this way, government efforts to better manage, recognise and respect the work and contribution of health professionals to the country may go a long way toward retaining its health professionals. Related to this was a need for the government to inform its health professionals more effectively regarding the relevant policies and bilateral agreements that have a direct effect on their practice. This could prevent the problem of health professionals misconstruing government's actions, which was found to further erode the relationship between the government and its health professionals.

Acknowledgements

The study was commissioned by the International Organization for Migration (IOM) and funded by the European Union. The authors would like to acknowledge Reiko Matsuyama and Natalie Ridgard from the IOM for their valuable input over the course of the study. We would also like to thank all the doctors and nurses who took time out of their busy schedules to share openly their views and opinions on the subject matter raised in this article.

Competing interests

The authors declare that they have no financial or personal relationship(s) which may have inappropriately influenced them in writing this article.

Authors' contributions

C.R. (University of KwaZulu-Natal) conceptualised the study, conducted the analysis and assisted in preparing the manuscript. G.G. (University of KwaZulu-Natal) conceptualised the study and prepared the manuscript.

References

1. World Health Organization. Everybody's business: Strengthening health systems to improve health outcomes. WHO framework for action [document on the Internet]. c2007 [cited 2013 Nov 15]. Available from: http://www.who.int/healthsystems/strategy/everybodys_business.pdf
2. World Health Organization. Global shortage of health care workers and its impact. Geneva, Switzerland: World Health Organization; 2006.
3. Wildschut A, Mgqolozana T. Nurses. In: Erasmus J, Breier M, editors. Skills shortage in South Africa: case studies of key professions. Cape Town: HSRC Press, 2009; pp. 132–151.
4. Department of Health. Human resources for health: HRH strategy for the health sector 2012/13–2016/17 [document on the Internet]. c2011 [cited 2013 Nov 15]. Available from: www.gov.za/documents/download.php?f=152486
5. Crush J, Pendleton W, Tevera DS. Degrees of uncertainty: Students and the brain drain in southern Africa. Southern African Migration Project, Migration Policy Series No. 35. Cape Town: Idasa and Kingston: Queen's University; 2005.
6. Pendleton W, Crush J, Lefko-Everett K. The hemorrhage of health professionals from South Africa: Medical opinions. Southern African Migration Project, Migration Policy Series No. 47. Cape Town: Idasa; 2007.
7. Bezuidenhout MM, Joubert G, Hiemstra LA, et al. Reasons for doctor migration from South Africa. SA Fam Pract. 2009;51(3):211–215. http://dx.doi.org/10.1080/20786204.2009.10873850
8. Maslin A. Databank of bilateral agreements. Washington: The Aspen Institute – Global Health and Development; 2003.
9. Oberoi SS, Lin V. Brain drain of doctors from southern Africa: Brain gain for Australia. Aust Health Rev. 2006;30(1):25–33.
10. George G, Reardon C. Preparing for export? Medical and nursing student migration intentions post-qualification in South Africa. Afr J Prm Health Care Fam Med. 2013;5(1), Art. #483, 9 pages.
11. Mahlathi P. Occupational specific dispensation for medical & dental practitioners, pharmaceutical and EMS Personnel (Presentation to the Select Committee on Social Services) [document on the Internet]. c2009 [cited 2013 Nov 15]. Available from: http://www.pmg.org.za/files/docs/090818health-edit.pdf
12. Reid S. Compulsory community service for doctors in South Africa – an evaluation of the first year. S Afr Med J. 2001;91(4):329–336.
13. Erasmus N. Slaves of the state – medical internship and CS in South Africa. S Afr Med J. 2012;102(8):655–658. http://dx.doi.org/10.7196/samj.5987
14. Nemutandani MS, Maluleke FRS, Rudolph MJ. Community service doctors in Limpopo province. S Afr Med J. 2006;96(3):180–182.
15. Rogerson CM. Medical recruits: The temptation of South African health care professionals. Southern African Migration Report. Migration Policy Series No. 45. Cape Town: Idasa; 2007.
16. Governments of UK and South Africa. Memorandum of Understanding between the Government of the United Kingdom of Great Britain and Northern Ireland and the Government of the Republic of South Africa on the reciprocal educational exchange of healthcare concepts and personnel [document on the Internet]. c2003 [cited 2013 Nov 15]. Available from: http://www.publications.parliament.uk/pa/cm200304/cmselect/cmfaff/117/4030208.htm
17. Robinson M, Clark P. Forging solutions to health worker migration. Lancet. 2008;371(9613):691–693. http://dx.doi.org/10.1016/S0140-6736(08)60310-4
18. Department of Health. Code of practice for the international recruitment of healthcare professionals [document on the Internet]. c2004 [cited 2013 Nov 15]. Available from: http://www.nursingleadership.org.uk/publications/codeofpractice.pdf
19. Hamilton K, Yau J. The global tug-of-war for health care workers [document on the Internet]. c2010 [cited 2014 Aug 27]. Available from: http://www.migrationpolicy.org/article/global-tug-war-health-care-workers
20. Day C, Gray A. Health and related indicators. In: Barron P, Roma-Reardon J, editors. South African Health Review 2008. Durban: Health Systems Trust; pp. 239–396.
21. Bogdan R, Biklen SK. Qualitative research for education: An introduction to theory and methods. 2nd ed. Boston: Allyn and Bacon; 1992.
22. Ryan GW, Bernard HR. Techniques to identify themes. Field Methods. 2003;15(1):85–109. http://dx.doi.org/10.1177/1525822X02239569
23. Gibbs G. Analysing qualitative data. California: Sage Publications Ltd; 2008.
24. Pagett C, Padarath A. A review of codes and protocols for the migration of health workers. Regional Network for Equity in Health in east and southern Africa. Discussion Paper No. 50 [document on the Internet]. c2007 [cited 2014 Aug 27]. Available from: http://www.aspeninstitute.org/sites/default/files/content/images/review%20of%20codes%20and%20protocols%20pagett.pdf
25. George G, Rhodes B. Is there really a pot of gold at the end of the rainbow? Has the Occupational Specific Dispensation, as a mechanism to attract and retain health workers in South Africa, leveled the playing field? BMC Public Health. 2012;12:613. http://dx.doi.org/10.1186/1471-2458-12-613
26. Wonca. A code of practice for the international recruitment of health care professionals: The Melbourne Manifesto [document on the Internet]. c2002 [cited 2013 Nov 15]. Available from: https://www.acrrm.org.au/files/uploads/pdf/advocacy/melbourne-manifesto_wonca.pdf

14

Risk factors for visual impairment and blindness amongst black adult diabetics receiving treatment at Government healthcare facilities in Mopani District, Limpopo province, South Africa

Authors:
Raymond G. Mabaso[1]
Olalekan A. Oduntan[2]

Affiliations:
[1]Department of Health Studies, University of South Africa, South Africa

[2]Discipline of Optometry, University of KwaZulu-Natal, South Africa

Correspondence to:
[1]Raymond Mabaso

Email:
mabaso@mweb.co.za

Postal address:
PO Box 392, UNISA 0003, South Africa

Background: Diabetes mellitus (DM) is a common systemic disease amongst Black South Africans. It may lead to diabetic retinopathy (DR), a common cause of visual impairment (VI) and blindness. DR may significantly increase the prevalence of VI and blindness.

Aim: To assess risk factors for VI and blindness amongst a black diabetic South African population aged ≥ 40 years.

Setting: The study was conducted in seven Government healthcare facilities (two hospitals, four clinics and one health centre) in Mopani District, Limpopo province, South Africa.

Methods: This was a cross-sectional health facility-based quantitative study. Structured interviews were used to obtain information, which included sociodemographic profile, knowledge about DM and its ocular complications, presence of hypertension and accessibility to health facilities. Subsequently participants were examined for VI and blindness using an autorefractor, pinhole disc, ophthalmoscope and logMAR visual acuity chart. Anthropometric measurements (height, weight and waist) were also taken. Associations between 31 risk factors and VI as well as blindness were statistically examined.

Results: Participants ($N = 225$) included 161 women and 64 men aged 40–90 years (mean 61.5 ± 10.49 years); 41.3% of them had VI and 3.6% were blind. Cataracts (76.8%) and DR (7.1%) were the common causes of compensated VI and blindness. Risk factors that were associated with VI and blindness were age, monthly income, compliance with losing weight and physical activity.

Conclusion: Findings suggest that lifestyle intervention and appropriate eyecare programmes may reduce VI and blindness in this population.

Facteurs de risques de déficiences visuelles et de cécité chez les adultes diabétiques noirs sud-africains recevant un traitement dans les établissements hospitaliers gouvernementaux du District de Mopani.

Historique: Le Diabète Mellitus (DM) est une maladie systémique commune chez les Sud-africains noirs. Cela peut entrainer la rétinopathie diabétique (DR), une cause commune de déficience visuelle (VI) et de cécité. La DR peut augmenter considérablement la prévalence de VI et de cécité.

Objectifs: Evaluer les facteurs à risque de VI et de cécité dans la population de diabétiques noirs sud-africains âgés de ≥ 40 ans.

Cadre: L'étude a été menée dans sept établissements de santé du gouvernement (deux hôpitaux, quatre cliniques et un centre de santé) dans le District de Mopani, dans la province du Limpopo, en Afrique du Sud.

Méthode: C'était une étude quantitative transversale au sein d'un établissement. On a utilisé des interviews structurées pour obtenir des informations, comprenant des profils sociodémographiques, des connaissances sur le DM et ses complications oculaires, la présence d'hypertension et l'accès aux services de santé. Ensuite, les participants ont été examinés pour détecter les problèmes de vision et la cécité à l'aide d'un appareil auto-réfracteur, un disque à trou, un ophtalmoscope, et un tableau logMAR d'acuité visuelle (VA). En outre, on a pris les mesures anthropométriques (taille, poids et tour de taille). On a examiné statistiquement le rapport entre 31 facteurs de risques et le VI ainsi que la cécité.

Résultats: Les participants ($N = 225$) comprenaient 161 femmes et 64 hommes âgés de 40 à 90 ans (moyen = 61.5 ± 10.49 ans), 41.3% d'entre eux avaient le VI et 3.6% étaient aveugles. La cataracte (76.8%) et le DR (7.1%) étaient les causes communes de VI compensé et de cécité. Les facteurs de risques associés au VI et à la cécité étaient l'âge, les revenus mensuels, l'acceptation de perdre du poids et l'activité physique.

Conclusion: les résultats suggèrent que le changement de mode vie et les programmes appropriés de soins visuels peut réduire le VI et la cécité dans cette population.

Introduction

Diabetes mellitus (DM) is a common metabolic disorder characterised by sustained hyperglycaemia of varying severity secondary to lack and/or diminished efficacy of endogenous insulin.[1] Based on aetiology DM can be classified into type 1 (insulin-dependent) DM, type 2 (non-insulin-dependent) DM, gestational DM, and other specific types of DM.[2] Type 1 DM (T1DM), which accounts for only 5% – 10% of all types of DM, results from a cellular-mediated auto-immune destruction of β-cells of the pancreas. This cell destruction leads to absolute insulin deficiency and dependence on exogenous insulin for survival.[3] Type 2 DM (T2DM) accounts for about 90% – 95% of all types of DM and results from insulin resistance and relative insulin deficiency.[3] T2DM can be controlled through healthy diet, participating in physical activities, losing excess weight and taking oral medication.[4] Gestational DM occurs only during pregnancy and is a risk factor for T2DM after pregnancy.[5] Other specific types of DM may be due to other causes such as genetic defects in β-cell function, insulin action, diseases of the pancreas, and drug-(such as HIV medication)or chemical-induced DM.[3]

Globally the number of people with DM is projected to double between the years 2000 and 2030, because of population aging, unhealthy diet, obesity and sedentary lifestyles.[6] According to the International Diabetes Federation[7] the number of people with DM in the sub-Saharan African region is projected to increase from 14.7million in 2011 to 28 million by 2030. In South Africa the number of adults (20–79 years) with DM is projected to increase from 1.9 million in 2011 to 2.5 million in 2030, with at least 78% of those with the condition being undiagnosed.[7] The long-term effects of DM include, amongst others, development of diabetic retinopathy (DR), a common cause of visual impairment (VI) and blindness amongst adults aged 20 to 65 years.[7] Some authors[8,9] have reported that people with DM are more likely to be visually impaired than those without it.

The World Health Organization (WHO)[10] defines a risk factor as any attribute, characteristic or exposure of an individual that increases the likelihood of developing a disease or injury. Several demographic and socio-economic risk factors have been reported to be significantly associated with VI and blindness in the general population, including age,[9] gender,[9] educational and economic status.[8,9] Sociodemographic profiles such as age,[11,12,13,14] female gender,[12,14] low level of education,[8,15] unemployment[12] and low income[9] have been reported to be positively associated with VI and blindness amongst DM patients. Further, types of DM,[16,17,18] insulin treatment[12,14] and hypertension[13,14] have been found to be positively associated with VI and blindness. A negative association has been found between DR and physical activity, weight loss and special diet compliance.[19] Smoking status[20] and anthropometric features[21] such as high waist circumference (WC) and high body mass index (BMI) have also been reported to be positively associated with DR.

Knowledge about DM and its complications has an effect on compliance with treatment and successful management of the disease.[22] Regular visits to medical clinics have been identified as a proxy indicator of better primary prevention of DM eye complications, and participants with irregular visits were found to be at higher risk of VI and blindness than those with regular visits.[23]

In a study conducted on 795 Taiwanese patients[24] the average duration from a state of absence of signs of DR to background DR and blindness was approximately 10 years and 23 years respectively, suggesting that longer duration could be a risk factor for VI and blindness. Early detection and treatment of DR may lead to 60% reduction in DR progression from preproliferative diabetic retinopathy (PPDR) to proliferative diabetic retinopathy (PDR), and 57% reduction in the progression from PDR to blindness.[24]

No previous literature report could be found on the risk factors for VI and blindness amongst people with DM in South Africa.[25] Such a report could be useful to the health authorities in planning for the prevention and elimination of modifiable risk factors associated with VI and blindness amongst people with DM. Therefore the purpose for this article was to investigate the risk factors for VI and blindness amongst black South Africans with DM aged ≥ 40 years who were receiving treatment at Government healthcare facilities in Mopani District.

Research methods and design

Study design

This was a cross-sectional health facility-based quantitative study.

Setting

The study was conducted in seven Government health facilities in Mopani District, which included four clinics (Carlota, Dan, Ga-kgapane and Tzaneen), two hospitals (Ga-kgapane and Letaba), and one health centre (Nkowankowa). During the period of this study (May–December 2011) the total number of black South Africans with DM recorded in the chronic diseases registers at these seven health facilities was 721. Of this number, 25 (3.5%) were < 40 years of age, which included 15 women and 10 men. The 696 (96.5%) others were ≥ 40 years of age and included 475 (68.2%) women and 221 (31.8%) men.

Study population and sampling strategy

The population was black South Africans of both sexes with DM, aged ≥ 40 years and receiving diabetes treatment from the targeted health facilities. The inclusion criteria included being black South African with DM, aged ≥ 40 years, willing to participate and signing the consent form. Convenience sampling was used to select participants from the targeted facilities. This method is non-probability sampling, which involves the use of the most conveniently available people as study participants. The advantages of this method include ease of recruitment, easier monitoring and follow-up, generally good response rates and retention of sample members.[26] All of the patients who came to receive DM treatment and who satisfied the inclusion criteria were requested to participate. The plan was to have an equal number of participants from each health facility, but that was not possible because the number of DM patients varied significantly from one facility to another. Based on an estimate of 15% prevalence of VI and blindness amongst the target population, the calculated sample size was 195:

$$N = \frac{z^{2*}[P(1-P)]}{D^2} \quad \text{[Eqn 1]}$$

where N = sample size required; 95% confidence level is z^2 (two-tail) = 1.96,
prevalence of VI and blindness is $P = 0.15$, and acceptable error is $D^2 = 0.0025$.

Whilst the calculated sample size requirement was 195, 225 participants were included in this study.

Data collection

First structured interviews were used to collect information which included sociodemographic profiles, knowledge of DM and its ocular complications, hypertension, smoking habits as well as accessibility to health facilities. Secondly, anthropometric measurements (height, waist and weight) were taken using a tape measure and bathroom scale. BMI (kg/m^2) was calculated as weight (kg) divided by height in square metres (m^2).[27] BMI was graded according to the WHO classification,[27] where 'normal' refers to a BMI of < 25 kg/m^2, being 'overweight' to a BMI of 25–29 kg/m^2, and 'obese' to a BMI of ≥ 30 kg/m^2. WC was measured by locating the upper hip bone of the participant and placing a measuring tape around the abdomen, ensuring that the tape was snug, but did not compress their skin and was parallel to the floor. The participant was asked to relax and exhale, and then the measurement was taken.[28] Three readings were taken for each of the anthropometric measurements and the average of each was recorded.

Thirdly, refractive errors were neutralised with optical correction from autorefraction values and visual acuity (VA) was measured with the participants wearing the optical correction. In cases where VA could not improve to better than 6/9.5, a pinhole disc was placed over the optical correction to rule out any residual uncorrected refractive error. An ophthalmoscope was used to determine the cause of VI or blindness. Thirteen participants were referred to the hospital ophthalmologist for a second opinion on diagnosis. All participants with treatable eye conditions and refractive error were referred to the ophthalmic nurses for treatment and/or for referral. Only the primary cause of VI was recorded. Where there were two or more primary disorders equally contributing to the visual loss, the WHO convention was followed, which is to record the cause that is easiest to treat and prevent.[29] VI was defined as VA of worse than 6/9.5, but equal to or better than 3/60, and blindness was defined as VA of worse than 3/60 to no light perception (NLP). Therefore, for the purposes of this study, VI and blindness refer to VA from worse than 6/9.5 to NLP. This definition was adapted from the definition of VI and blindness by the WHO.[30]

Finally, 31 risk factors were statistically tested for association with VI and blindness.

Data analysis

Data were analysed using the Statistical Analysis System (SAS) version 9.2 software package. Chi-square tests of association as well as logistical regression were performed, and odds ratios were calculated and interpreted. The level of significance was set at 0.05. There was no significant difference between the means of the VAs of the two eyes (t-value = 0.47, df = 224, p = 0.638). Therefore data from the right eyes only were used to study the associations. This is in keeping with usual practice for statistical research, where one eye from each subject is used to avoid a lack of independence of data.[31]

Ethical considerations

This study was approved by the Health Studies Research and Ethics Committee of the University of South Africa (Project number: 0729-138-8), and permissions were obtained from the relevant authorities before commencement of the study. All the relevant ethics protocols were observed before, during and after the study.

Results

Of the 225 participants, 161 (71.6%) were women and 64 (28.9%) were men. Their ages ranged from 40 to 90 years (mean 61.5 ± 10.49 years), and 41.3% had VI and 3.6% were blind. Cataracts (76.8%) and DR (7.1%) were the most common causes of compensated VI and blindness. The prevalence of VI and blindness ranged from 0.9% amongst those aged 40–44 years to 29.3% amongst those aged ≥ 60 years (Figure 1). There was a significant association between age and VI and blindness (df = 4, χ^2 = 11.2, p = 0.02).

Table 1 shows the demographic risk factors for VI and blindness that were examined, and results of chi-square tests.

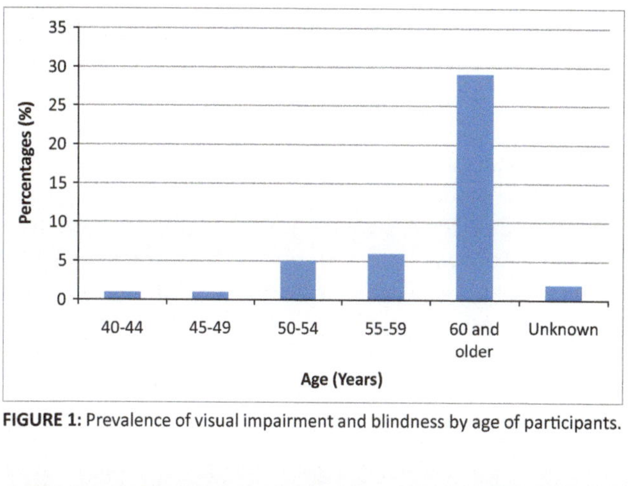

FIGURE 1: Prevalence of visual impairment and blindness by age of participants.

TABLE 1: Demographic and anthropometric risk factors examined.

Risk factors	VI/blind			Variables	
	Df	χ^2	*P*-value	*N*	%
Age	4	11.2	0.02*	225	100
Monthly income	4	14.0	0.007*	225	100
Gender	1	0.1	0.799	224	99.6
Marital status	3	3.8	0.285	225	100
Educational level	3	5.2	0.156	223	99.1
Residence	1	1.1	0.299	219	97.3
BMI	2	0.0	0.994	200	88.9
WC	5	0.6	0.990	224	99.6

*, Only age and monthly income were statistically associated with VI and blindness.
VI, visual impairment; BMI, body mass index; WC, waist circumference.

TABLE 2: Prevalence and distribution of visual status by monthly income.

Monthly income	VI/blind		Not VI		Total	
	N	%	*N*	%	*N*	%
No income	17	7.6	17	7.6	34	15.1
≤ R500	4	1.8	11	4.9	15	6.7
R501 – R1000	4	1.8	11	4.9	15	6.7
R1001 – R2000	67	29.8	58	25.8	125	55.6
➤ R2000	9	4	27	12	36	16.0
Total	**101**	**44.9**	**124**	**55.1**	**225**	**100**

VI, visual impairment.

Only age and monthly income were statistically associated with VI and blindness (Table 1). The prevalence of VI and blindness was higher (33.4%) amongst those earning ≤ R2000 a month than amongst those earning > R2000 (4%) (Table 2). In addition, the probability of those earning ≤ R2000 a month being visually impaired is 3.14 times that of those earning > R2000. Monthly income was statistically associated with VI and blindness (df = 4, χ^2 = 14.0, *p* = 0.007).

For brevity, only statistics on risk factors that are statistically associated with VI and blindness are elaborated upon in this article; others are briefly presented. Gender was not statistically significant (*p* = 0.799). The prevalence of VI and blindness amongst those who were single, married, divorced and/or separated, and widowed was 51.6%, 41.1%, 42.9% and 61.2% respectively, and marital status was not associated with VI and blindness (*p* = 0.285).

Amongst the 57 participants with no formal education, 54.4% had VI and blindness. VI and blindness prevalence was higher amongst those with primary (19.3%) than those with tertiary (2.7%) education, but the difference was not statistically significant (*p* = 0.156). The prevalence amongst those living in rural and semi-urban areas was 43.9% and 51.6% respectively, but place of residence was not associated with VI and blindness (*p* = 0.299).

VI and blindness was highest (18.5%) amongst those who were obese and lowest (1%) amongst those who were underweight. However, there was no association between VI and blindness and BMI (*p* = 0.994). The prevalence amongst male participants with WC > 94 cm was 46% and 36.4% amongst those with WC ≤ 94 cm. Amongst the female participants, the prevalence was 53.9% amongst those with WC > 80 cm, and there was no female with a WC of ≤ 80 cm. There was no association with WC (*p* = 0.990).

Table 3 shows the clinical risk factors for VI and blindness and the results of chi-square tests. Only physical activity and compliance with losing weight were statistically associated with VI and blindness.

The prevalence of VI and blindness amongst those who engaged in physical activity was 22.7% and it was 20.3% amongst those who did not; there was a significant association between VI and blindness and physical activity (df = 1, χ^2 = 6, *p* = 0.014, odds ratio 0.51). The prevalence of VI and blindness was 7.7%, 17.1% and 16.2% respectively amongst those who reported engaging in weight loss activities always, not always and those who did not. There was a significant association between compliance with losing weight and VI and blindness (df = 2, χ^2 = 9.4, *p* = 0.009).

Prevalence of VI and blindness was highest (16.4%) amongst those who had had DM diagnosed for < 5 years and lowest (1.3%) amongst those who had had it for longer periods (16–20 years). However, this association was not significant (p = 0.614). Prevalence of VI and blindness was 33.7% amongst participants who were not aware of the existence of different types of DM, 6.6% and 7.6% amongst those who knew one type and two types respectively. The prevalence amongst type 1 and type 2 patients was 4.1% and 40.5% respectively. Both knowledge and the types of DM were not associated with VI and blindness (*p* = 0.920 and *p* = 0.714 respectively).

Prevalence of VI and blindness was highest (21.9%) amongst those who had an eye examination within a period of one year or more before the study, and the lowest (0.8%) amongst those who were examined less than one month earlier (Table 4). There was no significant association between date of last eye examination and VI and blindness (df = 4, χ^2 = 9.1, *p* = 0.059). The period of the last eye examination in relation to VI is shown in Table 4.

Prevalence of VI and blindness amongst participants with and without hypertension was 35.5% and 8.6% respectively; however, the association was not significant (*p* = 0.652). Most (80.6%) of the participants had never smoked cigars, cigarettes or a pipe. Prevalence amongst those who never smoked, smoked occasionally, smoked regularly and always smoked was 37.1%, 3.3%, 0% and 5.2% respectively. There was no association between VI and blindness and smoking status (*p* = 0.214). The prevalence amongst those who walked < 30 minutes and for > 1 hour to the health facility was 16% and 3.2% respectively, with no significant association with accessibility (*p* = 0.693).

When the Proc Logistic of the SAS was used to fit models of all the above variables, only monthly income (df = 4, χ^2 = 10.75, *p* = 0.03) and physical activity (df = 2, χ^2 = 14.96, *p* = 0.00) remained significantly associated with VI and blindness. Age and compliance with losing weight were not associated in the multivariate analysis.

TABLE 3: Clinically related risk factors examined.

Risk factors	VI/blind			Variables	
	df	χ^2	*P*-value	*N*	%
Physical activity	1	6.0	0.014	207	92.0
Weight loss compliance	2	9.4	0.009	117	52
Duration of DM	3	1.8	0.614	225	100
Knowledge of types of DM	2	0.2	0.920	222	98.7
DM type	1	0.1	0.714	222	98.7
Special diet	1	0.1	0.705	220	97.8
Losing weight	1	1.0	0.314	204	90.7
Special diet compliance	1	0.5	0.468	213	94.7
Physical activity compliance	2	2.6	0.278	145	64.4
Date of last DM check-up	1	1.4	0.238	224	99.6
DM family history	2	2.4	0.305	220	97.8
Knowledge that DM can cause VI	1	0.8	0.359	224	99.6
Knowledge that DM can cause DR	1	0.3	0.601	223	99.1
Knowledge that DM can cause glaucoma	1	0.0	0.973	224	99.6
Eye examination history	1	1.3	0.255	217	96.4
Last eye examination	4	9.1	0.059	119	52.9
Family members with VI	2	0.3	0.859	169	75.1
Date for last blood pressure check-up	1	0.5	0.469	225	100
Hypertension	1	0.2	0.652	217	96.4
Hypertension treatment	1	0.5	0.463	177	78.7
Smoking status	3	4.4	0.214	213	94.7
Age when started smoking	4	2.4	0.660	225	100
Accessibility to health services	4	2.2	0.693	219	97.3

VI, visual impairment; DM, Diabetes mellitus; DR, diabetic retinopathy.

TABLE 4: Period since last eye examination in relation to visual status.

Period since last eye examination	VI/blind		Not VI/blind		Total	
	N	%	*N*	%	*N*	%
< 1 week	0	-	0	-	0	-
< 1 month	1	0.8	12	10	13	10.9
< 6 month	11	9.2	8	6.7	19	16
< 1 year	8	6.7	8	6.7	16	13.5
≥ 1 year	26	21.9	28	23.5	54	45.4
Unknown	7	5.9	10	8.4	17	14.3
Total	**53**	**44.5**	**66**	**55.5**	**119**	**100**

VI, visual impairment.

Discussion

VI and blindness due to DM is largely preventable through early detection, monitoring and management of diabetic eye diseases.[24] Risk factors that were individually associated with VI and blindness in this study were age, monthly income and compliance with losing weight and physical activity. However, only monthly income and physical activity remained significantly associated following multivariate analysis. Some of the risk factors reported in this article are not necessarily specific for persons with DM alone, but are also risk factors for VI and blindness in the general population.

The positive association of increasing age with VI and blindness found in this study is in agreement with findings from several previous studies.[12,13,14,15,32,33] The probable explanation for the association is that many blinding eye diseases, such as cataract, glaucoma and DR, are age-related. The fact that a larger percentage of the participants were ≥ 60 years of age may explain the association between age and VI and blindness in this study. It is therefore important that people in this age group have regular eye examinations so that conditions (DM- and non-DM-related) that may result in VI and blindness may be detected early.

In addition, low monthly income was significantly associated with VI and blindness. This agrees with the findings of a previous study[9] that low income earners in the general population were twice as likely to have VI as those with higher income. Low socio-economic status[14] has also been reported to be significantly associated with increased risk of VI. However, findings in this study disagree with those of another study[32] where no association was reported.

That the prevalence of VI and blindness was high amongst the participants with a monthly income of ≤ R2000 may be explained by the fact that many of them were elderly and receiving the Government old-age pension of about R1200. They therefore may not be able to afford eyecare services. A contributory factor may be poor access to cataract surgery and affordable spectacles provided by Limpopo province; these are available only at Elim and Mankweng Hospitals, which are about 150km from the site of this study. Some studies[12,15,24] found a positive association between female gender and VI and blindness. However, in agreement with previous reports,[13,34] no association between these variables was found in this study.

Previous authors[8,9,12,35] have reported that the prevalence of VI tends to decrease significantly with increasing level of education. This is because people with higher levels of education are more likely than those with low levels to seek medical intervention before they are visually impaired or blind, as they are better informed about the related risk factors. In addition, persons with tertiary education are likely to have higher income than those with primary education, and could therefore afford spectacles and cataract surgery.[35] Further, a higher level of education is associated with a greater likelihood of seeking eyecare services, better knowledge and more reasonable health-seeking behaviour.[35] Contrary to those reports, there was no association between educational qualification and VI and blindness in this study. This was the case despite the fact that the prevalence of VI and blindness was lower amongst those with tertiary education than those with primary education.

The higher prevalence of VI and blindness amongst those living in rural areas compared with those living in other places may be because most (68.9%) of the participants in this study were from rural areas. Another possible explanation is that there is a lack or shortage of eyecare services in the rural areas, a common situation in South Africa. In addition, services provided in the urban areas are often better than those that are available in the rural areas.[36] Poor economic status, lack of transportation, low literacy level, lack of awareness and traditional beliefs of rural dwellers have been reported to be responsible for underutilisation of available eyecare services.[36] It has been recommended that eyecare services for disadvantaged communities should include education and eye health promotion as preventive measures.[37]

Although a previous study[13] found that higher BMI was positively associated with VI and blindness, others[33,38,39] found low BMI to be positively associated with VI and blindness. In this study there was no significant association between VI and BMI, although VI and blindness was more common amongst obese participants (BMI ≥ 30 kg/m^2) than those who were not obese. This may be attributed to the fact that most of the participants in this study were obese. This finding is in agreement with those of other studies[11,14] which did not find any significant association.

A WC of > 94 cm for men or > 80 cm for women has been reported to be associated with an increased risk of diseases of lifestyle[27] such as DM and hypertension. A WC of > 102 cm for men or > 88 cm for women has been reported to be associated with a substantially increased risk of diseases of lifestyle.[27] Although the prevalence of VI and blindness amongst the participants in this study was higher in those with a WC of > 94 cm and > 80 cm, for 46% versus 36.4% (for men) and 53.9% versus 0% (for women) respectively, there was no association between VI and blindness and WC. The prevalence of VI and blindness was lowest amongst those who reported trying to lose weight. In addition, the risk of being visually impaired amongst those who engaged in physical activity is 0.51 that of those who did not. The association between losing weight as well as physical activity with VI can be explained by the fact that those factors help in glycaemic control, which is important in the control of DM and therefore prevention of diabetic eye diseases that can result in VI and blindness.

Several studies[12,32,33,34,35] have found longer duration of DM to be positively associated with high prevalence of VI. This is expected because the severity of DR increases with duration of DM. However, there was no association between duration of DM and development of VI in this study. This could be due to the fact that a larger percentage (39.6%) of the participants was diagnosed with DM within < 5 years of this study. Further, more than half (54.7%) of the participants were aged ≥ 60 years, suggesting that their VI might be due to age-related eye diseases.

The higher prevalence of VI and blindness amongst the T2DM patients than amongst the T1DM patients in this study agrees with findings from other studies.[15,17] However, there was no association between the types of DM and VI and blindness in this study. An obvious explanation for the higher prevalence of VI and blindness in the T2DM category is the greater number of T2DM participants (90.1%). In addition, T2DM patients are generally older than T1DM patients, which suggests that some of the VI and blindness may be age-related.

The non-association of prevalence of VI and blindness with smoking in this study agrees with the findings of previous studies,[12,34] but disagrees with that of another study[22] in which smoking was associated with DR. This may be because most (80.6%) of participants in this study had never smoked cigars, cigarettes, or a tobacco pipe. The higher prevalence of VI and blindness amongst participants who lived closer to the facilities rather than far away may be attributed to the fact that there were more participants in the former group than in the latter. Accessibility to health facilities was not associated with VI and blindness ($p = 0.693$). The prevalence of VI and blindness was higher amongst those last examined > 1 year ago compared to those last examined < 1 year ago ($p = 0.059$). More participants in the former group probably had undiagnosed or untreated eye conditions prior to the research study. This agrees with the views of other authors[18] who reported that a regular visit to medical clinics was a proxy indicator of better primary prevention of DM eye complications.

Strengths and limitations

This study is the first to describe the risk factors for VI and blindness amongst black South Africans with DM in a predominantly rural district of Limpopo province, and therefore provides valuable data on these risk factors in the community. The fact that this study was conducted in Government health facilities and not population-based could have introduced a health-seeking bias. The larger proportion of older, unemployed and poor participants, and there being more women than men in this study, could also introduce some bias. This could be due to the fact that those who were employed (mostly men) might have been at work when the study was conducted, or it might mean that men do not survive DM as well as women. In addition, individuals in formal employment (mostly men) tend to have medical aid schemes and therefore use private health services. It is acknowledged that the study population is not representative of the entire population of persons with DM in the district.

Recommendations

Based on the findings in this study it is recommended that a qualitative study be conducted to shed light on some of the findings amongst rural Africans with DM in Limpopo province. For example, could there be personal, social or cultural barriers to exercise, compliance to a special diet and use of eyecare services in this population? If such a study reveals no barriers, it would then be recommended that efficient and targeted lifestyle intervention programmes that focus on physical activity and losing weight be initiated to reduce the modifiable risk factors for VI and blindness in this population. An awareness-raising campaign should also be established to educate this population about control of DM and early detection of DR, as well as other causes of VI amongst diabetics, including refractive errors, cataract and glaucoma. In addition, refraction and cataract surgical services should be made available and accessible to this and other rural populations of Limpopo province.

Conclusion

This study demonstrated that age, monthly income, compliance with losing weight and physical activity were individually associated with VI and blindness; however, only monthly income and physical activity remained significantly associated following the multivariate analysis. Findings in this study may be useful to health authorities in planning for prevention of VI and blindness, as well as DM intervention programmes in the province.

Acknowledgements

The work reported in this article is part of a D.Litt et Phil project. The authors would like to thank Mr Idon Sibuyi (optometrist) for helping with data collection. We express our gratitude to Professor P. Ndlovu and Ms M.A. Managa (statisticians) for helping with data analysis. Also, we wish to thank the peer reviewers of this article.

Competing interests

The authors declare that they have no financial or personal relationship(s) that may have inappropriately influenced them in writing this article.

Authors' contributions

R.G.M. (University of South Africa) was responsible for the project design, collection of data, analysis and writing of the manuscript under the supervision of O.A.O. (University of KwaZulu-Natal).

References

1. Kanski JJ. Clinical ophthalmology: A systematic approach. 5th ed. London: Butterworth-Heinemann; 2003.
2. World Health Organization. Laboratory diagnosis and monitoring of diabetes mellitus. Bull WHO. 2002;1–26 [cited 2012 January 13]. Available from: http://whqlibdoc.who.int/hq/2002/9241590483.pdf
3. American Diabetes Association. Diagnosis and classification of diabetes mellitus. Diabetes Care. 2010;33:S62–S69. http://dx.doi.org/10.2337/dc10-S062
4. Centers for Disease Control and Prevention. National diabetes fact sheet: National estimates and general information on diabetes and pre-diabetes in the United States. 2012 [cited 2012 January 20]. Available from: http://www.cdc.gov/diabetes/pubs/pdf/ndfs_2011
5. Buchanan TA, Xiangh AH. Gestational diabetes mellitus. Clin Invest. 2005;115:485–491. http://dx.doi.org/10.1172/JCI200524531
6. Wild S, Roglic G, Green A, et al. Global prevalence of diabetes: Estimates for the year 2000 and projections for 2030. Diab Care. 2004;27:1047–1053. http://dx.doi.org/10.2337/diacare.27.5.1047
7. International Diabetes Federation. Diabetes: A global threat.Diabetes Atlas. 5th ed. 2011 [cited 2011 November 05]. Available from: http://www.eatlas.idf.org/print/diabetesatlas/5e/the-global-burden
8. Zhang X, Gregg EW, Cheng YJ, et al. Diabetes mellitus and visual impairment; National Health and Nutrition Examination Survey, 1999–2004. Arch Ophthalmol. 2008;126:1421–1142. http://dx.doi.org/10.1001/archopht.126.10.1421
9. Ryskulova A, Turczyn K, Makuc DM, et al. Self-reported age-related eye diseases and visual impairment in the US: Results of the 2002 National Health Interview Survey. Am J Pub Health. 2008; 98:454–461. http://dx.doi.org/10.2105/AJPH.2006.098202
10. World Health Organization. Risk factors. 2013 [cited 2013 September 12]. Available from: http://www.who.int/topics/risk_factors/en/
11. Roy MS, Skurnick J. Six-year incidence of visual loss in African Americans with type 1 diabetes mellitus: The New Jersey 725. Arch Ophthalmol. 2007;125:1061–1067. http://dx.doi.org/10.1001/archopht.125.8.1061
12. Saaddine JB, Narayan KMV, Engelgau MM, et al. Prevalence of self-rated visual impairment among adults with diabetes. Am J Pub Health. 1999;89:1200–1205. http://dx.doi.org/10.2105/AJPH.89.8.1200
13. Horri N, Farmani M, Ghassami M, et al. Visual acuity in an Iranian cohort of patients with type 2 diabetes: The role of nephropathy and ischemic heart disease. J Res Med Sci. 2011;16:S419–s426.
14. Rani PK, Raman R, Gella L, et al. Prevalence of visual impairment and associated risk factors in subjects with type 2 diabetes mellitus: Sankara Nelthralaya Diabetic Retinopathy Epidemiology and Molecular genetics Study (NN-DREAMS, Report 16). Middle East Afr J Ophthalmol. 2012;19:129–134. http://dx.doi.org/10.4103/0974-9233.92129
15. Mvitu Muata M, Longo-Mbenza B. Causes of visual disability among Central Africans with diabetes mellitus. Afr Health Sci. 2012;12:193–197.
16. Jeppesen P, Bek T. The occurrence and causes of registered blindness in diabetes patients in Arhus County, Denmark. Acta Ophthalmol Scand. 2004;82:526–530. http://dx.doi.org/10.1111/j.1600-0420.2004.00313.x
17. Arun CS, Al-Bermani A, Stannard K, Taylor R. Long-term impact of retinal screening on significant diabetes-related visual impairment in the working age population. Diab Med. 2009;26:48–492. http://dx.doi.org/10.1111/j.1464-5491.2009.02718.x
18. Sivaprasad S, Gupta B, Gulliford MC, et al. Ethnic variation in the prevalence of visual impairment in people attending diabetic retinopathy screening in the United Kingdom (DRIVE UK). PloS One. 2012; 7:e39608.DOI:10.1371/journal.pone.0039608 [cited 2012 July 20]. Available from: http://www.plosone.org. http://dx.doi.org/10.1371/journal.pone.0039608
19. Pan XR, Li GW, Hu YH, et al. Effects of diet and exercise in preventing NIDDM in people with impaired glucose tolerance. Diab Care. 1997;20:537–544. http://dx.doi.org/10.2337/diacare.20.4.537
20. Esteves JF, Kramer CK, de Azevedo MJ, et al. Prevalence of diabetic retinopathy in patients with type 1 diabetes mellitus. Rev da Assoc Méd Bras. 2009;55:268–273. http://dx.doi.org/10.1590/S0104-42302009000300017
21. Dirani M, Xie J, Fenwick E, et al. Are obesity and anthropometry risk factors for diabetic retinopathy? The Diabetes Management Project. Invest Ophthalmol. Vis Sci. 2011;52:4416–4421. http://dx.doi.org/10.1167/iovs.11-7208
22. Phillips KC, Mashige KP, Clarke-Farr PC. Knowledge of diabetes mellitus in privately-funded diabetic patients attending a rural optometric practice in Malmesbury, South Africa. S Afr Optom. 2012;71:70–77.
23. Al-Akily SA, Bamashmus MA, Gunaid AA. Causes of visual impairment and blindness among Yemenis with diabetes: A hospital-based study. East Mediterr Health J. 2011;17:831–837.
24. Liu W-J, Lee L-T, Yent M-F, et al. Assessing progression and efficacy of treatment for diabetic retinopathy following the proliferative pathway to blindness: Implication for diabetic retinopathy screening in Taiwan. Diab Med. 2003;20:727–733. http://dx.doi.org/10.1046/j.1464-5491.2003.01019.x
25. Burgess PI, Msukwa G, Beare NAV. Diabetic retinopathy in sub-Saharan Africa: Meeting the challenges of an emerging epidemic. BMC Med. 2013;11:157. http://dx.doi.org/10.1186/1741-7015-11-157
26. Bowling A. Research methods in health: Investigating health and health studies. 2nd ed. Berkshire: Open University Press; 2002.
27. World Health Organization. BMI classification. 2004 [cited 2011 November 13]. Available from: http://apps.who.int/bmi/index.jsp?intropage=intro_3.html
28. Eustice C. How to measure your body mass index and waist circumference. 2012 [cited 2012 November 09]. Available from: http://arthritis.about.com/od/preventionandriskfactors/ht/bodymassindex.htm
29. Wei M, Chen H, Fan YC, *et al.* Prevalence and causes of visual impairment and blindness in Sichuan Province of China. Int J Ophthalmol. 2010;3:83–88.
30. World Health Organization. 2011. ICD update and revision platform: change definition of blindness. 2011 [cited 2014 April 04]. Available from: http://www.who.int/blindness/Change%20the%20Definition%20of%20Blindness.pdf?ua=1

31. Ciolin JB, Khachikian SS, Belin MW. Comparison of corneal thickness measurements by ultrasound and Scheimpflug photography in eyes that have undergone laser *in situ* keratomileusis. Am J Ophthalmol. 2008;145:75–80. http://dx.doi.org/10.1016/j.ajo.2007.08.026

32. Roy MS. Diabetic retinopathy in African Americans with type 1 diabetes: The New Jersey 725. Arch Ophthalmol. 2000;118:97–104. http://dx.doi.org/10.1001/archopht.118.1.97

33. Olafsdottir E, Andersson DK, Stefánsson E. Visual acuity in a population with regular screening for type 2 diabetes mellitus and eye disease. Acta Ophthalmol Scand. 2007;85:40–45. http://dx.doi.org/10.1111/j.1600-0420.2006.00753.x

34. Henricsson M, Tyrberg M, Heijl A, Janzon L. Incidence of blindness and visual impairment in diabetic patients participating in an ophthalmolgical control and screening programme. Acta Ophthalmol Scand. 1996;74:533–538. http://dx.doi.org/10.1111/j.1600-0420.1996.tb00729.x

35. Fotouhi A, Hashemi H, Mohammad K. Eye care utilization patterns in Tehran population: A population-based cross-sectional study. BMC Ophthalmology. 2006;6:4. http://dx.doi.org/10.1186/1471-2415-6-4

36. Sacharowitz HS. Visual impairment in South Africa: achievements and challenges. S Afr Optom. 2005;64:139–149.

37. Oduntan OA, Raliavhegwa M. An evaluation of the impact of the eye care services delivered to the rural communities in the Mankweng health sub-district of the Northern Province. S Afr Optom. 2001;60:71–76.

38. Raman R, Rani PK, Gnanamoorthy P, et al. Association of obesity with diabetic retinopathy: Sankara Nethralaya Diabetic Retinopathy Epidemiology and Molecular genetics Study (SN-DREAMS, Report 8). Acta Diabetologica. 2010;47:209–215. http://dx.doi.org/10.1007/s00592-009-0113-8

39. Klein R, Klein BEK. Vision disorders in diabetes. In: Harris MI, editor. Diabetes in America, 2nd ed. National Diabetes Data Group. 1995 [cited 2010 March 19]. Available from: http://diabetes.niddk.nih.gov/dm/pubs/america/pdf/chapter14.pdf

An analysis of blood pressure measurement in a primary care hospital in Swaziland

Authors:
Ganizani Mlawanda[1,2]
Michael Pather[1]
Srini Govender[1,3]

Affiliations:
[1]Faculty of Medicine and Health Sciences, Department of Interdisciplinary Health Sciences, Division of Family Medicine and Primary Care, University of Stellenbosch, Tygerberg, South Africa

[2]Royal Swaziland Sugar Corporation (RSSC) Medical Services, Mhlume, Swaziland

[3]Khayelitsha Community Health Centre, Khayelitsha, South Africa

Correspondence to:
Ganizani Mlawanda

Email:
mlawandag@yahoo.co.uk

Postal address:
PO Box 3973, Stanger 4450, South Africa

Background: Measurement of blood pressure (BP) is done poorly because of both human and machine errors.

Aim: To assess the difference between BP recorded in a pragmatic way and that recorded using standard guidelines; to assess differences between wrist- and mercury sphygmomanometer-based readings; and to assess the impact on clinical decision-making.

Setting: Royal Swaziland Sugar Corporation Mhlume hospital, Swaziland.

Method: After obtaining consent, BP was measured in a pragmatic way by a nurse practitioner who made treatment decisions. Thereafter, patients had their BP re-assessed using standard guidelines by mercury (gold standard) and wrist sphygmomanometer.

Results: The prevalence of hypertension was 25%. The mean systolic BP was 143 mmHg (pragmatic) and 133 mmHg (standard) using a mercury sphygmomanometer; and 140 mmHg for standard BP assessed using wrist device. The mean diastolic BP was 90 mmHg, 87 mmHg and 91 mmHg for pragmatic, standard mercury and wrist, respectively. Bland Altman analyses showed that pragmatic and standard BP measurements were different and could not be interchanged clinically. Treatment decisions between those based on pragmatic BP and standard BP agreed in 83.3% of cases, whilst 16.7% of participants had their treatment outcomes misclassified. A total of 19.5% of patients were started erroneously on anti-hypertensive therapy based on pragmatic BP.

Conclusion: Clinicians need to revert to basic good clinical practice and measure BP more accurately in order to avoid unnecessary additional costs and morbidity associated with incorrect treatment resulting from disease misclassification. Contrary to existing research, wrist devices need to be used with caution.

Une analyse de la mesure de la tension artérielle dans un hôpital de soins primaires au Swaziland.

Contexte: La tension artérielle (BP) est mal mesurée à cause de l'erreur humaine et des machines.

Objectif: Evaluer la différence entre la BP mesurée d'une façon pragmatique et celle mesurée à l'aide des directives classiques; pour évaluer les différences entre les mesures prises au tensiomètre de poignet et celles prises au tensiomètre à colonne de mercure; et pour évaluer l'impact sur la prise de décision clinique.

Cadre: L'hôpital Mhlume de la Royal Swaziland Sugar Corporation, au Swaziland.

Méthode: Après avoir obtenu le consentement, la BP a été mesurée d'une façon pragmatique par une infirmière qui a décidé du traitement. Ensuite, on a remesuré la BP des patients avec le tensiomètre à colonne de mercure et le tensiomètre de poignet.

Résultats: La prévalence de l'hypertension était de 25%. La tension artérielle systolique moyenne était 143 mmHg (pragmatique) et 133 mmHg (standard) avec un tensiomètre à mercure et 140 mmHg pour la BP standard évaluée avec un tensiomètre de poignet. La BP diastolique moyenne était 90 mmHg, 87 mmHg et 91 mmHg respectivement pour la mesure pragmatique, la standard au mercure et celle au poignet. Les analyses de Bland Altman ont montré que les mesures de BP pragmatiques et standard étaient différentes et ne pouvaient pas être cliniquement interverties. Les décisions de traitement entre les mesures basées sur la BP pragmatique et la BP standard correspondaient dans 83.3% des cas, alors que les résultats des traitements de 16.7% des participants étaient mal classés. 19.5% des patients avaient été mis sous un traitement erroné antihypertenseur basé sur la BP pragmatique.

Conclusion: Les cliniciens doivent revenir aux bonne pratiques cliniques de base et mesurer la BP avec plus de précision afin d'éviter les coûts supplémentaires superflus et la morbidité liée au traitement incorrect dû à la mauvaise classification de la maladie. Contrairement aux recherches existantes, les tensiomètres de poignet doivent être utilisés avec précaution.

Introduction

Hypertension is a consistent, powerful and independent risk factor for cardiovascular disease, stroke and renal disease.[1] Diagnosis of hypertension is based on measurement of blood pressure (BP). Obtaining accurate BP readings has been noted to be a challenge faced by health professionals at all levels.[2] A large number of surveys have shown that physicians, along with other healthcare providers, seldom follow established guidelines for measurement of BP.[3] This study analysed variations between pragmatic ('real-life') and standardised (as per protocol) BP measurement. Technology has brought in various BP measuring devices, a common one in primary care being the wrist sphygmomanometer as opposed to the 'gold standard', but environmentally unfriendly, mercury sphygmomanometer. How does BP measurement from wrist device compare with the gold standard?

Literature review

Hypertension is a common health burden affecting both developed and developing nations.[4] The prevalence of high BP increases dramatically with age, with the lifetime risk of high BP approaching 100%.[5] Extensive data have shown beyond doubt the benefit of controlling hypertension.[6]

Control of BP begins with accurate measurement that leads to appropriate diagnosis, assessment of cardiovascular risk and treatment decisions.[1,2,3,4,5,6] The target BP for patients using anti-hypertensive treatment has been lowered for those with diabetes or renal disease,[1] thus, it has become increasingly important to be able to detect small differences in BP. Whilst BP measurement is a vital clinical skill, it is performed poorly by all categories of healthcare professional.[4] There are, in general, three sources of error in the indirect measurement of BP: (1) observer bias; (2) faulty equipment; and (3) failure on the part of clinicians to standardise the measurement techniques.[7]

The mercury sphygmomanometer, because of its accuracy and reliability, is widely regarded as being the gold standard against which all other devices for BP measurement should be compared.[5] As a result of environmental awareness, there has been increasing pressure to remove medical devices containing mercury from clinical areas, which is leading to the gradual decline in use of the mercury sphygmomanometer and, as a result, automated BP devices have been adopted by clinicians for their convenience and ease of use.[8]

Rose suggested that the observer was the most critical component of accurate BP measurement.[9] Petrie et al. declared that only an observer who is aware of the factors that lead to false readings should measure BP, because 'wrong readings obtained through failure to use the proper technique often lead to the wrong diagnosis, which may result in unnecessary or inappropriate treatment and follow up'.[10]

In a study by Roubsanthisuk, Wongsurin and Saravich, physicians and trained nurses were compared, showing that trained nurses overestimated, rather than underestimated, blood pressure, but systolic BP underestimation was very common in participants with moderate to severe hypertension.[11] 'Systolic BP underestimation of > 5 mmHg was as high as 57.5% by trained nurses [using the traditional device] versus 33.8% by the automatic device, indicating that nurses tended to underestimate BP in participants with more severe hypertension'.[11] The BP measurements done by nurses were found to be consistently higher than those recorded by doctors.[11] McKay et al. noted that few physicians ask their patients to rest for at least five minutes before BP measurement as recommended and, as a consequence, BP done by doctors was consistently high because of the 'white-coat' effect.[12] Contrary to the recommended five minutes of rest, it appears that 10 minutes rest before clinic BP evaluation could improve further the precision and accuracy of the measurement and implies that the optimal time at rest before clinic BP measurement is still undefined.[13]

Clinicians should also be aware that BP in human beings is affected by multiple stimuli, such as respiration, temperature, body posture, emotional or physical stress, meals, alcohol, or caffeine and smoking and hence these factors should be taken into consideration during measurement of BP.[14] For some patients, BP measurements taken in a doctor's rooms may not be an accurate representation of their typical BP. In up to 25% of patients, this measurement is higher than their typical BP – a phenomenon known as 'white-coat hypertension'.[14]

From the literature reviewed, it is clear that BP measurement is subject to errors, thus there are still some social and scientific questions which need clarity and further research, especially in resource-limited settings. Literature review concluded that with proper measurement technique, machine variation between the gold standard mercury sphygmomanometer and the wrist is minimal.[3,7,10] In addition there are problems associated with pragmatic-nature BP measurement and other observer-related errors.[1,2,3,4,5,6,7,8,9,10]

Nearly all the articles found on literature review are from developed countries with a good patient-to-health-worker ratio. In a developing country setting, where the patient-to-health-worker ratio is low and resources limited, the potential for BP measurement errors may be worse. One obvious question was on assessment of the reliability of BP measurement methods, looking at both sphygmomanometer and observer differences in resource-limited settings. In so doing, such research will further enlighten health workers about the trustworthiness of BP readings and ensure that health workers are treating BP optimally. Problems related to over- or under-treatment may be serious and, if identified early, could reduce unnecessary morbidity and mortality. Most of the prior studies have focused mainly on sphygmomanometer-related differences.

Study rationale and motivation

An analysis of variations between pragmatic or 'real-life' and standard BP measurement based on the 'gold standard' would be useful in improving chronic disease management and ensuring effective use of already-strained resources in primary care. This study will have an impact on increasing awareness of human-induced variation in BP measurement and its impact on therapeutic decisions; hence, it may motivate clinicians to follow protocol. In the long run, it may have some economic advantages in saving cost of drugs erroneously prescribed to those who, if BP had been recorded properly, would not need treatment.

Aims and objectives

Research question

Is there a difference between pragmatic and standard BP measurement in primary care?

Aims

1. To ascertain variations between standard and pragmatic BP measurements and comparison of wrist BP and mercury sphygmomanometer-based BP.
2. To assess the impact of any differences on treatment decision.

Objectives

1. To quantify the existence of any differences between BP recorded in a pragmatic way and that recorded using standard BP measurement protocols.
2. To quantify any discrepancy between BP measurements done by wrist sphygmomanometer when compared to mercury sphygmomanometers.
3. To assess if the differences in BP measurement have impact on treatment decisions: whether or not to treat, to start anti-hypertensive treatment or to adjust hypertension treatment.

Research methods and design

Study design

A cross-sectional study design was used.

Study setting

This study was done at Royal Swaziland Sugar Corporation (RSSC) Mhlume hospital, targeting outpatients. RSSC Mhlume hospital is a rural primary care facility in the eastern part of Swaziland The facility has a turnover of about 5000 patients per month and offers mostly primary care with minor office procedures. It serves a catchment area of about 30 000.

Study population

The study population comprised adult (> 18 years) patients, with or without hypertension, who accessed primary care at the RSSC hospital during the study period June 2011 to December 2011 and who gave consent to participate in the study.

Sample size and sampling method

Every fourth patient who had attended the outpatient clinic was eligible for selection. A sample size of 60 was used, based on statistical calculations and sample size from similar studies.[15] Statistically, two observations per subject achieves an 80% power to detect an intra-class correlation difference of 0.15 using an *F*-test with a significance level of 0.05. In a similar study of agreement, Bland recommends a sample size of 30 as a 'good sample' and 60 as 'excellent', as it gives a 95% confidence interval of +/-0.34s, where s is the standard deviation of the differences between measurements by the two methods.[15]

Data collection and measurement method

Informed consent was obtained from eligible patients. Participants had BP assessed in a pragmatic way by nurse practitioners who would give their therapeutic decision based on their readings. Participants had BP re-assessed according to the standard protocol, using mercury sphygmomanometer and wrist sphygmomanometer alternately. To reduce bias, the order of measurement for pragmatic or standard BP measurements was alternated for successive patients. Finally, demographic and relevant clinical data were collected into a 'Data Collection' form, which was subsequently entered into a Microsoft® Excel spreadsheet for analysis.

Reduction of bias

To improve internal validity, the potential biases were handled as laid out below.

Selection bias

For the reduction of selection bias, a systematic random sample (every fourth patient) was used.

Measurement bias

This level of bias could occur at any stage during the measurement, recording, management or analysis of the data. Notable biases were the Hawthorne effect (nurses could change their BP measurement routine because they were aware of the investigation underway) and observer diagnostic suspicion bias. These were reduced by blinding the nurse researcher to results from the nurse practitioners and nurse practitioners were blinded to the ongoing study. Use of validated, standardised and calibrated sphygmomanometers reduced instrument variation. Batteries for the wrist devices were replaced regularly. To reduce subject physiologic variation, as well as the known regression to mean with repeated BP measurement phenomenon,[16] the standard BP was measured within a few minutes before or after the pragmatic BP.

Confounding

Time between performing the BP measurements was an important confounder. Blood pressure tends to come down with time, which is known as regression to the mean. The time between pragmatic and standard BP assessment was kept at a minimum so as to reduce the possibility of confounding bias. Previous studies indicate that a time lag of less than 10 minutes does not have any significant effect on the BP result.[13]

Data/statistical analysis

Microsoft® Excel was used to capture the data and the data analysis software system, STATISTICA version 9 (StatSoft Inc., 2009), was used to analyse the data. The statistical analysis comprised both descriptive and analytical statistics. For descriptive statistics, summary statistics were used to describe the variables. The Wilcoxon sign rank test was used to assess differences between means of BP. For analytical statistics, simple logistic regression, Pearson correlation (*r*), intra-class correlation coefficient (ICC) and Kappa were used appropriately. Standard reference scales were used for Pearson, ICC and Kappa. The Bland and Altman (BA) method of analysis of agreement was used for further assessment of agreement. Reference ranges for comparison of BA analysis were within 10 mmHg for diastolic BP and within 20 mmHg for systolic BP, because these are known ranges for hypertension severity grading.[4,5,6] Throughout the analysis, a *p*-value of $p < 0.05$ represented statistical significance in hypothesis testing and 95% confidence intervals were used to describe the estimation of unknown parameters.

Ethical considerations

Ethical approval for the study was granted by the University of Stellenbosch Human Research Ethics Committee (reference number N10/11/394) on 13 May 2011. Institutional ethical approval was also obtained.

Results

Sixty outpatients consented to participate in the study, of which 32 were men. The mean age of the participants was 42.6 years, the mean weight 77.8 kg and the mean height 1.6 metres. The prevalence of hypertension was 25%. Twenty-eight per cent of the participants had co-morbid diseases.

TABLE 1a: Demographic characteristics of participants.

Characteristics	Variables	s.d.
Males (*n*)	32	-
Females (*n*)	28	-
Mean age in years (standard deviation)	43	14.2
Mean weight in kilograms (standard deviation)	78	19.4
Mean height in centimetres (standard deviation)	164	8.5
Mean body mass index	29	-
Prevalence of hypertension	25%	-
Co-morbid conditions	28%	-
Mid-upper arm circumference (in centimetres)	32	-

TABLE 1b: Clinical characteristics of participants.

Treatment decision	No treatment		Treat		Change treatment	
	n	%	*n*	%	*n*	%
Based on pragmatic blood pressure	32	53	18	30	10	17
Based on standard blood pressure	41	68	11	18	8	13

The mean systolic BP was 143 mmHg for pragmatic BP, 133 mmHg for standard BP using mercury sphygmomanometer and 140 mmHg for standard BP assessed using wrist device. The mean diastolic BPs were 90 mmHg, 87 mmHg and 91 mmHg for pragmatic, standard mercury and wrist, respectively. It took an average of 4.2 minutes between pragmatic and standard BP measurement.

Three participants reported either having a full bladder or having eaten within 30 minutes before BP assessment, five had exercised, one had smoked and taken coffee and seven reported some degree of psychological stress. Table 1 summarises the findings.

Analytical statistical results

The Pearson correlation coefficient (*r*) was the same, 0.9, for systolic and diastolic BP for all BP methods which were being compared, corresponding to 'good association' between pairs being compared. The ICC (model 2) was consistent with 'almost perfect agreement' for all methods compared. Thus *r* and ICC could not differentiate further the level of agreement between the methods in study. Adjustment for confounding was done: neither psychological stress, full bladder, eating a meal, exercise, smoking nor taking coffee within 30 minutes before BP assessment were confounding factors based on less than 10% difference of *r*, ICC, Kappa and BA results. The key results are presented in Tables 2 and 3.

Comparison of pragmatic and standard blood pressure

For systolic BP, the regression relationship was summarised as SBPMc (systolic BP, mercury) = −10.7 + 1.2 SBPPr (systolic BP, pragmatic). For agreement, the bias was 9.6 mmHg with limits of agreement of −17.4 mmHg to 36.6 mmHg. Using the bias alone, 9.6 mmHg, this would equate to excellent clinical inter-changeability based on a clinically-significant BP range of within 20 mmHg. However, the limits of agreement were too wide for the two methods to be regarded as agreeing clinically. Figure 1 illustrates the distribution on a BA plot. For diastolic BP, the regression equation DBPPr (diastolic BP, pragmatic) = −0.7 + 1.0 DBPMc (diastolic BP, mercury) summarised the relationship of diastolic BP between pragmatic and standard mercury-based BPs. The BA bias of 3.0 could have meant excellent

TABLE 1c: Clinical characteristics of participants.

Blood pressure	Method	Observation	Mean	25th percentile	50th percentile	75th percentile
Systolic blood pressure in mmHg	Pragmatic	60	143	120	140	163
	Standard using mercury device	60	133	110	130	151
	Standard using wrist device	60	140	123	138	155
Diastolic blood pressure in mmHg	Pragmatic	60	90	73	90	105
	Standard using mercury device	60	87	75	85	102
	Standard using wrist device	60	91	77	86	106
	Mean time between pragmatic and standard blood pressure measurements (minutes)	4	-	-	-	-

agreement but the limits of agreement were again too wide (−16.6 mmHg to 22.6 mmHg) for agreement based on comparison to a clinically-interchangeable BP range of within 10 mmHg.

Comparison of wrist and mercury blood pressure

For systolic BP, the corresponding regression equation was SBPMc = −2.5 + 1.0 SBPWr (systolic BP, wrist). The BA analysis showed a bias of 7.1 mmHg and limits of agreement, −15.4 mmHg (lower) and 29.6 mmHg (upper), which were outside the clinical reference range for inter-changeability, within 20 mmHg. For diastolic regression the equation was linear, with DBPMc = 10.6 + 0.7 DBPWr (diastolic BP, wrist), a sign of good positive association. The limits of agreement, −19.0 mmHg (lower) to 11.7 mmHg (upper), confirmed poor clinical agreement when compared to the clinically-acceptable range of agreement, within 10 mmHg. Figure 2 illustrates the regression line and BA plots.

Comparison of wrist and pragmatic blood pressure

Finally, pragmatic BP and wrist-based standard BP were also compared for completeness. For systolic BP, r had a positive association. The BA plot in Figure 3 shows that the two methods could not be used interchangeably because the limits of agreement were wider than the within-20 mmHg clinical reference range. Similarly, for diastolic BP, the limits of agreement precluded exchangeable use as they were outside the within-10 mmHg clinical reference range.

TABLE 2: Pearson (r), Intra-class coefficient (ICC) and regression equations for blood pressure (BP) measurement methods.

Blood pressure	Methods in comparison	Pearson coefficient, r (*interpretation)	Intra-class coefficient (†interpretation)	Regression equations for relationship between blood pressure methods (‡ interpretation)
Systolic blood pressure	Standard/pragmatic	0.9 (good association)	0.8 (almost perfect)	SBPMc = −10.7 + 1.2 SBPPr (gradient 1.2; intercept 10.7)
	Standard/wrist	0.9 (good association)	0.9 (almost perfect)	SBPMc = 20 + 0.8 SBPWr (gradient 0.8; intercept 20)
	Pragmatic/wrist	0.9 (good association)	0.9 (almost perfect)	SBPPr = −2.5 + 1.0 SBPWr (gradient 1.0; intercept -2.5)
Diastolic blood pressure	Standard/pragmatic	0.9 (good association)	0.9 (almost perfect)	DBPPr = −0.7 + 1.0 DBPMc (gradient 1; intercept -0.7)
	Standard/wrist	0.9 (good association)	0.9 (almost perfect)	DBPMc = 10.6 + 0.8 DBPWr (gradient 0.8; intercept 10.6)
	Pragmatic/wrist	0.9 (good association)	0.9 (almost perfect)	DBPPr = 2.5 + 1.0 DBPWr (gradient 1; intercept 2.5)

*, Interpretation based on: −1.0 to −0.7 strong negative association; −0.7 to −0.3 weak negative association; −0.3 to +0.3 little or no association; +0.3 to +0.7 weak positive association; +0.7 to +1.0 strong positive association.
†, Interpretation based on: ICC can be interpreted as follows: 0–0.2 indicates poor agreement: 0.3–0.4 indicates fair agreement; 0.5–0.6 indicates moderate agreement; 0.7–0.8 indicates strong agreement; and > 0.8 indicates almost perfect agreement.
‡, Abbreviations: SBPMc, Sytolic BP Mercury; SBPPr, systolic BP Pragmatic; SBPWr, systolic BP wrist; DBPPr, diastolic BP Pragmatic; DBPMc, diastolic BP Mercury; DBPWr, diastolic BP wrist.

TABLE 3: Bland Altman analyses: Results and interpretation.

Blood pressure	Measurements	Limits of agreement between methods under study			Do the methods agree clinically?
		Bias (95% CI)	Lower (95% CI)	Upper (95% CI)	
Systolic blood pressure	Pragmatic/ideal	-9.6 (-13.2 to -6.1)	-36.6 (-42.7 to -30.5)	17.4 (11.2 to 23.5)	No
	Wrist/ideal	7.1 (4.1 to 10.0)	-15.4 (-20.5 to -10.3)	29.6 (24.5 to 34.7)	No
	Pragmatic/wrist	-2.6 (-5.8 to 0.7)	-26.9 (-32.4 to -21.4)	21.8 (16.3 to 27.3)	No
Diastolic blood pressure	Pragmatic/ideal	-3.0 (-5.6 to -0.4)	-22.6 (-27.0 to -18.1)	16.6 (12.1 to 21.0)	No
	Wrist/ideal	3.7 (1.6 to 5.7)	-11.7 (-15.1 to -8.2)	19.0 (15.5 to 22.5)	No
	Pragmatic/wrist	0.7 (-1.8 to 3.2)	-18.4 (-22.7 to -14.1)	19.8 (15.4 to 24.1)	No

CI, confidence interval.
Interpretation based on comparison of limits of agreement to clinically-acceptable range of blood pressure (BP), within 10 mmHg for diastolic BP and 20 mmHg for systolic BP.

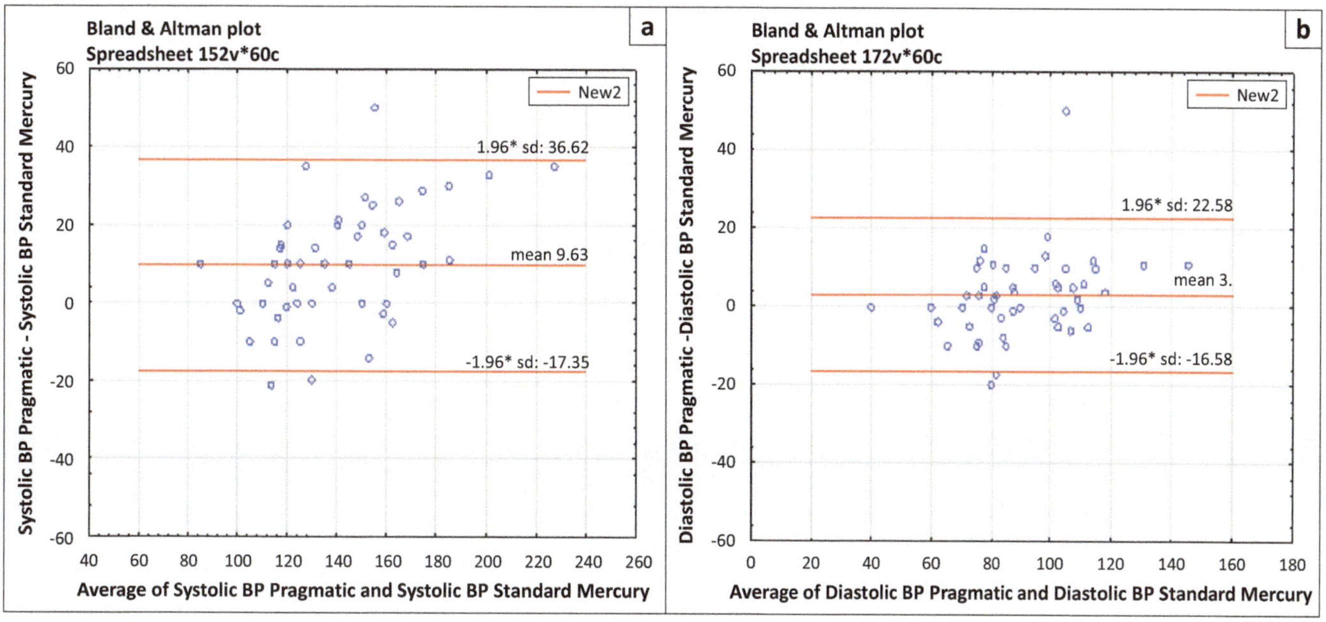

FIGURE 1: Bland Altman plot for (a) systolic and (b) diastolic blood pressure (BP): standard mercury compared with pragmatic BP.

Comparison of treatment decisions

Scores for treatment decisions (whether to start anti-hypertensive = 1; alter anti-hypertensive treatment = 2; or defer treatment = 0) were subsequently compared between decisions based on pragmatic BP and those based on standard mercury-based BP. The Kappa score was 0.7 which equates to 'good agreement' based on the widely-accepted Byrt's criteria (see Note under B). Overall (without stratifying), the treatment outcomes concurred in 83.8% of the cases, hence 16.7% were misclassified when compared with the standard BP. For the decision not to start treatment 78% of instances concurred; for the decision to start treatment, 90.9% agreed; and for the decision to adjust treatment, the agreement was 100%. Of the patients who were not supposed to start treatment (basing on the standard mercury-based BP), 19.5% ($n = 8/41$), were classified erroneously as requiring anti-hypertensive therapy when using pragmatic BP. Of those who needed to change treatment, the two BPs concurred (100%). Table 4 summarises the overall agreement level and Box 1 gives the stratified treatment outcomes.

Discussion

With hypertension defined as BP 140/90 mmHg, one in five (20%) South Africans have hypertension,[4] a prevalence which was lower than the 25% from this study. Since hypertension is more common in black people,[4] the higher prevalence was most likely a result of the black-ethnic predominance of the study population.

The next step was a comparison of pragmatic and standard BP measurements. Health workers generally do not follow BP

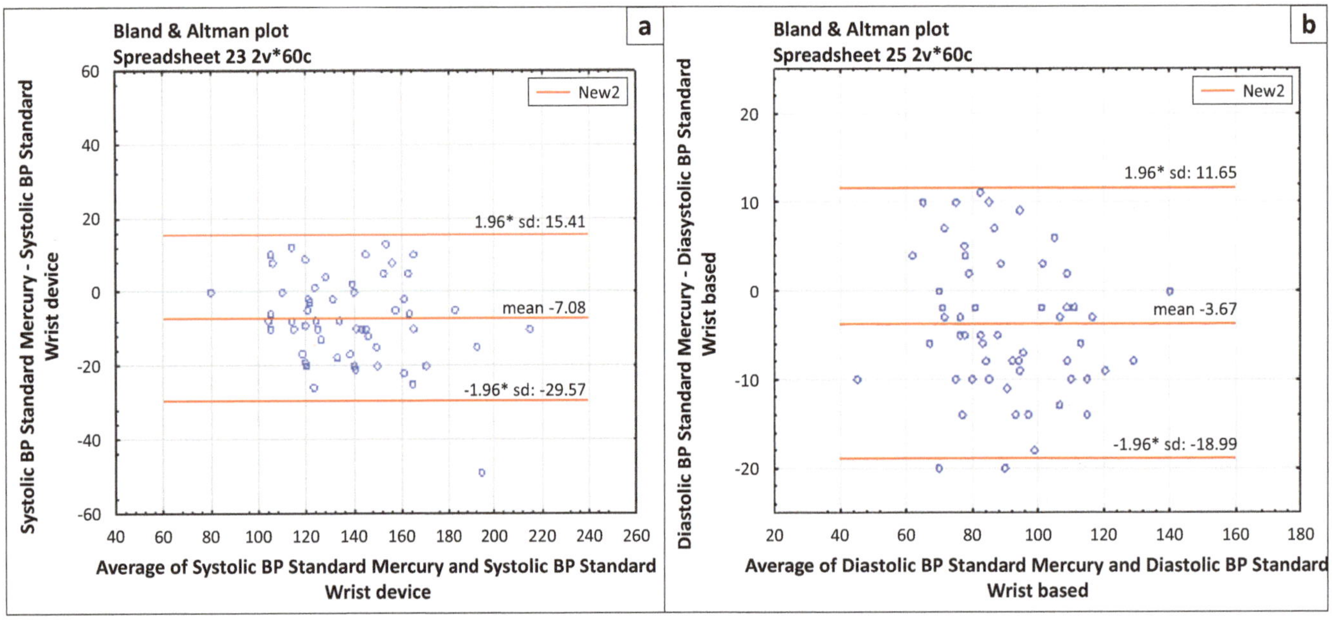

FIGURE 2: Bland Altman plot for (a) systolic and (b) diastolic blood pressure (BP): standard mercury compared with wrist BP.

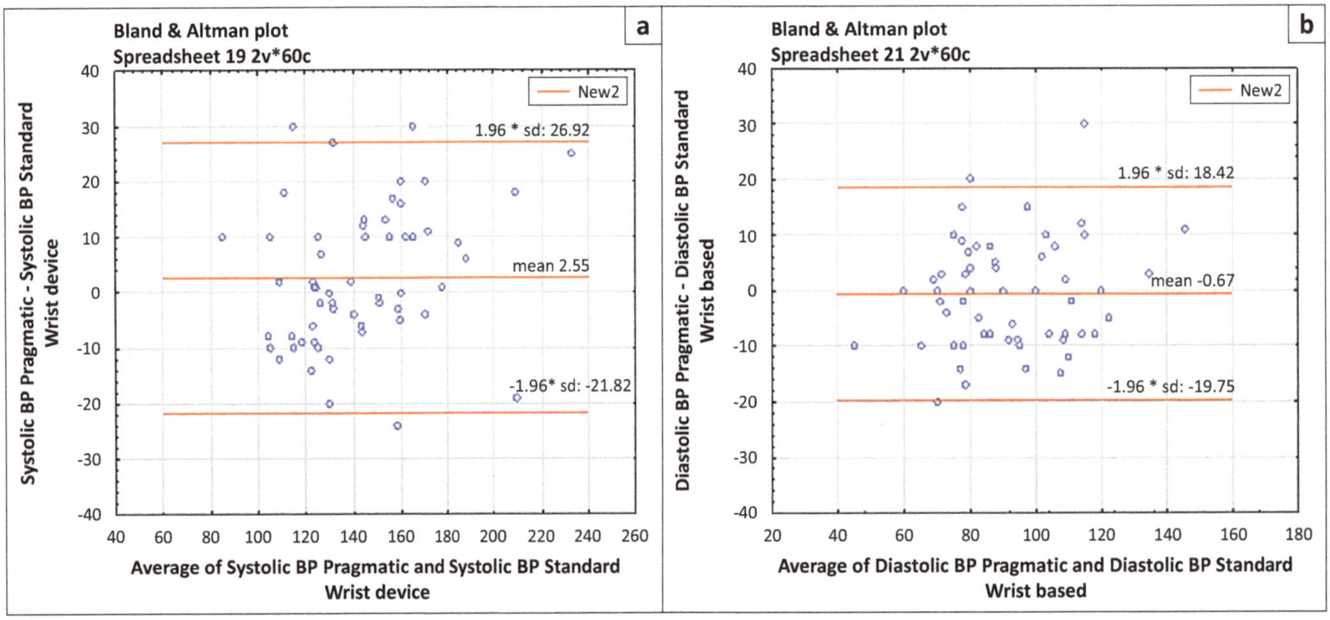

FIGURE 3: Bland Altman plot for (a) systolic and (b) diastolic blood pressure (BP): standard wrist compared with pragmatic BP.

TABLE 4: Comparison of treatment decisions between pragmatic and standard blood pressure measurements.

Agreement	Expected agreement	Kappa	Lower 95% CI	Upper 95% CI	*p*-value*
83.8	44.2	0.7	0.5	0.9	0

CI, confidence interval.
*, Byrt criteria: Excellent agreement 0.93–1.00; very good agreement 0.81–0.92; good agreement 0.61–0.80; fair agreement 0.41–0.60; slight agreement 0.21–0.40; poor agreement 0.01–0.20; no agreement ≤ 0.00.

BOX 1: Contingency table for per-stratum treatment outcomes comparing pragmatic to standard blood pressure.

		Treatment plan based on standard mercury blood pressure			
		0	1	2	Total
Treatment plan based on pragmatic blood pressure	0	32	0	0	*32*
		78.10%	0%	0%	
	1	8	10	0	*18*
		19.50%	90.90%	0%	
	2	1	1	8	*10*
		2.40%	9.10%	100.00%	
	Total	*41*	*11*	*8*	*60*

0, no treatment; 1, treatment; 2, treatment changed.

measurement guidelines. In a study on the BP measurement behaviour of clinicians done by Villegas et al., none of the physicians tested followed all the recommendations of the American Heart Association when measuring BP and a few recommendations were only followed by a minority of the physicians studied.[17] In this study, there was no clinical agreement between pragmatic and standard BP measurements for both systolic and diastolic BP. Pragmatic systolic BP was at least 10.7 mmHg higher than standard mercury BP. For diastolic BP, pragmatic readings were at least 3 mmHg higher than the standard mercury readings. These results were similar to those from a study by Myers et al. which found that when the primary care physician recorded BP using a mercury or anaeroid device, the resulting value frequently tended to be higher than what it would be if measurement guidelines were adhered to strictly.[18] Similarly Campbell and McKay concluded that pragmatic readings, namely, those obtained with little regard for patient factors or recommended technique, cause errors in BP assessment and do not correlate effectively with target organ damage; as such, no evidence exists to support the use of pragmatic readings in assessing a patient's need for pharmacologic treatment.[19] However, standardised readings, namely, those that follow recommended protocols, demonstrate high correlation with hypertensive target organ damage and were used in the major randomised controlled trials that showed the benefits of pharmacotherapy.[19]

The clinical consequences of poor BP measurement are well documented in literature: consistent overestimation of diastolic BP by as little as 5 mmHg may more than double the number of patients with hypertension in a physician's practice.[20] People who are identified incorrectly as having hypertension may experience adverse effects of medication and have increased medical insurance and treatment costs.[21] Conversely, consistent underestimation of diastolic pressure by the same margin would reduce by 62% the number of patients perceived as being hypertensive.[21] These errors could deprive patients of therapy which has been proven to be beneficial, thus leading to possible increases in serious medical and social complications.[21]

In this study, 19.5% of patients who were started on anti-hypertensive therapy based on pragmatic BP actually did not need any treatment. This trend was similar to many studies which showed increased diagnosis of hypertension if BP was not measured according to guidelines.[5,6,10,11,17,19,20] Overall, 16.7% of participants had their treatment outcomes misclassified. Of those who needed treatment, there was a concordance of 91% between pragmatic and standard BP-based decisions. However, for those hypertensive patients who needed to have their treatment adjusted, pragmatic and standard BP had 100% concordance. The likely explanation for this is that when BP was markedly elevated, there was no difference between pragmatic and standard BP.

Comparison of wrist and mercury BP measurements was subsequently performed. Standard mercury diastolic and systolic BPs were consistently higher when using a wrist device. For systolic BP, the difference was as much as 20 mmHg, whilst it was approximately 10 mmHg for diastolic BP, a sharp contrast to previous studies which found similarities between mercury and wrist devices.[3,7,10,22] We suspected that the difference was mostly because of the precise arm position and a known problematic phenomenon of wrist devices in which there is a systematic error introduced by the hydrostatic effect of differences in the position of the wrist relative to the heart.[22] This can be avoided if the wrist is always at heart level when the readings are taken, but there is no way of knowing retrospectively whether this was performed when a series of readings are reviewed.[22]

The mercury sphygmomanometer is generally regarded as the gold standard against which all other devices for BP measurement should be compared.[5] However, recent studies have shown that ambulatory BP measurements correlate better with the exact BP. Hodgkinson et al. have recently concluded that ambulatory BP was more cost effective than clinic or home BP.[23] However, guidelines for diagnosis and treatment of hypertension are still based on clinic BP measurements.[4,10]

Finally, a statistical lesson! Statistical methods for comparison methods have been subject of discussion amongst clinicians. The BA method is regarded as the gold standard.[23] Several papers have challenged the shortfalls of BA analysis,[24] but Bland and Altman have stated that the use of correlation coefficients is wrong for these types of studies.[25] In this study, intra-class correlation, Pearson's coefficient and linear regression both fell short of explicitly analysing the research question.

Strengths and weaknesses of the study

The main strength was that this study design was fast and inexpensive and was done in a resource-limited setting approximating most third-world institutions. It gave a useful initial overview of the problem, including the community prevalence. The statistical methods used were appropriate for studies of this nature.

There was very limited potential to make causal inference of any differences, an obvious weakness of this study. Secondly, we could not claim success with minimising regression to mean with the serial BP measurements as the exact time to ensure that regression to mean is rectified, is unknown. In addition, it was impossible to totally eliminate observer bias despite 'blinding' the nurses as there was always room for discussion when they meet outside the study centre; hence, the 'pragmatic' BPs might not have been as pragmatic as we expected. The other potential confounder was that the pragmatic BP was done by different nurse practitioner. No adjustments were made for this as surely their BP measurement techniques would differ. The other problem was diagnostic on the part of nurses: the clinical decision to start treatment. Usually, a number of readings are required to start treatment unless there are risk factors, significant target organ damage or BP was markedly elevated. The nurse practitioners might have over-diagnosed hypertension as they relied erroneously on one reading, even when BP was mildly elevated.

What is already known on this topic?

There are differences between pragmatic and standard BP but wrist and mercury BP readings are usually comparable.

What this study adds

This study further confirmed the existence of differences between pragmatic and standard BP measurements in a resource-limited setting. The difference leads to 16.7% disease status misclassification. Wrist and mercury devices potentially lead to conflicting results, which is contrary to earlier studies. Pearson and Intra-class correlation coefficients are weak statistical methods in studies of this nature.

Conclusion

There is a difference between pragmatic and standard BP measurements which affect the decision to start treatment and the decision to initiate treatment, but not the decision regarding alteration of regime for those already on treatment. There are also marked differences between wrist- and standard mercury-based BP devices which also affect treatment decision-making. In future, when assessing agreement between clinical methods, the BA method is more conclusive than correlation coefficients. Clinicians need to revert to basic good practice and measure BP more accurately so as to avoid unnecessary additional costs and morbidity associated with incorrect treatment resulting from disease misclassification. Wrist devices need to be used with caution.

Acknowledgements

Our thanks go to University of Stellenbosch statistician, Professor Justin Harvey, for verification of statistical analyses presented in this article.

Competing interests

The authors declare that they have no financial or personal relationship(s) that may have inappropriately influenced them in writing this article.

Authors' contributions

G.M. (University of Stellenbosch; RSCC) conceived the study, formulated the study design, did literature research, compiled the study protocol, performed the data collection statistical analysis, originated figures and graphs and was responsible for overall manuscript design. M.P. (University of Stellenbosch) was an active academic supervisor, strongly motivated the author, edited and actively contributed relevant input to this research from conception to publication, approved the final manuscript, closely followed up with the author to meet deadlines and submitted the manuscript on behalf of author and communicated with journal. S.G. (Khayelitsha Community Health Centre) was an academic co-supervisor and authorised ethical approval. Both G.M and M.P. approved the final manuscript for publication.

References

1. Neaton JD, Wentworth D. Serum cholesterol, blood pressure, cigarette smoking, and death from coronary heart disease. Overall findings and differences by age for 316,099 white men. Multiple Risk Factor Intervention Trial Research Group. Arch Intern Med. 1992;152(1):56–64. http://dx.doi.org/10.1001/archinte.1992.00400130082009
2. Kim JW, Bosworth HB, Voils CI, et al. How well do clinic-based blood pressure measurements agree with the mercury standard? J Gen Intern Med. 2005;20(7):647–649. http://dx.doi.org/10.1007/s11606-005-0112-6
3. Angeli F, Sardone M, Angeli E, et al. Validation of the A&D wrist-cuff UB-511 (UB-512) device for self-measurement of blood pressure. Blood Press Monit. 2006;11(6):349–354. http://dx.doi.org/10.1097/01.mbp.0000217995.12215.f2
4. Seedat YK, Croasdale MA, Milne FJ, et al. South African hypertension guideline 2006. S Afr Med J. 2006;96(4 Pt 2):337–362.
5. Jones DW, Appel LJ, Sheps SG, et al. Measuring blood pressure accurately: New and persistent challenges. JAMA. 2003;289(8):1027–1030. http://dx.doi.org/10.1001/jama.289.8.1027
6. Schwartz AR, Haas DC, Gerin W, et al. Accurate measurement of blood pressure. JAMA. 2003;289(21):2792. http://dx.doi.org/10.1001/jama.289.21.2792-a
7. Alexis O. Providing best practice in manual blood pressure measurement. Br J Nurs. 2009;18(7):410–415. http://dx.doi.org/10.12968/bjon.2009.18.7.41654
8. Wedgbury K, Valler-Jones T. Measuring blood pressure using an automated sphygmomanometer. Br J Nurs. 2008;17(11):714–718. http://dx.doi.org/10.12968/bjon.2008.17.11.29642
9. Rose G. Standardisation of observers in blood pressure measurement. Lancet. 1965;285(7387):673–674. http://dx.doi.org/10.1016/S0140-6736(65)91827-1
10. Petrie JC, O'Brien ET, Littler WA, et al. Recommendations on blood pressure measurement. Br Med J. 1986;293:611. http://dx.doi.org/10.1136/bmj.293.6547.611
11. Roubsanthisuk W, Wongsurin U, Saravich S, et al. Blood pressure determination by traditionally trained personnel is less reliable and tends to underestimate the severity of moderate to severe hypertension. Blood Press Monit. 2007;12(2):61–68. http://dx.doi.org/10.1097/MBP.0b013e3280b08317
12. McKay DW, Campbell NR, Parab LS, et al. Clinical assessment of blood pressure. J Hum Hypertens. 1990;4(6):639–645.
13. Sala C, Santin E, Rescaldani M, et al. How long shall the patient rest before clinic blood pressure measurement? Am J Hypertens. 2009;19(7):713–717. http://dx.doi.org/10.1016/j.amjhyper.2005.08.021
14. Jhalani J, Goyal T, Clemow L, et al. Anxiety and outcome expectations predict the white-coat effect. Blood Press Monit. 2005;10(6):317–319. http://dx.doi.org/10.1097/00126097-200512000-00006
15. Bland M. Frequently asked questions on the design and analysis of measurement studies: How can I decide the sample size for a study of agreement between two methods of measurement? [page on the Internet]. c2004 [cited 21 Sept. 2014]. Available from: http://www-users.york.ac.uk/~mb55/meas/sizemeth.htm
16. Bland M. Regression towards mean, or, Why was Terminator III such a disappointment? [page on the Internet]. c2004 [cited 21 Sept. 2014]. Available from: http://www-users.york.ac.uk/~mb55/talks/regmean.htm

17. Villegas I, Arias IC, Botero A, et al. Evaluation of the technique used by health-care workers for taking blood pressure. Hypertension. 1995;26(6 Pt 2):1204–1206. http://dx.doi.org/10.1161/01.HYP.26.6.1204

18. Myers MG, Godwin M, Dawes M, et al. Measurement of blood pressure in the office: Recognizing the problem and proposing the solution. Hypertension. 2010;55(2):195–200. http://dx.doi.org/10.1161/HYPERTENSIONAHA.109.141879

19. Campbell NR, McKay DW. Accurate blood pressure measurement: Why does it matter? CMAJ. 1999;161(3):277–278.

20. Haynes RB, Sackett DL, Taylor DW, et al. Increased absenteeism from work after detection and labeling of hypertensive patients. N Engl J Med. 1978; 299(14):741–744. http://dx.doi.org/10.1056/NEJM197810052991403

21. Joffres MR, Hamet P, Rabkin SW, et al. Prevalence, control and awareness of high blood pressure among Canadian adults. CMAJ. 1992;146(11):1997–2005.

22. Wonka F, Thümmler M, Schöppe A. Clinical test of a blood pressure measurement device with a wrist cuff. Blood Press Monit. 1996;1(4):361–366.

23. Hodgkinson J, Mant J, Martin U, et al. Relative effectiveness of clinic and home blood pressure monitoring compared with ambulatory blood pressure monitoring in diagnosis of hypertension: Systematic review. BMJ. 2011;342d3621.

24. Bland JM, Altman DG. Statistical methods for assessing agreement between two methods of clinical measurement. Lancet, 1986;i:307–310. http://dx.doi.org/10.1016/S0140-6736(86)90837-8

25. Pollock MA, Jefferson SG, Kane JW, et al. Method comparison – a different approach. Ann Clin Biochem. 1992;29(Pt 5):556–560. http://dx.doi.org/10.1177/000456329202900512

16

An audit of diagnosis and treatment of tuberculosis in Ethiopia

Authors:
Valerie J. Ehlers[1]
Getahun S. Aragaw[1]

Affiliations
[1]Department of Health Studies, University of South Africa, South Africa

Correspondence to:
Valerie Ehlers

Email:
ehlersjh@mweb.co.za

Postal address:
PO Box 65075, Erasmusrand, Pretoria 0165, South Africa

Background: Despite the existence of national tuberculosis guidelines (NTG) in Ethiopia, the incidence and prevalence of tuberculosis did not decline markedly. Audits could attempt to determine whether or not healthcare professionals actually implemented these guidelines, as non-implementation could contribute to suboptimal tuberculosis treatment outcomes.

Aim: To evaluate healthcare providers' implementation of Ethiopia's NTG during the diagnosis and treatment of tuberculosis in order to enhance tuberculosis treatment outcomes.

Methods: A descriptive, cross-sectional study design was used.

Results: Healthcare providers implemented the NTG during tuberculosis diagnosis for female (60.9%; n = 67) and male (56.1%; n = 69) patients. The correct numbers of anti-tuberculosis pills, complying with the NTG recommendations, were prescribed for 91.8% (n = 101) of the women and for 90.2% (n = 111) of the men. However, both over- and under-prescriptions of anti-tuberculosis drugs occurred. There was an over-diagnosis of smear-negative pulmonary tuberculosis. Only 2.6% (n = 2) of the 76 smear-negative pulmonary tuberculosis patients had been diagnosed correctly.

Conclusion: Implementation of the NTG should be enhanced, especially with regard to the diagnosis of smear-negative pulmonary tuberculosis patients and the correct prescription of anti-tuberculosis drugs. This would help to increase the number of correctly-diagnosed and -treated tuberculosis patients, improve tuberculosis treatment outcomes, decrease the spread of tuberculosis and prevent the development of multi-drug-resistant tuberculosis strains.

Application par les prestataires de soins des Directives nationales de l'Ethiopie pour la lutte contre la tuberculose.

Contexte: Malgré l'existence de Directives nationales contre la tuberculose (DNT) en Ethiopie, l'incidence et la prévalence de la tuberculose n'ont pas beaucoup diminué. On pourrait déterminer par des contrôles si oui ou non les professionnels de la santé ont appliqué ces directives, car la non-exécution de celles-ci pourrait avoir un effet sur les résultats sous-optimaux du traitement de la tuberculose.

Objectif: Evaluer l'application des DNT de l'Ethiopie par les prestataires de soins au cours du diagnostique et du traitement de la tuberculose afin de rehausser les résultats du traitement de celle-ci.

Méthodes: On a utilisé une conception d'étude transversale et descriptive.

Résultats: Les prestataires de soins ont appliqué les DNT au cours du diagnostique de la tuberculose chez les femmes (60.9%; n = 67) et chez les hommes (56.1%; n = 69). On a prescrit la quantité correcte de comprimés contre la tuberculose, conformément aux recommandations des DNT, à 91.8% (n = 101) des femmes et 90.2% (n = 111) des hommes. Cependant, il y a eu des cas de prescriptions excessives et insuffisantes de médicaments antituberculeux. Il y a eu un diagnostique excessif de tuberculose pulmonaire à frottis négatif. Seuls 2.6% (n = 2) des 76 patients avec une tuberculose pulmonaire à frottis négatif avaient été diagnostiqués correctement.

Conclusion: L'application des DNT devra être augmentée, en particulier en ce qui concerne le diagnostique des patients avec une tuberculose pulmonaire à frottis négatif et la prescription correcte des médicaments antituberculeux. Cela permettrait d'augmenter le nombre de patients tuberculeux bien diagnostiqués et bien traités, d'améliorer les résultats du traitement de la tuberculose, de diminuer la progression de la tuberculose et d'éviter le développement des souches de tuberculose multi-résistante aux médicaments.

Introduction

Tuberculosis (TB) poses major public health challenges and its incidence continues to increase in many parts of the world, especially in countries in sub-Saharan Africa (SSA). Based on estimates by the World Health Organization[1] (WHO), 9.27 million new TB cases (139 per 100 000 population) were diagnosed globally during 2007. It was estimated that 44% (4.1 million) of these cases

(61 per 100 000 population) were smear positive. Asia accounted for 55% of the global TB cases during 2007,[1] whilst Africa accounted for 31%.

In low-income countries with high rates of human immunodeficiency virus (HIV) infection, TB prevalence remains high. Although most countries have implemented the internationally-recommended directly-observed treatment short course strategy (DOTS), SSA continued to report high TB incidence and prevalence rates. Thirteen of the 15 countries with the highest estimated global TB incidence are in Africa.[1] Limited healthcare seeking behaviours on the part of the patients and shortages of healthcare professionals contribute to the TB prevalence rates in Africa.[2]

According to the 2008 WHO estimate,[1] Ethiopia ranks seventh amongst the countries with a high TB burden. According to Ethiopia's Ministry of Health,[3] TB is the major cause of morbidity in Ethiopia and the second-highest cause of mortality, superseded only by malaria. The incidence of all types of TB in Ethiopia totaled 379 diagnoses per 100 000 population in 2008, but only 40 794 smear-positive PTB cases were detected.[1] The highest case detection rate (76.7%) in Ethiopia was documented in the Gambella region and the lowest (20.3%) in the Somali region, whilst it was 68.3% in Addis Ababa, Ethiopia's capital city, during 2008. Mengiste et al.[4] also reported ineffective diagnosis and treatment of TB in the Tigray region of northern Ethiopia.

Understanding on the part of healthcare workers about the need for three sputum analyses for the diagnosis of TB, as well as its public health significance, is affected by their educational background, previous TB experience and knowledge of the national tuberculosis guidelines (NTG).[5] Healthcare providers' non-compliance with the NTG could contribute to discontent amongst patients and healthcare providers, misuse of scarce resources, a waste of time and missed opportunities for the early diagnosis of TB.[6]

A study conducted in Thailand revealed that 30% of TB patients were not diagnosed according to that country's NTG.[6,7] Non-adherence to the NTG included: (1) missing sputum smear examinations (6.8%); (2) TB diagnoses based on three sputum smear-negative results and chest x-ray abnormalities but without any antibiotic trials (12.5%); and (3) TB diagnoses based on fewer than three negative sputum smear results and chest x-ray findings (8.6%). Failure to adhere to NTG during the diagnosis and treatment of TB will increase the TB burden since there will be a higher risk of TB transmission, deterioration of TB patients and more cases of multi-drug resistant TB (MDR-TB).[7]

As many as 97.0% of the smear-negative PTB patients had diagnoses that did not comply with the NTG diagnostic procedures.[8] This author also reported that of these patients, 24.2% in one region of Ethiopia and 43.4% in another were treated as smear-negative PTB patients, without acid-fast bacillus (AFB) sputum microscopic examinations and without antibiotic trials.

Reportedly, 42.8% of TB diagnoses at Ethiopian hospitals and 60.8% of those at health centres were based on the NTG diagnostic criteria.[8] Complicated TB cases should be referred to hospitals since hospitals have better resources than clinics. If healthcare providers at hospitals fail to comply with the NTG, the patients' clinical condition might deteriorate, with the resultant increased risk of spreading TB and MDR-TB throughout Ethiopia.[7]

The recommended weight band classifications for the treatment of TB patients in Ethiopia are: 20 kg – 29 kg, 30 kg – 39 kg, 40 kg – 54 kg, 55 kg – 70 kg and ≥ 70 kg; and anti-TB drugs for all TB patients should be prescribed according to this classification.[9] In Malawi, a study revealed that 7% of TB patients were prescribed the incorrect number of pills in their anti-TB regimen.[10]

Problem statement

The Ethiopian Ministry of Health[2] reported that the national TB case detection rate in 2008 was only 33.9%. This was lower than the WHO's[1] global target of 70%. Ethiopia's 2008 case detection and treatment success rates were 33.9% and 84%, respectively.[2] This indicates the necessity of a prompt assessment of healthcare providers' implementation of the NTG, which could increase TB case detection rates, enhance timely and effective anti-TB treatment and reduce the prevalence of TB and MDR-TB in Ethiopia. Not only would the incidence and prevalence of TB in Ethiopia be decreased, but it would also reduce healthcare expenditure in this resource-limited country.

Aim of the study

The aim of this study was to assess implementation of the NTG by healthcare providers during diagnosis and treatment of TB patients; to recommend ways to improve TB treatment outcomes; and to reduce the number of patients suffering from TB and MDR-TB.

Research methods and design

Approach and design

A descriptive, cross-sectional, retrospective diagnostic audit of TB patients' medical records was undertaken in four public health facilities, namely, two hospitals and two health centres in Addis Ababa, the capital city of Ethiopia.

Study site

At the time of the data collection phase of this study, Addis Ababa had five public hospitals and 26 health centres, of which all 26 health centres and two of the regional hospitals were treating TB patients on the DOTS programme. The two participating health centres were selected randomly, whereas the two hospitals were selected purposively, as only those two regional hospitals provided DOTS services.

Study population and sample

The study population comprised newly-diagnosed TB patients who were at least 15 years old and who had commenced anti-TB treatment at the selected hospitals and clinics from March to November 2010. TB patients who had been diagnosed at other facilities were excluded because the procedures followed during diagnosis were unavailable. Known HIV-positive TB patients were excluded from the study since all HIV-positive persons are screened routinely for TB.

The sample size of 233 was calculated using a simple size determination for single proportion, using the following equation:

$$n = P(1-P)z^2/d^2 \quad \text{[Eqn 1]}$$

where,

n = sample size
P = the reliability coefficient 95%
d = 0.05 for the precision (based on providers' reported 45% adherence to the NTG during diagnosis and treatment in Tigray, Ethiopia[10])
z = confidence level or z-score of 1.96

These calculations indicated that a total of 212 patients' records needed to be audited. As some patients' medical records were expected to be unavailable, a 10% contingency was added, resulting in a final sample size of 233.

Proportionate sampling was used to allocate the records amongst the four participating public health facilities, based on the number of TB patients' records that met the inclusion criteria. The medical records that met all eligibility criteria were selected randomly, using a table of random numbers. Data were collected using a checklist based on the Ethiopian NTG. The checklist was pre-tested on 10 TB medical records that were excluded from the actual study. No problems were encountered during the pilot testing.

Data analysis

Data were transcribed anonymously from each TB patient's medical record, using the specifically-designed checklist. Transcribed information included symptoms suggesting TB; physical examinations and findings; laboratory and x-ray tests and their results; treatment with broad-spectrum antibiotics; age; sex; weight; and the types and dosages of drugs prescribed. Based on the documented clinical, physical and laboratory evidence, the diagnosis of each patient was compared with the diagnostic criteria specified by Ethiopia's NTG.

Ethical considerations

Permission to conduct the study was granted by the Research and Ethics Committee of the Department of Health Studies of the University of South Africa (certificate number 4205-680-2), the Addis Ababa Regional Health Bureau and each participating hospital or clinic, before data collection commenced.

Results

Of the 233 TB patients, 52.8% (n = 123) were men and 47.2% (n = 110) were women. Presenting complaints were recorded in 91% (n = 212), but the TB diagnoses had only been recorded in 9% (n = 21) of these patients' medical files. Coughs (71.2%; n = 151), chest pains (30.2%; n = 64), night sweats (29.2%; n = 62), fever (27.4%; n = 58) and loss of appetite (23.1%; n = 49) were the patients' most frequent reasons for visiting a healthcare facility, according to the other 212 patients' medical files.

The physical examination findings of only 53.2% (n = 124) of the patients had been recorded, implying that nothing had been recorded about the findings from the physical examination findings in the other patients' files (46.8%; n = 109).

The duration of illness was recorded in 80.8% (n = 122) of the files of the 151 patients who complained of coughing, showing that 68.9% (n = 104) had coughed for more than two weeks. Sputum smear examinations were done for 80.8% (n = 84) of these 104 patients, with 48.8% (n = 41) being sputum smear positive on two or more slides.

Healthcare providers correctly diagnosed 56.1% (n = 69) of the male and 60.9% (n = 67) of the female TB patients, according to the NTG. Of the 233 patients, 65.2% (n = 152) were diagnosed in hospitals and 34.8% (n = 81) at health centres. The diagnostic procedures followed the NTG criteria in 51.3% (n = 78) of the hospitals' patients. The percentage of correctly-diagnosed TB patients, complying with the NTG diagnostic criteria in hospitals, were, by type of TB: smear-positive PTB (93.3%; n = 14); smear-negative PTB (4.0%; n = 2); and extra-pulmonary TB (EPTB) (71.3%; n = 62). Similarly, in health centres, 97.5% (n = 39) of smear-positive PTB; 0% (n = 0) of smear-negative PTB and 60% (n = 9) of EPTB patients were diagnosed correctly in terms of the NTG diagnostic criteria (see Table 1). Of the smear-negative PTB patients, 25% (n = 19) were diagnosed using only radiological (x-ray) evidence.

TABLE 1a: Correctly-diagnosed new tuberculosis patients by type of health facility (n = 233).

Type of TB	Number of records reviewed		
	Hospital	Health centre	Total
Smear-positive PTB	15	40	55
Smear-negative PTB	50	26	76
EPTB	87	15	102
Total	**152**	**81**	**233**

TB, tuberculosis; PTB, pulmonary TB; EPTB, extra-pulmonary TB.

TABLE 1b: Correctly-diagnosed new tuberculosis patients by type of health facility (n = 233).

Type of TB	Diagnosed correctly					
	Hospital		Health centre		Total	
	f	%	*f*	%	*f*	%
Smear-positive PTB	14	93.3	39	97.5	53	96.4
Smear-negative PTB	2	4	0	0	2	2.6
EPTB	62	71.3	9	60	71	69.6
Total	**78**	**51.3**	**48**	**59.3**	**126**	**54.1**

f, frequency; TB, tuberculosis; PTB, pulmonary TB; EPTB, extra-pulmonary TB.

Of the 152 TB patients treated at hospitals, 88.2% (n = 134) had been prescribed the correct number of anti-TB pills. At health centres, 96.3% (n = 78) of the 81 patients had been prescribed the correct number of pills during the initial treatment, as is shown in Table 2.

Of the 21 TB patients who had been prescribed the incorrect number of anti-TB pills, 85.7% (n = 18) were from hospitals and of these, 77.8% (n = 14) had been prescribed doses lower than the NTG's recommendations. In health centres, 14.3% (n = 3) of the patients had been prescribed the incorrect number of pills, with 66.7% (n = 2) of these being prescribed anti-TB pills exceeding the NTG's recommended dosages.

The correct numbers of anti-TB pills, in compliance with the NTG treatment recommendations, were prescribed for 91.8% (n=101) of the 110 female TB patients and for 90.2% (n=111) of the 123 male patients. Of the 233 TB patients, 9% (n = 21) were prescribed the incorrect number of pills and of these, 71.4% (n = 15) were prescribed anti-TB pills below the recommended dose. The NTG recommends the prescription of anti-TB pills based on the TB patient's body weight and the guideline recommends one and a half, two, three, four or five anti-TB pills for a body weight of 20–29, 30–39, 40–54, 55–70 and over 70 kg, respectively.[1]

Mistakes with regard to the prescription of anti-TB medication were frequent in those TB patients whose pre-treatment weight band ranged from 55 kg to 70 kg – 22.6% (n = 14) of these 62 patients had been prescribed incorrect numbers of anti-TB pills. Of the 21 TB patients who had been prescribed incorrect anti-TB medication, 28.6% (n = 6) were over-prescribed, enhancing the possibilities of potential drug toxicities; and 71.4% (n = 15) were under-prescribed, which could have resulted in treatment failure.

Discussion

In 9% (n = 21) of the TB patients in the study, only their diagnosis had been recorded in the files. Such a dearth of information could impact negatively on communication amongst healthcare providers with regard to patients' continued care, treatment and follow-up examinations. This lack of information makes it impossible to compare TB patients' symptoms during and after treatment with their baseline symptoms. In addition, some records failed to portray the duration of the patients' complaints. The WHO[11,12] recommended 100% recording of patients' presenting complaints and physical examination findings in order to diagnose TB patients correctly. Failure to record patients' presenting complaints, the duration of illness and physical examination findings might affect the TB patient's treatment and prognosis.

Out of the 212 TB patients whose presenting complaints had been recorded, coughing was the most frequently occurring symptom (71.2%; n = 151), which finding was similar to the results of other studies.[13,14,15]

Bacteriological examination is the gold standard for TB diagnosis.[16,17] Ethiopia's NTG recommends that sputum smear examinations should be repeated in the following situations: (1) three sputum smear examinations were negative; or (2) only one sputum smear was positive before the diagnosis of PTB.[9] However, in this study, 3.6% (n = 2) of the TB patients were diagnosed with smear-positive PTB based on only one sputum smear-positive result, indicating non-adherence with the NTG and resulting in the potential for wrong diagnoses, treatments and the uncontrolled spread of TB.

Of the smear-negative PTB patients, 25% (n = 19) were diagnosed using only radiological evidence. This percentage was higher than the 6.9% reported in the Tigray region, but

TABLE 2: Prescription of initial anti-tuberculosis drugs by type of facility (n = 233).

Type of facility	TB patients prescribed incorrect numbers of anti-TB pills			Number and % of TB patients prescribed the correct number of anti-TB pills		Total	
	Dose too high	Dose too low	Total	*f*	%	*f*	%
Health centre	2	1	3	78	96.3	81	34.8
Hospital	4	14	18	134	88.2	152	65.2
Total	**6**	**15**	**21**	**212**	**91.0**	**233**	**100.0**

f, frequency; TB, tuberculosis.

TABLE 3: Prescription of initial anti-tuberculosis pills by weight band (n = 233).

Weight band in kg	Number of TB patients prescribed incorrect numbers of anti-TB pills			Number and % of TB patients prescribed correct numbers of anti-TB pills		Total	
	Dose too high	Dose too low	Total	*f*	%	*f*	%
20–29	0	0	0	0	0.0	0	0.0
30–39	4	0	4	14	77.8	18	7.7
40–54	2	0	2	150	98.7	152	65.2
55–70	0	14	14	48	77.4	62	26.6
Over 70	0	1	1	0	0.0	1	0.4
Total	**6**	**15**	**21**	**212**	**91.0**	**233**	**100.0**

f, frequency; TB, tuberculosis.

lower than the 41.4% reported in the Amhara region.[4,8,10] In 39.5% (n = 30) of the 76 smear-negative PTB patients, no sputum smear examinations were done. This might have resulted in wrong diagnoses of PTB because of the low specificity of clinical signs and radiological findings.[7]

There were no significant variations in the healthcare providers' level of implementation of the NTG during the diagnosis of TB patients in hospitals or clinics. There was also no major difference in implementation of the NTG treatment recommendations during the initial treatment of TB patients, irrespective of the TB patients' gender.

Implementation of the NTG initial anti-TB prescriptions of 91% (n = 212) was better than the 57.1% reported by a study in Thailand,[10] but lower than the 93% reported by a study in Malawi.[18]

Fewer healthcare providers at hospitals implemented the NTG during the initial prescribing of anti-TB medication than those at health centres. This could increase the risk of MDR-TB because of the inadequate administration of anti-TB drugs.[7] Both over- and under-prescription of TB drugs occurred which could lead to treatment failure, the spread of TB throughout communities and the development of MDR-TB. Over-prescription might aggravate the potential side effects of anti-TB drugs, especially hepatotoxicity, which could influence patients to discontinue their treatment, whilst under-prescription would not cure TB and could increase the number of MDR-TB sufferers in the specific communities and in Ethiopia in general.

Healthcare providers who do not implement the NTG treatment recommendations could cause increased numbers of MDR-TB cases in the country, which would have serious healthcare and budgetary consequences. MDR-TB patients require more sophisticated diagnostic and treatment facilities, posing affordability challenges in developing countries.[9] TB patients whose anti-TB drug dosages exceeded the NTG's recommendations, might encounter severe side effects, increasing the patients' risk of discontinuing their treatment and increasing the risk of MDR-TB.[19] Effective implementation of the NTG treatment recommendations could minimise the chances of TB patients progressing to MDR-TB.[1]

Conclusion

Healthcare providers' implementation levels of the NTG were low, as only 54.1% (n = 126) of diagnoses followed the NTG which could, in turn, contribute to the over-diagnosis of smear-negative PTB and EPTB. Although healthcare providers prescribed the correct regimens and types of anti-TB drugs, 9% (n = 21) of the 233 TB patients were prescribed an incorrect number of pills. Under-prescription could result in the increased transmission of TB and MDR-TB, whilst over-prescription could aggravate the drugs' side effects and cause patients to discontinue their treatment, potentially contributing to the number of MDR-TB cases in Ethiopia.

The healthcare providers' implementation of the NTG guidelines should be enhanced and sustained in order to prevent TB patients from developing and spreading MDR-TB. Reasons why healthcare professionals fail to implement the NTG should be investigated and addressed. For example, if laboratory or radiographic resources pose challenges to such implementation, these should be discussed with the local and regional healthcare authorities. The NTG might need to be adapted to make its implementation feasible within some resource-limited facilities, specifying referral guidelines to facilities with better resources.

A checklist should be included in every TB patient's file. This could save recording time as the healthcare provider would merely need to indicate the date and result of any test. The numbers and types of anti-TB pills to be prescribed for each weight band should also be indicated on this checklist. Then the healthcare provider would only need to identify the correct treatment (in terms of the patient's weight) and sign in the appropriate place. This could save much time in prescribing the correct treatment for uncomplicated PTB cases. The completion of the checklist, instead of writing paragraphs, could also facilitate and standardise future audits of patient records.

All patients' TB treatment outcomes should be audited on a regular basis. Identified shortcomings should be addressed during in-service education sessions. Regular audits of TB patients' medical records could contribute toward enhancing the healthcare professionals' implementation of the NTG. In addition, they could enhance the effectiveness of TB diagnosis and treatment in Ethiopia. This should contribute to early effective TB diagnoses and treatment, limiting the spread of TB in communities, enhancing the TB treatment outcomes, reducing the number of MDR-TB cases in Ethiopia and reducing healthcare costs.

Acknowledgements

We thank the Ethiopian authorities for permission to conduct this study. We also thank the managers of the participating healthcare facilities for making the patients' records available for data collection. In addition, we would like to acknowledge the fact that this article is based on the following unpublished dissertation of limited scope: Aragaw GS. 2011. Adherence by healthcare providers to Ethiopia's national tuberculosis guidelines. Master of Public Health dissertation. Pretoria: University of South Africa, College of Human Sciences, Department of Health Sciences.

Competing interests

The authors declare that they have no financial or personal relationship(s) which may have inappropriately influenced them in writing this article.

Authors' contributions

G.S.A. (University of South Africa) was the principal researcher who conceptualised the idea. V.J.E. (University of

South Africa) assisted with compiling the research proposal, literature review and instrument. G.S.A. collected the data, which were analysed with the assistance of a statistician. Both V.J.E. and G.S.A. interpreted and discussed the statistical findings and jointly wrote the article.

References

1. World Health Organization. Guideline for the programmatic management of drug-resistant tuberculosis. Emergency update [document on the Internet]. c2008 [cited 2009 Sep 05]. Available from: http://whqlibdoc.who.int/publications/2008/9789241547581_eng.pdf
2. Chaisson RE, Martinson NA. Tuberculosis in Africa – combating an HIV- driven crisis. NEJM. 2008;358:1089–1092. http://dx.doi.org/10.1056/NEJMp0800809
3. Abraha MW, Nigatu TH. Modeling trends of health and health related indicators in Ethiopia (1995–2008): a time-series study. Health Res Policy Syst. 2009;7:29. http://dx.doi.org/10.1186/1478-4505-7-29
4. Mengiste M, Tesfay T, Madeley R. The quality of tuberculosis diagnosis in districts of Tigray region of northern Ethiopia. Ethiop J Health Dev. 2005;7:13–20.
5. Shimeles E, Aseffa A, Yamuah H, et al. Knowledge and practice of private practitioners in TB control in Addis Ababa, Ethiopia. Int J Tuberc Lung Dis. 2006;10(10):1172–1177.
6. Marquez L. Helping healthcare providers perform according to standards [document on the Internet]. c2001 [cited 2014 Jun 06]. Available from: http://pdf.usaid.gov/pdf_docs/PNACN246.pdf
7. World Health Organization. Diagnostic and treatment delay in tuberculosis: an in-depth analysis of the health-seeking behaviour of patients and health system response in seven countries of the Eastern Mediterranean Region [document on the Internet]. c2006 [cited 2009 Sep 05]. Available from: http://www.emro.who.int/dsaf/dsa710.pdf
8. Birara T. Process evaluation of quality of care in the diagnosis and treatment of TB in Noth Wollo Zone of the Amhara region, Northern Ethiopia. Unpublished master's dissertation. Faculty of Science, Department of Health Studies. Jimma: Jimma University: 2007.
9. Ministry of Health (Ethiopia). Guideline for program and clinical management of drug resistant tuberculosis [document on the Internet]. c2009 [cited 2014 Jun 14]. Available from: www.etharc.org/resources/downloads/finish/66/367
10. Harries AD, Gausi F, Salaniponi FM. Prescriptions and dosages of anti-tuberculosis drugs in the National Tuberculosis Control Programme of Malawi. Int J Tuberc Lung Dis. 2004;8(6):724–729.
11. World Health Organization. Brief guide on tuberculosis control for primary health care providers [document on the Internet]. c2004 [cited 2009 Oct 24]. Available from: http://www.euro.who.int/document/e82858.pdf
12. World Health Organization. Pathway to better diagnostics for tuberculosis: a blueprint for the development of TB diagnostics [document on the Internet]. c2009 [cited 2010 Mar 05]. Available from: http://www.stoptb.org/wg/new_diagnostics/assets/documents/BluePrintTB_annex_web.pdf
13. Cambanis A, Ramsay A, Wirkom V, et al. Investing time in microscopy: an opportunity to optimise smear-based case detection of tuberculosis. Int J Tuberc Lung Dis. 2007;11(1):40–45.
14. Chung WS, Chang RE, Guo HR. Variations of care quality for infectious pulmonary tuberculosis in Taiwan: a population based cohort study. BMC Public Health. 2007;7:107. http://dx.doi.org/10.1186/1471-2458-7-107
15. Farah MG, Rygh JH, Steen TW, et al. Patient and health care system delays in the start of tuberculosis treatment in Norway. BMC Infect Dis. 2006;6:33. http://dx.doi.org/10.1186/1471-2334-6-33
16. Canan ED, Tanrikulu AC, Acemoglu H, et al. A multicentre study of doctors' approaches to the diagnosis and treatment of tuberculosis in Turkey. J Infect Dev Ctries. 2009;3(5):357–364.
17. World Health Organization. International standards for tuberculosis care [document on the Internet]. c2006 [cited 2009 Nov 21]. Available from: http://www.who.int/management/quality/standards/InternationalStandardsTBCare.pdf
18. Thongraung W, Chongsuvivatwong V, Pungrassamee P. Multilevel factors affecting tuberculosis diagnosis and initial treatment. J Eval Clin Pract. 2008;14(3):378–384. http://dx.doi.org/10.1111/j.1365-2753.2007.00871.x
19. Jittimanee SX, Madigan EA, Jittimanee S, et al. Treatment default among urban tuberculosis patients, Thailand. Int J Nurs Pract. 2007;13(6):354–362. http://dx.doi.org/10.1111/j.1440-172X.2007.00650.x

Patient satisfaction at accredited antiretroviral treatment sites in the Gert Sibande District

Authors:
Selente Bezuidenhout[1]
Damilola A. Ogunsanwo[1]
Elvera A. Helberg[1]

Affiliations:
[1]Department of Pharmacy, University of Limpopo, Medunsa Campus, South Africa

Correspondence to:
Selente Bezuidenhout

Email:
selente.bezuidenhout@ul.ac.za

Postal address:
PO Box 218, Department of Pharmacy, Medunsa 0204, South Africa

Background: Patient satisfaction has been used as a significant indicator of quality services provided by healthcare personnel. With the largest antiretroviral therapy (ART) programme in the world, the healthcare industry is struggling increasingly with challenges of meeting patients' requirements and expectations for quality ART service provision. This study was conducted in order to identify the importance of factors contributing to satisfaction or dissatisfaction.

Aim: This study sought to explore and describe the general satisfaction or dissatisfaction of patients with accredited ART hospital sites at public health facilities in the Gert Sibande District, Mpumalanga and to identify factors contributing to either satisfaction or dissatisfaction.
Setting: Six hospitals that initiated ART in the district, participated in the study.

Method: The study was conducted using a sample of 300 patients. Proportional random sampling was used in selecting the number of patients from each facility. A structured interview with each participating patient was conducted using a standardised structured questionnaire. The first available required number of patients that complied with requirements from each of the six hospitals was selected for the interview. Descriptive statistics were used to analyse data and data with qualitative aspects were captured and categorised manually.

Results: The major factors contributing to satisfaction included the availability of medicines and knowledge regarding how to take medication. Factors contributing to dissatisfaction on the part of the patients included confidentiality issues, long waiting periods, shortage of staff and dirty toilets.

Conclusion: This study indicated general satisfaction with the ART-related services at the accredited ART hospital sites in the Gert Sibande District. Regular monitoring and evaluation are recommended.

Satisfaction des patients aux centres de traitement antiviral accrédités dans le District Gert Sibande, dans la Province du Mpumalanga.

Contexte: La satisfaction des patients a été utilisée comme indicateur principal des services de qualité donnés par le personnel soignant. Avec le programme le plus vaste de thérapie antirétrovirale (ART) du monde, le secteur médical se trouve confronté de plus en plus aux défis de satisfaire les besoins et les attentes des patients demandant des prestations de service ART de qualité. Cette étude a été menée afin d'identifier l'importance des facteurs contribuant à la satisfaction ou au mécontentement des patients.

Objectifs: Cette étude s'est efforcée d'étudier et de décrire la satisfaction ou le mécontentement général des patients dans les services de santé publique avec des services ART accrédités dans le District Gert Sibande au Mpumalanga et d'identifier les facteurs qui contribuent à la satisfaction ou au mécontentement des patients.

Lieu: Six hôpitaux qui ont mis en place ART dans le district, ont participé à l'enquête.

Méthode: L'enquête s'est faite sur un échantillon de 300 patients. On a utilisé l'échantillonnage aléatoire proportionnel pour sélectionner le nombre de patients de chaque endroit. On a eu une entrevue structurée avec chaque patient participant à l'aide d'un questionnaire normalisé et structuré. On a sélectionné pour les entrevues le nombre requis de patients conformes aux exigences dans chacun des six hôpitaux. On a utilise les statistiques descriptives pour analyser les données, puis on a saisi les données aux aspects qualitatifs et on les a classées manuellement par catégories.

Résultats: Les facteurs principaux contribuant à la satisfaction des patients comprenaient la disponibilité des médicaments et les connaissances de base sur la façon de les utiliser. Les facteurs contribuant au mécontentement des patients comprenaient les questions de confidentialité, les longues attentes, la pénurie de personnel et les toilettes sales.

Conclusion: Cette étude a montré une satisfaction générale envers les services ART aux hôpitaux accrédités d'ART dans le district Gert Sibande. Il est recommandé de faire des évaluations et des contrôles réguliers.

Introduction

The Operational Plan for Comprehensive Human Immunodeficiency Virus (HIV) and Acquired Immune Deficiency Syndrome (AIDS) Care, Management and Treatment (CCMT), was approved by the South African government in 2003. This plan provided for free antiretroviral treatment (ART) at public health facilities.[1] According to the 2013 Global Update on HIV Treatment, more than 2.1 million people were receiving ART in South Africa.[2] This high number of patients who qualify for ART increases the workload of the public healthcare system.[3]

Patient satisfaction has become an important performance and outcome measure of healthcare. In a debilitated healthcare system, it is important to ensure quality of care and patient satisfaction in order to make the best use of limited resources.[4,5] The provision of ART using the public health system can transform HIV infection from a fast, deadly disease into a manageable chronic illness.[6] However, in resource-limited settings, there are many challenges to successfully scaling-up ART and reorienting service delivery toward chronic disease care. Patient satisfaction surveys can be of benefit to health professionals with regard to identifying areas where service delivery and health expenditure can be improved.[7] South Africa has the largest ART programme in the world and, as ART treatment access is improving, public health benefits are also increased. Six-month mortality amongst patients at a HIV treatment centre in the Western Cape Province was reduced from 12.7% to 6.6% between 2003 and 2005.[8]

Mpumalanga has the second-highest prevalence of HIV in South Africa. It is estimated that about 10% of the overall population in the Mpumalanga Province lives with HIV. The Gert Sibande District has an HIV prevalence of 40.5%, which is the highest in the Mpumalanga Province. By the end of November 2011, 32 979 patients were receiving ART in the Gert Sibande District.[9]

All Primary Health Care (PHC) clinics and Community Health Centres (CHCs) in the District have been prepared for ART readiness by the provincial government since April 2010.

Although previous studies conducted in the Free State[10] and KwaZulu-Natal[11] showed high patient satisfaction with ART-accredited sites, the aim of this study was to determine patient satisfaction with ART-accredited hospital-based sites in the Gert Sibande District, Mpumalanga Province and to identify the factors contributing to either satisfaction or dissatisfaction. This was important in order to define service areas that required improvement and to assist hospital management with regard to targeting interventions for quality improvement.

Research methods and design

Study design

The study adopted a quantitative approach using a cross-sectional descriptive design, where data were collected in the form of researcher-administered questionnaires.

Study sites

The study was conducted at all five district hospitals (Embhuleni, Piet Retief, Carolina, Bethal and Standerton) and at one regional hospital (Ermelo) in the Gert Sibande District.

Study population

The target population included all patients on ART who attended the six hospitals.

Sample selection

According to 2011 hospital statistics supplied by the different hospital administration departments, a total number of 695 patients on ART attended these six hospitals on a daily basis. Sample size estimation was performed using nQueryAdvisor, Release 6.0 (Elashoff 2005). The required sample size for 695 patients was at least 248. A sample of 300 patients was studied. With a sample size of 300, a two-sided 95% confidence interval for the proportion of satisfied subjects, using the normal approximation, extended a distance of 0.05 from the observed proportion (calculated from the sample). The expected proportion of satisfied subjects was in the range of 0.65–0.75 (65% – 75%). Proportional random sampling was used to determine the number of patients to be included in the study from each hospital site according to the number of patients attending each hospital site daily. Convenience sampling was used further in order to recruit the required number of patients from each hospital site.

Inclusion criteria

Patients over 18 years who had received ART for at least four months or longer and were collecting repeat medication were included in the study. The first available required number of patients (sample of convenience) that complied with the criteria from each of the six hospitals, who were willing to participate and who provided consent, completed the questionnaire.

Data collection

An interview with each participating patient was conducted by using a standardised structured questionnaire. The data collection tool was adapted from a patient exit interview questionnaire that the Pharmacy Department uses and updates every year in order to collect data from PHC Clinics as part of the Research Module in the BPharm curriculum.[12] However, validity of this questionnaire was again tested during a pilot study that was conducted before the actual research data collection, just to be sure that all questions asked were understood correctly and that the trained data collectors were satisfied with the responses to the questions. The method of data collection from participating patients was selected because of the possibility of differences in patients' literacy levels. The questionnaire comprised sections on sociodemographics, general facility and healthcare provision, communication and medicine management.

The required number of patients was recruited whilst they were waiting for medication at the pharmacy waiting area. Information leaflets were distributed in the waiting area and the interview took place in the pharmacy's private consulting room prior to the patients receiving their medication. The study was explained to the patients and consent forms were provided. Patient questionnaires, information leaflets and consent forms were translated into siSwati (translation–back-translation process). The questionnaire was administered in English. A data collector was trained in data collection and interviewing and administered a translated version in siSwati (the main language spoken in Gert Sibande) to the patients when necessary. The sequence of events was practised so as to ensure that all questionnaires were administered in the same way. All responses in siSwati were translated to English through the translation-back-translation process. All the included patients participated both voluntarily and anonymously.

Data analysis

The data that were collected during the study were captured in a Microsoft Excel® 2010 spreadsheet. Data capturing was verified and validity checks were performed. Data were then analysed using descriptive statistics. Responses to categorical variables were summarised as frequency counts and percentages. All statistical procedures were performed on the Statistical Analysis System (SAS), Release 9.2 or higher (SAS Institute Inc. 2008), running on Microsoft Windows Vista®. Responses to open-ended questions were captured and categorised, which allowed for the counting of responses where appropriate.

Ethical considerations

Ethical approval was obtained from the Medunsa Research and Ethics Committee (MREC/H/14/2011: PG). Approval was also obtained from the Chief Executive Officers at each of the different hospitals, the District Manager of the Gert Sibande District and the Mpumalanga Ethics and Research Committee.

Informed consent was obtained from the patients before participation in the study and the patients were informed that they may withdraw from the study without negative consequences. Interviews were conducted in a private consultation area in order to ensure privacy, safety and confidentiality. The questionnaires were anonymous – the identity of patients was not disclosed and patients were informed of this fact. Data were handled with confidentiality and controlled access to data forms was ensured by keeping the completed questionnaires locked away.

Results

The majority of the patients (n = 165; 55%) fell within the 31–45 year age category. Gender distribution showed that there were 202 women on treatment (69%) compared with 91 (31%) men. The patients had an education level ranging from Grades 8 to 12 and the majority of patients (n = 244; 82%) could both read and write. However, 61% (n = 181) were unemployed (Table 1).

Of the total number of patients interviewed, 169 (56%) reported not seeing the same healthcare provider whilst 131 (44%) consulted with the same healthcare provider each time. Of all the patients interviewed, 290 (97%) reported that they had privacy during their clinic consultation and the majority (n = 293; 98%) of patients also reported that their medical records were kept confidential. A high number of the patients surveyed (n = 284; 95%) found their ART site to be convenient to them and 258 (86%) of patients found the waiting area suitable for them whilst waiting for their appointment (Table 2).

TABLE 1: Socio-demographic characteristics of patients.

Characteristics	Frequency	Percentage
Age (n = 299)*		
18–30	90	30.1
31–45	165	55.2
46–60	42	14.0
61 +	2	0.7
Gender (n = 293)*		
Male	91	31.1
Female	202	68.9
Education level (n = 299)*		
Below Grade 7	81	27.1
Grades 8–12	208	69.6
Tertiary education	10	3.3
Literacy level (n = 298)*		
Cannot read or write	42	14.1
Only read	4	1.3
Only write	8	2.7
Read and write	244	81.9
Socio-economic status (n = 296)*		
Employed	115	38.9
Unemployed	181	61.1
Patients with a disability (physical, intellectual and/or mental) (n = 298)*		
Yes	24	8.1
No	274	91.9

*, n < 300 – not all patients answered the specific question.

TABLE 2: General facility and healthcare provision.

Characteristics	Frequency	Percentage
Attended by the same healthcare provider each time (n = 300)		
Yes	131	43.7
No	169	56.3
Privacy during examination (n = 300)		
Yes	290	96.7
No	10	3.3
Confidentiality of medical records (n = 300)		
Yes	293	97.7
No	7	2.3
Convenience of ART hospital site (n = 300)		
Yes	284	94.7
No	16	5.3
Attendance to patients on a first come, first help basis (n = 300)		
Yes	268	89
No	32	11
Suitability of waiting area (n = 299)*		
Yes	258	86.3
No	41	13.7

ART, antiretroviral therapy.
*, n < 300 – not all patients answered the specific question.

The majority of the patients (n = 289; 96%) reported that their healthcare provider spoke their language. Most of the patients interviewed (n = 293; 98%) agreed that their healthcare provider listened to their problems. Table 3 shows that 93% (n = 279) of the patients had an opportunity to ask their healthcare provider questions and 98% (n = 292) of the patients were satisfied with the explanations provided. Table 3 also indicates that 293 (98%) of the patients reported that the healthcare provider who attended to them was polite and 294 (98%) of the patients were asked to return to the hospital site at a specific time.

Of the patients surveyed, 297 (99%) reported that medicines are always available to them every time they visit the hospital for their repeat treatment. The majority (n = 252; 85%) of the patients collected their tuberculosis (TB) and/or other chronic medication on the same day as their visit to the ART clinic. All the patients across the ART facilities indicated that the pharmacist was the dispenser of their medicines during consultation and the majority (n = 294; 99%) of the patients understood the directions on the labels of the medicines. Table 4 also indicates that 244 (81%) of the patients preferred to collect their medication at the main pharmacy and 292 (97%) found their medicines easy to administer.

Over all, reflections from the patients interviewed on satisfaction of care in the facilities showed that the majority (n = 297; 98%) of the patients were satisfied with the care they receive from the ART sites and 95% (n = 283) said that they would come again. However, 180 (61%) of the patients would like to be referred to institutions closer to them and 232 (78%) found transport to be difficult.

Discussion

Patient satisfaction is one of the vital components for the success of any healthcare service, especially in ART units which play a vital role in the lives of thousands of HIV patients.

The majority of patients were between the ages of 31 and 45, which represents a large percentage of the active South African workforce.[13] This emphasises the importance of ensuring adequate ART coverage in this population in order to maintain South Africa's economic integrity. Almost 69% of the patients interviewed were women, which is consistent with previous studies showing that more women than men are receiving ART. Biologically, women are twice more likely to become infected with HIV through unprotected heterosexual intercourse than men and therefore more women present at treatment centres.[14] In addition, a review of the literature has indicated that men attend ART clinics less frequently than women and they are generally initiated on ART later in the course of their infection. However, the main causes for this gender gap have not yet been explained in full.[15]

The educational level of patients revealed that 70% had between Grade 8 and Grade 12 formal educational levels.

TABLE 3: Communication.

Characteristics	Frequency	Percentage
Healthcare provider speak your language (n = 300)		
Yes	289	96.3
No	11	3.7
Healthcare provider listens to problems (n = 300)		
Yes	293	97.7
No	7	2.3
Healthcare provider gives opportunity to patients to ask questions (n = 299)*		
Yes	279	93.3
No	20	6.7
Patient satisfaction with answers by healthcare provider (n = 299)*		
Yes	292	97.7
No	7	2.3
Politeness of healthcare provider (n = 300)		
Yes	293	97.7
No	7	2.3
Explanation of CD4 + count to patients (n = 300)		
Yes	276	92.0
No	24	8.0
Healthcare provider asks patient to return to hospital site at a specific time (n = 300)		
Yes	294	98
No	6	2

*, n < 300 – not all patients answered the specific question.

TABLE 4: Medicine management.

Characteristics	Frequency	Percentage
Patients receiving medication on time (n = 300)		
Yes	297	99
No	3	1
Collection of tuberculosis and/or chronic medicines at the same time (n = 297)*		
Yes	252	84.8
No	45	15.2
Person dispensing medicines (n = 298)*		
Pharmacist	298	100
Other	0	0
Clear directions on label (n = 298)*		
Yes	294	98.7
No	4	1.3
Knowledge regarding the administration of medication (n = 300)		
Yes	292	97
No	8	3
Collection of medication from the main pharmacy preferred (n = 300)		
Yes	244	81.3
No	56	18.7

*, n < 300 – not all patients answered the specific question.

TABLE 5: Satisfaction or dissatisfaction with care.

Characteristics	Frequency	Percentage
Would you come to this facility again? (n = 299)*		
Yes	283	94.6
No	16	5.3
Transport to facility difficult (n = 297)*		
Yes	232	78.1
No	65	21.9
Patients who want to be transferred to other institutions (n = 296)*		
Yes	180	60.8
No	116	39.2
General satisfaction or dissatisfaction with care at facility (n = 297)*		
Satisfied	290	97.6
Dissatisfied	7	2.4

*, n < 300 – not all patients answered the specific question.

Almost 82% of patients could read and write. This high literacy level may be a result of the fact that about 70% of patients had formal education. A high rate of unemployment (61%) was also found amongst the patients and this is more than double the average unemployment rate for South Africa (25%) as revealed by the Statistics South Africa Report in 2011.[16] However, reasons for unemployment, whether it was the disease or a disability grant or something else, were not investigated.

General facility and healthcare provision

Less than half of the patients were seen by the same healthcare provider each time they visited the ART hospital sites. This might be because, in most cases, human resource shortages are experienced at the ART hospital sites as there are no specific doctors dedicated to the ART sites in some facilities. However, all the patients interviewed at Carolina Hospital (100%) *did* consult with the same healthcare provider, who was specifically employed for the ART site by a non-governmental organisation (NGO) partnering with government.

Privacy during medical examination and confidentiality of medical records are factors that are of utmost importance to patients. Table 2 showed that 97% of the patients indicated privacy during medical examinations and 98% of patients perceived that their medical records were kept confidential. Confidentiality is very important as it promotes confidence between the patient and the doctor. Patients are most likely to provide accurate information when they are not worried about public exposure.

Patients were attended to in the clinics on a first-come-first-serve basis and 86% found the waiting area of the hospital site to be both suitable and comfortable. The reason attributed to this high rate of suitability is the fact that most of the ART site structures were either renovated or donated by NGOs via the USA President's Emergency Plan for AIDS Relief (PEPFAR) funds.

The majority of the patients surveyed indicated that they had to wait for at least one hour before being attended to. Human resource shortages such as doctors and nurses were a factor highlighted by the patients who complained about long waiting times at the clinics. This result is comparable to a previous study carried out by Wouters et al.[10] which identified lack of human resources as being a causal factor for long waiting times.

Communication

The majority of the patients reported that they were, in general, satisfied regarding communication with the attending healthcare provider. Almost all patients (98%) interviewed responded that their healthcare providers were polite to them during their consultation. These results are similar to another South African study by Magoro et al.[17] where patients reported that doctors and nurses were kind, polite, respectful, and attentive during consultations. A patient satisfaction survey conducted in Singapore by Molina et al.[18] reported that the courtesy and respect displayed by doctors has a positive impact on patient satisfaction. Also, patients are more likely to miss appointments or to fail to follow medical advice when poor communication exists.[18]

Medicine management

All but three patients across all the ART hospital sites received their medication on time every month at the pharmacy with few or no complaints. The results of this study agree with a similar study carried out by Karunamoorthi et al. in Addis Ababa, where 73% of the patients were very satisfied with the pharmacy service.[19]

Eighty-five percent of the patients collected their TB and/or other chronic medication on the same day at the same pharmacy, as the services at these sites are integrated. This result implied that patients would not have to come to the clinic twice which saved them time and money, an important consideration in their socio-economic background.

An additional factor that could also be linked to the patient satisfaction at ART hospital sites is that the majority of patients (98%) understood the directions on the labels clearly, which implied that they knew how to take their medication. This might be linked to the high literacy levels of the patients. From the individual questions, patients from all the ART sites showed adequate knowledge regarding all their treatment regimen categories. The patients described the exact quantities and frequency of usage of their treatment regimens. The high literacy level of the patients and clear directions on the medicine labels may be responsible for this trend.

The majority of the patients (81%) preferred to collect their medicines from the main pharmacy rather than a pharmacy that is separated from the general outpatient pharmacy.

Satisfaction or dissatisfaction with care

The overall satisfaction of patients included in this study was very high (98%), as is seen with respect to the general ART care provided by the facilities. This result is similar to that obtained in a study of an ART programme in the Free State.[10]

A study carried out by Chimbindi, Bärnighausen and Newell[11] on patient satisfaction with HIV treatment and TB care in rural KwaZulu-Natal, South Africa showed that overall patient satisfaction was high but patients expressed some dissatisfaction with certain dimensions of the quality of care, including an inability to talk to health workers about their treatment and problems, time spent in queues waiting to be examined and facility cleanliness.

In this study, although 95% of the patients found their ART hospital site to be convenient and were happy with the services they received at the ART hospital sites, 78% experienced transport problems and 61% indicated that they would rather transfer to a facility closer to their home.

The reasons why seven (2%) patients indicated dissatisfaction with services included human resource shortages (especially doctors and nurses), bad staff attitude (such as impoliteness on the part of the nurses), non-protection of their confidentiality and dirty toilets.

Limitations to the study

The fact that participants in this study may have answered questions to please the interviewer is acknowledged. It is also acknowledged that at another time or under other circumstances, the outcomes may be different. Although proportional random sampling was used to determine the number of patients at each ART hospital site, convenience sampling was used to select the required number of patients at the ART hospital site and the sample might not be representative.

Conclusion

The findings of this study indicated general high satisfaction of patients with the ART-related services at the accredited ART sites in the Gert Sibande District. The major factors contributing to satisfaction included the availability of medicines, knowledge regarding how to take their medication and general satisfaction with providers. The major factors contributing to dissatisfaction (mentioned by seven respondents) included waiting too long, confidentiality issues, shortage of staff and dirty toilets.

Despite many efforts and successes with satisfaction measurement, evidence shows that more work in this area is still needed. One of the primary challenges has been in sustaining patient/customer satisfaction improvement initiatives in the face of competing priorities and diminishing resources. Patient satisfaction is important if service improvement is to be translated into outcomes meaningful to patients, especially improved quality of life.

It is therefore recommended that the results of this study be analysed and incorporated into the service planning process of the department and the departmental policy makers integrate the learning opportunities from patient feedback into their quality improvement plans. This, together with a successful down-referral system where a large population of stable ART patients at treatment-initiation sites could be down-referred, will increase capacity and will also reduce long waiting times and save the patient money. A regular monitoring and evaluation plan is also recommended.

Acknowledgements

The authors would like to thank Prof Rob Summers for reviewing the draft manuscript.

Competing interests

The authors declare that they have no financial or personal relationship(s) which may have inappropriately influenced them in writing this article.

Authors' contributions

S.B. (University of Limpopo) was the supervisor and was responsible for manuscript preparation. D.O. (Pharmaceutical Services, Gert Sibande District) was the data collector and E.H. (University of Limpopo) was responsible for the editing of the draft manuscript.

References

1. Department of Health. Monitoring and evaluation framework for the comprehensive HIV and AIDS care, management and treatment plan for South Africa. Pretoria: Department of Health; 2004.
2. World Health Organization, UNAIDS, UNICEF. Global update on HIV treatment 2013: results, impact and opportunities. [document on the Internet]. 2013 [cited 2014 Apr 23]. Available from: http://www.unaids.org/en/media/unaids/contentassets/documents/unaidspublication/2013/20130630_treatment_report_en.pdf
3. Dieleman M, Bwete V, Maniple E, et al. 'I believe that the staff have reduced their closeness to patients': an exploratory study on the impact of HIV/AIDS on staff in four rural hospitals in Uganda. BMC Health Serv Res. 2007;7:205. http://dx.doi.org/10.1186/1472-6963-7-205
4. Cowing M, Davino-Ramaya CM, Ramaya K, et al. Health care delivery performance: Service, outcomes, and resource stewardship. Perm J. 2009;13(4):72–78.
5. The Health Boards Executive. Measurement of patient satisfaction guidelines: health strategy implementation project 2003. [page on the Internet] 2003 [cited 2010 Aug 10]. Available from: http://www.lenus.ie/hse/handle/10147/43559?locale=ga
6. Abdool Karim SS, Abdool Karim Q, Baxter C. Overview of the book. In: Abdool Karim SS, Abdool Karim Q, editors. HIV/AIDS in South Africa. Cambridge: Cambridge University Press, 2005; pp. 37–47.
7. Ilioudi S, Lazakidou A, Tsironi M. Importance of patient satisfaction measurement and electronic surveys: methodology and potential benefits. International Journal of Health Research and Innovation. 2013;1(1):67–87.
8. Boulle A, Bock P, Osler M, et al. Antiretroviral therapy and early mortality in South Africa. Bull World Health Organ. 2008;86(9):678–687. http://dx.doi.org/10.2471/BLT.07.045294
9. Mpumalanga Department of Health. Gert Sibande District Health Plan 2011/2012. Gert Sibande District: Mpumalanga Province; 2010.
10. Wouters E, Heunis C, Van Rensburg D, et al. Patient satisfaction with antiretroviral services at primary health-care facilities in the Free State, South Africa – a two-year study using four waves of cross-sectional data. BMC Health Serv Res. 2008;8:210. http://dx.doi.org/10.1186/1472-6963-8-210
11. Chimbindi N, Bärnighausen T, Newell M-L. Patient satisfaction with HIV treatment and TB care in rural KwaZulu-Natal, South Africa: a Researching Equity in Access to Healthcare (REACH) study. [document on the Internet] 2009 [cited 2014 Apr 23]. Available from: http://www.africacentre.ac.za/Portals/0/News%20Archive/SA%20AIDS%20Conf%202011/10%20NatsayiChimbindi.pdf
12. Department of Pharmacy: University of Limpopo (Medunsa Campus), Department of Pharmaceutical Sciences: Tshwane University of Technology. Module 1.7: Experiential learning: research methodology and primary health care. Staff Guide; 2011.
13. Carapinha R. South Africa: Statistical Profile. [document on the Internet: password access only] 2009 [cited 2014 Apr 19]. Available from: http://www.bc.edu.proxy.bc.edu/content/dam/files/research_sites/agingandwork/pdf/publications/CP11_Workforce_SouthAfrica.pdf
14. Sachdeva RK, Wanchu A. Women's issues in HIV infection. JK Science, 2008;8(3):129–132.
15. Cornell M. Gender inequality: bad for men's health. S Afr J HIV Med. 2013;14(1):12–14. http://dx.doi.org/10.7196/sajhivmed.894
16. Statistics South Africa. Mid-year population estimates. Statistical release P0302. Pretoria: Stats SA; 2011.
17. Magoro MT, Hoque, ME, Van der Heever H. ART patients' satisfaction level regarding comprehensive HIV and AIDS care management and antiretroviral treatment programme in Pretoria. South Afr J Epidemiol Infect. 2012;27(2):71–75.
18. Molina JA, Lim GH, Seow E, et al. Effects of survey mode on results of a patient satisfaction survey at the observation unit of an acute care hospital in Singapore. Ann Acad Med Singapore. 2009;38(6):487–493.
19. Karunamoorthi K, Rajalakshmi M, Babu SM, et al. HIV/AIDS patient's satisfactory and their expectations with pharmacy service at specialist antiretroviral therapy (ART) units. Eur Rev Med Pharmacol Sci. 2009;13(5):331–339.

18

African Primary Care Research: Qualitative interviewing in primary care

Authors:
Steve Reid[1]
Bob Mash[2]

Affiliations:
[1]Primary Health Care Directorate, University of Cape Town, South Africa

[2]Family Medicine and Primary Care, Stellenbosch University, South Africa

Correspondence to:
Steve Reid

Email:
steve.reid@uct.ac.za

Postal address:
Primary Health Care Directorate, Old Main Building, Groote Schuur Hospital E47-66, Observatory 7925, Cape Town, South Africa

This article is part of a series on African Primary Care Research and focuses on the topic of qualitative interviewing in primary care. In particular it looks at issues of study design, sample size, sampling and interviewing in relation to individual and focus group interviews. There is a particular focus on helping postgraduate students at a Masters level to write their research proposals.

Recherche africaine dans le domaine des soins primaires: interviews qualitatives dans le domaine des soins primaires. Cet article fait partie d'une série sur la Recherche africaine dans le Domaine des Soins primaires et se concentre sur le thème des interviews qualitatives dans le domaine des soins primaires. On y examine la conception de l'étude, la taille des échantillons, les échantillons et les interviews des individus et groupes cibles. On s'efforce particulièrement à aider les étudiants licenciés au niveau de la Maitrise à rédiger leurs propositions de recherche.

Introduction

This article is part of a series on Primary Care Research and deals with qualitative interviewing and the issues to consider when writing your research proposal. Other articles in the series outline how to write a proposal, ethical considerations, how to perform a literature review and qualitative data analysis, amongst other topics.

Qualitative research is helpful with regard to exploring a phenomenon or a behaviour that is poorly understood, in order to interpret it from the perspective of those who have a direct involvement.[1] In contrast to quantitative studies, in which certain variables are controlled and others compared, qualitative studies create deeper understanding by allowing for contextual issues to be included in the data, even including the background and person of the researcher and the process of data collection itself.

Mixed-methods research, in which both quantitative and qualitative methods are used, combines the strengths of both approaches by describing the whole picture as fully as possible.[2] The sequence is debatable: exploratory qualitative studies can provide insight into a phenomenon and the important variables in that context that can then be quantified in a subsequent study. Qualitative process evaluation can also provide insight into why a particular intervention, that might have been observed originally or measured quantitatively, works or does not work in that context. The two types of studies produce different data: quantitative studies produce numerical data and statistics that are illustrated in tables and graphs, whereas qualitative studies produce textual data and themes that can be illustrated by selected quotes and conceptual diagrams.

Study design

Most qualitative studies are descriptive in nature and use interviews, participant observation or ethnography (the study of a phenomenon or disease in a particular cultural framework, usually over a period of time) to gain an in-depth understanding of behaviour.[3,4]

The two interview methods used in qualitative research are individual interviews of key informants and focus group discussions (FGDs). The same principles of the qualitative approach apply to both forms of interview, which aim to explore the interviewee's perspective of the world and the meaning that they make of it.[5]

FGDs are a form of group interview that capitalise on communication between research participants in order to generate data on collective views, as well as the meanings that lie behind those views. They are used widely to examine people's experiences of disease and of health services and are an effective technique for exploring the attitudes or needs of staff. Although group interviews are often used simply as a quick and convenient way to collect data from several people simultaneously, focus groups explicitly use group interaction as part of the method. This means that instead of the researcher asking each person to respond to a question in turn, people are encouraged to talk to one another: asking questions, exchanging anecdotes and commenting on each other's experiences and points of view. The method is particularly useful for exploring people's knowledge and experiences and can be used to examine not only *what* people think, but *how* they think and *why* they think that way. They also have advantages for researchers in the field of health and medicine since they do not discriminate against people who cannot read or write and they can encourage participation from people who are reluctant to be interviewed on their own or who feel they have nothing to say.

Another aspect of study design is the degree of structure one chooses, from structured to semi-structured, to unstructured or open-ended interviews. Structured interviews are, essentially, verbally-administered questionnaires in which a list of predetermined questions are asked, with little or no variation and with no scope for follow-up questions to responses that warrant further elaboration.

Most qualitative researchers design semi-structured interviews using a predetermined interview guide that sets out the broad issues that are assumed to be important through a sequence of open-ended questions. Developing an interview guide requires careful consideration of the main research question and its constituent parts; and particular attention needs to be given to their phrasing. The initial open question in the interview guide can reflect the overall research question of the study almost directly, whilst subsequent questions will probe specific aspects of the issue under discussion. Questions should move from general to more specific questions and the order should be relative to the importance of issues in the research agenda. It is important that each question is structured in an open-ended way so as to avoid one-word answers and encourage elaboration.

Unstructured or open-ended interviews do not reflect any preconceived theories or ideas and require greater skill. Such an interview may simply start with an opening question such as *'Can you tell me about your experience of x?'* and will then progress, based primarily upon the initial response, using techniques described below under the heading 'The Interview'.

Sample size

The number of interviewees does not need to be as large as in quantitative studies. The idea is to try to get an in-depth understanding of a phenomenon from a few perspectives, each of which is unique, as opposed to determining the average and the range for a predetermined set of variables. A sample size of one has even been used, since one person's particular experience can raise a wide range of issues that may not have been considered previously.

Generally for individual interviews, a sample size of between five and 15 interviewees is adequate to obtain a sufficient range of responses and experiences, until a level of so-called data 'saturation' is reached, beyond which no significantly new information is being produced. This can be discussed by the research team after each batch of five interviews has been completed and a decision can be made regarding whether or not to continue. An alternative approach to the size of the sample is to perform a preliminary analysis of the data after each interview, developing new ideas and hypotheses in an iterative process which can then be tested in subsequent interviews.

For FGDs, a group size of between five and eight people is advised, but they can work successfully with as few as three and as many as 15 participants. It may, however, be necessary to invite more than eight in case some do not come. A diversity of views is useful, but it is important to be aware of power dynamics in a group, such as between nurses and doctors. With gender-sensitive issues, for example, it may be better to hold FGDs with women and men separately. The profile and diversity of interviewees needs to be carefully considered, as it is important to recruit key informants who have the position and experience that will enable you to gain a perspective of a whole system.

When writing your research proposal it is usual to state at least the initial number of interviews you plan to perform and the rationale for this, as well as how you will determine if you have interviewed sufficient people in order to explore the phenomenon and meet your objectives.

Sampling

Representivity is not the issue in qualitative research, so random sampling is unnecessary. Convenience sampling can be used, as determined by the context of the recruitment process, but a more directed approach gives better results. Purposive sampling allows you to choose to interview those who are key informants by virtue of their position, or who are known for their opinions and views and are not afraid to voice them. These are so-called 'information-rich' participants, as compared with those who are known to be quiet or withdrawn. Examples of purposive sampling include:[6]

- *Extreme case sampling:* A controversial figure in a particular group or community, for example, is useful in drawing out divergent views on an issue and should be specifically sought out for an FGD or interview. Learning from unusual manifestations of the phenomenon can be helpful, for example, when selecting outstanding successes or notable failures to interview.
- *Criterion sampling:* Inclusion and exclusion criteria can be drawn up according to the purposes of the study and purposive sampling allows one to choose participants who will potentially be the most informative.
- *Snowball sampling:* A 'snow-balling' technique can be used to find further participants through those recruited initially, asking particularly for those known to have

strong views on the topic under study. It is also possible to 'sample as you go', purposively choosing further subjects as you learn more about the issues.
- *Purposeful random sampling:* This is useful when the potential number of people who could be interviewed is too many to cope with practically and all are of equal interest. Remember, though, that in this case random sampling is being used for a different purpose than in quantitative study designs. The aim is not to produce data that is representative of a larger population, but rather to understand a few instances that help us to appreciate the variety and limits of a phenomenon.

It is important that the process of recruitment of interviewees is entirely voluntary and without coercion, as this may affect the quality of the information collected.

In considering who could be interviewed for a particular research question, a number of criteria should be borne in mind:

- The total number of interviewees.
- The profile and diversity of the interviewees.
- The likelihood of obtaining useful information on the phenomenon in which you are interested.

When writing your research proposal you should describe your sampling strategy and the specific criteria used to select people in purposive sampling. The practical way in which these criteria will be applied in the field should also be described.

Data collection

The interviewer

Qualitative interviewing requires specific skills which can be developed and learnt, but not everyone makes a good interviewer. Do not make the assumption that it is an easy task, or that the researcher should necessarily be the interviewer. Specific training in qualitative interviewing may be required by members of the research team who plan to do the interviewing themselves; this should be arranged in good time. At the very least, the interview guide and process of interviewing should be piloted or role-played by the interviewers. Alternatively, it may be preferable to engage the services of a professional interviewer who has no vested interest in the research topic, particularly if there is a language barrier between the researcher and the interviewees.

The person who is the researcher or interviewer is important in qualitative research and should be 'visible' in the report. Participants asked the same question will give different responses to different people depending on who they are, or who they perceive them to be. So the actual results of a qualitative study are influenced directly by the person of the researcher, not only their level of skills but also their background and pre-existing views. Every interviewer, however skilled or professional, brings a certain bias with regard to the topic under discussion into an interview, which is a recognised feature of qualitative research. One method for minimising this bias is for the principal investigator or academic supervisor to interview the interviewer(s) on what they expect to find in response to the research question and to record this interview. This then forms part of the dataset and is used in the analysis, along with the interviews of the research participants. The effect of this process is to make explicit the existing ideas, position and bias of the interviewer(s) with respect to the topic under discussion, so that they are more consciously aware of the moments in the interviews when they have strong feelings or opinions, positive or negative, in response to what the participants are saying.

The facilitation of FGDs requires a greater level of skill, as they are more complex than individual interviews and, again, specific training and practice are helpful. It is often necessary to hold several opposing or conflicting views in the group in tension during the discussion and to create a space for those who feel less confident to express themselves clearly. When there are divergent views or opinions within a group, it is important to acknowledge these clearly when summarising, without assuming that there should be consensus or agreement. These are high order skills that require equanimity or balance, particularly when the discussion becomes heated or emotional, whilst at the same time keeping in mind the overall direction of the discussion. When to intervene with a participant who is dominating the discussion, for example, or how to encourage those who are reticent with regard to expressing their views, are skills that can only be acquired through practice and reflection. Reviewing the transcripts or the actual videos of FGDs is a powerful method of reflection and learning, which is best done through non-judgemental feedback by peers or an experienced interviewer. As with any skill, the more often one practises it, the more comfortable one becomes with the process and the better the quality of information that can be collected which truly reflects the participants' views.

Inviting the participants

Participants should be invited well in advance and given the clear option of declining the invitation without prejudice. It is important to state up front that refusing to participate in the interview will not influence the way that they are dealt with, for example, as patients or members of staff who may be reticent to speak freely about issues that could potentially affect them personally. Each potential participant should be sent an information sheet about the study, as well as the consent form, in advance, including the standard details of confidentiality and protection of privacy. It is important to note, however, that FGDs cannot guarantee anonymity, because the other members of the FGD cannot be bound by confidentiality agreements. If it is appropriate, transport costs for attending the interview can be reimbursed at a standard rate, but no other incentives are usually offered, apart from tea or refreshments when they arrive.

Setting up the interviews

It is useful to devote some attention to setting up the venue for the interviews optimally, as this may have a direct effect on the quality of the data collected. A venue that is neutral is preferable, separate from the environment of the issues under discussion, so that it does not set up unnatural power dynamics (e.g. a board room that intimidates participants) or provoke potentially uncomfortable feelings or reactions. Participants need to be invited well in advance so that they are able to clear their schedules for the interview. In a work environment, it is often good to use a lunch hour or an after-hours timeslot, unless it has been clearly negotiated and approved by their managers, so that participants are not anxious about getting back to work. If you are interviewing patients, make sure that they are not inconvenienced in terms of missing their appointments or losing their place in a queue.

The logistical arrangements are crucial, including the seating arrangements in the venue, the tea or refreshments and the setting up of audio- or video-recording apparatus. With FGDs, a circle of chairs in a flat venue without desks or tables is optimal. For individual interviews, it is better to avoid talking across a desk, rather sitting alongside the interviewee. It is preferable not to take notes as this can distract the interviewees' attention, apart from very brief reminders for effective summary. Ask participants to switch off cellphones and try to minimise other possible interruptions.

It is worth investing in good recording equipment and to check it properly before and during the interview. There is nothing worse than finding that the interview or FGD which took an enormous amount of effort to set up, failed to be recorded adequately for technical reasons, with the result that the data is lost.

The interviews

After welcoming the interviewees, start by explaining the procedure and the length of time that it is expected that the interview will take, as well as the purpose of the study. You will need 60 minutes for a focus group and between 30 and 60 minutes for an individual interview. Give enough information about the study, repeating what is written in the information sheet, without actually asking the research question before the discussion begins, and allow for questions of clarification. Once participants are satisfied and prepared to continue, ask them to sign the consent form. At the same time, it is useful for each participant to complete a basic demographic identification form, without names, so that the profile of the participants can be described when writing up the study.

Explain the role of an observer or camera operator, if there is someone helping with the recording, and request that cellphones be put on silent mode.

Begin the interview or focus group by requesting everyone in the room to contribute to open discussion without restriction in response to the questions, including examples or personal experiences. As some participants will not be accustomed to open-ended interviews, they will need to be encouraged to voice their opinions spontaneously rather than waiting to respond to a specific question.

Start with the main overall research question that is phrased in as open a way as possible, so as to allow the participants to understand the ultimate aim of the interview before going into detail. Wait for the initial responses without interrupting. Facilitate the discussion by summarising these initial responses in your own words, which gives you an opportunity to restate the research question. Don't be in a rush to go on to the next question in the interview guide, but rather wait for the participants to produce their own priorities in their own words, using encouraging body language. Ask for examples to illustrate what they have been saying, or ask a question such as: '*Can you tell us more about that?*' or '*Can you give us an example from your own experience?*'. Don't be afraid of short silences, as people are often just thinking about what has been said or catching up in their heads.

The two main tools of facilitation are clarifying and summarising. Clarification seeks to expand a notion by giving it different words and descriptions, as in: '*If I understand you correctly, you mean …*' or '*Can you explain what you mean by … ?*'. It also includes requesting examples or experiences to elaborate on a point. Asking 'why' can stimulate people to think about an issue at a deeper level, for example, '*When you said you felt x, why was that?*'.

Summarising means bringing together a series of inputs and reflecting them back to the participants, using their own words as far as possible: '*So to summarise what we have heard so far, it seems that …* '. This is also an opportunity in a FGD to reflect divergent views, as in: '*It appears that there are two different perspectives on this issue in the group: …* '. Summarising is also a technique of reflective listening. The facilitator should summarise the discussion at several points in the course of the interview, trying to capture as accurately as possible the main issues that have been put forward. The first summary reflection should be given within 10 minutes of the start of the interview and a final summary reviewing all the issues should be given toward the end. An accurate summary by the facilitator reassures the participants that what they have said has been heard, received and understood. If it is not accurate, they then have an opportunity to correct it, or they can add to it or embellish it with an example. Reflecting back an accurate summary releases the participants to think about what has not been said so far and to offer further information or a whole new idea. In other words, summaries should not close off the discussion, but rather invite more input, so they should be phrased in a tentative way rather than in a definitive manner that cannot be challenged.

An interview guide can be both useful and a hindrance. In inexperienced hands it can be turned into a questionnaire that becomes a barrier to free discussion between the interviewer and participants and may shape the discussion toward the researcher's bias. It should rather be seen as a supportive tool, for reference if the discussion needs some stimulation, but only after the techniques of clarifying and summarising have been used to elaborate on the main research question. Above all, it should only contain open-ended questions that help to remind the interviewer of important components of the research question that are likely to be raised. But it is better if the main issues are brought up spontaneously by the participants through active facilitation. If they do not arise spontaneously, it could be deduced that the participants did not regard them as important enough to mention.

Stay with the ideas and experiences of the interviewees until they have been understood and explored even if they are not what you expected, as long as it is within the focus of the study. Pay particular attention to viewpoints that contradict your own views or others in the group, as there is a tendency to not hear these. Similarly, when interviewees bring up issues that you feel strongly about yourself, be aware of your own responses that may bias the discussion in one particular direction. Never correct an interviewee during an interview, or offer advice. Also, avoid answering direct questions from the interviewees about the content. Rather reflect these back to them by asking: '*What is your opinion on that issue?*'.

In an FGD, it is often necessary to spread the questions around the group, or to use body language to turn to members of the group who have been silent up to that point, anticipating their input with a reflection such as: '*What do the rest of you think of this issue?*'. Invite specific participants' contributions by name or, after a strong contribution by one participant, ask the question: '*Does everyone else feel that way, or are there others who feel differently?*'. Look for issues in which there is a divergence of opinion in order to stimulate more discussion, as in: '*So Mr X says this and Ms Y maintains that: what is the actual situation?*'.

The final summary by the facilitator, if well done, may not be the actual end of the interview, because participants may be reminded of other points that have not been raised at all. So be prepared to be flexible, but at the same time stick to the agreed time for the interview. When the allotted time is up, thank all the participants for their participation and give them some idea of what the next steps are. If a feedback session is planned, then that is an opportunity to arrange it.

Conclude interviews with care and respect for the issues and emotions that may have been raised. Any unresolved emotional issues need to be dealt with through appropriate referral or another suitable process. It is often necessary to clarify how the information will be analysed and used, with a commitment to feeding back the reports or papers that arise from the study.

In your research proposal it is important to describe your interview guide and often to include it in full as an appendix. The practical details of who will conduct the interview, how language issues will be dealt with, how we can be sure that they will be a skillful interviewer, how they will be reflexive about their own prior perspective, how people will be invited, where the interviews will be held, how they will be recorded and any other practical arrangements (see Box 1) should be described in the data collection section of your research proposal.

Open-ended interviewing in primary care

There is much to learn from qualitative research that has relevance to clinical practice in primary care.[7] In contrast to the closed questions of traditional history-taking, as is taught to medical students, the open-ended interview style used in qualitative research resonates with the more relational approach in family medicine and primary care.

Open-ended interviewing skills as practised in qualitative research can add a rigour to the consultation process in primary care by teaching practitioners who undertake interviews how to listen actively to what the patient is saying. The attitude of tuning in to the patient without interruption, giving one's full attention to exactly what is being said and meant, as well as what is not being said, can reveal the patient's real agenda within the first few minutes of an interaction.[8] In contrast to expectations, active listening does not necessarily take more time and the qualitative interviewing techniques outlined above, namely, careful listening, clarifying and summarising, can actually lead to shorter and more efficient consultations, since the real issues of concern to the patient become apparent early on. Clarifying the patient's experience of the illness or problem by following their lead, avoids the interrogative style of standard history-taking that uses closed questions and puts the patient on the defensive. Summarising the patient's subjective experience of the illness in the practitioner's words can be extremely reassuring to those who feel distressed or alienated, as they

BOX 1: Practical checklist for conducting qualitative interviews.

1.	Use purposive sampling to choose information-rich participants.
2.	Invite the participants well in advance.
3.	Send them the information sheet and consent form.
4.	Offer to reimburse transport costs if appropriate.
5.	Set aside adequate time for the interview.
6.	Choose and secure a neutral venue where there will be no interruptions.
7.	Set up the audio- or video-recording apparatus and test it.
8.	Offer tea or refreshments when the participant(s) arrive(s).
9.	Request their full attention without interruptions (e.g. cellphones).
10.	Explain the purpose of the study and the process of the interview.
11.	Obtain their signed consent including for recording.
12.	Request participants to complete an anonymous demographics sheet.
13.	If there is an observer, clarify their role with the group.
14.	Start with the main research question.
15.	Develop and use an interview guide of open-ended questions.
16.	Clarify responses and issues as they arise.
17.	In an FGD, spread the questions around the group.
18.	Summarise frequently, as well as toward the end of the time.
19.	Conclude the interview or FGD with care and respect for the participants.
20.	Refer participants with any unresolved issues appropriately, if necessary.

FGD, focus group discussion.

finally feel that someone has listened and understood them. A skilled listener is far more efficient than a practitioner who asks all the correct routine questions, because they are able to understand the patient's agenda more quickly and can make a better assessment and plan.

Conclusion

This article has outlined the key issues to consider when planning a qualitative study using individual or focus group interviews. The article should assist you with writing the methods section of your research proposal, particularly the study design, sample size, sampling and data collection section. Qualitative data analysis is covered in another article in this series on Primary Care Research.

Acknowledgements

The authors gratefully acknowledge funding received from the U.S. President's Emergency Plan for AIDS Relief (PEPFAR), through the Health Resources and Services Administration (HRSA) under the terms of award T84HA21652; and via the Stellenbosch University Rural Medical Education Partnership Initiative (SURMEPI).

Competing interests

The authors declare that they have no financial or personal relationship(s) which may have inappropriately influenced them in writing this article.

Authors' contributions

S.R. (University of Cape Town) wrote the initial manuscript, which B.M. (Stellenbosch University) then revised. Both authors agreed on the final manuscript.

References

1. Creswell J. Qualitative inquiry & research design: choosing among five approaches. 2nd ed. Thousand Oaks, CA: Sage Publications, Inc.; 2006.
2. Creswell J. Research design: qualitative, quantitative, and mixed methods approaches. 3rd ed. Thousand Oaks, CA: Sage Publications, Inc.; 2008.
3. Lincoln YS, Guba EG. Naturalistic inquiry. Newbury Park, CA: Sage Publications; 1985.
4. Denscombe M. The good research guide: for small-scale social research projects. 4th ed. Maidenhead: Open University Press; 2010.
5. Denzin NK, Lincoln YS. The Sage handbook of qualitative research. 3rd ed. Thousand Oaks, CA: Sage Publications, Inc.; 2005.
6. Patton MQ. Qualitative research & evaluation methods. 3rd ed. London: Sage Publications Ltd; 2002.
7. Enelow AJ, Swisher SN. Interviewing & patient care. 4th ed. New York: Oxford University Press; 1996.
8. Barry CA, Bradley CP, Britten N, et al. Patients' unvoiced agendas in general practice consultations: qualitative study. BMJ. 2000;320:1246. http://dx.doi.org/10.1136/bmj.320.7244.1246

19

African Primary Care Research: Performing a programme evaluation

Author:
Lilian Dudley[1]

Affiliation:
[1]Community Health Division, Faculty of Medicine and Health Sciences, Stellenbosch University, South Africa

Correspondence to:
Lilian Dudley

Email:
ldudley@sun.ac.za

Postal address:
Faculty of Medicine and Health Sciences, Stellenbosch University, PO Box 19063, Francie van Zijl Drive, Tygerberg 7505, South Africa

This article is part of a series on Primary Care Research in the African context and focuses on programme evaluation. Different types of programme evaluation are outlined: developmental, process, outcome and impact. Eight steps to follow in designing your programme evaluation are then described in some detail: engage stakeholders; establish what is known; describe the programme; define the evaluation and select a study design; define the indicators; plan and manage data collection and analysis; make judgements and recommendations; and disseminate the findings. Other articles in the series cover related topics such as writing your research proposal, performing a literature review, conducting surveys with questionnaires, qualitative interviewing and approaches to quantitative and qualitative data analysis.

Recherche africaine de soins primaires: Evaluation des Programmes. Cet article fait partie d'une série sur la Recherche sur les soins primaires dans le contexte africain et se concentre sur l'évaluation des programmes. On y décrit différents types d'évaluation de programmes: développement, processus, résultats et impact. Les huit étapes à suivre pour organiser votre programme d'évaluation sont décrites en détail: nommer des parties prenantes; établir ce que l'on sait; décrire le programme; définir l'évaluation et choisir un plan d'étude; définir les indicateurs; planifier et gérer la collecte et l'analyse des données; faire des jugements et des recommandations; et disséminer les résultats. Les autres articles dans la série couvrent des sujets connexes comme la rédaction d'une proposition de recherche, la rédaction de revues d'articles, faire des enquêtes avec des questionnaires, des interviews qualitatives et les méthodes d'analyse de données quantitatives et qualitatives.

Introduction

This article is part of a series on Primary Care Research and focuses on programme evaluation. This overview of programme evaluation provides a framework to guide health professionals and postgraduate health sciences students as to the type of programme evaluation that is relevant or required and the choice of research methods that would be appropriate in different contexts. The framework is based on the theory and practice of evaluation as described in scientific literature, which has been adapted for a postgraduate programme for health sciences students in South Africa. Some of the specific methods are described in detail in other articles in the series, such as surveys, questionnaires and qualitative interviewing, whilst others, such as randomised controlled trials, would require further reading and may not be feasible at a Masters level.

Evaluation is:

> [*t*]he systematic collection of information about activities, characteristics, and outcomes of a program, services, policy or processes, in order to make judgements about the program/process, improve effectiveness, and/or inform decisions about future development.[1]

A wide range of health-related activities, including community mobilisation and communication campaigns, laboratory diagnostic services, training and education, direct service interventions, policy processes, surveillance systems and infrastructure programmes, can be evaluated. In this article, the term 'programme evaluation' will include evaluations of all such health-related interventions, processes and services. Further, it provides a framework for the performance of such evaluations, drawing on the theory and practice of evaluation in the literature and the experience and materials used in teaching evaluation methods for postgraduate health professionals at Stellenbosch University.

Evaluations are action oriented and inform judgements on whether a proposed programme should be started, how well an existing programme is functioning, or whether an established programme is achieving the desired effects. An evaluation therefore provides information so as to plan, correct, adapt and improve practices to enhance the likelihood of achieving the desired effects and to make decisions regarding the continuation, expansion or termination of a programme. An evaluation can also be used to build capacity, by enhancing the skills of health professionals and other stakeholders involved in a programme and by strengthening internal processes and accountability.

Types of evaluation

Traditionally, evaluations were conducted at the end of the programme. Often this meant that problems, which arose during the planning and implementation, were not detected and corrected timeously. To be most beneficial and instrumental, evaluations should be conducted at all phases of the life of a programme.[2]

Evaluations during the planning of a new programme can ensure that what is being planned is appropriate. It clarifies whether it has merit and is acceptable to stakeholders affected by it. Thus, an evaluation can inform the conceptualisation of a programme by assessing the motivation for starting such a programme, define the need for the programme and inform decision makers about what the programme should look like. Such a *developmental evaluation* therefore assesses whether a new programme makes sense and assists in making decisions on whether or how it should be implemented.

An evaluation conducted during the implementation of a programme assesses whether the planned activities are indeed occurring and the intensity at which they are occurring. Such a *process or performance evaluation* also assesses the extent to which the selected target groups are being reached and whether the resources are available and being used efficiently in the delivery of the activities.

In well-established programmes, an *outcome or impact evaluation* provides evidence regarding whether the desired effects are being achieved. It answers the questions of whether the programme is meeting the stated goals and objectives, whether the target group or community has experienced any benefits or adverse effects and how effective it has been in bringing about the planned changes in healthcare or health status. Effects of a programme may be immediate, or may be longer term. Effects that occur soon after the programme delivery are generally described as 'outcomes' (e.g. changes in patient behaviour). Longer-term broader societal effects are described as 'impacts' (e.g. reduction in morbidity or mortality).[3] It helps to distinguish the early outcomes from the longer-term impacts so as to identify the direct effects of the programme, which should be measured in the programme evaluation. An outcome evaluation could also include a costing of the resources used by conducting a cost analysis or a full economic evaluation to assess whether the benefits are worth the costs.[4]

A *comprehensive evaluation* includes all phases of a programme life cycle from the planning stages to the impact evaluation. Such a comprehensive approach ensures the alignment of the programme with the needs and desires of target groups and important stakeholders and continually informs adjustments to improve the delivery of the planned activities, increasing the likelihood of producing the desired outputs and achieving the planned outcomes and longer-term impact.

Eight steps in conducting programme evaluation

The following eight steps are described as a guide for conducting a performance evaluation.

Step 1: Engage stakeholders

Stakeholders are people with a vested interest, either as supporters or sceptics, who may potentially be affected by the programme and its evaluation.[2] They could include community members, patients, health facility staff, health managers and other decision makers in the health system such as funders and politicians. Engaging stakeholders assists in the planning of the evaluation, by clarifying their interest and the extent to which they will either affect or use the evaluation.

A stakeholder mapping exercise is useful in identifying these individuals or groups and in categorising them into: (1) those involved in the delivery of the programme; (2) those served or affected by the programme; and (3) the intended users of evaluation findings.[2] It is important to identify the interest in, perspective on and potential effect of the programme and the proposed evaluation on the different stakeholder groups, in order to select key stakeholders who should be engaged throughout the evaluation process.

Step 2: Establish what is known

A well-designed evaluation should be informed by a critical review and synthesis of the literature, including local and contextual data.[5] Evaluators should be apprised of current knowledge regarding the problem that the programme is seeking to address, best practices and the effectiveness of similar programmes and evaluations. Establishing a practice of evidence-informed processes in planning the evaluation will promote an approach of evidence-informed decisions throughout the evaluation.

Step 3: Describe the programme

A clear programme description provides a frame of reference for all subsequent decisions, connects programme components to their effects and enables comparisons with similar programmes. The first step is to clarify the *stage of development of the programme* and the purpose of the evaluation. Will the evaluation be used to assist with planning during the conceptualisation of a new programme, to assess processes during implementation of a programme, to measure the effects of a mature programme, or will it be used for all stages of the programme? Then, clarify *the need for the programme* by defining clearly the problem that the programme seeks to address, identifying who the problem affects, as well as the causes of the problem. It is also important to understand how the need for the programme was determined and to assess whether the programme intent is appropriate.

Describe the *context of the programme*, particularly the setting and local influences (e.g. geography, history, politics, social and economic conditions, as well as related activities of organisations) within which the programme operates.[6] Understanding these influences can assist in the design of a context-sensitive evaluation, as well as in the interpretation and assessment of the generalisability of the results.

The *expected effects* of the programme should indicate what the programme should achieve in order to be considered successful. The mission, goals and objectives of the programme should be described in sufficient detail so as to ensure an understanding of the expected effects. Goals generally provide a broad statement of a desired, long-term outcome of the programme, whereas objectives are statements of desired, specific, realistic and measurable programme results. As different stakeholders may have different views of the goals and objectives of the programme, this should be clarified with the different groups at the outset of the evaluation.

The available *resources* such as the human resources, time, equipment, information, money and other assets available to conduct programme activities should also be ascertained.

Lastly, consider the programme's capacity to effect the desired change, based on the problem, the intervention, the context and resources. In short, why should this intervention work? A description of the *'programme design'* or *'programme logic'* assists by explaining why and how an intervention works. The logic model should clearly specify the resources required (inputs) for the programme, the activities that will be undertaken, the measurable products of the programme activities (outputs) and the benefits to clients, communities, systems or organisations (outcomes). The programme logic can be represented graphically through a 'logic model' which details the activities of a programme and the links between each phase, to assist in the planning, implementation, monitoring and evaluation of the programme (Figure 1). Logic models can be represented in different ways, including graphic displays of boxes and arrows, matrices in tables, or narratives which set out the logical arguments for a programme.[7] Thus, the logic model assists in detailing and clarifying the relationship between different components of the programme, as well as assisting in an evaluation by identifying important components to be measured and appropriate indicators to be used at the different stages of the programme. The programme description and logic model's accuracy should be confirmed by consulting with stakeholders, or by direct observation of activities in the field.

Step 4: Define the evaluation question and select a study design

The evaluation question determines the selection of the study design to be used for the evaluation. Without knowing what question(s) the evaluation is intending to answer, you cannot begin to consider methods or data sources. Engage the stakeholders in clarifying the questions of concern to decision makers through guided probes such as 'what do you hope to know at the end of this evaluation that you don't know now?', rather than 'what are the evaluation questions?'.

Habicht presents two considerations for selecting an appropriate study design to address evaluation questions: firstly, the stage of the programme and secondly, the inferences to be made by the evaluation.[8] In the programme planning stage, a developmental evaluation answers questions regarding whether the planned programme addresses the causes of the problem for the affected persons or groups, in a way which is likely to be effective and is acceptable and appropriate to the context. Whereas a process evaluation typically addresses questions such as whether services are available and accessible, of a suitable standard or quality and are being used (utilisation), as well as whether the target population is being reached (coverage). An outcome or impact evaluation answers questions regarding whether improvements in health-related behaviours, disease patterns and health status occurred. It therefore seeks to assess the effects of a programme, as well as its impact on stakeholders or participants.

The second important consideration relates to the type of inference to be made. Do decision makers simply want to

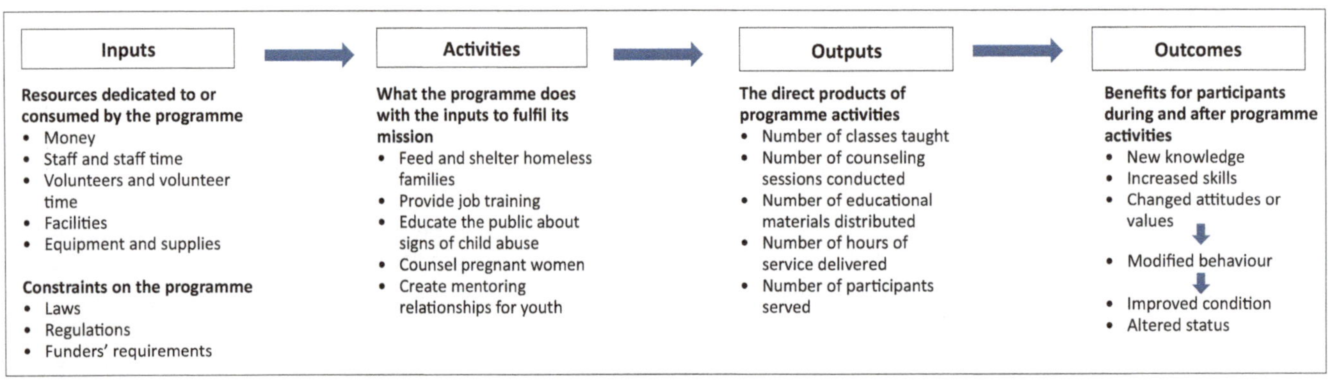

Source: Hatry 1996[16]

FIGURE 1: A programme logic model.

know whether the programme goals and expected changes have been achieved, or do they want to establish whether the programme was the cause of the outcomes achieved? This differentiates between 'contribution' of the programme and direct 'attribution' of the effects to the programme. Is it important to establish a causal relationship; and how confident do you need to be that observed effects were as a result of the programme interventions?

The three types of evaluation based on the inferences and 'level of certainty' required from an evaluation are: (1) adequacy, (2) plausibility and (3) probability assessments. At the lowest level of inference and certainty, an *adequacy assessment* simply answers the question, 'Did the expected changes occur?', without establishing any causal relationship between the programme activities and the changes. An adequacy assessment can indicate if activities were performed as planned, whether objectives were met and if the expected changes occurred, without inferring that the observed changes were because of the programme. It can also indicate whether resources were utilised efficiently or not. A *plausibility assessment* establishes if there was some form of a causal relationship between the programme and the outcomes and answers the question, 'Did the programme seem to have an effect above and beyond other external influences?'.[8] A *probability assessment* evaluates whether there was a direct causal relationship between the programme and the outcomes, as well as the strength of this relationship. Such an assessment aims at ensuring that there is only a small known probability that the difference between programme and control groups is a result of confounding problems, bias, or chance.

Study designs for evaluation are drawn from scientific research methods, particularly those developed in the social, behavioural and health sciences.[1,6] A broad classification of design types includes experimental, quasi-experimental and observational designs. Of these, observational study designs, which do not require controls but may have before-and-after comparisons, are suitable for an adequacy assessment. Quasi-experimental designs are best suited for a plausibility assessment. They include before-and-after comparisons, have control groups and seek to identify and manage the effects of confounding factors. Such quasi-experimental study designs include before-and-after controlled studies, or time series analysis.[9] Probability assessments require randomisation of intervention and control activities and thus require an experimental study design such as a randomised controlled trial.

Study designs should be selected during the programme planning, before implementation of the interventions, to allow for allocation of intervention and controls, including possible randomisation. Often this is not feasible, ethical or desirable, or does not occur for political or pragmatic reasons, so many evaluations of 'effect' are based ultimately on observational studies.[10] Failure to plan the evaluation early, however, limits the choice of study designs and the ability of an evaluation to answer questions, which may be important for decision making.

In addition to ascertaining whether an intervention worked (and to measure accurately any difference it made), it may be important to understand why the intervention worked, including characteristics associated with success or failure, as well as the pathways through which effects are generated.[5] The evaluation methods may thus require both quantitative approaches to measure effects, as well as qualitative approaches to understand why it worked. Such mixed-method approaches are able to address different evaluation questions and provide a comprehensive perspective of the programme.[11]

Lastly, in selecting a study design, consider the feasibility and ethical aspects of the proposed evaluation question and study design. How realistic are the proposed evaluation activities given the available time, resources and expertise? Is there adequate focus, or are you trying to do too much? Identify the ethical issues related to the context, participants and type of evaluation you are conducting in order to ensure that the evaluation is conducted ethically, legally, and considers the welfare of those involved and those affected.[12] Approvals from research ethics committees or from institutions to access routine data, staff, facilities or internal reports may be required. As these applications take time to be processed, it is advisable to commence applications early in the planning of the evaluation.

Step 5: Define the indicators

Having clarified the evaluation questions and study design, the next step is to select suitable indicators to measure the inputs, activities and outcomes of interest in the evaluation. Indicators are informed by the criteria that will be used to judge the programme. Thus, they should be meaningful with regard to addressing the evaluation questions and should align with and provide measures of the stated goals and objectives of the programme. Indicators can include measures of programme inputs (e.g. staff time, financial resources, materials and tools), activities (e.g. the participation rate, coverage rates and the efficiency of resource use) and measures of programme effects (e.g. changes in participant behaviour or practices, health status, quality of life or policies).

Characteristics of good indicators are that they:

> [s]hould actually measure what they are intended to (validity); they should provide the same answer if measured by different people in similar circumstances (reliability); they should be able to measure change (sensitivity); and, they should reflect changes only in the situation concerned (specificity). In reality, these criteria are difficult to achieve, and indicators, at best, are indirect or partial measures of a complex situation.[13]

Multiple indicators may be needed for tracking the implementation and effects of a programme. The programme logic model (or other conceptual frameworks) provides a useful structured approach to defining key indicators leading from programme inputs to activities to expected effects.[7,14] By relating indicators to the logic model, the early detection of small changes in performance is possible, rather than if a single outcome were the only measure used.

Step 6: Plan and manage data collection and analysis

The first step is to identify appropriate data sources for measurement of the indicators. Sources may include persons, documents or observations, which provide narrative (qualitative) or numeric (quantitative) data. Persons may provide information through surveys, interviews, focus group discussions or consensus development processes such as Delphi techniques. Documentary sources include routine health information systems, health service reports, grant proposals, press releases, meeting minutes, data records, presentations, articles, charts, photographs and videotapes. Routine health data sources are an important source of evaluation data as they are easily accessible, inexpensive and reflect directly on service activities and outputs. However, routine data are often incomplete or of poor quality and may need to be complemented by other sources such as survey data, for instance population census data, demographic or health surveys and facility surveys. Primary collection of new quantitative data may also be required for important indicators or to validate routine or survey data sources. Observations may include patient–provider interactions, service delivery, meetings, special events and other activities. The integration of data from different sources provides for a balanced evidence base, to respond to the needs and expectations of a diverse set of users.

A credible evaluation requires good quality data which are reliable, valid and appropriate for the intended use. Factors which affect the quality of the data collected include the indicator definitions, instrument design, data-collection procedures, training of data collectors, data source selection, coding, data management and routine error checking. Although all types of data have limitations, an evaluation's overall credibility can be improved by using multiple sources and procedures for gathering, analysing and interpreting data. A clear data collection and management plan assists by defining the processes, logistics and resources required for, as well as procedures to ensure quality control of, the data collection.

As part of the data management plan, describe how the data will be analysed in order to provide information to address the evaluation questions and to measure whether the programme has achieved its goals and objectives. Demonstrate how data sets, such as surveys or focus groups, will be analysed separately, as well as how the different sources of information will be combined or synthesised so as to reach a larger understanding of the programme performance. Mixed-method evaluations thus require the separate analysis of each element and a synthesis of different sources in order to examine patterns of agreement, convergence or complexity.[11]

Ultimately, the evidence generated by the evaluation needs to be credible to decision makers and other stakeholders. Credibility is affected by the extent to which stakeholders perceive it to be responsive to their needs and concerns; and by whether the study design is able to answer the evaluation questions. Other important factors include compliance with ethical practice, the quality of the data collected, the appropriateness and rigour of the data analysis and the approach used to interpret the results. Encouraging participation by stakeholders throughout the evaluation process can enhance perceived credibility. Stakeholders will be more likely to accept the evaluation's findings and to act on its recommendations, when they have been involved in defining, gathering and interpreting data that they find credible.[1]

Step 7: Make judgements and recommendations

The main purpose of an evaluation is to inform judgements of programme merit, worth or significance and thereby to contribute to decisions and actions on continuation, expansion or termination of a programme. Such judgements are made by comparing the findings and interpretations of the evaluation to the stated goals and objectives of the programme and to selected standards determined with stakeholders. Involving stakeholders in processes to interpret the data, assists by drawing on their information and perspectives to inform the judgements made about the programme. This, in turn, enhances stakeholders' perceptions regarding the credibility of the judgements and can influence the extent to which the evaluation will give effect to decisions and actions.

Recommendations on actions for consideration by decision makers should be based on the findings, their interpretation, the judgements made regarding programme performance and the context of the programme and its evaluation. Sharing draft recommendations, obtaining responses from multiple stakeholders and presenting options instead of directives ensures that recommendations will be relevant and well-received.

Step 8: Disseminate the findings

Finally, dissemination of findings of the programme evaluation can facilitate their use to inform programme decisions and practices and further knowledge generation. Mechanisms for dissemination include reports to decision makers, presentations to health service, community and other forums, scientific publications, the use of electronic and other media.[15]

Conclusion

These eight steps provide an introduction to important processes and considerations in performing a programme evaluation. However, they are not a comprehensive study of the theory and practice of evaluation methods and readers are encouraged to source additional resources when planning and conducting a programme evaluation.

Acknowledgments

The author gratefully acknowledge funding received from the U.S. President's Emergency Plan for AIDS Relief (PEPFAR), through HRSA under the terms of T84HA21652 and via the Stellenbosch University Rural Medical Education Partnership Initiative (SURMEPI).

Competing interests

The author declares that she has no financial or personal relationship(s) that may have inappropriately influenced her in writing this article.

References

1. Patton MQ. Utilization-focused evaluation: the new century text. 3rd ed. Thousand Oaks, CA: Sage Publications; 1997.
2. Centres for Disease Control and Prevention. Framework for program evaluation in public health. MMWR. 1999;48(RR11):1–40.
3. Louw J. Improving practice through evaluation. In: Donald DA, Dawes A, Louw J, editors. Addressing childhood adversity. Cape Town: David Philip, 2000; p. 62–73.
4. Drummond MF, O'Brien B, Stoddart GL, et al. Methods for the economic evaluation of health care programmes. 2nd ed. Oxford: Oxford University Press; 1997.
5. Bowen S. A guide to evaluation in health research. Department of Public Health Sciences, School of Public Health, University of Alberta. Canadian Institutes of Health Research. [document on the Internet] 2012 [cited 2013 Nov 25]. Available from: http://bit.ly/LwDITX
6. Worthen BR, Sanders JR, Fitzpatrick JL. Program evaluation: alternative approaches and practical guidelines. 2nd ed. New York, NY: Longman, Inc.; 1996.
7. McLaughlin JA, Jordan GB. Logic models: a tool for telling your program's performance story. Evaluation and Program Planning. 1999;22(1):65–72. http://dx.doi.org/10.1016/S0149-7189(98)00042-1
8. Habicht JP, Victora CG, Vaughan JP. Evaluation designs for adequacy, plausibility and probability of public health programme performance and impact. Int J Epidemiol. 1999;28(1):10–18. http://dx.doi.org/10.1093/ije/28.1.10
9. Cook TD, Campbell DT. Quasi-experimentation: design & analysis issues for field settings. Boston, MA: Houghton Mifflin; 1979.
10. Black N. Why we need observational studies to evaluate the effectiveness of health care. BMJ. 1996;312(7040):1215–1218. http://dx.doi.org/10.1136/bmj.312.7040.1215
11. Green JC, Caracelli V. Advances in mixed-method evaluation: the challenges and benefits of integrating diverse paradigms. New Directions for Program Evaluation, vol 74; San Francisco, CA: Jossey-Bass Inc.; 1997.
12. American Evaluation Association. Guiding principles for evaluators [page on the Internet] 2004 [cited 2014 Apr 26]. Available from: http://www.eval.org/p/cm/ld/fid=51
13. Alberta Heritage Foundation for Medical Research. SEARCH. A snapshot of the level of indicator development in Alberta health authorities. Toward a common set of health indicators for Alberta (Phase One). Edmonton: AHFMR; 1998.
14. Marsh D, Alegre JC, Waltensperger KZ. A results framework serves both program design and delivery science. J. Nutr. 2008;138(3):630–633.
15. Canadian Foundation for Healthcare Improvement. Resources and tools. [page on the Internet] n.d. [cited 2013 Nov 25]. Available from: http://www.cfhi-fcass.ca/PublicationsAndResources/ResourcesAndTools.aspx
16. Hatry HP. Measuring program outcomes: a practical approach. Alexandria, VA: United Way of America; 1996.

20

African Primary Care Research: Reviewing the literature

Authors:
Andrew Ross[1]
Bob Mash[2]

Affiliations:
[1]Department of Family Medicine, Nelson R. Mandela School of Medicine, University of KwaZulu-Natal, South Africa

[2]Family Medicine and Primary Care, Stellenbosch University, South Africa

Correspondence to:
Andrew Ross

Email:
rossa@ukzn.ac.za

Postal address:
Private Bag 7, Congella, Durban 7013, South Africa

This is the second article in the series on African primary care research. The article focuses on how to search for relevant evidence in the published literature that can be used in the development of a research proposal. The article addresses the style of writing required and the nature of the arguments for the social and scientific value of the proposed study, as well as the use of literature in conceptual frameworks and in the methods. Finally, the article looks at how to keep track of the literature used and to reference it appropriately.

La recherche sur les soins de santé primaire en Afrique: Étude documentaire. Cet article est le deuxième de la série consacrée à la recherche sur les soins de santé primaire en Afrique. Il se penche sur la marche à suivre pour rechercher des faits probants pertinents dans la littérature publiée qui puissent être utilisés dans l'élaboration d'une proposition de recherche. L'article traite du style d'écrit requis et de la nature des arguments en faveur de la valeur sociale et scientifique de l'étude proposée, ainsi que de l'utilisation de la littérature dans les cadres conceptuels et les méthodes. Enfin, l'article se penche sur la marche à suivre pour se tenir informé de la littérature utilisée et y faire référence de manière appropriée.

Introduction

The previous article introduced the topic of primary care research in an African context.[1] The various types of research were outlined and guidelines on choosing a topic were suggested. Before any research can be conducted, a proposal has to be approved by an institutional research and ethics committee. Headings for the development of a proposal were outlined in the previous article. It is helpful to use these headings as a formula. If you go step by step, from heading to heading, you will cover all the important aspects of the proposal and will usually have no problem with your institutional research and ethics committee. This second article in the series focuses on how to obtain and use the literature in preparing your proposal.

Before beginning to look for relevant literature, it is important to ensure that you are reasonably clear about your research question, aim and objectives. What is it that you are studying? What are you trying to investigate? Keep this at the front of your mind at all times. It is possible to read extensively and become overwhelmed by all the information. It is also possible to use too much background information and not focus clearly enough on your specific research question. Remember that you are not expected to read everything that has been written on the topic, but you should craft your arguments using the most relevant and important evidence.

Begin by reading generally around the topic. What have others said? As you familiarise yourself with the work that has been done previously on your topic you may start to focus or even redefine your research question. For example, you may become clearer as to what the gap in knowledge really is and what unanswered questions have been identified in the existing literature.

Hart[2] suggested that the purpose of a literature review should be to:

- establish the context of the current study
- rationalise the significance of the study
- synthesise and gain new insights
- distinguish what has been done from what needs to be done
- discover important variables relevant to the current study
- relate ideas and theory to applications
- identify methodologies that have been used.

Searching for the literature

Useful information will usually come from scholarly journals, books, internet sources and even unpublished theses. Articles from peer-reviewed journals are more likely to be methodologically sound than those from non-peer-reviewed journals. Try to find recent review articles, which already summarise the research on the topic of interest. Relevant systematic reviews that synthesise the evidence on a specific question should also be looked for. The Cochrane Library is a particularly useful source of systematic reviews. Try to include references from high impact journals, but also remember that African research is not always found in such European and American journals. You may need to conduct a specific search for African literature. For example, SABINET has an Index of South African Periodicals (ISAP) and a Union Catalogue of Theses and Dissertations (UCTD). EBSCOHOST also has Africa Wide NIPAD looking at African scholarship.

Broadly speaking, there are three entry points to the forest of scholarship. The most common is to use key words within search engines and databases so as to identify relevant and appropriate readings for your study. Useful search engines include Medline, Pubmed, EBSCO, Science Direct and Google scholar.

A second strategy, however, is to identify a few of the key scholars and their critical publications in your field of interest and to then follow their later publications and see who else is citing and using their work. Many search engines link you to work by the same author as well as other work that cites the article. Examining the references used by critical publications may also identify other key scholars and literature.

The third strategy is to locate the key journals or places where scholars publish in your field of interest and search specifically these journals for additional work that is relevant. In the discipline of family medicine, do not forget to look at our regional journals such as the African Primary Health Care and Family Medicine Journal or the South African Family Practice Journal.

It is important to use current literature. The bulk of your literature should be from the last five years and, ideally, none of your references should be more than 10 years old. The only exception is historical research which, for obvious reasons, traces patterns of scholarship and practice over time.

Be systematic as you search for relevant literature. Remember that you want to perform a smart, targeted search. As you locate the relevant articles, read the abstracts, assess their importance and relatedness to your work (discard any that you feel are not useful or related). If the abstract seems relevant, access and read the whole article.

Style of writing

The style of writing should go beyond just summarising the literature (i.e. listing the studies you have read in a series of paragraphs), or even synthesising the literature (i.e. grouping the studies chronologically or by topic), to a critical appraisal of the literature (i.e. interpreting the quality of the evidence and what is relevant to your own research question) and finally to the use of the literature to authorise the arguments that you are making.[2,3] Therefore, the literature review is a critical synthesis, not simply a description of 'who said what'. It should be a critical engagement with the established research on your topic. You must read and evaluate critically the strengths and weaknesses of the studies in relation to your research and determine which literature makes a significant contribution to the topic

When constructing your arguments, it may be helpful to first outline the logical flow by the use of headings and subheadings. Each paragraph should establish a key point in your argument and be linked together in a logical sequence. Within the argument it is often helpful to move from the general to the more specific, for example, from discussion of global evidence to regional or national and finally to local.

Try to obtain original or primary sources and do not support a point by citing a reference out of context. Do not copy and paste material from the internet into your writing. To prevent your inadvertently plagiarising material, it is better to make notes from the literature to capture the salient points and then use your notes to write your argument. If you do quote or copy material from other authors then use inverted commas to indicate this and always reference the source.

It is important that you do a spelling and grammar check once your writing is complete. It is also helpful to ask someone else to read through your completed writing to ensure that it flows and is coherent. It is always a good idea to submit your work via Turnitin or another anti-plagiarism software programmes to ensure that you have not inadvertently plagiarised the work of others.

Using the literature in your proposal

The structure of the proposal has been outlined in the first article of this series.[1] You will have seen from this article that we do not advocate for a section entitled 'literature review' as this does not make the purpose of your writing clear in terms of the proposal. Rather, we have suggested that you have an introduction or background section to your proposal that makes an argument, both consciously and explicitly, for the social and scientific value of your study.

Making an argument for the social value of your study

The social value speaks to the importance or relevance of the proposed research study in your context. This often includes information about the size or scale of the problem to be addressed, the importance of the issue to improving care and the likely benefits to the healthcare system, patients or society of performing this research study.

For example, in a study on pain in children with HIV, you may argue that HIV and pain are common and important problems in children taking antiretroviral medication in South Africa and that understanding the different types of pain and how to assess them will improve the quality of care for such children. Each of these points should be established by use of the evidence.

Making an argument for the scientific value of your study

The scientific value speaks to the original contribution that this study will make. This requires a critical appraisal of what is already known about the specific topic or problem and clarification of the knowledge gap that this study will address. The argument is focused on your research question and specific topic and should not involve a lengthy summary of general background information. At a Master's level the originality may often be contextual, in the sense that the study has not been done in the researcher's specific location before. The aim and objectives of the study should usually flow logically from the argument for the scientific value of the study.

Constructing a conceptual framework

In some research proposals, it is also necessary to describe the theoretical foundation for your study. Sometimes these theories or underlying concepts are linked together into a model of the relationships between them, which is also called a conceptual framework. The conceptual framework provides an explicit framework that helps to order your thinking, provides internal cohesion to your proposal and may guide your methodological choices. This framework is not static and may evolve as you conduct your research. Trafford and Leschem state that:

> [*d*]eveloping a conceptual framework forces you to be explicit about what you think you are doing. It also helps you to be selective; to decide which are the important features; which relationships are likely to be of importance or meaning; and hence, what data you are going to collect and analyse.[4]

For example, a study on the health benefits of family physicians to the district health services developed the conceptual framework shown in Figure 1 to guide the study design.[5,6] The framework shows how family physicians can be considered to be a generic intervention that will potentially impact on health system performance, clinical processes and eventually health outcomes. Any evaluation of their impact should also monitor other policy, targeted and clinical interventions that may also impact on these areas. The model helps decide what to measure and how to conceptually link together the different concepts.

Informing study design and methods

As you familiarise yourself with the literature, you may also obtain useful guidance on the study design and methods. Think about how other researchers studied this issue and what would be an appropriate way for you to study your research question? You may gain useful insights into methodological problems such as confounding variables, sample selection, calculating sample size, allocation of control groups or statistical analyses. Sometimes you may

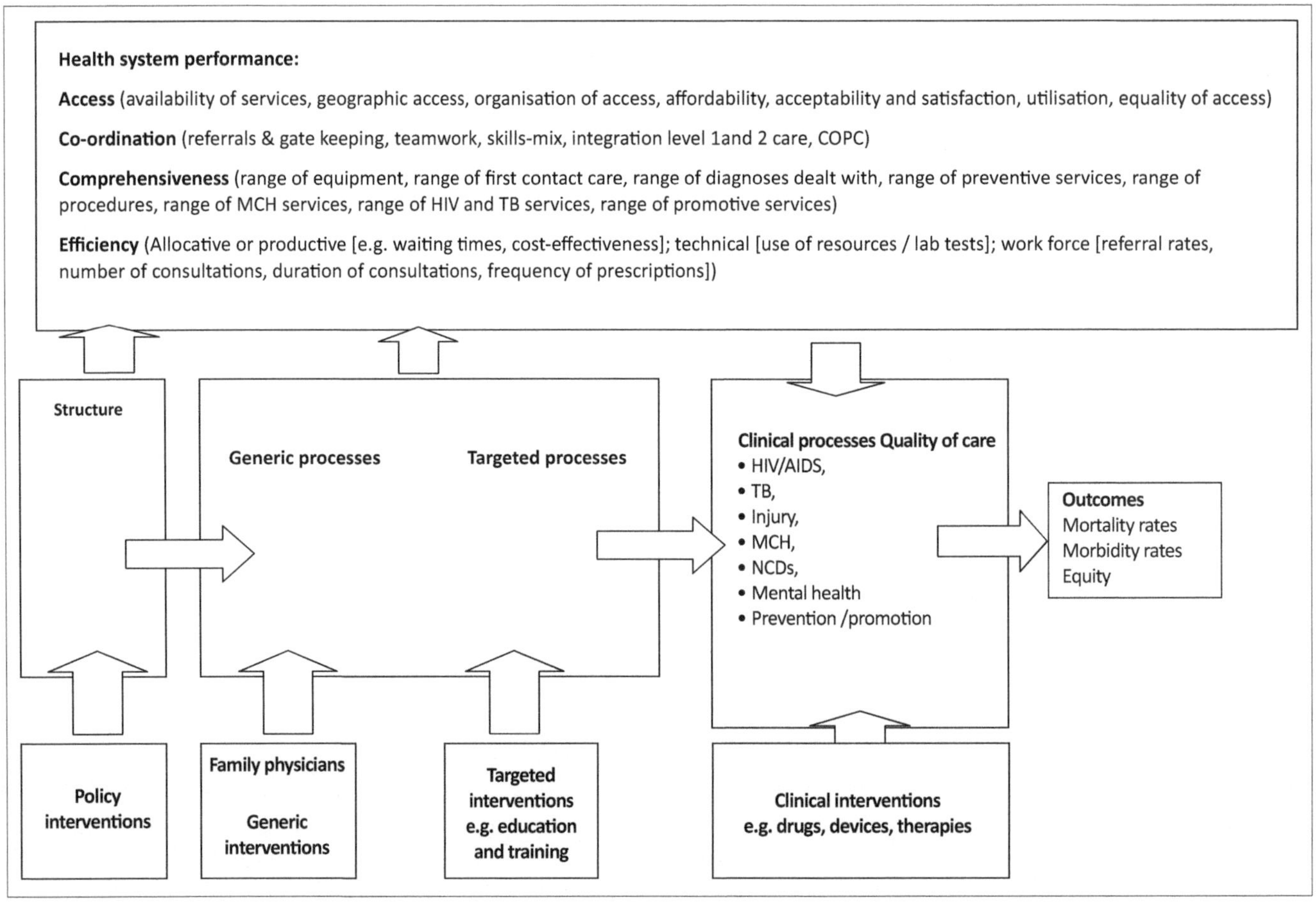

COPC, community-oriented primary care; MCH, maternal and child health; TB, tuberculosis; NCDs, non-communicable diseases.

FIGURE 1: Conceptual framework of the health benefits of employing a Family Physician in the district.

identify specific tools, such as questionnaires, that could be adapted to your own study. Using validated tools may not only improve the scientific validity of your own study but also enable you to compare your results more easily to other published work.

Keeping track of information and referencing

After reading an article, make a critical summary of its salient points and how they relate to your research study in terms of helping you with the argument for social value, scientific value, conceptual framework or methodological issues.[3] Many of these articles will also be useful when you discuss the results of your study later on.

It is critically important to record the full details of each article you have read and summarised – the title of the article, author(s) name(s), source and date of publication – all of which are required when drawing up a reference list. Keeping good records will save you hours of effort and frustration at the end of your literature review. There are a number of software programmes that help you to store the essential information (e.g. Ref Works, Reference Manager or EndNote) and to then automatically cite the references and generate reference lists in different styles. It is a good idea to invest in the time and energy required to learn how to use one of these programmes and to systematically enter the literature you use.

Referencing is an important way of acknowledging where ideas have come from. References must be accurate and complete so as to enable readers to follow up on sources. Reference are made in the text at the relevant place (usually a number or author's surname and date), as well as at the end of the article, where full bibliographic details are provided. All references noted in the text should appear in the reference list and all references in this list must be cited in the text. The two most common ways to reference are:

- Vancouver system (number sequence): Each reference is given a consecutive number in the text and in the reference list at the end of the document there is a list of the full references arranged in *numerical order* (i.e.. the order in which they have been cited in the text) .
- Harvard scheme (author-date): Each reference uses the name of the author(s) and date of publication in the text and the reference list is arranged *alphabetically by author*.

Whichever style you choose, it is important, above all, to be consistent in your approach.

Acknowledgements

The authors gratefully acknowledge funding received from the U.S. President's Emergency Plan for AIDS Relief (PEPFAR), through HRSA under the terms of T84HA21652., and via the Stellenbosch University Rural Medical Education Partnership Initiative (SURMEPI).

Competing interests

The authors declare that they have no financial or personal relationship(s) which may have inappropriately influenced them in writing this article.

Authors' contributions

A.R. (Nelson R. Mandela School of Medicine) developed the first draft of the manuscript which was then developed jointly by A.R. and B.M. (Stellenbosch University).

References

1. Mash R. African primary care research: choosing a topic and developing a proposal. Afr J Prm Health Care & Fam Med. 2013. In Press.
2. Hart C. Doing a literature review: releasing the social science research imagination (2nd ed.). California: SAGE; 1999.
3. Cresswell J. Educational research: planning, conducting, and evaluating quantitative and qualitative research (3rd ed.). New Jersey: Pearson Education; 2008.
4. Trafford V, Leshem S. Stepping stones to achieving your doctorate. Maidenhead: Open University; 2008.
5. Lilford R, Chilton P, Hemming K, et al. Evaluating policy and service interventions: framework to guide selection and interpretation of study end points. BMJ. 2010;341:c4413. http://dx.doi.org/10.1136/bmj.c4413, PMid:20802000
6. Kringos DS, Boerma WGW, Hutchinson A, et al. The breadth of primary care: a systematic literature review of its core dimensions. BMC Health Services Research. 2010;10:65. http://dx.doi.org/10.1186/1472-6963-10-65, PMid:20226084, PMCid:PMC2848652

21

African Primary Care Research: Quantitative analysis and presentation of results

Authors:
Bob Mash[1]
Gboyega A. Ogunbanjo[2]

Affiliations:
[1]Division of Family Medicine and Primary Care, Stellenbosch University, South Africa

[2]Department of Family Medicine, University of Limpopo, Medunsa Campus, South Africa

Correspondence to:
Bob Mash

Email:
rm@sun.ac.za

Postal address:
Box 19063, Tygerberg 7505, South Africa

This article is part of a series on Primary Care Research Methods. The article describes types of continuous and categorical data, how to capture data in a spreadsheet, how to use descriptive and inferential statistics and, finally, gives advice on how to present the results in text, figures and tables. The article intends to help Master's level students with writing the data analysis section of their research proposal and presenting their results in their final research report.

Recherche africaine dans le Domaine des Soins primaires: Analyse quantitative et présentation des résultats. Cet article fait partie d'une série sur les Méthodes de Recherche dans le Domaine des Soins primaires. L'article décrit les types de données continues et catégoriques, comment saisir les données dans un tableur, comment utiliser les statistiques descriptives et déductives et, finalement, donne des conseils sur la présentation des résultats dans un texte, des figures ou des tableaux. L'article a pour but d'aider les étudiants au niveau de la Maitrise à rédiger l'analyse des données de leur proposition de recherche et à présenter leurs résultats dans leur rapport de recherche final.

Introduction

This article is part of a series on Primary Care Research and focuses on how to capture, clean and analyse quantitative data, as well as how to present your results. Other articles in the series focus on how to write your research proposal, research report and how to collect quantitative data, typically through a survey with a questionnaire. The series is written to support Master's level research in family medicine and primary care in the African context. Your research proposal should contain an analysis plan that explains how you will capture and analyse your data.

Types of data

When planning your data collection, for example, choosing or designing a questionnaire, it is important to be aware of the type of quantitative data that you will obtain and how this will be analysed. If you do not intend to analyse the data or if it does not directly contribute to answering your aim and objectives, then you should re-consider whether it is worth collecting at all. The selection of statistical approaches varies depending on the type of data and you should describe the different types you will be using in the data analysis section of your research proposal. The following broad types of data exist:[1,2]

Continuous data: This is when the numbers are on a continuous scale, such as weight, age or blood pressure. In other words, they are data that can be measured on a scale and compared with other data. Whenever possible, data should be collected as a continuous variable, rather than as a categorical variable, as you have more statistical power and flexibility during the analysis. For example, it is better to collect the actual age rather than asking people to select which age category they fall within. In addition, it makes it easier to determine the mean, mode, median or standard deviation when the actual ages are collected. Some continuous datasets are distributed normally (with a symmetrical bell-shaped curve when plotted on a graph) and others are not distributed normally (asymmetrical bell-shaped curve when plotted on a graph). Whether the distribution is normal or not makes a difference to the selection of statistical approaches.

Categorical data: These are numeric data, which represent different categories or a set of data sorted or divided into different categories, according to the attributes thereof:

- Nominal data: used for categories that are mutually exclusive, but without any specific order or progression in size. Binary data is when there are just two categories such as (yes) and (no), or (male) and (female). Other nominal data categories could be marital status or employment where there are multiple options.

- Ordinal data: when the categories have some kind of order or relationship to each other, such as on a Likert scale or with a progression of income categories.

Capturing quantitative data

Data are often captured on an Excel® spreadsheet which can then be imported into a statistical software package for analysis. When capturing data, each row is usually a patient or data source and each column a variable. The first row can be used to give each column a brief one word title that will be used in the analysis to refer to that variable. Each column deals with only one variable and the cells should contain either a number (e.g. 1 for male and 2 for female) or a symbol (e.g. M for male and F for female), but should not use both simultaneously. If there are no data available for that cell, it is usual to leave it blank. In a question that has multiple possible responses, each option will need to be treated as a separate column in the spreadsheet. Table 1 gives an example of data captured in an Excel® spreadsheet from a study on diabetes.[3]

Once all data are entered, they should be checked and cleaned. One way of doing this is to use the filter tool in Excel® and look at the range of entries in each column. Obvious mistakes can then be recognised, such as numbers outside the expected range or which are clinically unlikely. Mistakes can then be addressed or cleaned up before analysing the data. This involves referring to the source document or questionnaire in order to recognise which information was entered incorrectly.

In your research proposal you should describe how you will capture, check and clean up your data. You should then describe the analytical software that you will be using and who may assist you, as well as the statistical tests that you expect to use. The rationale for selecting the various tests is outlined below.

Data analysis

It is important to consider how many variables you want to analyse at the same time. 'Univariate' analysis involves only one variable, 'bivariate' analysis looks at the relationship between two variables and, when you have more than two variables, this is referred to as 'multivariate' analysis. The most common application of univariate analysis is in descriptive studies or when describing a sample that has been selected for a study. The most common application of bivariate or multivariate analysis is in observational or experimental studies where groups are being compared and the researcher wants to make inferences about any significant differences. Descriptive and inferential statistics are described below.

Descriptive statistics

Categorical data can be analysed and presented as frequencies and percentages. These results can be described in the text, if very simple, such as the frequency and percentage of people that were male and female or, if more complicated, they can be presented in a table. When there are multiple categories, such as an age distribution, then a histogram can be helpful (see Figure 1).

Continuous data that are normally distributed can be analysed as a mean with a range, standard deviation or confidence interval. The standard deviation gives an idea of

TABLE 1: Example of data entered into an Excel® spreadsheet.

Study code	Age	Sex	HbA1c	Chol	Wt	WC	DBP	SBP
BEVDH1	59	F	10.9	6.5	83.6	96.0	101.0	193.5
BEVDH2	61	F	-	-	82.5	118.0	79.0	157.5
BEVDH3	52	F	10.3	5.3	83.5	101.0	87.5	125.0
BEVDH4	56	F	11.0	7.1	75.0	108.0	93.0	135.5
BEVDH5	53	F	9.4	8.1	77.6	100.0	103.5	158.0
BEVDH6	55	F	5.1	6.7	92.3	108.0	116.0	186.0
BEVDH7	54	F	6.7	6.2	58.0	86.0	92.0	147.5
BEVDH8	68	F	7.8	4.0	81.5	104.0	71.5	118.5
BEVDH9	52	F	8.8	5.0	88.1	104.0	82.5	140.0
BEVDH10	68	M	9.4	4.3	107.0	121.0	87.0	173.5
BEVDH11	66	M	8.9	4.8	96.7	112.0	67.5	134.5
BEVDH12	72	F	6.2	6.1	81.0	97.0	80.5	136.5
BEVDH13	51	F	10.3	4.2	79.6	93.0	79.0	139.5
BEVDH14	46	M	6.3	5.3	62.1	81.0	98.5	156.0
BEVDH15	66	F	7.0	5.1	48.5	74.0	80.0	137.5
BEVDH16	64	F	8.7	5.7	68.4	95.0	79.0	145.5
BEVDH17	47	M	7.1	4.6	85.0	101.0	101.5	158.0
BEVDH18	64	M	5.9	5.6	75.0	102.0	86.0	132.5
BEVDH19	48	F	7.8	4.4	65.5	89.0	76.5	130.5
BEVDH20	55	F	6.9	7.6	61.3	86.0	101.5	154.0
BEVDH21	59	M	6.0	5.4	103.7	111.0	83.5	134.5
BEVDH22	28	F	12.3	3.4	59.0	80.0	81.0	104.5
BEVDH23	66	F	6.4	6.3	53.7	81.0	75.5	118.0
BEVDH24	48	F	9.8	5.1	92.5	94.0	99.5	140.5

HbA1c, Glycated haemoglobin; Chol, total cholesterol; Wt, weight; WC, waist circumference; DBP, diastolic blood pressure; SBP, systolic blood pressure.

the spread of the total dataset from the mean (it is calculated as the square root of the variance). A small standard deviation implies that the data fall closely around the mean, whereas a large standard deviation implies that the data are more widely dispersed around the mean. The 95% confidence interval tells you that the real mean for the population is 95% likely to fall between the upper and lower limits of the interval. For purely descriptive purposes, the standard deviation would be preferred, whilst the confidence interval is more helpful when comparing data.

Continuous data that are not normally distributed can be analysed as a median with an interquartile range.

Data can be presented in text if very simple, such as the mean age with a standard deviation, or in a table, or in a histogram (normally distributed data) or a box and whisker plot (if not normally distributed). Table 2 gives an example from a study on diabetes of how such descriptive data can be presented in your research report, whilst Figures 1 and 2 give an example of a histogram and a box-and-whisker plot.

TABLE 2: Example of descriptive statistical results from a study on people with diabetes (N = 860).[3]

Results	*n* (%)
Level of control	
HbA1c < 7%	134 (15.6)
Cholesterol < 5.0 mmol/L	458 (53.3)
Diastolic BP < 80 mmHg	289 (33.6)
Systolic BP < 130 mmHg	345 (40.1)
Waist circumference –Women < 82 cm	40/650 (6.2)
Waist circumference – Men < 94 cm	80/209 (38.3)
Clinical measurements	**Mean (95% CI)**
HbA1c (%)	9.3 (9.2–9.5)
Cholesterol (mmol/L)	4.9 (4.8–5.0)
Weight (kg)	83.9 (82.7–85.2)
Waist circumference (cm)	100.3 (99.3–101.3)
Diastolic blood pressure (mmHg)	85.6 (84.7–86.5)
Systolic blood pressure (mmHg)	137.1 (135.4–138.7)
Self-care activities	**Mean (SD)**
Use of diet plan – days/week	4.7 (2.0)
Exercise – days/week	3.0 (2.3)
Foot care – days/week	5.6 (2.1)
Use of medication – days/week	6.9 (0.5)

HbA1c, Glycated haemoglobin; BP, blood pressure; CI, confidence interval; SD, standard deviation.

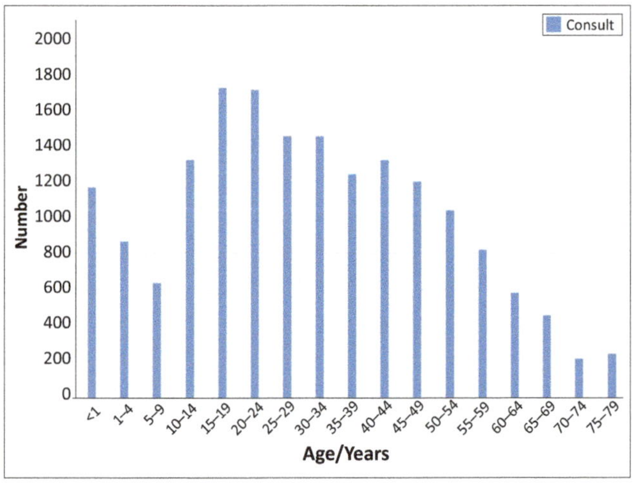

FIGURE 1: Example of a histogram showing the distribution of primary care consultations by age categories.

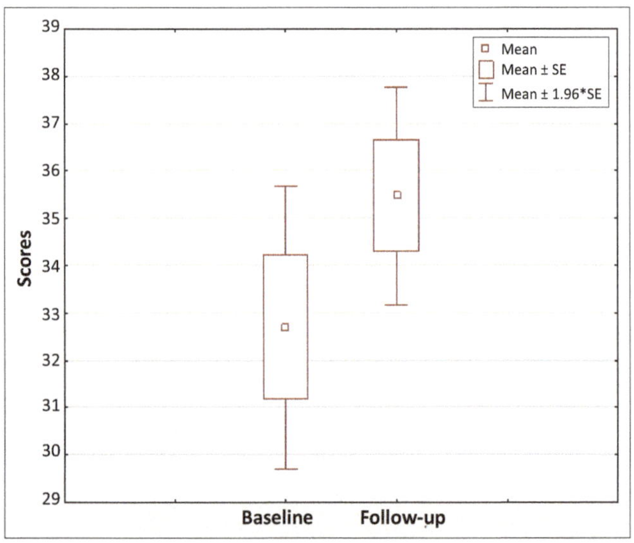

FIGURE 2: Example of a box-and-whisker plot for scores on the Kentucky Inventory of Mindfulness before and after a course on mindfulness-based stress interventions.

Inferential statistics

Inferential statistics are used when you intend to compare groups and draw inferences about any statistically-significant differences. In broad terms, the following types of data can be compared:

- Continuous data versus categorical data.
- Categorical data versus categorical data.
- Continuous data versus continuous data.

In some comparisons, independent groups are compared with each other (i.e. two different groups), whilst in other situations, paired groups are compared over time (i.e. the same group at baseline and follow up). The following examples are based on the comparison of different independent groups.

Continuous data versus categorical data

Analysis of variance (ANOVA) is used to determine whether the mean of the continuous variable differs between the different categories or groups. Again, different tests are used depending on whether the data is normally distributed (parametric tests such as t-test or F-test) or not normally distributed (non-parametric tests such as Mann-Whitney test for binary data, Kruskal-Wallis test for multiple categories). When in doubt, use a non-parametric test on the assumption that the data is not normally distributed. The analysis should give you a p-value that represents the likelihood of making a type 1 error (which infers that there is a difference, when in fact no difference really exists in the population). A statistically-significant p-value is usually set as less than 0.05 (less than a 5% chance of making a type 1 error).

Figure 3 compares the mean age of high school students in Grades 8–10 who abuse illicit substances with those that do not.[4] The graph shows the mean and 95% confidence intervals as well as the p-value derived from a Mann-Whitney test. This graph is produced by the analytical software and does not have to be copied in your results section when writing a research report. The p-value of < 0.01 in the example tells us that the two groups are significantly different. Table 3 demonstrates how these results could be presented in a table in your research report. One could also present this as the means and then the confidence interval for the difference between the means.

Categorical data versus categorical data

The two sets of categories are compared in a contingency table (also called a cross-tabulation table or a '2 by 2' table) and a chi-square test is used to determine whether there is any significant difference. When values in the cells of the table are very small (typically less than 5 or below 10 when there is only one degree of freedom), the Fisher Exact test is then used instead. Table 4 is an example of such a table, in which smoking habits are compared between high school students in Grades 8 and 10.[4] The chi-square test gave a p-value of 0.772, indicating that there was no significant difference between smoking habits in Grade 8 when compared with Grade 10. Results can be presented in a table in your research report (Table 5) where the frequencies and percentages are compared and the p-value given to indicate whether there is any statistical difference.

Continuous data versus continuous data

Regression and correlation analysis are used to determine whether one continuous variable has a significant influence over or correlation with another continuous variable. This relationship can be plotted on a graph and if the regression line differs significantly from zero then there is a correlation. A correlation coefficient is usually calculated between 0 (no correlation) and ± 1 (complete correlation). The square of the correlation coefficient tells you what percentage of the dependent variable is determined by the variation of the independent variable being tested. These results are often best presented graphically, using a scatterplot and regression line.

Figure 4 gives an example of such a scatterplot and regression line in which results for glycated haemoglobin (HbA1c) are correlated with random blood glucose results in the same group of diabetic patients.[5] The correlation coefficient (r) was 0.67, indicating a moderate correlation and the square of the correlation (r^2) was 0.45, indicating that 45% of the variability of the random blood glucose can be explained by the HbA1c reading. The p-value was < 0.001, indicating that the relationship has statistical significance. This graph from the analysis is probably also the best way of presenting your results.

Clearly, the selection of a statistical test is not always easy and in many situations it is essential to consult a statistician. Table 6 gives a simplified guide to the commonly-used tests and comparisons.

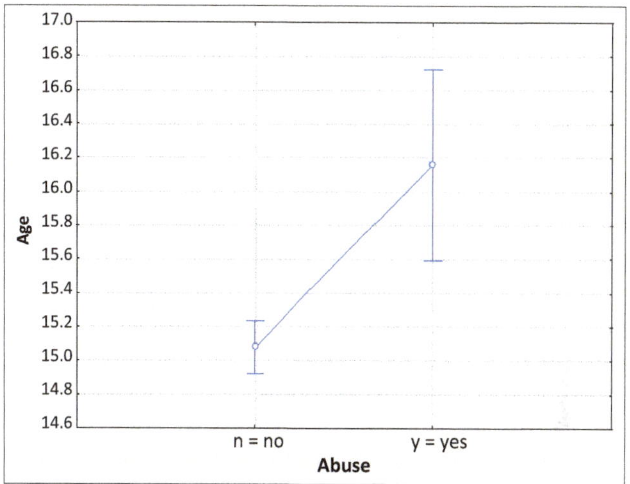

FIGURE 3: Example of analysis of variance (ANOVA) using a Mann-Whitney test to compare the age of high school students that use illicit substances with those that do not.

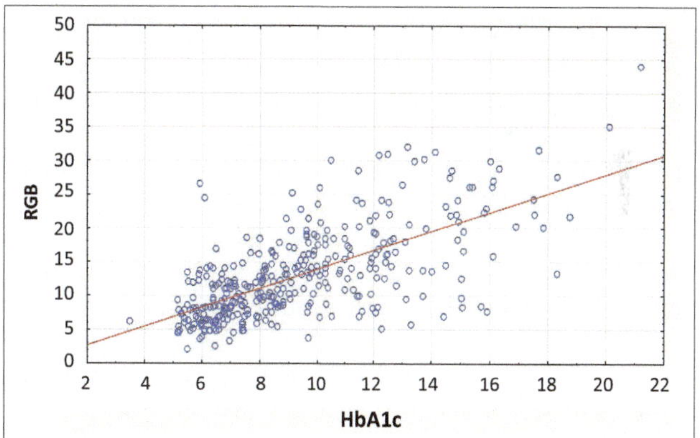

FIGURE 4: Example of a scatterplot and regression line for random blood glucose versus glycated haemoglobin values.

TABLE 3: Example of presentation of results shown in Figure 1 (N = 435).

Variables	Substance abuse N = 32 Mean (95% CI)	No substance abuse N = 403 Mean (95% CI)	p-value
Age (years)	16.2 (15.6-16.7)	15.1 (14.9–15.2)	< 0.01

CI, Confidence interval.

TABLE 4: Example of a contingency (cross-tabulation) table.

Please insert heading	Non-smoker	Smoker	Row total
Grade 8	66	38	104
Row %	63.46%	36.54%	100.00%
Grade 10	74	47	121
Row %	61.16%	38.84%	100.00%
Total	140	85	225

TABLE 5: Example of presentation of results from analysis shown in Table 4.

Variables	Grade 8 students N = 104 n (%)	Grade 10 students N = 121 n (%)	p-value
Tobacco smoking	38 (36.5)	47 (38.8)	0.772

TABLE 6: Selection of statistical tests for comparing data types between different groups in bivariate analysis.

Independent variable	Dependent variable			
	Categorical – binary	Categorical - nominal	Continuous – normally distributed	Continuous – non-normally distributed
Categorical – binary	Fisher exact†/chi square	Chi square	Independent samples *t*-test	Mann-Whitney test
Categorical – nominal	Chi square	Chi square	ANOVA	Kruskal-Wallis test
Continuous – normally distributed	Independent samples *t*-test	ANOVA	Pearson's correlation/linear regression	Spearman's correlation
Continuous – non-normally distributed	Mann-Whitney test	Kruskal-Wallis test	Spearman's correlation	Spearman's correlation

†, Fisher exact test is used when one or more of the expected counts in a 2 x 2 table is small i.e. less than five.

Presenting your results

The results section usually starts with the presentation of descriptive statistics that describe the sample or comparison groups. After this, inferential statistical results can be presented for the key comparisons that have been outlined in your objectives. Make use of subheadings to structure the presentation of your results.

It is important to stay aligned with your objectives and original intentions in performing your analysis and presenting your results. Do not start comparing everything with everything or performing more and more subgroup analyses in the hope of finding something significant. This 'data dredging' is frowned upon, because you are testing hypotheses that your study was never designed for.

Usually, the bulk of your results can be presented most clearly in a few well-designed tables (see Tables 3 and 4). You will usually have to extract the relevant results from your analysis document and re-organise them in tables designed for this purpose. It is seldom possible to just copy and paste tables from your analysis documents. Do not present endless figures (e.g. histograms, pie charts) for each variable and do not present the same results in both tables and figures unless there is a specific reason to do so. For example, you may want to highlight an important result that is more obvious when shown in a figure (see Figure 4). Take care when cutting and pasting graphs from your analytical software package as they may need editing and formatting in order to be clear to another reader.

Once you have constructed your tables and any additional figures you will need to provide the text to go with them. Each table and figure should be numbered sequentially and given a title. Tables are traditionally numbered with Roman numerals (e.g. I, II, III, IV) and the title placed above the table, although it is always important to consult the house style when converting from a thesis to an article, as the requirements may change, depending on the publication. Figures, on the other hand, use Arabic numbers (e.g. 1, 2, 3, 4) and the title is placed below the figure. Always take care when formulating the titles and legends of your figures and tables. Many readers will only have a look at the figures and tables, without reading your text. They should be able to pick up and understand the most important messages on the basis of title, figures and tables only.

It is usual to introduce and refer to each table beforehand in the text, in order to make sure your reader knows what the table is about and how to make sense of it, especially if there is anything that needs additional explanation. You can provide some interpretation of the results for the reader, without discussing them more broadly, for example, by highlighting the most significant findings. However do not be tempted to repeat all the results in the text. If there are any additional related results that are not in the table, these can also be given in the text.

Conclusion

Researchers should identify the type of quantitative data they will be collecting and ensure that they are captured cleanly and accurately in a spreadsheet. The data can then be analysed using any of the commercially-available statistical software. Descriptive statistics can be presented as frequencies with percentages, means with standard deviations or confidence intervals, or as medians with an interquartile range. Inferential statistics can compare continuous and categorical data types so as to determine whether there is a statistically-significant difference using a variety of carefully-selected statistical tests. The final results should be presented in tables, supported by the text and, if necessary, additional figures.

Acknowledgements

The authors gratefully acknowledge funding received from the U.S. President's Emergency Plan for AIDS Relief (PEPFAR), through HRSA under the terms of T84HA21652 and via the Stellenbosch University Rural Medical Education Partnership Initiative (SURMEPI).

Competing interests

The authors declare that they have no financial or personal relationship(s) that may have inappropriately influenced them in writing this article

Authors' contributions

B.M. (Stellenbosch University) wrote the original manuscript and G.O. (University of Limpopo, Medunsa Campus) made revisions. Both authors approved the final manuscript.

References

1. Aldous C, Rheeder P, Esterhuizen T. Writing your first clinical research protocol. Cape Town: Juta; 2011.
2. Denscombe M. The good research guide: for small-scale social research projects. 4th ed. Maidenhead: Open University Press; 2010.
3. Mash B, Levitt N, Steyn K, et al. Effectiveness of a group diabetes education programme in underserved communities in South Africa: pragmatic cluster randomized control trial. Presentation at 16th SA National Family Practitioners Conference 10–11 May 2013. [abstract on the Internet] 2013 [cited 2013 Dec 13]. Available from: http://saafp.org/conferences/index.php/ANFPC/2013/paper/view/286
4. Hamdulay AK, Mash R. The prevalence of substance use and its associations amongst students attending high school in Mitchells Plain, Cape Town. S Afr Fam Pract. 2011;53(1):83–90.
5. Daramola OF, Mash R. The validity of monitoring the control of diabetes with random blood glucose testing. SA Fam Pract. 2013;55(6):579–580.

22

African Primary Care Research: Qualitative data analysis and writing results

Authors:
Langalibalele H. Mabuza[1]
Indiran Govender[1]
Gboyega A. Ogunbanjo[1]
Bob Mash[2]

Affiliations:
[1]Department of Family Medicine, Medunsa Campus, University of Limpopo, South Africa

[2]Family Medicine and Primary Care, Stellenbosch University, South Africa

Correspondence to:
Langalibalele Mabuza

Email:
honeymanyosi@gmail.com

Postal address:
PO Box 222, Medunsa 0204, South Africa

This article is part of a series on African primary care research and gives practical guidance on qualitative data analysis and the presentation of qualitative findings. After an overview of qualitative methods and analytical approaches, the article focuses particularly on content analysis, using the framework method as an example. The steps of familiarisation, creating a thematic index, indexing, charting, interpretation and confirmation are described. Key concepts with regard to establishing the quality and trustworthiness of data analysis are described. Finally, an approach to the presentation of qualitative findings is given.

Recherche en Soins primaires africains: analyse de données qualitatives et rédaction des résultats. Cet article fait partie d'une série sur la recherche en soins primaires africains et offre des conseils pratiques pour l'analyse des données qualitatives et la présentation des résultats qualitatifs. Après un survol des méthodes qualitatives et des approches analytiques, l'article se penche particulièrement sur l'analyse du contenu, en utilisant comme exemple la méthode du cadre logique. On y décrit les étapes de familiarisation, la création d'un index thématique, l'indexage, le répertoriage, l'interprétation et la confirmation. Les concepts clés concernant la détermination de la qualité et de la fiabilité de l'analyse des données sont définis. Finalement, on y donne une méthode de présentation des résultats qualitatifs.

Introduction

This article is part of a series on African primary care research and addresses the topics of qualitative data analysis and writing results. Over the last few decades there have been several improvements in the scientific rigour of qualitative research methods, which had previously been regarded as being less scientific than more established quantitative approaches.[1,2]

In the discipline of family medicine and primary care, most researchers have been using focus group or in-depth interviews to collect qualitative data. Few researchers engage with participant or non-participant observation or immerse themselves for prolonged periods in other social groups or cultures. Research questions often focus on the need to gain a better understanding of the experiences of people regarding health-related topics or the experiences of patients regarding health services. The need to explore or understand people's perceptions, attitudes, beliefs, concerns, feelings or expectations are often mentioned in the aim and objectives. Whilst the qualitative research field is a broad one (see Table 1), this article will focus mainly on the analysis and reporting of qualitative data derived from interviews. This article complements the other article in this series on qualitative interviewing and methods.

Qualitative data

Qualitative data is usually text that has been derived from interviews, observations or already-existing documents. Interviews are usually audio- or video-recorded and must be transcribed verbatim in order to create data that can be analysed further.[3,4,5,6,7,8,9,10] The transcript should therefore be a word-by-word account and not paraphrased. Transcripts should include page and line numbers and should have sufficiently large margins to allow for coding.[11,12] Before analysing the data the transcript should be checked for accuracy and any mistakes in the transcription corrected against the original recording. If the interview must be translated, then the accuracy of the translation must also be verified. These steps in preparing the data for analysis must be described in the research proposal.

Approach to qualitative data analysis

Most primary care researchers use content analysis to make sense of their data and most approaches to content analysis follow the same basic stages of familiarisation, coding and formation of categories, interpretation of themes, confirmation of the interpretation and presentation of the

TABLE 1: Range of qualitative methodological approaches and analysis.

Type of qualitative research	Description
Ethnography[3]	This refers to the study of culture or cultures shared by a group of people. The investigator immerses him- or herself in the group for a long period of time (a year or more), gradually establishing trust and experience in the social world of the participants.
Netnography (Cyberethnography/virtual ethnography)[4]	This is a method that investigates communities created by a network (e.g. online communities), which are distant from the investigator and dispersed in their nature. Like physical communities, the researcher can study online communities through immersion in the group for an extended period of time.
Ethnomethodology[5]	This focuses on the way that participants construct the social world in which they live (how they 'create their own reality') – unlike ethnography which seeks to describe the social world as the participants see it.
Conversation analysis[6]	This focuses on how reality is constructed, rather than what it is. The moment-by-moment conversational interchange of a group of participants is analysed line-by-line to bring about the subtle meaning which the participants may not even be fully aware of.
Narrative analysis[7]	The focus of this analytical method is on understanding the bigger story or 'narrative' that people use to make sense of their experiences and events. 'Narratives must have a point (a "so what?" factor), which often takes the form of a moral message'.
Grounded theory[8,9]	'A systematic theory developed inductively, based on observations that are summarized into conceptual categories, re-evaluated in the research setting, and gradually refined and linked to other conceptual categories'.[8] Often involves a constant comparative analytical method, culminating in the production of a substantive theory.[9]

results.[13] Attention must also be given throughout to the trustworthiness of the data and data analysis process, as is discussed below. In order to provide a practical approach to qualitative data analysis, the Framework Method is described in some detail below as one commonly-used example.[14] In your research proposal, you should outline the steps that you will follow in your analysis.

Familiarisation

If you are performing your own data collection, this process may start in the field when you collected your data and made field notes. Once the data is available, however, the researcher(s) will make themselves familiar with the qualitative data as a whole by reading the transcripts and observation notes or listening to the tapes. During this process they should take note of key ideas and recurrent themes as they emerge, their own reactions to the data (see 'Reflexivity' below) and any remarks on the quality of the data or methodological issues. If there is a large amount of data then it may be necessary to select a representative sample of the data for this stage.[15]

BOX 1: Example of a thematic index.

1. How patients incorporate the taking of ARVs into their lifestyle
1.1 Use of technology (e.g. cellphone alarm, clock/watch alarm)
1.2 Reminders from family members or treatment supporters
1.3 Intuition (they just feel it is the right time)
1.4 Et cetera
2. Beliefs and feelings of patients/treatment supporter regarding their ARVs
2.1 Believe that they make them better (not get AIDS)
2.2 Believe that they increase life expectancy
2.3 Use of ARVs is form of unintended disclosure (that leads to stigma)
2.4 Et cetera
3. Positive experiences of patients/treatment supporters attending the ARV clinic at the district hospital
3.1 Caring and supportive staff
3.2 Sharing experiences with other patients
3.3 Regular supply of medication (vs. not regular at local clinic)
3.4 Et cetera
4. Negative experiences of patients/treatment supporters attending the ARV clinic at the district hospital
4.1 Uncaring and unsupportive staff
4.2 Blaming or judging person for their problems
4.3 Long queues and waiting times
4.4 Et cetera

ARV, antiretroviral.

Development of a thematic index

A list of codes is created based on the familiarisation process mentioned above and organised into categories. Codes and categories should be developed from the data (an inductive process),[16] but with the aim and objectives of the study in mind, as sometimes the data contains material that is irrelevant. Sometimes the objectives also provide an overall structure for the categories. The final list of codes and categories is called a 'thematic index'[14,17] and an example is given in Box 1 from a study looking at how people experienced the use of anti-retroviral medication. The thematic index can then be tested and refined on a small number of the transcripts or data sources.

Your codes should enable you to organise your data into manageable 'bites' that can be interpreted with ease in the next step. The range of opinions, for example, can be captured during interpretation, so you do not need a code for every viewpoint. However, once coding is completed it is easy to join codes together, but very difficult to divide up a code without re-analysing all the coded text. Codes, therefore, should be close to the data and not too broadly defined. The researcher should give the code a short descriptive label and be clear as to what data belong to this code and what is excluded. This can be defined with examples in the thematic index. Codes should be mutually exclusive,[18] although the same passage of text can have multiple codes attached.

Indexing

In this step, the codes in the thematic index are applied systematically to all the qualitative data. Text is annotated with all the codes that are being applied to it, usually by highlighting the passage and noting the code used in the margin.[14] This is not a mechanical process and often requires the use of judgement to decide on the most appropriate code.

Charting

In this step, the data are re-arranged into a series of charts that bring all the data with the same code together in one place from all the data sources.[14,17] Charts are often constructed using the framework of the thematic index (i.e. one chart per major category) or can be aligned with another conceptual framework that makes sense of the study aim and objectives. Each chart will usually be a matrix in which each column is a particular code and each row a particular data source. The cells of the chart may contain the highlighted quotation or a summary of the point being made. Each cell should be traceable back to the original data source, page and line number. One can use tables in a Word document, cells in an Excel spreadsheet or specially designed software to create charts.

Interpretation

The researcher will now read each chart and interpret the data. As the charts bring all the data related to a particular category or concept together in one place, it is easy to establish the range and nature of the phenomenon of interest.[16] Depending on the research aim and objectives, the following interpretations may also be necessary: how respondents defined the characteristics of key concepts, how emerging themes can be organised into a typology (a range of types of cases), or how patterns in the data suggest associations or explanations. In interpreting the data, it may be useful to pay particular attention to 'deviant cases' that contradict or negate the main findings.[15] Contradictory and deviant experiences may be a rich source of information allowing for a further understanding of the phenomenon and should not be discarded just because they are a minority view.

Confirmation

It can be helpful to confirm your interpretation of the findings with your respondents – so-called 'respondent validation'.[19] This is, however, not feasible or even desirable in all studies. Triangulation (see below) of findings with data from different sources and methods can help confirm the validity of the interpretation. Having several researchers independently analyse and confirm their interpretation with each other can also assist.[15]

Checking for trustworthiness

Qualitative research should be written up with enough clarity regarding the processes that were employed so as to enable the reader to evaluate the scientific rigour of the study, hence enabling acceptance or refutation of the findings.[20] The concepts and terminology used to describe the trustworthiness of qualitative research findings are different from quantitative research. The criteria for trustworthiness (verification) are credibility (for internal validity), transferability (external validity), dependability (reliability) and confirmability (objectivity).[21] Table 2 displays the various strategies employed to achieve each criterion.

TABLE 2: Criteria for trustworthiness of qualitative research.

Criterion	Strategy employed
Credibility	• Prolonged engagement • Peer briefing • Triangulation • Member checks
Transferability	• Providing thick description • Purposive sampling
Dependability	• Create an audit trail • Triangulation
Confirmability	• Triangulation • Practise reflexivity

Credibility

Credibility is concerned with the validity of the conclusions that are drawn from the data and how these conclusions match the reality being reported on. There are many aspects of the study design and reporting that affect the credibility of the work: recognised research methods, sufficient engagement with the phenomenon of interest, checking the transcriptions and emerging themes with the informants (so called 'member checking' and 'respondent validation'), debriefing of the researcher with their mentor or supervisor, peer scrutiny of the process and triangulation.

Triangulation has been described as 'the process of corroborating evidence from different individuals, types of data, or methods of data collection'.[20] For example, data sources could be interviews, observations of events in the field (including the informants' non-verbal expressions), information obtained from semi-structured questionnaires or other relevant documents. Triangulation could also refer to obtaining information from various different types of informants on the same phenomenon.[20,22] The effect of triangulation is to render a more holistic picture of the phenomenon under study and to prevent undue reliance on a single data collection method or source.[23]

Transferability

Transferability refers to how well the study conclusions can be applied to other similar settings. The ability of others to judge whether the findings can be transferred depends on a detailed description of the study setting, the selection of participants and the findings. This is often referred to as a 'thick description'.

Dependability

Dependability refers to the extent to which similar findings would be obtained if the study were repeated.[24] However, variability should be expected in qualitative studies as the focus is on 'the range of experience rather than the average experience'.[25] The best way of supporting the dependability of the research is to ensure that the methods are described in sufficient detail that they could be replicated by someone else (a step-by-step 'audit trail') and any limitations are discussed. Triangulation of methods will also improve the dependability of the findings.

Confirmability

Confirmability refers to the degree of objectivity of the researcher in data collection and reporting. The reader wants to ensure that the results are truly based on the data and not the characteristics or preferences of the researcher. Triangulation of the findings with other researchers and methods can help with this, but all qualitative researchers must also account for their own reflexivity.

Reflexivity refers to the researcher's awareness of the self as a research instrument.[26] The quality of the data obtained through interviewing or observation will, to some extent, depend on the nature of the interviewer. The extent to which they are open, detached, curious and unprejudiced will affect the responses that they receive and/or what they observe. Issues such as power, hierarchy, class, culture and language may also influence the responses.[27] The researchers should be aware of their own reactions (thoughts, feelings, judgements etc.) and pet theories that may influence how they interpret the data during the analytical process. Qualitative research does not claim to be free of subjectivity, but should strive to be conscious thereof and to describe how the researchers have accounted for the subjectivity as part of the research process.[27] Describing the researcher's credentials, training, occupation and prior relationship to the subjects of the research helps to demonstrate in the proposal that you are thinking about reflexivity.

Computer-assisted qualitative data analysis

These enhance the analytical process by making it easier and quicker to code, collate, interpret your data and select quotations for the final report.[28] The most popular programmes are HyperRESEARCH (ResearchWare, Inc.), NVivo (QSR International) and ATLAS.ti (ATLAS.ti Scientific Software Development GmbH). It should be noted that these programmes do not interpret the data for you, but simply speed up the process and make the handling of large amounts of data both manageable and systematic.[15,29]

Presentation of findings

A checklist for explicit and comprehensive reporting of qualitative studies has been suggested by Tong, Sainsburg and Craig in order to promote complete and transparent reporting amongst researchers of interview and focus group studies.[30] The checklist is based on three domains: research team and reflexivity, study design and reporting on findings. The study design has been described in another article in this series and reflexivity has been described above.

You should start writing up your findings as soon as you have completed the interpretation of your data. It is customary to start the results section of your thesis with an overview or profile of your research subjects or respondents. Sometimes this can be narrative, but a table may also help to clarify who they were along with their key characteristics. It is important to remember to collect this information (e.g. sex, age, qualifications or whatever is relevant to your study) when you interview or observe them.

The presentation of results will depend on the level of analysis. For example, a simple narrative may be presented chronologically or according to key topics, subheadings may be used to present a series of emergent themes or results may be presented to establish a new theory. In primary care research it is common to present a series of themes. In this example, the main theme may be given as a subheading and then the subthemes and main points are described in your own words according to your interpretation of the data. It is important to remember that these are not quantitative data and should not usually be reported in terms of the number of people who expressed a particular viewpoint.[15] Each main point is usually supported by a quotation from the raw data that speaks to the trustworthiness of your analysis. Quotations also help to connect the reader to the phenomenon that you are describing and to bring it alive.[16] The voice behind each quotation can be identified in brackets, as long as this does not clash with the need for confidentiality. It is, however, helpful to the reader to know in general terms whose voice the quote represents (e.g. patients or health workers). It is also helpful to number or code the different sources so that

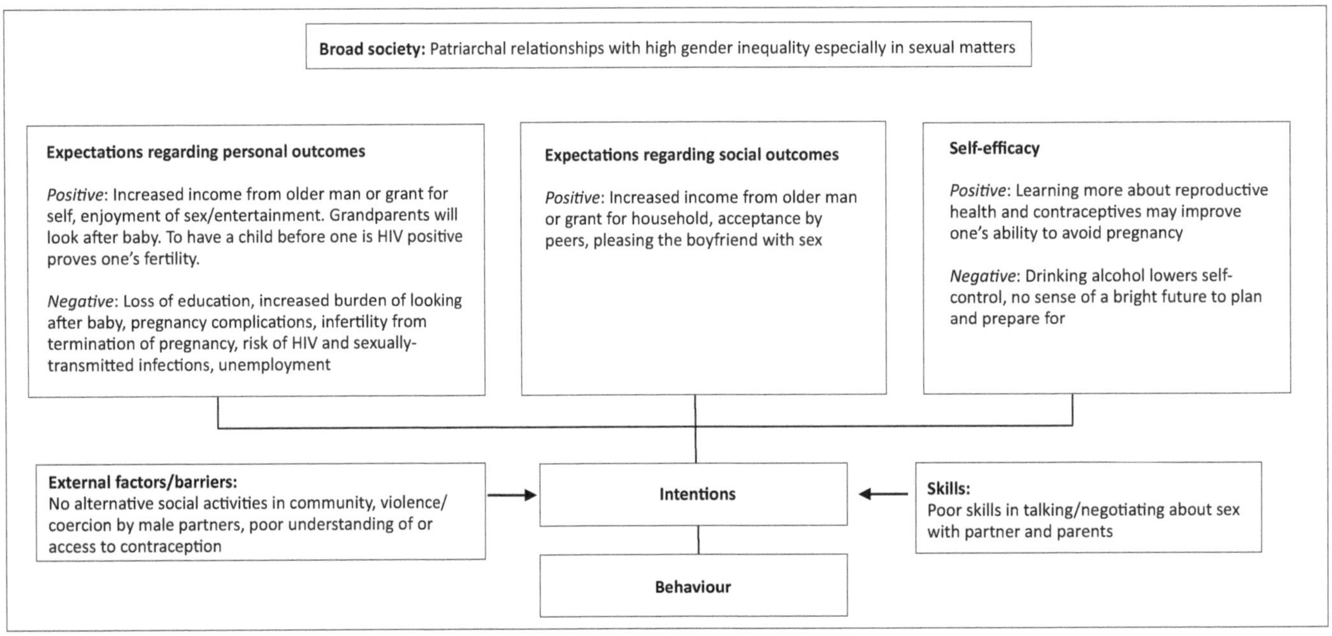

FIGURE 1: Example of a conceptual framework.

BOX 2: Example of how to present qualitative results.[31]

Participants did not identify their skin condition in terms of Western medical knowledge and did not view it as serious:
'I do not know [*what it is*], but every child has it and we do not see it as a problem. I also have it on my body, but it is not causing any problems [*for*] me.' (TN, Female, 23 years)
'Yes, I always see it on the bodies of the children, but I do not know anything about it.' (BM, Female, 77 years)

the reader can see you have used a wide variety of sources in supporting your findings.

An example of presentation of results from a study by Ifebuzor et al., conducted on the perceptions of parents about the skin conditions of their children in Francistown, Botswana, is given in Box 2.[31]

At the end of the results section, it can be helpful to try and summarise the key findings for the reader using a conceptual framework. For example, this could be in the form of a picture, a diagram such as a fishbone (e.g. for factors influencing an adverse event), a table (e.g. a strengths–weaknesses–opportunities–threats [SWOT] matrix) or a theoretical framework taken from the literature (see Figure 1 for an example from a study exploring the factors that influence teenage pregnancy, where social cognitive theory was used for the conceptual framework).[32]

Conclusion

This article has described the broad range of qualitative methods and types of analysis and then focused on a stepwise approach to content analysis using the framework method as a specific example. It has described the factors involved in determining the trustworthiness of qualitative data analysis and, finally, has outlined how to present your findings in a thesis or scientific article.

Acknowledgements

The authors gratefully acknowledge funding received from the U.S. President's Emergency Plan for AIDS Relief (PEPFAR), through HRSA under the terms of T84HA21652 and via the Stellenbosch University Rural Medical Education Partnership Initiative (SURMEPI).

Competing interests

The authors declare that they have no financial or personal relationship(s) which may have inappropriately influenced them in writing this article.

Authors' contributions

LM (University of Limpopo) wrote the original manuscript with assistance from IG (University of Limpopo) and GO (University of Limpopo). The manuscript was revised with feedback and contributions from BM (Stellenbosch University). All authors approved the final manuscript.

References

1. Patton MQ. Enhancing the quality and credibility of qualitative analysis. Health Serv Res. 1999;34(5 Pt 2):1189–1208.
2. Meyer J. Using qualitative methods in health related action research. BMJ. 2000;320:178.1.
3. Van Maanen J (editor). Representation in ethnography. Thousand Oaks, CA: Sage Publications; 1995.
4. Rybas N, Gajjala R. Developing cyberethnographic research methods for understanding digitally mediated identities. Forum Qual Soc Res. 2007;8(3):Art. 35.
5. Garfinkel H. Studies in ethnomethodology. Englewood Cliffs, NJ: Prentice-Hall; 1967.Antaki C. Discourse analysis and conversation analysis. In: Alasuutari P, Bickman L, Brannan J (editors). The SAGE Handbook of Social Research Methods. London: Sage Publications Ltd 2008; p.431–446. http://dx.doi.org/10.4135/9781446212165.n25
6. Griffin C. Narrative analysis [document on the Internet]. No date [cited 2013 Oct 23]. Available from: staff.bath.ac.uk/psscg/QM-Nar-lec.htm
7. Shutt RK. Investigating the social world: the process and practice of research. 7th ed. Thousand Oaks, CA: Sage Publications; 2012.
8. Sbaraini A, Carter SM, Evans RW, et al. How to do a grounded theory study: a worked example of a study of dental practices. BMC Med Res Methodol. 2011;11:128. http://dx.doi.org/10.1186/1471-2288-11-128
9. DiCicco-Bloom B, Crabtree BF. Making sense of qualitative research: the qualitative research interview. Medical Education. 2006;40:314–321. http://dx.doi.org/10.1111/j.1365-2929.2006.02418.x
10. Denzin NK, Lincoln YS. The SAGE Handbook of qualitative research. 4th ed. Los Angeles: Sage Publications; 2011.
11. Gläser J, Laudel G. Life with and without coding: two methods for early-stage data analysis in qualitative research aiming at causal explanations. Forum Qual Soc Res. 2013;14(2):Art 5.
12. Mayring P. Qualitative content analysis. Forum Qual Soc Res. 2000;1(2): Art 20.
13. Ritchie J, Spencer L. Qualitative data analysis for applied policy research. In: Bryman A, Burgess R (editors). Qualitative data analysis. London: Routledge, 1994; p.173–194.
14. Pope C, Ziebland S, Mays N. Qualitative research in health care: analysing qualitative data. BMJ. 2000;320(7227):114–116. http://dx.doi.org/10.1136/bmj.320.7227.114
15. Elo S, Kynga SH. The qualitative content analysis process. J Adv Nurs. 2008;62(1):107–115. http://dx.doi.org/10.1111/j.1365-2648.2007.04569.x
16. Attride-Stirling J. Thematic networks: an analytic tool for qualitative research. Qualitative Research. 2001;1(3):385–405. http://dx.doi.org/10.1177/146879410100100307
17. Glaser BG, Strauss AL. The discovery of grounded theory: strategies for qualitative research. Chicago: Aldine; 1967.
18. Riessman CK. Narrative methods for the human sciences. Thousand Oaks, CA: Sage Publications, Inc; 2008.
19. Creswell J. Educational research: planning, conducting, and evaluating quantitative and qualitative research. Upper Saddle River, NJ: Merrill Prentice Hall; 2002.
20. Anfara VA, Brown KM, Mangione TL. Qualitative analysis on stage: making the research process more public. Educ Res. 2002;31(7):28–38. http://dx.doi.org/10.3102/0013189X031007028
21. Huberman AM, Miles MB. Data management and analysis methods. In: Denzin NK, Lincoln YS (editors). Collecting and interpreting qualitative materials. Thousand Oaks, CA: Sage Publications, Inc, 2000; p.179–210.
22. Miles MB, Huberman AM. Qualitative data analysis: an expanded source book. 2nd ed. London: Sage Publications, Inc; 1994.
23. Shenton AK. Strategies for ensuring trustworthiness in qualitative research projects. Education for Information. 2004;22:63–75.
24. Guba EG. Criteria for assessing the trustworthiness of naturalistic inquiries. ECTJ. 1981;29(2):75-91.
25. Jootun D, McGhee G, Marland GR. Reflexivity: promoting rigour in qualitative research. Nurs Stand. 2009;23(23):42–46. http://dx.doi.org/10.7748/ns2009.02.23.23.42.c6800
26. Seale C, Silverman D. Ensuring rigour in qualitative research. Eur J Public Health. 1997;7(4):379–384. http://dx.doi.org/10.1093/eurpub/7.4.379
27. Richards L, Richards T. From filing cabinet to computer. In: Bryman A, Burgess RG (editors). Analysing qualitative data. London: Routledge, 1994; p.146–172. http://dx.doi.org/10.4324/9780203413081_chapter_8
28. Rambaree K. Bringing rigour in qualitative social research: the use of a CAQDAS. UoM Research Journal. 2007;13A (Special ed.):1–16.
29. Tong A, Sainsbury P, Craig J. Consolidated criteria for reporting qualitative research (COREQ): a 32-item checklist for interviews and focus groups. Int J Qual Health Care. 2007;19 (6):349–357. http://dx.doi.org/10.1093/intqhc/mzm042
30. Ifebuzor DC, Mabuza LH, Malete NH, et al. The perceptions of parents about the skin conditions of their children presenting with comorbid fungal skin infections in Francistown, Botswana. Afr J Prm Health Care Fam Med. 2013;5(1), Art. #459, 6 pages. http://dx.doi.org/10.4102/phcfm.v5i1.459
31. Kanku T, Mash R. Attitudes, perceptions and understanding amongst teenagers regarding teenage pregnancy, sexuality and contraception in Taung. SA Fam Pract. 2010;52(6):563–572.

Knowledge, attitude and practice regarding lifestyle modification in type 2 diabetic patients

Authors:
Henry I. Okonta[1]
John B. Ikombele[2]
Gboyega A. Ogunbanjo[1]

Affiliations:
[1]Department of Family Medicine and Primary Health Care, University of Limpopo, Medunsa Campus, Pretoria

[2]Mamelodi District Hospital, Pretoria

Correspondence to:
Henry Okonta

Email:
okonta@mweb.co.za

Postal address:
PO Box 222, Medunsa 0204, South Africa

Background: The number of persons suffering from type 2 diabetes mellitus continues to rise worldwide and causes significant morbidity and mortality, especially in the developing world. Behaviour change and adoption of healthy lifestyle habits help to prevent or slow down the complications of type 2 diabetes mellitus. However, the knowledge and practice of healthy lifestyles in many diabetic patients have been inadequate.

Aim: This study sought to establish the knowledge, attitude and practice regarding lifestyle modification amongst type 2 diabetic patients.

Setting: The diabetic clinic of Mamelodi hospital, Pretoria, Gauteng Province, South Africa.

Methods: A cross-sectional study was done using a structured questionnaire amongst 217 type 2 diabetic patients seen at the diabetic clinic of Mamelodi hospital. Baseline characteristics of the participants were obtained and their knowledge, attitude and practice regarding lifestyle modification were assessed.

Results: Of the 217 participants, 154 (71%) were obese and 15 (7%) were morbidly obese. The majority of respondents (92.2%) had poor knowledge of the benefits of exercise, weight loss and a healthy diet. What is interesting is that the majority (97.7%) demonstrated bad practices in relation to lifestyle modifications, although over four-fifths (84.3%) had a positive attitude toward healthy lifestyle modifications.

Conclusion: Despite the positive attitudes of respondents toward healthy lifestyle modifications, the knowledge and practice regarding lifestyle modifications amongst type 2 diabetes mellitus participants seen at Mamelodi hospital were generally poor.

Connaissances, attitudes et pratiques concernant le changement du mode de vie des diabétiques de type 2.

Contexte: Le nombre de personnes souffrant du diabète sucré de type 2 continue à augmenter dans le monde entier et est une cause importante de morbidité et de décès, surtout dans les pays en voie de développement. Les changements de comportement et l'adoption d'un mode de vie sain permet de prévenir ou de ralentir les complications du diabète sucré de type 2. Cependant, la connaissance et la pratique d'un mode de vie sain sont insuffisantes chez de nombreux diabétiques.

Objectif: Cette étude a cherché à déterminer les connaissances, attitudes et pratiques relatives à la modification du mode de vie des diabétiques de type 2.

Lieu: La clinique pour diabètes de l'hôpital de Mamelodi, à Pretoria, Province de Gauteng, Afrique du Sud.

Méthodes: On a effectué une étude transversale au moyen d'un questionnaire structuré parmi 217 diabétiques de type 2 examinés à la clinique du diabète de l'hôpital de Mamelodi. On a collecté les caractéristiques de base des participants et évalué leurs connaissances, attitudes et pratiques relatives à la modification de leur mode de vie.

Résultats: Des 217 participants, 154 (71%) étaient obèses et 15 (7%) étaient d'une obésité excessive. La majorité des répondants (92.2%) ne savaient presque rien des bienfaits de l'exercice physique, de la perte de poids et d'un régime alimentaire sain. Il est intéressant de noter que la majorité (97.7%) n'avait pas modifié son mode vie tandis que plus des quatre cinquième d'entre eux (84.3%) avaient une attitude positive envers les modifications relatives à un mode de vie sain.

Conclusion: En dépit des attitudes positives des répondants envers les modifications relatives à un mode vie sain, les participants diabétiques de type 2 examinés à l'hôpital de Mamelodi avaient une mauvaise connaissance et pratique de la modification du mode de vie.

Introduction

Social value

The burden of type 2 diabetes mellitus is becoming an epidemic and is a cause of morbidity and mortality, especially in the developing world. Worldwide, the prevalence of type 2 diabetes mellitus was 382 million in 2013 and it is estimated to rise to 592 million by 2035.[1] The prevalence of people living with type 2 diabetes mellitus in Africa was 20 million in 2013 and is projected to go through a two-fold increase over the next 22 years (i.e., by 2035).[1] The prevalence of type 2 diabetes mellitus in South Africa is amongst the highest in sub-Saharan Africa, with 2 million people known to have the condition and more than 1.5 million people with undiagnosed diabetes mellitus.[2] In a South African study in 2006, the greatest prevalence of type 2 diabetes mellitus was found amongst the Indian community of Durban (13%) and the elderly (mixed-race) community of Cape Town (28.7%).[3] Another study in South Africa confirmed the high prevalence of 28.2% of type 2 diabetes mellitus amongst the South African mixed-race population.[4] The main driving force for this current worldwide epidemic of type 2 diabetes mellitus is environmental. Urbanisation encourages a sedentary lifestyle, with a lack of participation in physical activities. This can lead to obesity, which is an important factor in developing type 2 diabetes mellitus through insulin resistance.[5]

Scientific value

Lifestyle modification is vital in the management of type 2 diabetes mellitus. Studies on the knowledge, attitude and practice of lifestyle modification, specifically with regard to type 2 diabetic patients, are very few, with varied results from various settings. In a study of 100 type 2 diabetic patients in Malaysia, 87% of the participants were knowledgeable, with a score of 50% or more on knowledge questions; 98% had a score of 50% or more on attitude questions; and 99% had a score of 50% or more on lifestyle modification practices scores.[6] However, in another study of 207 type 2 diabetic patients in India, 83.3% of participants had poor knowledge of lifestyle modification as a non-pharmacologic treatment for diabetes mellitus.[7] Furthermore, in a study of 1982 diabetic patients in Kenya, 28% of the participants had a good attitude toward lifestyle modification; 75% had poor dietary practice; and 72% did not exercise regularly.[8]

Conceptual framework

We observed that most patients seen at the diabetic clinic of Mamelodi hospital were obese, with suboptimal control of their blood glucose levels. In addition, some also had hypertension, diabetic retinopathy and diabetic feet. Encounters with these patients revealed that most of them had poor dietary and physical exercise habits despite the fact that they had been counseled at least once about lifestyle modification.

Aim and objectives

Within our context, there was no previous study on this topic in this black-populated setting of Mamelodi Township in South Africa. The aim of this study was to explore the knowledge, attitude and practice regarding lifestyle modifications amongst type 2 diabetic patients seen at Mamelodi hospital, east of Pretoria.

Research methods and design

Setting

We conducted this study in the diabetic clinic at Mamelodi hospital, a district hospital east of Pretoria in Gauteng Province, South Africa. At the time of this study there was no organised medical nutrition programme to support diabetic patients at Mamelodi hospital.

Study design

This was a cross-sectional study. The study population was all diagnosed type 2 diabetes mellitus patients seen at the diabetic clinic of Mamelodi hospital from 05 December 2010 to 05 January 2011.The inclusion criteria were type 2 diabetic patients aged 30 years and above seen at Mamelodi hospital for regular follow-ups and who consented to participate in the study.

Sample population and sampling structure

The sample size was calculated using Epi Info™ version 3.2 (US Centers for Disease Control and Prevention, Atlanta, GA 2004). With an estimated total of 500 type 2 diabetes mellitus patients who attend the diabetic clinic monthly, an expected prevalence of 50% type 2 diabetes mellitus patients with good knowledge, positive attitude and good practice of lifestyle modification, using a 95% confidence level and a 5% degree of error, the sample size was 217. The patients who met the inclusion criteria were selected through systematic sampling of every second patient until the last patient in the sample was selected.

Data collection

The data for this study were collected using a structured questionnaire. The questionnaire used in this study was created by using questions from existing validated questionnaires in the 'spoken knowledge in low literacy in diabetes knowledge assessment scale' (SKILLD[9]) and similar researches by Ambigapathy et al.[6] in 2003 and Palaian et al.[10] in 2006. Knowledge questions were obtained from the SKILLD questionnaire,[9] whilst attitude and practice questions were obtained from the questionnaires developed by Ambigapathy[6] and Palaian.[10] Identifying information, such as names of participants, was omitted from the questionnaires.

The questionnaire was administered by the researcher and two qualified professional nurses trained as research assistants and who were proficient in Sepedi and Isizulu (local languages predominantly spoken in Mamelodi Township). Participants who agreed to participate in the study signed informed consent. The data collected from the participants included baseline demographic characteristics, their average monthly income, anthropometric measurements and information on lifestyle modification knowledge, attitude and practice.

Scoring on the questionnaires

The lifestyle modification knowledge, attitude and practice questionnaire had 6 questions on knowledge regarding the benefits of exercise and weight loss, 12 questions on knowledge about healthy diet, 4 questions on attitudes toward lifestyle modifications and 3 questions on lifestyle modification practices. Each correct answer by the participant for a question earned a score of '1' and each incorrect answer earned a score of '0'.

Reliability and validity

A pilot study on 10 type 2 diabetes mellitus patients who were not included in the study was done and the questionnaire was refined according to the feedback received from the pilot study.

The Isizulu and Sepedi versions of the questionnaire were tested by translation back to English by a different accredited translator and were found to be comparable.

Data analysis

The data from the questionnaires were captured in Microsoft® Excel 2007 and exported to SPSS Statistics for Windows, Version 17.0 (SPSS Inc., Chicago 2008) where they were analysed by a statistician using descriptive statistics. Linear correlation and *p*-values were calculated to ascertain the statistical significance of key findings.

The results of the analysis were presented in frequency distribution tables. For the 6 questions on knowledge regarding the benefits of exercise and weight loss, participants who had zero to 2 correct answers out of the 6 were assumed to have poor knowledge about the benefits of exercise and weight loss. This score range of 0–2 was labeled as 'poor knowledge' in the frequency distribution table. Participants who had between 3 and 4 correct answers were assumed to have average knowledge about the benefits of exercise and weight loss and this score range of 3–4 was labeled as 'average knowledge'. Participants with 5 to 6 correct answers were assumed to have good knowledge about the benefits of exercise and weight loss, with this score range of 5–6 being labeled as 'good knowledge'.

Similarly, for the 12 questions on knowledge regarding a healthy diet, score ranges of 0–5, 6–9 and 10–12 were labeled as poor knowledge, average knowledge and good knowledge, respectively. For the 18 global knowledge questions, score ranges of 0–8, 9–13 and 14–18 were labeled as poor knowledge, average knowledge and good knowledge, respectively. For the 3 practice of lifestyle modification questions, scores of 0, 1, 2 and 3 were labeled as very poor practice, poor practice, good practice and very good practice, respectively.

Ethical considerations

The Medunsa Research Ethics Committee (MREC) provided ethical clearance for our study (clearance certificate number: MREC/M/224/2010:PG). The management of Mamelodi hospital provided permission to conduct the study. Informed consent was obtained from the participants; both the administration and collection of the questionnaires were anonymous and all information volunteered was kept in strict confidence.

Results

Baseline characteristics of the respondents

Two hundred and seventeen type 2 diabetes mellitus patients were recruited for the study. Table 1 shows the age group distribution of the participants with the 51- to 60-year age group, within which the majority of the participants fell ($n = 93$, 42.9%). It also shows that a majority of the participants either had no formal education ($n = 108$, 49.5%) or primary school education ($n = 95$, 43.9%); and they had a very low average monthly income – only 1 (0.5%) earning above R4000 (approximately USD 400) per month. Only 7.4% ($n = 16$) had a normal body mass index (BMI); for the others, some were overweight ($n = 47$, 21.7%) and 70.9% ($n = 154$) were obese, with 15 (6.9%) falling in the class 3 obesity subgroup.

TABLE 1: Baseline characteristics of participants.

Baseline characteristic	Number	Percentage
Age group (years)		
30–40	16	7.4
41–50	47	21.6
51–60	93	42.9
61–70	46	21.2
>70	15	6.9
Total	**217**	**100**
Level of education		
No formal education	108	49.5
Primary school	95	43.9
High school	14	6.6
Tertiary education	0	0.0
Total	**217**	**100**
Average monthly income (Rands)		
< 500	40	17.9
500–999	55	24.5
1000–1999	111	52.4
2000–4000	10	4.7
> 4000	1	0.5
Total	**217**	**100**
BMI (Kg/m^2)		
Normal (18.5–24.9)	16	7.4
Overweight (25.0–29.9)	47	21.7
Obese class 1 (30.0–34.9)	94	43.3
Obese class 2 (35.0–39.9)	45	20.7
Obese class 3 (40 or more)	15	6.9
Total	**217**	**100**

BMI, body mass index.

TABLE 2: Frequency distribution of knowledge about lifestyle modification, diet and global knowledge scores.

Variable	Number	Percentage
Score on knowledge about benefits of exercise and weight loss		
0–2 (Poor knowledge)	200	92.1
3–4 (Average knowledge)	16	7.4
5–6 (Good knowledge)	1	0.5
Total	**217**	**100**
Score on knowledge about healthy diet		
0–5 (Poor knowledge)	159	73.3
6–9 (Average knowledge)	58	26.7
10–12 (Good knowledge)	0	0.0
Total	**217**	**100**
Global knowledge score		
0–8 (Poor knowledge)	201	92.6
9–13 (Average knowledge)	16	7.4
14–18 (Good knowledge)	0	0.0
Total	**217**	**100**

TABLE 3: Frequency distribution of participants according to attitude score for lifestyle modifications.

Attitude score	Number of respondents	Percentage
0 (Strongly negative)	1	0.5
1 (Negative)	5	2.3
2 (Neutral)	28	12.9
3 (Positive)	71	32.7
4 (Strongly positive)	112	51.6
Total	**217**	**100**

Knowledge about lifestyle modification

Table 2 shows that 92.1% (n = 200) of the participants had poor knowledge regarding the benefits of exercise and weight loss; 73.3% (n = 159) had poor knowledge regarding a healthy diet and 92.6% (n = 201) had poor global knowledge regarding the value of exercise, weight loss and a healthy diet.

Attitude towards lifestyle modification

A majority of participants either had a strongly positive attitude (n = 112, 51.6%) or a positive attitude (n = 71, 32.7%) toward lifestyle modifications – a total of 183 (84.3%) with positive attitudes (Table 3).

Practice of lifestyle modification

Regarding healthy lifestyle practices, 91.7% (n = 199) of the participants reported that they did not exercise regularly; of the 8.3% (n = 18) that exercised regularly, the majority (n = 17, 94.4%) exercised less than 30 minutes per day or less than 150 minutes per week. Most of the participants (n = 217, 99.1%) did not follow a controlled and planned diet and 212 (97.7%) did not monitor their body weight. Table 4 shows the distribution of participants according to their lifestyle modification practice score.

Correlation between knowledge, attitude and practice of lifestyle modification

Table 5 shows a positive Pearson correlation of 0.170 (p = 0.012) between the global knowledge level and attitude level; a weak, insignificant positive Pearson correlation of 0.037 (p = 0.587) between the global knowledge level and practice level; and a weak, positive Pearson correlation of 0.102 (p = 0.132) between the attitude level and practice level.

TABLE 4: Frequency distribution of participants according to lifestyle modification practice score.

Practice score	Number of respondents	Percentage
0 (Very poor practice)	199	91.7
1 (Poor practice)	13	6.0
2 (Good practice)	3	1.4
3 (Very good practice)	2	0.9
Total	**217**	**100**

TABLE 5: Correlations between global knowledge, attitude and practice level regarding lifestyle modifications (N = 217).

Correlation	Pearson correlation	p-value
Global knowledge and attitudes	0.17	0.012
Global knowledge and practice	0.04	0.587
Attitudes and practice	0.10	0.132

Discussion

The majority of participants in this study were in the age groups of 41–50 years (21.6%), 51–60 years (42.9%) and 61–70 years (21.2%). This reflects the fact that type 2 diabetes mellitus usually has its onset after the age of 40 years.[11] The preponderance of these age groups is also consistent with the findings of the 2003 South African demographic and health surveys in which the majority of South Africans who attended public health facilities in the preceding 30-day period were in the over-45-year age group.[12]

Participants with no formal education (49.5%) and participants with primary school education (43.9%) together constitute an overwhelming 93.4% of the participants in this study. This indicates that most participants have little or no education, a finding which is similar to the results of another South African study which found that 70.6% of black South Africans with type 2 diabetes mellitus had less than a Standard 8 (Grade 10) education.[13] A majority of the participants were poverty-stricken, with 52.4% earning (ZA) R1000 – R1999, 24.5% earning R500 – R999 and 17.9% earning less than R500 per month. Poverty could limit accessibility to and affordability of a well-balanced diet and healthy food and this could explain why the majority of participants had a less-than-acceptable lifestyle modification practice score despite having a positive attitude. This finding is in keeping with the results from a South African income distribution and poverty study where 64% of black South Africans were shown to have a low income.[14]

The high prevalence of overweight (21.6%) and obesity (71%) amongst the participants is similar to the findings in 2009 by another South African study which found that 23% of women were overweight and 41.6% were obese compared with 14.6% and 7.5% of men, respectively, in their study.[15] Obesity is a major risk factor for type 2 diabetes mellitus and the sedentary lifestyle and lack of physical activity amongst the participants seem to contribute to the high proportion of overweight and obese persons in this study.

The patients' extremely poor knowledge of lifestyle modification has been replicated in a study in India, in which a majority of respondents (83.3%) had poor knowledge of the advantages of lifestyle modification.[7] The low level of education amongst the participants, as well as the lack of a well-organised medical nutrition therapy programme within the hospital, may have contributed to this result. In contrast, another study using the same questions found that the majority of respondents in their study (67%) were knowledgeable about lifestyle modifications.[6] These different finding may be because of the differences in literacy level, training received and availability of information on type 2 diabetes mellitus for their study patients. In this other study, 47% of their respondents had secondary-level education and had access to a well-organised awareness programme on diabetes mellitus.[6] This may have accounted for the good lifestyle modification knowledge found in their study participant.

In terms of attitude assessment, the 51.6% of participants with strongly positive attitudes toward lifestyle modification and the 32.7% with positive attitudes jointly constitute a majority 84.3% of the participants with positive attitudes in this study. This is also reflected in other studies, in which the majority of respondents had positive attitudes towards lifestyle modifications.[16,17] The proportion of participants with very poor lifestyle practices is similar to a study done in which 75.6% of respondents had bad practices in relation to lifestyle modifications.[8] This has not been found consistently, as was shown in a study done in India where a majority (99%) of their participants had good lifestyle modification practices.[6]

The positive correlation (p = 0.012) between the global knowledge level and the attitude level of participants indicates that the more knowledgeable the participants, the more willing they were to observe lifestyle habits. The very weak and insignificant positive correlation (p = 0587) between the global knowledge level and practice level of participants is indicative that being knowledgeable did not necessarily translate into healthy lifestyle practices. In the same vein, the weak insignificant positive correlation (p = 0.132) between attitude level and practice level of participants demonstrates that positive attitude did not necessarily translate to good lifestyle modification practices. The correlation trend in this study matches the trend in other studies which found a significant positive correlation ($p < 0.01$) between knowledge and attitude scores.[6,8] As there is evidence in the literature that good knowledge can be translated into healthy lifestyle practices by promoting behavior change using motivational interview approach,[18,19] the lack of knowledge and skills of Mamelodi healthcare workers with regard to motivational behaviour change facilitation might have contributed to this result.

Limitations of the study

The design of the study did not allow the researchers to determine any causality of the research findings. Secondly, patients at the diabetic clinic of Mamelodi hospital may not be representative of patients with type 2 diabetes mellitus in the general South African population. These limitations notwithstanding, the study revealed important trends that need to be factored into the management of type 2 diabetes mellitus patients, especially in peri-urban black townships.

Recommendation

A hospital-based lifestyle intervention programme should be implemented in order to improve the knowledge and practice of patients regarding healthy lifestyle. This should be extended to the primary healthcare clinics where the majority of patients are seen.

Conclusion

The knowledge and practice levels of lifestyle modifications amongst type 2 diabetes mellitus patients attending Mamelodi hospital were generally poor. Nevertheless, majority of these patients have positive attitude toward healthy lifestyle habits which could potentially be harnessed and translated into healthy lifestyle practices.

Acknowledgements

We thank all the participants who took part in this study, the clinic nurses who assisted in data collection and Ms Annah M. Mulalo of the statistics department for the data analysis.

Competing interests

The authors declare that they have no financial or personal relationship(s) that may have inappropriately influenced them in writing this article.

Authors' contributions

J.B.I. (Mamelodi District Hospital, Pretoria) was involved in the conceptualisation of the study, data collection, data analysis and report. H.I.O. (University of Limpopo) was involved in the conceptualisation, data verification and writing of the manuscript. G.A.O. (University of Limpopo) was involved in the data verification, writing of the manuscript and review of the manuscript for important intellectual content. All authors approved the final version of the manuscript.

References

1. International Diabetes Federation. IDF diabetes atlas, sixth edition [document on the Internet]. c2013 [cited 2014 Jan 25]. Available from: http://www.idf.org/sites/default/files/EN_6E_Atlas_Full_0.pdf
2. International Diabetes Federation. IDF diabetes atlas, 5th edition [document on the Internet]. c2012 [cited 2014 Jan 25. Available from: http://www.idf.org/sites/default/files/5E_IDFAtlasPoster_2012_EN.pdf
3. Rheeder P. Type 2 diabetes: the emerging epidemic. SA Fam Pract. 2006;48(10):20. http://dx.doi.org/10.1080/20786204.2006.10873480
4. Erasmus RT, Soita DJ, Hassan MS, et al. High prevalence of diabetes mellitus and metabolic syndrome in a South African coloured population: Baseline data of a study in Bellville, Cape Town. S Afr Med J. 2012;102(11 Pt 1):841–844.
5. Hicks J. A sedentary lifestyle and diabetes [page on the Internet]. c2008 [cited 2014 Jan 25. Available from: http://diabetes.about.com/od/benefitsofexercise/a/sedentary7.htm

6. Ambigapathy R, Ambigapathy S, Ling HM. A knowledge, attitude and practice (KAP) study of diabetes mellitus among patients attending Klinik Kesihatan Seri Manjung. NCD Malaysia. 2003;2(2):6–16.

7. Malathy R, Narmadha M, Ramesh S, et al. Effect of a diabetes counseling programme on knowledge, attitude and practice among diabetic patients in Erode district of South India. J Young Pharm. 2011;3(1):65–72. http://dx.doi.org/10.4103/0975-1483.76422

8. Kiberenge WM, Ndegwa ZM, Njenga EW, et al. Knowledge, attitude and practices related to diabetes among community members in four provinces in Kenya: A cross-sectional study. Pan Afr Med J. 2010;7:2.

9. Rothman RL, Malone R, Bryant B, et al. The spoken knowledge in low literacy in diabetes scale: a diabetes knowledge scale for vulnerable patients. Diabetes Educ. 2005;31(2):215–224. http://dx.doi.org/10.1177/0145721705275002

10. Palaian S, Acharya LD, Rao PGM, et al. Knowledge, attitude and practice outcomes: Evaluating the impact of counseling in hospitalized diabetic patients in India. P&T Around the World. 2006;31(7):383–396.

11. Hansraj P, Ragunathan S, Zhu T. Endocrinology: Diabetes Mellitus. In: Klostranec JM, Kolin DL. The essential med notes for medical students; 2012; pp. E6–E11.

12. Department of Health, Republic of South Africa). South Africa democratic and health survey 2003 [document on the Internet]. c2003 [cited 2014 Oct 26]. Available from: http://www.mrc.ac.za/bod/sadhs.htm

13. Erasmus R, Blanco E, Okesina A, et al. Assessment of glycemic control in stable type 2 black South African diabetics attending a peri-urban clinic. Postgrad Med J. 1999;75(888):603–606.

14. Leibbrandt M, Woolard I, Finn A, et al. Trends in South African income distribution and poverty since the fall of apartheid. OECD Social, Employment and Migration Working Papers, No. 101, OECD Publishing.

15. Groenewald AJ, van Wyk HJ, Walsh CM, et al. Prevalence of diabetes mellitus in the rural southern Free State. SA Fam Pract. 2009;51(6):502–505. http://dx.doi.org/10.1080/20786204.2009.10873914

16. Mukhopadhyay P, Paul B, Das D, et al. Perceptions and practices of type 2 diabetics: A cross-sectional study in a tertiary care hospital in Kolkata. Int J Diab Dev Ctries. 2010;30(3):143–149. http://dx.doi.org/10.4103/0973-3930.66510

17. Upadhyay DK, Palaian S, Shankar PR, et al. Knowledge, attitude and practice about diabetes among diabetes patients in Western Nepal. RMJ. 2008;33(1):8–11.

18. Calhoun D, Brod R, Kirlin K, et al. Effectiveness of motivational interviewing for improving self-care among Northern Plains Indians with type 2 diabetes. Diabetes Spectrum. 2010;23(2):107–114. http://dx.doi.org/10.2337/diaspect.23.2.107

19. West SD, DiLillo V, Bursac Z, et al. Motivational interviewing improves weight loss in women with type 2 diabetes. Diabetes Care. 2007;30(5):1081–1087. http://dx.doi.org/10.2337/dc06-1966

24

Maternal complication prevention: evidence from a case-control study in southwest Nigeria

Authors:
Kayode O. Osungbade[1,2]
Olubunmi O. Ayinde[3]

Affiliations:
[1]Faculty of Public Health, College of Medicine, University of Ibadan, Ibadan, Nigeria

[2]University College Hospital, Ibadan, Nigeria

[3]Oyo State Ministry of Health, Ibadan, Nigeria

Correspondence to:
Kayode Osungbade

Email:
koosungbade@yahoo.com

Postal address:
PMB 5017, General Post Office, Ibadan, Nigeria

Background: The importance of strengthening maternal health services as a preventive intervention for morbidities and complications during pregnancy and delivery in developing countries cannot be over-emphasised, since use of prenatal health services improves maternal health outcomes.

Aim: This study investigated differences in risk factors for maternal complications in booked and unbooked pregnant women in Nigeria, and provided evidence for their prevention.

Setting: The study was carried out in a postnatal ward in a secondary health facility.

Methods: This was a case-control study involving booked and unbooked pregnant women who had delivered. Consecutive enrolment of all unbooked pregnant women (cases) was done, and one booked pregnant woman (control) was enrolled and matched for age with each of these. Both groups were interviewed using a questionnaire, whilst records of delivery were extracted from the hospital files. Findings were subjected to logistical regression at a significance level of $p < 0.05$.

Results: Booked women had a lower median length of labour (10 hours) compared to unbooked women (13 hours). More women in the booked control group (139; 35.1%) than in the unbooked case group (96; 23.6%) reported at least one type of morbidity during the index pregnancy ($p = 0.0004$). Booking status was associated with a likelihood of spontaneous vaginal delivery. Young maternal age, low education, rural residence and low socio-economic status were associated with less likelihood of using prenatal services. Young maternal age, low education and intervention in the delivery were associated with a likelihood of experiencing a complication of delivery.

Conclusion: Strengthening antenatal and secondary healthcare services as short- and medium-term measures might be cost-effective as a preventive strategy in complications of pregnancy, whilst socio-economic dimensions of health are accorded priority in the long term.

Prévention des complications maternelles au sud-ouest du Nigeria.

Historique: L'utilisation des services de santé prénatals améliore la santé maternelle.

But: Cette étude examine les facteurs de risques de complications maternelles chez les femmes enceintes prises en charge et celles qui ne le sont pas au Nigeria et apporte des preuves pour prévenir ces complications.

Cadre: un service maternité dans un établissement de santé secondaire.

Méthodes: Une étude de contrôle des cas impliquant des femmes enceintes prises en charge et non prises en charge qui avaient accouché. L'inscription de tous les (cas de) grossesses non pris en charge ont eu lieu consécutivement tandis qu'une femme enceinte prise en charge (contrôle) a été inscrite et appariée selon l'âge avec chacun des (cas) de grossesse non pris en charge. Les deux groupes de participantes ont été interviewés à l'aide d'un questionnaire tandis que des dossiers des accouchements ont été obtenus à partir de la carte de renseignements personnels de chaque participante. Les résultats ont été soumis à la régression logistique à un haut niveau de $P < 0.05$.

Résultats: Les femmes prises en charge avaient aient un accouchement plus court (10 heures) comparé aux 13 heures des femmes non prises en charges. Plus de femmes dans le groupe de 'contrôle' pris en charge que dans le groupe de 'cas' non pris en charge ont signalé au moins un type de morbidité pendant l'indice de grossesse (139 [35.1%] contre 96 [23.6%]; $P = 0.0004$). La prise en charge allait de pair avec la possibilité d'un accouchement vaginal spontané. Le jeune âge de la mère, le bas niveau d'éducation, le milieu de résidence rural et le faible état socio-économique allaient de pair avec une probabilité moindre d'utilisation des services prénatals. Le jeune âge de la mère, le bas niveau d'éducation et l'accouchement avec intervention extérieure allaient de pair avec la probabilité de complications à l'accouchement.

Conclusion: Le renforcement des services de santé anténatals et secondaires comme mesure à court-et moyen-terme pourrait réduire les prix en tant que stratégie préventive tandis que les dimensions socio-économiques de la santé pourront avoir la priorité à long-terme.

Introduction

Although recent evidence has shown that not all components of antenatal care are useful in improving maternal and perinatal outcomes,[1,2] the role of antenatal care utilisation in achievement of the Millennium Development Goals cannot be under-estimated. Hence the introduction of the concept of focused antenatal care by the World Health Organisation (WHO) and a recommendation of at least four antenatal visits during pregnancy.[3,4] However, antenatal care utilisation through a trained health worker has remained far from optimal in developing countries, both in terms of rate of utilisation and quality of services provided. In Nigeria, for example, the antenatal care utilisation rate (i.e. antenatal care clinic attendance at least once during most recent pregnancy) is estimated at only 58% – 60%,[5,6] and the rate is much lower when using the WHO standard of antenatal care utilisation. A previous study reported at least four antenatal care visits in 56.6% of women in northern Nigeria during their last pregnancy.[7]

Furthermore, previous studies consistently reported poor quality of maternal health services.[8,9,10] Poor quality of care is one of the most common reasons why women do not choose to use available maternal health services. One study found that perceived quality of service was the most important factor influencing choice of facility for obstetric care.[11] Similarly, perceived lack of quality in antenatal care was associated with a late first antenatal visit in Kenya.[8] Therefore low or non-utilisation and declining quality of maternal health services are interwoven challenges which are working against efforts aimed at improving maternal health outcome in developing countries. Apart from quality of care other factors are responsible for low utilisation of the maternal health service, amongst which age, education and socio-economic status are prominent. Young maternal age, low education and low socio-economic status have been associated with lower likelihood of using maternity health services.[6,8]

Evidence abounds on the relationship between the use of prenatal care services and improved maternal and birth outcomes,[12,13,14] with the maternal mortality rate for unbooked pregnant women reported at 24/1000 and for booked women at 1/1000 in a study in northern Nigeria.[12] Other researchers reported that unbooked women were 13 times more likely to die in the hospital than booked women.[13] Likewise, unbooked mothers were twice as likely to deliver preterm babies and three times more likely to have babies with birth asphyxia than booked mothers,[14] whilst perinatal mortality occurs three times less in booked mothers than in unbooked mothers.[12] Furthermore, researchers have reported that maternal deaths could be reduced by promoting the availability of, access to and utilisation of basic and comprehensive emergency obstetric care services for women with complications of pregnancy and childbirth.[15] Effective implementation of such services resulted in a reduction in case fatality rate for direct maternal deaths from 7.2% to 4.6%.[15] Similarly, adequate use of prenatal care has been linked to higher birthweight and reduced neonatal tetanus; unbooked mothers have been shown to be three times more likely to have low birthweight babies than booked mothers, whilst two or more tetanus immunisations received during prenatal care were protective (adjusted odds ratio [AOR]0.78) against neonatal mortality in sub-Saharan African countries.[16–18]

Despite the potential benefits of maternal health services, pregnant women in developing countries do not utilise these services maximally. This constitutes a barrier to ameliorating maternal morbidity and mortality in such settings. Furthermore, efforts aimed at addressing this challenge are thwarted by lack of commitment of national governments to improve quality of service and also address socio-economic dimensions of health. In view of the foregoing, the importance of strengthening maternal health services as a preventive intervention for dealing with morbidities and complications during pregnancy and delivery in developing countries cannot be over-emphasised. This study therefore investigated differences in risk factors for maternal complications between booked and unbooked pregnant women in Nigeria, and the findings provided evidence on measures for preventing maternal complications and consequently reducing the unacceptably high maternal mortality in developing countries.

Research methods and design

We carried out a case-control study amongst women who delivered in a secondary healthcare facility over a period of six months.

Setting

The secondary healthcare facility was the first in Ibadan metropolis, south-west of Nigeria. This area has about 1 million people, and the facility takes referrals from surrounding public and private health facilities. It has a bed capacity of 247 and a health staff comprising 60 physicians (including specialists and medical officers) and 247 nurses. The hospital's records showed that about 410 deliveries occur per month and of these 75 (18.3%) of the women would present with no record of an antenatal visit.

Study population and sampling strategy

Our study population consisted of all booked (controls) and unbooked (cases) pregnant women who had a delivery (either live or stillbirth) in the health facility within the six months preceding the study. A pregnant woman was categorised as booked (control) if she had made at least two antenatal visits (the second less than two weeks before delivery) or was referred to the hospital with a record of antenatal care. On the other hand, a pregnant woman was categorised as unbooked (case) if she had not made any antenatal visits before delivery or made one or two visits (the second visit more than two weeks before date of delivery), or was referred to the hospital as an emergency for delivery and without any antenatal records at presentation.[19]

Using a prevalence of 58% as the proportion of pregnant women who would attend the antenatal service at least once during their current pregnancy,[5] 377 booked and 377 unbooked pregnant women were required for the study. All participants were recruited and interviewed in the lying-in ward of the health facility immediately as they arrived and not more two days after delivery, before discharge. All unbooked women who delivered in the hospital during the six-month period were consecutively enrolled. For the purpose of comparison each unbooked woman was matched for age with one booked woman, who was systematically enrolled using a sampling fraction of one-fifth. Written consent was obtained from each participant after providing them with detailed information about the study.

Data collection

This was carried out using a questionnaire which was developed and pretested in the lying-in ward of a similar health facility. The questionnaire had two parts: the first was used to document sociodemographic characteristics such as marital status, age, parity, socio-economic status, level of education and booking status, and was interviewer-administered in the local language of Yoruba. The second part was used to document delivery records extracted from health facility case notes for each participant. Extracted information comprised obstetric history, age of pregnancy at delivery, duration of labour in hours, method of delivery, complications (during and after delivery) and outcome of pregnancy. A 'bidding game approach' was used to obtain estimates of weekly income.[20] Each participant was asked about her weekly income by providing a yes/no answer to a suggested amount of money in the local currency. If the answer was 'no' to a first suggested amount, which was arbitrarily fixed at 6500 Naira (≈$45) per week, the interviewer made enquiries from the participant as to whether it was an under-estimation or over-estimation in order to determine the direction of bidding. The interviewer then either increased or decreased the bid by increments or decrements of 5000 Naira (≈$35) respectively until the participant said yes. The last sum of money receiving a 'yes' response was used as the estimated weekly income for that participant. This was found useful, as it is always difficult for respondents in an informal sector to provide accurate information on weekly income.

Data analysis

The Statistical Package for the Social Sciences (SPSS 12) was used for data analysis. Mean and standard deviations were estimated for continuous variables and number and percentage were estimated for categorical variables. Students' t-test was used to compare continuous variables and the chi-square test for categorical variables. The comparison of sociodemographic characteristics, maternal morbidity during pregnancy, mode of delivery and complications of delivery between cases and controls was tested using the chi- square test. Two sets of logistical regression analysis were done, one examining the effect of sociodemographic characteristics (as the independent variables) on booking status (as the dependent variable) and other models examining the effect of booking status (as the independent variable) on outcomes such as mode of delivery, maternal morbidity during pregnancy and complications of delivery (as dependent), with adjustments made for differences in sociodemographic characteristics between cases and controls. For the effect of sociodemographic characteristics on booking status, univariable logistical regression was done, followed by multiple logistical regression analysis including those variables significant at 10% on univariable logistical regression. The unadjusted (univariable) and adjusted (multivariable) odds ratios are presented. The odds ratios comparing unbooked with booked women concerning the outcomes (mode of delivery, maternal morbidity and complications at delivery) after adjusting for differences in sociodemographic characteristics are also stated. Level of significance for all tests was 5%.

Ethical considerations

Prior to data collection the researchers sought and received approval from the Ethical Research Committee of the State Ministry of Health (AD13/262/114). We also received permission from the authorities of the hospital in which the study was conducted.

Results

Records showed that 2610 pregnant women delivered in the hospital during the period of the study. Of these, 406 (15.5%) presented in labour as unbooked pregnancies (cases) and were delivered of their babies. Another 406 who also presented in labour, but as booked women, and delivered were enrolled as the comparison group (control). Ten of the booked women were either discharged or referred before they could be interviewed.

The ages of all the studied women were between 16 and 44 years, with a mean of 26.6 ± 5 years. The mean age of booked women was 26.9 ± 4 years compared to 26.4 ± 5.2 years for unbooked women (p = 0.12). Most of the studied women, 724 (90.2%), were aged 20 to 35 years; others were either less than 19 or more than 36 years old (Table 1). More of the unbooked pregnant women (307 or 75.6%) were semi-urban and rural residents, with 276 (69.7%) booked women of similar residence (p = 0.0326). Seventy-two (18.2%) of the booked women were single mothers compared to 116 (28.6%) of the unbooked women (p = 0.0008). More than half of the women (484 or 60.3%) had a secondary education, 189 (23.6%) had primary and 84 (10.5%) a tertiary education. A significantly lower proportion of booked women (15 or 3.8%) had no formal education compared to 30 (7.4%) of unbooked women. Concerning tertiary education, a significantly higher proportion of booked women (56 or 14.1%) had a tertiary education compared to 28 (6.9%) of unbooked women (p = 0.0009) (Table 1). The parity of all the studied women was between 0 and 6 children, with a mean of 2.3 ± 1.4 children. The mean parity of booked women was 2.3 ± 1.4 children compared to 2.3 ± 1.5 children for unbooked women (p = 0.5). Almost all of the women, 775 (96.6%), self-reported a lower weekly income category of N6500 (≈$45) per week (Table 1).

TABLE 1: Characteristics of the studied women.

Characteristics	Sub-category	Booking status				Total		*p* value
		Booked (*n* = 396)		Unbooked (*n* = 406)		*n*	%	
		n	%	*n*	%			
Age group (yrs)	≤ 19	15	3.8	24	5.9	39	4.9	0.3264
	20–29	261	65.9	269	66.3	530	66.0	
	30–35	103	26.0	91	22.4	194	24.2	
	≥ 36	17	4.3	22	5.4	39	4.9	
Residence	Urban	120	30.3	99	24.4	219	27.3	0.0326
	Semi-urban	269	68.0	290	71.4	559	69.7	
	Rural	7	1.7	17	4.2	24	3.0	
Marital status	Single	72	18.2	116	28.6	188	23.4	0.0008
	Married	317	80.0	288	70.9	605	75.4	
	Divorced	7	1.8	2	0.5	9	1.2	
Educational Status*	No education	15	3.8	30	7.4	45	5.6	0.0009
	Primary	84	21.2	105	25.9	189	23.6	
	Secondary	241	60.8	243	59.8	484	60.3	
	Tertiary	56	14.1	28	6.9	84	10.5	
Weekly Income (1 US $ ≈ N143)	≤N6500	376	94.9	399	98.3	775	96.6	0.009
	>N6500	20	5.1	7	1.7	27	3.4	
Disease	Any antenatal morbidity	**139**	**35.1**	**96**	**23.6**	**235**	**29.3**	**0.0004**
	Malaria	93	23.5	47	11.6	140	17.5	
	Hypertension	10	2.5	7	1.7	17	2.1	
	Antepartum haemorrhage	6	1.5	18	4.4	24	3.0	
	Infections†	17	4.3	7	4.4	24	3.0	
	Premature rupture of membranes	13	3.3	17	4.2	30	3.7	
Methods of delivery	Spontaneous vaginal delivery	364	91.9	348	85.7	712	88.8	0.0176
	Caesarean section	23	5.8	45	11.1	68	8.5	
	Assisted vaginal delivery‡	9	2.3	13	3.2	22	2.7	
Complications at delivery	Any delivery complication	**92**	**23.2**	**93**	**22.9**	**185**	**23.1**	**0.9128**
	Perineal tears	59	14.9	16	3.9	75	9.4	
	Retained placenta	7	1.8	31	7.6	38	4.7	
	Intrapartum haemorrhage	12	3.0	21	5.2	33	4.1	
	Eclampsia	8	2.0	10	2.5	18	2.2	
	Foot drop§	5	1.3	9	2.2	14	1.7	
	Malaria	2	0.5	7	1.7	9	1.1	
	Sepsis	3	0.8	9	2.2	12	1.5	
	Anaemia	5	1.3	18	4.4	23	2.9	

*, Educational status – highest educational level attained.
†, Infections – urinary tract infection, respiratory tract infection, vaginal candidiasis.
‡, Assisted vaginal deliveries – forceps, vacuum, assisted breech.
§, Foot drop – this is usually a temporary condition caused by compression of the nerve that controls the muscles involved in lifting the foot especially following a difficult labour. It causes weakness or paralysis of the muscles and makes it difficult or impossible for women to walk after child delivery.

Overall the number of hours in labour ranged from 3 to 23 hours, with a median of 12 hours. Booked women had a lower median of hours of labour (10 hours) compared to 13 hours recorded for unbooked women. More women in the booked 'control' group than in the unbooked 'case' group reported at least one type of morbidity during the index pregnancy (139 [35.1%] versus 96 [(23.6%]; p = 0.0004). Reported morbidities during pregnancy included malaria, hypertension, antepartum haemorrhage, other infections (bacterial or fungal) and premature rupture of the membranes (Table 1). Most of the women (712 or 88.8%) had a spontaneous vaginal delivery, whilst 90 (11.2%) had an intervention delivery. Of the 712 women who had a spontaneous vaginal delivery, 364 (91.9%) were booked and 348 (85.7%) were unbooked women; likewise, of the 68 women who had a caesarean section, 23 (5.8%) were booked compared to 45 (11.1%) women who were unbooked; these differences were statistically significant (p = 0.0176). Similarly, of the 22 women who had an assisted vaginal delivery, 9 (2.3%) were booked compared to 13 (3.2%) who were unbooked; however, this difference was not statistically significant (p = 0.42).

During delivery 209 women were given an episiotomy; of these, 137 (34.6%) were booked and 72 (17.7%) were unbooked. About equal proportions of women in the two groups (92[23.2%] booked versus 93 [22.9%] unbooked; p = 0.9128) reported at least one type of complication during delivery of the index pregnancy. These complications included perineal tears, retained placenta, intrapartum haemorrhage, eclampsia, foot drop, sepsis and anaemia (Table 1). One maternal death resulting from prolonged obstructed labour was reported amongst the unbooked women.

Pregnant women who were rural residents were half as likely to book for antenatal care as those who resided in urban and semi-urban areas (AOR = 0.45; 95% confidence interval [CI] 0.17–1.18) (Table 2). Pregnant women in the reproductive age group were more likely to use prenatal services than adolescent or elderly gravida women (OR for those ≤ 19 years old 0.64 [95% CI 0.33–1.26] and 0.80[0.41–1.53] for those aged ≥ 36 years). Single pregnant women were less likely to use prenatal services than married or divorced women (AOR = 0.58; 95% CI 0.41–0.81). Women of low education were less likely to use prenatal services than women with at least secondary education (AOR for women with no formal education 0.46 (95% CI 0.24–0.90) and for women with primary education 0.82 (0.58–1.15)). Women with a higher weekly income of 6500 Naira (≈$45) and above were twice as likely to use prenatal services than those who earned less (AOR = 2.07; 95% CI 0.84–5.13).

Table 3 shows that pregnant women who used prenatal services were about one and a half times more likely to experience at least one morbidity during pregnancy than women who did not use them (AOR = 1.69; CI 1.23–2.32). Women of low education were less likely to experience a morbidity during pregnancy than women with at least secondary education (AOR for women with no formal education 0.89 [95% CI 0.42–1.88] and 0.90 [0.61–1.34] for women with primary education). There were no significant differences between booked and unbooked groups in terms of tendency to experience complications during delivery (Table 1), although certain sociodemographic characteristics were found to influence this tendency. Adolescent pregnant

TABLE 2: Univariate and multivariate analyses of factors associated with booking for antenatal care by women.

Variable category	Sub-category	Booking for antenatal care	
		Univariate logistical regression, unadjusted OR (95% CI)	Multivariable logistical regression, adjusted OR (95% CI)
Residence	Urban	1.00	1.00
	Semi-urban	1.31 (0.96–1.79)	1.36 (0.98–1.87)
	Rural	0.50 (0.19–1.25)	0.45 (0.17–1.18)
Age group (yrs)	20–29	1.00	
	≤ 19	0.64 (0.33–1.26)	
	30–35	1.17 (0.84–1.62)	
	≥ 36	0.80 (0.41–1.53)	
Marital status	Married	1.00	1.00
	Single	0.56 (0.40–0.79)	0.58 (0.41–0.81)
	Divorced	6.36 (0.78–52.0)	4.83 (0.94–24.6)
Educational status	Secondary education	1.00	1.00
	No formal education	0.52 (0.27–0.99)	0.46 (0.24–0.90)
	Primary education	0.81 (0.58–1.13)	0.82 (0.58–1.15)
	Tertiary education	2.01 (1.24–3.28)	1.64 (0.99–2.74)
Minimum wage	≤ N6500	1.00	1.00
	> N6500	3.03 (1.27–7.25)	2.07 (0.84–5.13)

TABLE 3a: Univariate and multivariate analyses of factors associated with experiencing any morbidity during pregnancy and complications during delivery.

Characteristics	Sub-category	Morbidity during pregnancy	
		Univariate logistical regression, unadjusted OR (95% CI)	Multivariable logistical regression adjusted OR (95% CI)
Booking status	Unbooked	1.00	1.00
	Booked	1.75 (1.28–2.38)	1.69 (1.23–2.32)
Educational status	Secondary education	1.00	1.00
	No formal education	0.81 (0.39–1.64)	0.89 (0.42–1.88)
	Primary education	0.85 (0.58–1.24)	0.90 (0.61–1.34)
	Tertiary education	1.82 (1.13–2.93)	1.85 (1.11–3.06)

TABLE 3b: Univariate and multivariate analyses of factors associated with experiencing any morbidity during pregnancy and complications during delivery.

Characteristics	Sub-category	Complications during delivery	
		Univariate logistical regression, unadjusted OR (95% CI)	Multivariable logistical regression adjusted OR (95% CI)
Age group (yrs)	20–29	1.00	1.00
	≤ 19	1.72 (0.87–3.41)	1.13 (0.52–2.42)
	30–35	0.58 (0.38–0.90)	0.57 (0.35–0.93)
	≥ 36	1.06 (0.50–2.23)	0.96 (0.42–2.18)
Mode of delivery	Spontaneous vaginal	1.00	1.00
	Assisted vaginal	1.49 (0.57–3.88)	1.37 (0.51–3.69)
	Caesarean section	4.47 (2.68–7.45)	5.96 (3.45–10.29)
Income group	≤ N6500	1.00	1.00
	> N6500	1.70 (0.75–3.85)	2.94 (1.20–7.20)
Educational status	Secondary education	1.00	1.00
	No formal education	0.87 (0.40–1.87)	
	Primary education	1.25 (0.85–1.84)	1.61 (1.06–2.44)
	Tertiary education	0.73 (0.40–1.34)	0.78 (0.40–1.51)

women were more likely to experience a complication during pregnancy than older women (AOR = 1.13; CI 0.52–2.42). Women who gave birth by assisted vaginal delivery (AOR 1.37; 95% CI 0.51–3.69) and caesarean section (AOR 5.96; 3.45–10.29) were about one and half and six times more likely to have experienced a complication during pregnancy respectively. Higher weekly income earners were three times more likely to experience a complication during pregnancy than women in the low weekly income group (AOR = 2.94; CI 1.20–7.20). Women of low education (AOR 1.46; 95% CI 0.62–3.41) were about one and half times more likely to experience a complication during pregnancy than women with at least secondary education (AOR 1.61; CI 1.06–2.44).

Discussion

This study reported a prevalence of unbooked pregnancies of 15.5%. This is evidence of low or non-utilisation of antenatal care as a persistent and common practice in the study setting, confirming previous reports of 17% – 29% from similar surveys.[13,14] This study reported a significantly higher occurrence of maternal morbidity amongst the booked control group than the unbooked cases. This finding could be considered to be one of the benefits of antenatal care received by booked women, as it might have made possible early detection and prompt management of the reported morbidities during pregnancy. Booked women would also have had their delivery plans discussed and instituted with healthcare workers. These interventions, coupled with skilled delivery care received and the higher socio-economic parameters of booked women, might have been responsible for the improved maternal and perinatal outcomes amongst the study participants. The low reporting of morbidities by unbooked women might have partly resulted from under-reporting and missed diagnosis of the conditions; for example, the reported considerable use and abuse of antimalaria drugs and antibiotics, which are easily purchased across the counter for self-treatment in the study setting,[21] might be responsible for the low rate of malaria and infections of the urinary, respiratory and vaginal tracts.

As observed above, low or non-utilisation of antenatal care is a common practice in the study setting; in addition, out-of-hospital delivery is high, as 62.1% of deliveries reportedly occurred at home.[5] These factors, amongst others, may contribute to the different experiences reported amongst the two groups of women with regard to normal and intervention deliveries. Caesarean section and assisted delivery occurred more frequently amongst the unbooked women than their booked counterparts. This finding could be viewed as a direct output of the skilled delivery care received by the unbooked women, as the procedures might have been interventions aimed at dealing with the above-reported maternal complications, thereby saving the lives of mother and child.

From the foregoing, the common occurrence of unbooked emergencies with their attendant complications and potential contribution to maternal mortality seem to justify the proposition that promoting the availability of, access to and utilisation of basic and comprehensive emergency obstetric care services for women with complications of pregnancy and childbirth should be emphasised more than routine antenatal care services as a means of reducing maternal mortality in developing countries.[15] Although the cost of this 'preventive' mitigating strategy could be enormous in a resource-poor setting, the number of lives of women expected to be saved would evidently outweigh the cost consideration, particularly as emergencies are highly prevalent in unbooked women.

In view of the above it is suggested that health planners and care providers should accord high priority to strengthening the health systems with capacity to provide prompt and effective interventions against pregnancy and labour complications, particularly for unbooked pregnancies. Consequently health facilities should be appropriately staffed with personnel who are capable of providing the desired services. Equipping healthcare facilities to provide basic and comprehensive emergency obstetric care services sufficient to deal with such complications in developing countries requires specific training for health workers and provision of state of the art equipment and facilities for detecting, resuscitating and managing life-threatening situations. The capacity of midwifery and nursing personnel could be enhanced through WHO training on life-saving skills;[22] likewise, medical personnel require skill building in cardiopulmonary resuscitation as well as assisted and operative delivery to be able to intervene when necessary. Staff training should be supported by provision and maintenance of appropriate equipment and facilities optimally required to provide the desired services, including blood transfusion services, in the health facilities.

In order to ensure efficiency in the health systems, the policy on human resources for health should address strategies (such as staff redeployment and retention) which are required to make available healthcare staff in a manner to favour rural residents in particular.[23] Furthermore, best practices dictate a continuous review of health systems, as such an exercise provides the opportunity for appraisal and identification of strengths and weaknesses requiring specific interventions. It is highly desirable to subject the above recommended measures to a periodical clinical audit for maintenance of quality care at all times.

Whilst the above recommendations could suffice as short- and medium-term measures, we further suggest that healthcare planners and providers institute long-term cost-effective measures aimed at addressing the high maternal mortality. It has previously been shown that antenatal care could positively influence a key strategy of maternal mortality reduction in developing countries – that is that all pregnant women deliver with the assistance of a skilled attendant.[24] Unfortunately the situation with regard to skilled delivery assistance in the study setting is poor; this was recently reported to be 39% – 44%.[5,6] Therefore strategies aimed at increasing the current antenatal care utilisation rate of 58% – 60% should be vigorously pursued alongside improving the quality of service. It is hoped that increasing the utilisation rate of antenatal care services would have a direct impact on use of delivery services manned by skilled health workers.

National governments and international development partners might place priority on other long-term strategies such as education of every girl child and improving household wealth in poor-resource settings, especially for female populations. It is expected that these measures will have multidimensional effects. Firstly, girls' education would help them to develop essential life skills, including self- confidence, ability to participate effectively in society, and to protect themselves from harmful sociocultural practices, including late or non-booking for antenatal care. Secondly, educational attainment of girls and improvement in household wealth would empower women economically and in decision making to seek health care. Thirdly, female education might help to keep women in school until they are of an age which would favourably use maternal health services.

Conclusion

Unbooked pregnant women presenting in labour is a common phenomenon amongst the study population, and might be contributing significantly to the high maternal mortality rates in developing countries. Whilst efforts at provision of basic and comprehensive emergency obstetric care services for such women are currently being emphasised as a means of reducing maternal mortality, strategies aimed at addressing the low or non-utilisation of maternal health services are equally important, and hence require adequate attention.

Acknowledgements

The authors are grateful to Oyo State Hospital's Management Board and the management of the secondary healthcare facility for the permission given to conduct the study.

Competing interests

The authors declare that they have no financial or personal relationship(s) that may have inappropriately influenced them in writing this article.

Authors' contributions

O.O.A. (Ministry of Health) took part in conceptualising and designing the study, collected, analysed and interpreted the data, and approved the final draft of the manuscript. K.O.O. (University of Ibadan and University College Hospital) took part in conceptualising and designing the study, prepared the first draft of the manuscript and approved the final draft.

References

1. Gagnon AJ. Individual or group antenatal education for childbirth parenthood. Cochrane Database of Systematic Reviews. 4: CD002869; 2000.
2. Villar J, Ba'aqeel H, Piaggio G, et al. WHO antenatal care randomised trial for the evaluation of a new model of routine antenatal care. Lancet. 2001;357:1551–1564. http://dx.doi.org/10.1016/S0140-6736(00)04722-X
3. World Health Organisation. WHO antenatal care randomised trial: Manual for the implementation of the new model. Geneva: WHO; 2001.
4. World Health Organisation. Antenatal care in developing countries: Promises, achievements and missed opportunities. Geneva: WHO; 2003.
5. National Population Commission, Nigeria and ICF Macro. Nigeria Demographic and Health Survey 2008. Abuja, Nigeria: National Population Commission and ICF Macro; 2009.
6. Babalola S, Fatusi A. Determinants of use of maternal health services in Nigeria – looking beyond individual and household factors. BMC Pregnancy Childbirth. 2009;9:43. http://dx.doi.org/10.1186/1471-2393-9-43
7. Galadanci HS, Ejembi CL, Iliyasu Z, Alagh B, Umar US. Maternal health in Northern Nigeria – a far cry from ideal. BJOG. 2007;114:448-452. http://dx.doi.org/10.1111/j.1471-0528.2007.01229.x
8. Van Ejik AM, Bles HM, Odhiambo F, et al. Use of antenatal services and delivery care among women in rural western Kenya: A community based survey. Reprod Health. 2006;3:2. http://dx.doi.org/10.1186/1742-4755-3-2
9. Sagay AS, Ekwempu CC, Kabiru M, Daru PC, Aisien AO. Audit of antenatal services in primary healthcare centers in Jos, Nigeria. Niger Med Pract. 2007;51:80–84.
10. Osungbade KO, Oginni SA, Olumide EA. Content of antenatal care services in secondary health care facilities in Nigeria: Implication for quality of maternal health care. Int J Qual Health Care. 2008;20:346–351. http://dx.doi.org/10.1093/intqhc/mzn026
11. Iyaniwura CA, Yussuf Q. Utilisation of antenatal care and delivery services in Sagamu, south western Nigeria. Afr J Reprod Health. 2009;13:111–122.
12. Ekwempu. The influence of antenatal care on pregnancy outcome. Trop J Obstet Gynaecol. 1988;1(1):67–71.
13. Chigbu B, Onwere S, Kamanu CI, Aluka C, Okoro O, Adibe E. Pregnancy outcome in booked and unbooked mothers in South Eastern Nigeria. East Afr Med J. 2009;86(6):267–71.
14. Owolabi AT, Fatusi AO, Kuti O, Adeyemi A, Faturoti SO, Obiajuwa PO. Maternal complications and perinatal outcomes in booked and unbooked Nigerian mothers. Singapore Med J. 2008;49(7):526–531.
15. Mekbib T, Kassaye E, Getachew A, Tadesse T, Debebe A. The FIGO save the mother's initiative: The Ethiopia-Sweden collaboration. Int J Gynaecol Obstet. 2003;81:93–102. http://dx.doi.org/10.1016/S0020-7292(03)00071-7
16. McCurdy RJ, Kjerulff KH, Zhu, J. Prenatal care associated with reduction of neonatal mortality in Sub-Saharan Africa: Evidence from Demographic and Health Surveys. Acta Obstet Gynaecol Scand. 2011;90(7):779–790. http://dx.doi.org/10.1111/j.1600-0412.2011.01133.x
17. Olowonyo T, Oshin S, Obasanjo-Bello I. Some factors associated with low birth weight in Ogun State, Nigeria. Niger Med Pract. 2006;49:154–157. http://dx.doi.org/10.4314/nmp.v49i6.28823
18. Tucker A, Ogutu D, Yoong W, Nauta M, Fakokunde A. The unbooked mother: A cohort study of maternal and foetal outcomes in a North London Hospital. Arch Gynaecol Obstet. 2010;281(4):613–616. http://dx.doi.org/10.1007/s00404-009-1152-7
19. Harrison KA. William Meredith Fletcher Shaw Memorial Lecture: Poverty, deprivation and maternal health. In: Studd J, editor. Yearbook of the Royal College of Obstetricians and Gynaecologists. London: Royal College of Obstetricians and Gynaecologists, 1995; pp. 33–44.
20. Dong H, Kouyate B, Cairns J, Mugisha F, Sauerborn R. Willingness-to-pay for community-based insurance in Burkina Faso. Health Econ. 2003;12:849–862. http://dx.doi.org/10.1002/hec.771
21. Agbaje EO, Uwakwe LO. Irrational use of antimicrobial agents in Surulere local government area of Lagos State, Nigeria. Niger J Med. 2003;13:1–2.
22. World Health Organisation. Making pregnancy safer: the critical role of the skilled attendant. A joint statement by WHO, ICM and FIGO. Department of Reproductive Health and Research [monograph online]. WHO; 2004. [cited 2008 Mar 5]. Available from: http://www.who.int/reproductive-health/publications/2004/skilled_attendant.pdf
23. Koblinsky M, Matthews Z, Hussein J, et al. Going to scale with professional skilled care. Lancet. 2006;368:1377–1186. http://dx.doi.org/10.1016/S0140-6736(06)69382-3
24. McDonagh M. Is antenatal care effective in reducing maternal morbidity and mortality? Health Policy Plan. 1996;11:1–15. http://dx.doi.org/10.1093/heapol/11.1.1

25

Attitudes, knowledge and practices of healthcare workers regarding occupational exposure of pulmonary tuberculosis

Authors:
Lesley T. Bhebhe[1]
Cornel Van Rooyen[2]
Wilhelm J. Steinberg[1]

Affiliations:
[1]Department of Family Medicine, Faculty of Health Sciences, University of the Free State, South Africa

[2]Department of Biostatistics, Faculty of Health Sciences, University of the Frees State, South Africa

Correspondence to:
Wilhelm J. Steinberg

Email:
steinbergwj@ufs.ac.za

Postal address:
PO Box 339, Bloemfontein 9300, South Africa

Background: Healthcare-associated tuberculosis (TB) has become a major occupational hazard for healthcare workers (HCWs). HCWs are inevitably exposed to TB, due to frequent interaction with patients with undiagnosed and potentially contagious TB. Whenever there is a possibility of exposure, implementation of infection prevention and control (IPC) practices is critical.

Objective: Following a high incidence of TB among HCWs at Maluti Adventist Hospital in Lesotho, a study was carried out to assess the knowledge, attitudes and practices of HCWs regarding healthcare-associated TB infection and infection controls.

Methods: This was a cross-sectional study performed in June 2011; it involved HCWs at Maluti Adventist Hospital who were involved with patients and/or sputum. Stratified sampling of 140 HCWs was performed, of whom, 129 (92.0%) took part. A self-administered, semi-structured questionnaire was used.

Results: Most respondents (89.2%) had appropriate knowledge of transmission, diagnosis and prevention of TB; however, only 22.0% of the respondents knew the appropriate method of sputum collection. All of the respondents (100.0%) were motivated and willing to implement IPC measures. A significant proportion of participants (36.4%) reported poor infection control practices, with the majority of inappropriate practices being the administrative infection controls (> 80.0%). Only 38.8% of the participants reported to be using the appropriate N-95 respirator.

Conclusion: Poor infection control practices regarding occupational TB exposure were demonstrated, the worst being the first-line administrative infection controls. Critical knowledge gaps were identified; however, there was encouraging willingness by HCWs to adapt to recommended infection control measures. Healthcare workers are inevitably exposed to TB, due to frequent interaction with patients with undiagnosed and potentially contagious TB. Implementation of infection prevention and control practices is critical whenever there is a possibility of exposure.

Attitudes, Connaissances et Pratiques des membres du personnel soignant relatives à l'exposition du personnel soignant à la Tuberculose pulmonaire.

Historique: La Tuberculose nosocomiale (TB) est devenue un risque professionnel important pour le personnel soignant (HCWs). Les membres du HCW sont forcément exposés à la Tuberculose, en raison de l'interaction fréquente avec les patients ayant une tuberculose non diagnostiquée et potentiellement contagieuse. Il est essentiel de mettre en œuvre la prévention de l'infection et de faire des contrôles (IPC) quand il y a un risque d'exposition.

Objectif: Suite à la haute incidence de Tuberculose parmi les HCW au Maluti Adventist Hospital du Lesotho, on a mené une enquête pour évaluer les connaissances, attitudes et pratiques des HCW en ce qui concerne la tuberculose nosocomiale et le contrôle des infections.

Méthodes: C'était une étude transversale réalisée en juin 2011 à laquelle ont participé les HCW du Maluti Adventist Hospital, qui s'occupent des patients et/ou du frottis d'expectoration. On a fait l'échantillonnage stratifié de 140 HCW auquel 129 (92%) ont pris part. On a utilisé un questionnaire auto-administré et semi-structuré.

Résultats: la majorité des répondants (89.2%) avaient une bonne connaissance de la transmission, du diagnostic et de la prévention de la Tuberculose, mais seuls 22% des répondants connaissaient la méthode appropriée de prélèvement des expectorations. Tous les répondants (100%) étaient motivés et désireux de mettre en œuvre les mesures de prévention et de contrôle des infections. Une proportion importante de participants (36.4%) a signalé de mauvaises pratiques de contrôle des infections où la majorité des pratiques inadéquates étaient les contrôles administratifs des infections (> 80%). Seuls 38.8% des participants ont signalé qu'ils utilisaient le respirateur approprié $N = 95$.

Conclusion: Les mauvaises pratiques de contrôle des infections relatives aux risques professionnels d'exposition à la Tuberculose ont été démontrées, les pires étant les contrôles administratifs de première ligne des infections. On a identifié aussi des lacunes dans les connaissances. Cependant, il est encourageant de constater la volonté des HCW d'adopter les mesures recommandées de contrôle des infections. Les HCW sont forcément exposés à la Tuberculose, en raison de l'interaction fréquente avec les patients souffrant de Tuberculose non-diagnostiquée et potentiellement contagieuse. La mise en œuvre des pratiques de contrôle et de prévention des infections (IPC) est essentielle quand il y a la possibilité d'exposition à la contagion.

Introduction

Tuberculosis (TB) has become a major, global public-health concern; in 2009,[1] it claimed an estimated 1.7 million lives. In 2008, the Sub-Saharan Africa incidence rate of TB was 350 cases per 100 000 population, and 640 per 100 000 in Lesotho alone. Exacerbating factors are: the HIV epidemic, lack of proper facilities and resources for TB prevention, and lack of political will.[2,3,4,5] In the light of this high burden of TB, healthcare workers (HCWs) in high TB prevalence areas are inadvertently and inevitably exposed to TB, due to their constant interaction with patients with undiagnosed, untreated and potentially contagious TB in healthcare settings. In Kwazulu-Natal in South Africa, the incidence of TB among HCWs in public sector hospitals was higher than community-acquired TB.[6]

Despite TB being curable with the use of drugs, TB control depends on more than just chemotherapy. The ultimate prevention requires the integration of chemotherapy with infection prevention and control (IPC) measures to reduce transmission of TB in the general population and in health facilities.[7] Knowledge and implementation of TB control measures by HCWs, and their compliance and willingness, remain the key factors in the effective management of healthcare-associated TB. Numerous comprehensive IPC guidelines have been designed for healthcare facilities, inclusive of low-resourced settings.[8,9,10]

In 2009, Maluti Adventist Rural District Hospital in Lesotho had seven HCWs diagnosed with healthcare-associated TB. That year, there were approximately 225 healthcare workers (inclusive of nursing students) working directly with patients and/or sputum. Thus, 3111 per 100 000 HCWs at Maluti Adventist hospital were newly infected with TB in that year. Those infected were of diverse profiles with one common factor: work-related exposure. Correct knowledge of the health problem, accompanied with the right attitude, can ultimately result in healthy practices and behaviour.[11] Hence, the present study to evaluate knowledge, practices and attitudes of HCWs regarding healthcare-associated TB.

Research methods and design

This was a cross-sectional descriptive study of knowledge, attitudes and practices of HCWs at Maluti Adventist Hospital in the Berea District of Lesotho, which is located 70 km south of the capital city, Maseru. These HCWs spent at least 2 h a day with patients in the ward or as outpatients, and were employed at the hospital for at least 6 months. All participants were 18 years and older, and gave written consent to participate in the study. The data were collected between June 01 and 30 2011. There were 337 workers at Maluti Adventist Hospital, of which, 225 were directly involved with patients and/or sputum at the time of the present study. A stratified sampling method was used to select 140 participants.

A self-administered questionnaire was used. This included: 13 demographic characteristics of the HCWs; 35 questions on knowledge (True/False or Yes/No type); 10 questions on attitudes (Yes/No type); and 12 questions on practices of HCWs regarding healthcare-associated TB infection (Yes/No type and two multiple choice-type questions). A pilot study was conducted on six participants, one from each of the six HCW population subgroups. No problems were identified and they were included in the study. The questionnaire was available in English and Sesotho, and distributed and collected by the researcher. The questionnaires were administered to each participant at different times, and participants were asked to be complete it without consulting a colleague. The study was approved by the Ethics Committee of the Faculty of Health Sciences of the University of the Free State (ECUFS NR 37/2011). Permission was granted by the Maluti Adventist Hospital Administration. Participation was on a voluntary basis and confidentiality was maintained throughout. Analysis of the data was performed by the Department of Biostatistics, University of the Free State. Total scores for each section for knowledge, attitude and practice were calculated and categorised as poor (< 39.0%), fair (40.0% – 69.0%) and good (70.0% +).

Results

Participant demographics

Of the 140 individuals selected for participation, 11 refused consent. This resulted in a final sample size of 129, which is a participation rate of 92.0% and corresponds to 57.3% of the HCW population. The distribution of the sample aligned well to the population strata of the HCWs at the hospital (see Table 1).

Of the 129 respondents, 11.6% were male and 88.4% were female. The age of the respondents ranged from 19 to 60 years, whilst the mean and median age was 31 and 27 years, respectively. The duration of employment ranged from 1 to 37 years, with a mean duration of 6.7 years and a median of 3 years. Table 1 summarises the baseline characteristics of the study population and confirms the representativeness of the sample.

Knowledge, attitudes and practices

In the knowledge section, 86.1% of the participants obtained a fair score (40.0% – 69.0%). Concerning attitudes, 93.0% of the respondents reflected good attitudes towards TB IPC

TABLE 1: Baseline characteristics of the sample (n = 129) of healthcare workers at Maluti Adventist Hospital.

Variable	Frequency (n)	%	Percentage in hospital
Gender			
Male	15	11.6	16.0
Female	114	88.4	84.0
Profession type in hospital			
General hand	7	5.4	4.0
Student nurse	70	54.3	55.1
Nurse assistant	29	22.5	20.9
Nurse attendant	9	7.0	10.2
Registered nurse	9	7.0	6.2
Medical doctor	5	3.9	3.6

measures, whilst 52.7% obtained a fair score for reported practices. Table 2 summarises the scores in the three respective areas.

Knowledge

Whilst the majority of respondents recognised pulmonary TB as being potentially contagious, 117 (90.7%) recognised airborne spread as the mode of transmission, whilst 12 (9.3%) gave other, inappropriate modes of transmission that included waterborne spread (1.6%) and direct contact (7.6%).

Most respondents were able to identify constitutional symptoms of TB; however, only 69 (53.5%) considered fever to be a symptom of TB. The majority of respondents recognised the link between HIV and TB, and knew that sputum examination was a major diagnostic tool; however, only 29 (22.0%) respondents were aware of the appropriate place for sputum collection. The majority of respondents were well acquainted with the circumstances around the treatment of PTB. The BCG (Bacille Calmette-Guérin) vaccination was identified by 75 (58.6%) respondents as not being a preventive measure against contracting pulmonary TB. Table 3 shows the participant responses on knowledge questions regarding transmission, predisposing factors, prevention, diagnosis and treatment of TB.

Attitudes

All respondents indicated that they were willing to change their habits and practices towards TB IPC methods, with 93.0% of them reporting positive attitudes. Table 4 contains the responses measuring HCW attitudes.

Practices

Forty-seven (36.4%) of the respondents self-reported inappropriate practices (Table 2). The majority of the respondents (> 50%) reported poor administrative IPC control practice. Screening of TB patients for HIV was the exception, with 93.8% reporting appropriate practice. Environmental control measures, which are second-line IPC practices, had mixed responses with 35 (27.1%) respondents observing controls to avoid air recirculation into other (non-TB) wards. On personal protective measures, 92 (71.3%) respondents reported that they used masks, of which 54.4% used the N95 respirator (accounting for 38.8% of the entire sample size). Other personal protective measure practices were fair (Table 5).

Discussion

All HCWs managing inpatients and outpatients with a risk of healthcare-associated TB infection at this hospital were represented in the present study. The sample was comparable in composition to the HCW population strata of the hospital. A thorough understanding of the way in which TB is contracted remains critical for the implementation of IPC measures. The respondents of the present study

TABLE 2: Levels of knowledge, attitudes and practices of Maluti Adventist Hospital healthcare workers towards tuberculosis infection control.

Variable	Frequency (n)	%
Knowledge scores (n = 129)		
≤ 39%	14	10.9
40% – 69%	111	86.1
≥ 70%	4	3.1
Attitudes scores (n = 129)		
≤ 39%	0	0.0
40% – 69%	9	7.0
≥ 70%	120	93.0
Practice scores (n = 129)		
≤ 39%	47	36.4
40% – 69%	68	52.7
≥ 70%	14	10.9

TB, tuberculosis.

TABLE 3: Knowledge on tuberculosis transmission, predisposing factors, prevention, diagnosis and treatment by Maluti Adventist Hospital healthcare workers.

Variable (n = 129)	Appropriate knowledge		
	Symptoms	n	%
Airborne mode of transmission	-	117	90.7
Pulmonary TB as contagious type of TB	-	122	94.7
Pulmonary TB constitutional symptoms	Chronic cough	122	94.7
	Weight loss	102	79.1
	Fever	69	53.5
	Night sweats	109	84.5
HIV predisposition to contracting TB	-	123	96.1
Diagnosis of pulmonary TB by sputum smear	-	125	96.9
Appropriate place for collection of sputum	-	29	22.0
Six-month treatment duration	-	128	99.2
TB curable	-	126	97.7
Preventability of contracting pulmonary TB	-	117	91.4
BCG vaccination not preventive to contracting pulmonary TB	-	75	58.6

TB, tuberculosis; BCG, Bacille Calmette-Guérin; n, respondents.

TABLE 4: Attitudes of healthcare workers towards preventive methods of nosocomial tuberculosis.

Variable (n = 129)	Yes		No		Not sure	
	n	%	n	%	n	%
Would you use a mask even though it is uncomfortable?	93	72.1	8	6.2	28	21.7
Would you be screened for TB if you had suggestive symptoms?	123	95.4	1	0.8	5	3.9
If diagnosed with TB, would you be willing to test for HIV?	113	87.6	7	5.4	9	7.0
If diagnosed with TB, would you be willing to complete treatment?	126	97.7	0	0.0	3	2.3
If you had a condition that predisposed you to contracting TB, would you be willing to change your work environment?	104	80.6	12	9.3	13	10.1
If malnourished, would you be willing to adjust your eating habits?	126	97.7	2	1.6	1	0.8
Would you be willing to provide adequate ventilation and sunlight, regardless of weather conditions?	116	89.9	1	0.8	12	9.3
Would you be willing to teach patients and co-workers about TB prevention?	124	96.1	0	0.0	5	3.9
Would you be willing to attend seminars for TB prevention?	122	94.6	2	1.6	5	3.9

TB, tuberculosis.

TABLE 5: Administrative, environmental and personal tuberculosis infection control practices by Maluti Adventist healthcare workers.

Variable (n = 129)	Appropriate practice Knowledge	
	n	%
Administrative control measures		
Appropriate collection of sputum	23	17.8
Screening of suspicious TB patients in waiting areas (n = 127)†	25	19.7
Prioritising TB suspects for prompt service (n = 127)*	23	18.11
Screening TB patients for HIV	121	93.8
TB infection control education	34	26.4
Environmental control measures		
Isolation of patients, use of separate TB ward	101	78.3
Avoidance of air recirculation in non-TB wards	35	27.1
Open windows for ventilation and sunlight	89	69.0
Personal protection measures		
Personal protection by use of a respirator	92*	71.3
Use of appropriate respirator N-95 (n = 92)‡	50	54.4
Protective clothing usage	64	46.9
Hand hygiene	98	76.0
Disposition of linen infection control (n = 126)*	72	57.1

†, 3 responses missing; ‡, of the 92 respondents who use masks, 54.4% use the correct mask; *, 2 responses missing; n respondents.

confirmed sufficient knowledge about the transmission of PTB. The risk for TB transmission should be evaluated in all of the departments and areas where infectious TB patients might access care.

Eighty-nine percent of the respondents reported satisfactory knowledge of TB transmission, predisposing factors, prevention, diagnosis and treatment. The knowledge findings are similar to those of surveys conducted elsewhere in developing countries. Kiefer et al., whose scope of knowledge questions was similar to that of the present study, found that most participants scored between 57.8% and 85.0%, which falls within the fair and excellent range of knowledge scale of this study.[12] Hoa et al.,[13] with a similar profile of knowledge questions, found that rural Vietnamese health providers had a mean knowledge score of 67.0%. The mean knowledge score in the present study was 61.5%. In Iraq, Hashin et al.[14] found the knowledge of TB among HCWs to be almost 100%. Most of the participants in their study had a diploma qualification as health professionals and the majority (73.0%) had been employed for more than 10 years. In contrast, the present study population included nursing students, and the median duration of employment was three years. In a Russian study by Woith et al.,[15] the overall knowledge scores on TB and IPC practices were low for HCWs, which is in contrast to the present study.

Early diagnosis of infectious patients should result in a reduction of exposure of the HCWs in hospitals. If HCWs are able to identify the symptoms of TB, in the event that they are infected, they can seek help early and prevent morbidity and mortality associated with the infection. No studies can be cited of HIV prevalence among HCWs in Lesotho, but studies performed in South Africa have shown the prevalence of HIV among HCWs to be 15.7% and 11.5 %.[16,17] The knowledge of HIV status and its association with TB is essential in order for susceptible HCWs to take relevant precautionary measures towards exposure reduction.

Knowledge gaps were identified in the present study, with only 22.0% of respondents knowing the appropriate sputum collection method. Critical knowledge gaps, despite good knowledge levels, were also found by Kiefer et al. in a study conducted in Peru.[12] However, the actual knowledge gaps were different to the ones found in the present study. HCWs are frequently in contact with infectious patients and they facilitate the collection of sputum for both inpatients and outpatients. Sputum collection could thus predispose HCWs, as well as other patients, to healthcare-associated infection. Only 17.8% of the respondents reported collecting sputum correctly from patients, as recommended by Centres for Disease Control and Prevention (CDC) guidelines.[8] This is likely a major risk for healthcare-associated infection.

TB control does not depend soley on chemotherapy, IPC measures and pathophysiology knowledge, but also on motivated HCWs with good attitudes towards IPC. Cooperation and team work is essential in the fight against TB, with HCWs who are willing to implement necessary changes and embrace new practices and recommendations. In the present study, 100% of the participants indicated that they were willing to implement preventive measures against healthcare-associated TB infection. A review study of several international studies support this finding of a high degree of willingness of HCWs to collaborate with TB national guidelines and infection controls.[18] It needs to be borne in mind that these studies, as well as the present study, only tested the self-reported willingness of the HCWs to implement changes, which may differ from actual (eventual) practices.

The World Health Organization (WHO) proposed guidelines for IPC measures that are effective, affordable and can be implemented in resource-limited settings.[19,10] The CDC and WHO guidelines proposed the implementation of IPC measures at three levels: administrative, environmental and personal respiratory protection.[8,10] In order for the IPC methods to be effective, an IPC plan should be endorsed. In the IPC strategy, administrative controls are the cornerstone and first priority, whilst the other two are entirely dependent on administrative control for their effectiveness. Administrative controls reduce HCW and patient exposures to healthcare-associated TB infection. Poor IPC practices (as high as 36.4%) were measured in the present study, with poor administrative IPC measures constituting the majority. Administrative IPC measure implementation levels of less than 20.0% were reported. This is a huge pitfall, since these should be implemented at first contact with an infectious patient at a health facility. Delays in screening, diagnosis and treatment of TB due to failure of implementation of these controls increase the risk of healthcare-associated infection. Environmental IPC measures are dependent on infrastructural design, the use of ventilation and irradiation, which all require capital investment; however, simpler effective methods have been proposed based on adequate ventilation through the opening of windows.[10] This is challenging, especially in Lesotho, where weather conditions are harsh, with winters that can record temperatures below 0 °C. This could possibly contribute to some HCWs not opening the windows for ventilation and keeping doors closed, explaining, to a degree, the low compliance reported with these IPC practices.

The findings regarding personal protective equipment were of concern. Biscotto et al. had similar findings, in which they found that HCWs infrequently used masks when performing procedures or attending patients with high risk of healthcare-associated infection. For example, of those attending TB isolation rooms, only 39.5% were observed to be using N95 respirators.[20] This is comparable to the 38.8% in the present study who reported to be using respirators. On the other hand, unavailability of respiratory protective equipment could limit their use in the hospital, which was something not measured in the present study. Widespread and constant use of appropriate N95 respirators is regarded as impractical at Maluti Adventist Hospital due to the financial constrains resulting in failure to acquire them. In other studies, it has been noted that prohibitive costs in low-income countries in Africa result in failure of widespread use of N95 respirators for healthcare-associated TB prevention and control.[21,22] At Maluti Adventist Hospital, it was also noted that in some departments, the use of N95 respirators was limited to areas of perceived high risk for healthcare-associated TB infection only. This could have also contributed to a low percentage of the respondents reporting their usage in the present study.

Limitations

The present study only measured variables that were self-reported by the HCWs and did not take into consideration the availability of resources (such as respirators) required for the implementation of IPC measures. This could have affected the results, as the respondents who reported not implementing these measures may have done so because of non-availability of resources. It is noteworthy to mention that the use of a self-administered questionnaire to measure practice is subject to response bias, as compared to the actual practices. Studies observing practices would yield more accurate data than using self-administered questionnaires.

Conclusion

Despite the good general knowledge about TB that was shown by the HCWs, knowledge gaps regarding safe sputum collection were demonstrated. The HCWs reported to be willing to implement IPC practices. In this resource-limited setting, environmental controls and respiratory protective equipment implementation rates were reportedly low. Further studies should investigate why this is the case, and consider the availability of resources and other possible infrastructure constrains.

Administrative IPC measures should be the first-line pillar of infection control, and should receive more recognition in the studied setting. In the absence of appropriate IPC practices, healthcare-associated infections will inevitably remain a risk.

Acknowledgements

We thank the administration of Maluti Adventist Hospital for permission to do the study. The results of this study have been presented at the combined RuDASA and Phasa Conference held in Bloemfontein, August 2013.

Competing interests

The authors declare that they have no financial or personal relationship(s) that may have inappropriately influenced them in writing this article.

Authors' contributions

L.T.B. (University of the Free State) initiated, designed and executed the protocol and project. W.J.S. (University of the Free State) was the supervisor and gave significant input and guidance to planning and execution of the study project as well as the write up. C.V.R. (University of the Free State) helped with the design of the data gathering tool and gave inputs on the methodology, analysed the data and reviewed versions of the write up.

References

1. World Health Organization. Global tuberculosis control: Epidemiology, strategy, financing 2009. [online] 2009 [cited 2011 Jan 14]. Available from: www.who.int/tb/publications/global_report/2009/pdf/full_report.pdf
2. Joshi R, Reingold AL, Menzies D, Pai M. Tuberculosis among Health-Care Workers in Low- and Middle-Income Countries: A Systematic Review. PLoS Med. 2006;3(12):e494. http://dx.doi.org/10.1371/journal.pmed.0030494
3. Nyangulu DS, Harries AD, Kang'ombe C, Yadidi AE, Chokani K, Cullinan T, et al. Tuberculosis in a prison population in Malawi. Lancet. 1997;350:1284–1287. http://dx.doi.org/10.1016/S0140-6736(97)05023-X
4. World Health Organization. Tuberculosis Fact Sheet [online] 2010 [cited 2010 Dec 14]. Available from: www.who.int/mediacentre/factsheets/fs104/en/
5. World Health Organization. Global Tuberculosis Database [online] 2011 [cited 2011 Feb 2]. Available from: http://www.who.int/tb/country/data/profiles/en/index.html
6. Naidoo S, Jinabhai CC. TB in healthcare workers in KwaZulu-Natal, South Africa. Int J Tuberc Lung Dis. 2006;10(6):676–682.
7. South African Department of Health. South African National Tuberculosis Management Guidelines, 2009. [online] 2009 [cited 2014 Apr 10]. Available from: http://familymedicine.ukzn.ac.za/Libraries/Guidelines_Protocols/TB_Guidelines_2009.sflb.shax
8. Centre for Disease Control and Prevention. Guidelines for preventing the transmission of Mycobacterium tuberculosis in health-care settings, 2005. MMWR. 2005;54 (No.RR-17).
9. California Division of Occupational Safety and Health (Cal/OSHA). Interim Tuberculosis Control Enforcement Guidelines, revised March 1, 1997. Policy and Procedure C-47.
10. World Health Organization. Guidelines for the prevention of tuberculosis in healthcare facilities in resource-limited settings. Geneva, Switzerland. WHO, 1999 [online] 2005 [cited 2010 Dec 14]. Available from: www.who.int/docstore/gtb/publications/healthcare/PDF/ WHO99-269.pdf
11. Achalu EI. Health education concept, method and planning. Lagos: Simarch Nig. Ltd; 2001:91–93.
12. Kiefer E, Shao T, Carasquillo O, Nabeta P, Seas C. Knowledge and attitudes of tuberculosis management in San Juan de Lurigancho district of Lima, Peru. J Infect Dev Ctries. 2009;3(10):783–788.
13. Hoa NP, Diwan VK, Thorson AE. Diagnosis and treatment of pulmonary tuberculosis at basic healthcare facilities in rural Vietnam: a survey of knowledge and reported practices among health staff. Health Policy. 2005;72(1):1–8. http://dx.doi.org/10.1016/j.healthpol.2004.02.013
14. Hashim DS, Al Kubaisy W, Al Dulayme A. Knowledge, attitudes and practices survey among healthcare workers and tuberculosis patients in Iraq. East Mediterr Health J. 2003;9(4):718–731.

15. Woith WM, Volchenkov G, Larson JL. Russian healthcare workers' knowledge of tuberculosis and infection control. Int J Tuberc Lung Dis. 2010; 14(11):1489–1492.

16. Shisana O, Hall EJ, Maluleke R, Chauveau J, Schwabe C. HIV/AIDS prevalence among South African health workers. S Afr Med J. 2004;94(10):846–850.

17. Connelly D, Veriava Y, Roberts S, Tsotetsi J, Jordan A, DeSilva E, et al. Prevalence of HIV infection and median CD4 counts among healthcare workers in South Africa. S Afr Med J. 2007;97(2):115–120.

18. Bell CA, Duncan G, Saini B. Knowledge, attitudes and practices of private sector providers of tuberculosis care: A scoping review. Int J Tuberc Lung Dis. 2011;15(8):1005–1017. http://dx.doi.org/10.5588/ijtld.10.0294

19. Harries AD, Maher D, Nunn P. Practical and affordable measures for protection of healthcare workers from tuberculosis in low-income countries. Bulletin of the World Health Organization. 1997;75(5):477–489.

20. Biscotto CR, Pedroso ER, Starling CE, Roth VR. Evaluation of N95 respirator use as a tuberculosis control measure in a resource-limited setting. Int J Tuberc Lung Dis. 2005;9(5):545–549.

21. Nettleman MD, Fredrickson M, Good NL, Hunter SA. Tuberculosis control strategies: The cost of particulate respirators. Ann Intern Med. 1994;121(1):37–40. http://dx.doi.org/10.7326/0003-4819-121-1-199407010-00007

22. Catanzaro A. Preventing nosocomial transmission of tuberculosis. Lancet. 1995;345:204–205. http://dx.doi.org/10.1016/S0140-6736(95)90216-3

Knowledge and attitudes of non-occupational HIV post-exposure prophylaxis amongst first- and second-year medical students at Stellenbosch University in South Africa

Authors:
Nondumiso B.Q. Ncube[1]
Willem A.J. Meintjes[2]
Lumbwe Chola[3]

Affiliations:
[1]Division of Community Health, Stellenbosch University, South Africa

[2]Unit for Infection Prevention and Control, Stellenbosch University and Tygerberg Hospital, and Division of Community Health, Stellenbosch University, South Africa

[3]Health Systems and Services Research, Division of Community Health, Stellenbosch University, South Africa

Correspondence to:
Nondumiso Ncube

Email:
ndumi10@yahoo.com

Postal address:
Unit F2 Rosedon Place, 7 Rosedon Road, Rondebosch East 7700, South Africa

Background: Human immunodeficiency virus (HIV) infection is a worldwide problem, with 68% of infected people residing in sub-Saharan Africa. Antiretroviral therapy is used as post-exposure prophylaxis (PEP) to prevent infection in cases of occupational exposure, and use has recently been expanded to non-occupational exposure. Studies have demonstrated a lack of awareness of non-occupational PEP (NO-PEP) in the general population.

Aim: The aim of this study was to evaluate knowledge and attitudes towards availability of, access to and use of NO-PEP amongst first- and second-year medical students.

Setting: Participants were medical undergraduates of Stellenbosch University in the Western Cape of South Africa who were registered in 2013.

Methods: A descriptive cross-sectional study of 169 students was performed. Data were collected using self-administered questionnaires handed out in a classroom in August 2013. Self-reported knowledge and attitudes towards NO-PEP and barriers to access to and use of NO-PEP were analysed using frequency tables. Associations between self-reported and objective knowledge of NO-PEP were analysed by odds ratios.

Results: Over 90% of students had good knowledge on HIV transmission, and about 75% knew how it can be prevented. Twenty eight per cent (n = 47) of students reported knowledge of NO-PEP; 67% reported hearing about it from lecturers, whilst 1% reported hearing about it from their partner. Students who knew the correct procedure to take when a dose is forgotten were 2.4 times more likely to report knowledge of NO-PEP than those who did not know what to do when a dose is forgotten (p = 0.029). No other associations were statistically significant.

Conclusion: Students had positive attitudes towards the use of NO-PEP and also identified barriers to its use. Despite good knowledge of HIV prevention and transmission, knowledge on NO-PEP was poor.

Contexte: Connaissances et Attitudes de la Prophylaxie non-professionnelle post-exposition au VIH chez les étudiants en médecine de première et seconde année à l'université de Stellenbosch en Afrique du Sud.

Objectif: Le virus de l'immunodéficience humaine (VIH) est un problème mondial avec 68% des personnes infectées résidant en Afrique sub-saharienne. La thérapie antirétrovirale est utilisée comme prophylaxie post-exposition (PEP) pour prévenir l'infection due à l'exposition professionnelle, et son utilisation a récemment été étendue aux expositions non professionnelles. Des études ont révélé un manque de sensibilisation de la PEP (NO-PEP) non professionnelle parmi la population en général. Le but de cette étude était d'évaluer les connaissances et attitudes envers la disponibilité, l'accès et l'utilisation des NO-PEP chez les étudiants en médecine de première et seconde année.

Méthodes: Une étude transversale et descriptive de 169 étudiants a été effectuée. On a collecté des données à l'aide de questionnaires auto-administrés distribués dans une salle classe en août 2013. Les connaissances déclarées et les attitudes envers le NO-PEP, ainsi que les barrières à l'accès et à l'utilisation du NO-PEP ont été analysées au moyen de tableaux de fréquence. Les associations entre les connaissances déclarées et les connaissances objectives du NO-PEP ont été analysées par rapports de risques.

Résultats: Plus de 90% des étudiants avaient de bonnes connaissances sur la transmission du VIH, et environ 75% savaient comment la prévenir. Vingt-huit pour cent (n = 47) des étudiants ont déclaré connaitre le NO-PEP. Soixante-sept pour cent des étudiants ont dit avoir eu connaissance du NO-PEP par leurs professeurs alors que 1% ont dit que leur partenaire leur en avait parlé. Les étudiants qui connaissaient la procédure correcte à suivre quand on oublie de prendre une dose, avaient 2.4 plus de chance de signaler leur connaissance du NO-PEP que ceux qui ne savaient pas quoi faire quand on oublie une dose (p = 0.029). Aucune autre association n'avait d'importance du point de vue statistique. Les étudiants avaient des attitudes positives envers l'utilisation du NO-PEP et pouvaient aussi identifier les barrières à son utilisation.

Conclusion: Malgré une bonne connaissance de la prévention et de la transmission du VIH, la connaissance du NO-PEP était mauvaise.

Introduction

HIV infection in sub-Saharan Africa and South Africa

The human immunodeficiency virus and/or acquired immunodeficiency syndrome (HIV/AIDS) epidemic continues to be a problem several decades after it was first discovered. According to the World Health Organisation (WHO) update on the global AIDS epidemic, '34 million people were living with HIV at the end of 2010'.[1] HIV infection is spreading at a fast pace, with over 2.7 million infections each year, and sub-Saharan Africa bearing most of these: 'In 2010, about 68% of people living with HIV in the world were residing in sub-Saharan Africa'.[1] In July 2008 the Joint United Nations Program on AIDS-WHO estimated that the number of people living with HIV infection in South Africa aged between 15 and 49 years was 5.3 million,[2] with the Western Cape province prevalence ranging from 1% to 4.9%.[9]

Antiretroviral therapy

There are several ways in which HIV infection can be prevented and treated. For treatment, the WHO recommends antiretroviral therapy (ART). ART is the use of a combination of antiretroviral (ARV) medicines taken orally to suppress HIV infection by controlling replication of the virus within the infected individual's body.[1] HIV makes the host's immune system weak, and hence the person is unable to fight infections. The use of ARV medicines therefore strengthens the immune system and helps it to regain the power to fight off infections. In South Africa the use of ARVs began in 2003,[3] and the WHO 'recommends that adults infected with HIV initiate ART at $CD4^+$ cell counts of ≤ 350 cells/μL'.[3]

First-line ART comprises a backbone of two nucleoside and/or nucleotide reverse transcriptase inhibitors (NRTIs, such as zidovudine, abacavir or tenofovir; plus lamivudine or emtricitabine); and a non-nucleoside reverse transcriptase inhibitor (NNRTIs, either nevirapine or efavirenz).[4] For second-line treatment the WHO Rapid ADVICE Guidelines recommend the use of two NRTIs (tenofovir plus lamivudine/emtricitabine, or zidovudine plus lamivudine) as the backbone together with a ritonavir-boosted protease inhibitor such as lopinavir or atazanavir.[5]

Amongst the various prevention measures for HIV, ART is recommended particularly in emergency situations. ART is mainly used by medical personnel after exposure to HIV-infected tissues and fluids. Recently the use of ART to prevent infection post non-occupational exposure to HIV has increased, with most countries developing guidelines for this. Clinical trials that prove the effectiveness of using ART to prevent HIV infection have not been carried out due to ethical reasons.

Post-exposure prophylaxis

First-aid is given post-occupational exposure to HIV-infected tissues or fluids, followed by emergency ART. The reason for giving first-aid before putting the individual on emergency ART is to lessen the time of contact with the infected bodily fluids and tissues, hence reducing the risk of infection. In situations where the skin is cut, the site is washed with soap and water and the wound is encouraged to bleed freely under running water for several minutes or until bleeding ceases, with no use of strong agents like alcohol. If there is no water, the area is cleaned with available gel or solution for cleaning hands. If, however, there is a splash with body fluids or blood and the skin is intact, the same procedure mentioned above is followed and use of a mild disinfectant like 2% – 4% chlorhexidine gluconate on the site is encouraged.[6]

The use of ART for occupational post-exposure prophylaxis (PEP) and its expansion for use in non-occupational exposures has caused a lot of uncertainty for providers of health care and policy makers.[5] Non-occupational exposure to HIV happens where an individual is exposed to the virus in ways other than whilst executing their professional duties. This could be the case where there is substantial risk of acquiring HIV infection when body openings such as the eye, vagina, mouth, rectum and/or other mucous membranes or non-intact skin are contaminated with any infected body fluids when the contaminating source is HIV positive.

Key issues amongst provision of non-occupational PEP are 'the appropriate indications for HIV-PEP, ART choices, and management strategies to accompany the use of PEP for HIV'.[5] As there is expansion in the use of ART, policy decisions and plans for delivering services even to settings that have poor resources are required in implementing ART programmes.

Depending on the severity of exposure, the exposed individual may take a combination of two drugs (zidovudine or tenofovir disoproxyl fumarate, and lamivudine) if the risk of exposure is low; or three drugs (zidovudine or tenofovir disoproxylfumarate, lamivudine and lopinavir/ritonavir) for high- risk exposure.[7] High-risk exposure to HIV is when a HIV-negative person comes into contact with the blood of somebody who is infected, tissues and body fluids where there is intramuscular injury, injury is caused by a device entering a blood vessel, injury with a hollow-bore needle, as well as when the mucous membranes of an uninfected person come into contact with the above-mentioned products from an infected person. The risk is also considered high if the infected person's viral load is high.[7]

Low-risk exposure to HIV, on the other hand, is when the skin of the HIV-negative person is not broken when it comes into contact with the infected person's tissues, blood and body fluids.

Literature review

This section discusses the literature on non-occupational PEP, including guidelines, knowledge, and its use. Non-occupational PEP for HIV infection is defined as 'a course of antiretroviral drug treatment taken for the prevention of HIV infection after a potential non-occupational exposure to the virus for example after unprotected sexual contact or sharing injecting drug equipment with an HIV positive person.'[8]

An extensive search was performed on Medline, Scopus, the WHO website and Google Scholar using the search string (awareness or knowledge or attitudes or beliefs) and (non-occupational HIV) and (post-exposure prophylaxis). The initial search provided about 950 articles, and 22 were used for the study. Each article was examined by reading its abstract, opening paragraph and conclusion and a general browse of the whole article to see the relevance of the material to this study. A working bibliography was hence generated. Then each of the articles was thoroughly investigated in terms of the depth and breadth of coverage of the topic to ascertain whether they were pertinent to this research. After deciding on the sources that were relevant, the quality of each article was assessed to see if the arguments presented were clearly stated, well researched and reasonable. Sources were also chosen on the basis of how old the information was and whether up to date and accurate in the field on non-occupational PEP. The search was not restricted by date, study design or language. However, only articles published in English were used. The following key words were used: human immunodeficiency virus, non-occupational PEP, knowledge, awareness, attitudes, beliefs, practices.

Guidelines on use of non-occupational post-exposure prophylaxis

Guidelines on provision of occupational and non-occupational PEP were developed by the International Labour Organisation and WHO in 2005 and became available in 2006.[5] These guidelines address healthcare workers' needs and non-healthcare workers who are exposed to blood and/or body fluids infected with HIV.

The guidelines on use of non-occupational PEP differ from one country to another. The National Australian PEP guidelines recommend that the exposed person be initiated on a four-week course of treatment,[8] and an HIV test must be done before initiation (within 72 hours of exposure). The HIV test must be repeated at '4 weeks, 3 months and 6 months after commencement of non-occupational PEP.'[8] This is in line with the WHO recommendations, which state that the exposed individual must be initiated on a 28-day course of ART within 72 hours of exposure, with follow-up care.[1]

South Africa also has guidelines recommending the use of PEP after sexual exposure to HIV which are similar to the WHO and Australian PEP guidelines.[9] However, there are few published studies that monitor follow-up of patients to completion of PEP. The first pioneering PEP provision initiatives in South Africa began around 1998, before the national PEP policy or guidelines were adopted.[10] However, without a transparent national directive with regard to PEP, these initiatives were not implemented successfully.

In 1999 the South African Medical Association released a statement which 'supported PEP provision for rape survivors, and subsequently publicised guidelines on support to rape survivors in liaison with the Minister of Health, local and international non-governmental organisations as well as the pharmaceutical industry.'[10] The South African Cabinet finally announced that it supported the provision of PEP for people that have been raped who attend South African healthcare facilities in 2002.[10] The PEP followed protocols established by other developing countries, which comprised a two-drug regimen of zidovudine and lamivudine.[10]

In countries where there has been implementation and use of official recommendations for non-occupational PEP, there has been a change in practitioners' attitudes towards non-occupational PEP as well as an increase in the number of prescriptions.[11]

Knowledge of post-exposure prophylaxis

Knowledge of PEP in the general population is quite scant. The topic has not been studied to a great extent, and the few studies that have been done highlight the magnitude of this lack of awareness. In a study of 2932 French people living with HIV infection with a median age of 40 years, a number of factors were found to be associated with no knowledge of PEP.[12] These were a CD4 cell count of below 200, low educational level, older age, and unemployment.[12] Of the 2932 participants recruited, 2280 were sexually active. Amongst sexually active participants, 16% were immigrants, 26% were females, and 41% were homosexual men. Homosexual men were more aware of PEP compared to the rest of the participants: 'Awareness was significantly higher in sexually active people (69.7% versus 52.6% in non-sexually active respondents; $p = 0.001$).'[12] Individuals who had used injectable drugs in the previous 12 months accounted for 2.1% of the whole sample; in this group PEP awareness was not significantly different in both sexually active and inactive intravenous drug users (66.7% versus 60.9%; $p = 0.645$).[12]

A study that sought to understand factors associated with knowledge of non-occupational PEP and pre-exposure prophylaxis (PrEP) in high-risk men who have sex with other men in New York City, found that these men had a low level of knowledge:

> Ethnicity, previous HIV testing, gay self-identification, higher educational level, having a primary provider aware of sexual orientation, reported interaction with healthcare system, and use of internet to meet sex partners were each significantly associated with awareness of PEP or PrEP.[13]

In the United Kingdom there has been a demonstrated increase in knowledge and awareness of non-occupational PEP. A study on nurses working in sexual health clinics showed that 72% (from a sample of 402) had experience of its use in their clinic, and 21% indicated existence of a specific HIV non-occupational PEP policy in their clinic.[14] Another study in the United Kingdom that assessed clinical practice and opinions on non-occupational PEP found that the number of prescriptions increased between 1997 and 1999. The study attributed this increase to a mix of factors, such as increasing public and physician awareness, increased risky sexual behaviour, as well as improved access to PEP.[15]

The findings of a study done in Western Australia showed that level of awareness increased after a multimodal communication strategy on PEP, and the need for ongoing activities to raise awareness on non-occupational PEP was identified.[8]

Use of non-occupational post-exposure prophylaxis

A few studies have been done on non-occupational PEP, and the use of medication to prevent HIV transmission in non-occupational exposure is still relatively new in South Africa. A study based on a review of literature on sexual violence and the use of PEP following occupational and non-occupational exposures was conducted in South Africa.[10] The study incorporated perspectives from in-depth interviews of people who had been raped, activists in HIV and gender, non-governmental domestic violence organisations, rape crisis centres, physicians, lawyers, researchers, and HIV and/or AIDS advisors in the Department of Health.[10] The study found that:

> … the public health and social justice rationale for implementing PEP was equal and actually exceeded industrialised countries. However, issues of delays in accessing PEP caused by the public justice system and lack of training for service providers were found to be significant obstacles to effective implementation.[10]

The increase in uptake of non-occupational PEP in many countries can be attributed to survivors of sexual assault being referred to specialised local clinics until the PEP treatment course is complete, and these people being followed up after initiation.[16] However, there still are challenges in ensuring effective uptake, particularly in low- and middle-income countries, where there usually is no formal way to track patients within and between such clinics, along with lack of an approach to ensure that patients complete their treatment.[16] A study in a rural hospital in South Africa showed that 'sexual assault survivors were three times more likely to complete the entire PEP course when they received care from specially trained nurses.'[17]

Although some countries have guidelines and recommendations in place, there still are conflicting attitudes and practices amongst physicians.[18]A factor that could be affecting the prescribing and uptake of non-occupational PEP is that some medical practitioners 'do not view rape as a serious medical condition'[16] A cross-sectional study on nurses and doctors in South Africa showed that 'a third of these practitioners did not view rape as a serious medical condition, and less than a third of them had been trained on caring for rape victims'.[16] Furthermore, around 60% of the practitioners reported that the facilities in which they worked had no protocol for rape care, and about half of the practitioners had referred rape survivors for counselling.[16]

Justification of the study

Studies on awareness of PEP are scant, but have been done in the United Kingdom, Mumbai in India and Nigeria, mainly focusing on assessing occupational exposure. These studies found that awareness was low amongst surgical residents and doctors (around 40%),[19,20] and higher in nurses (around 72%).[14] Studies on social exposure have been done in New York City on high-risk men who have sex with men,[13] and in California on homosexual and bisexual men.[21] Generally, there is a lack of literature on PEP and its use, particularly in low- and middle-income countries.

In South Africa non-occupational PEP has mainly been used in cases of sexual violence. There is little published literature documenting its use and the knowledge that both patients and health practitioners have with regard to non-occupational PEP. This is particularly worrying, since the studies have shown that rape is not viewed as a medical condition requiring critical care by most medical professionals, and that many of them lack training on how to give proper medical and supportive treatment to rape survivors.[16] Also, information gathered from Tygerberg Hospital casualty department in the Western Cape showed that few people are initiated on non-occupational PEP, and a larger number is initiated on occupational PEP. Apparently there is no functional system that ensures that the people initiated on PEP are referred to specialised clinics for supportive care that will ensure that they complete their course of treatment. Hence little is known about treatment completion and follow-up. As the country continues to contain the HIV and/or AIDS epidemic, this issue is of concern because it could help to reduce new infections.

This exploratory study was performed to provide baseline information to fill the gap on knowledge and attitudes towards NO-PEP. This study aimed to evaluate knowledge and attitudes towards the availability of, access to and use of NO-PEP at Tygerberg medical campus in South Africa amongst aspiring medical professionals. The secondary objectives were to describe barriers to the access and use of NO-PEP, and to evaluate the association between specific knowledge items and self-reported knowledge of NO-PEP.

Medical students were chosen as the target population for this study because they are future health workers and are at risk of both occupational and non-occupational HIV infection. Ensuring that they are equipped with the necessary information on what NO-PEP is and how to access it in cases of exposure is critical in sustaining human resources in the health sector. The university is a relatively closed community. However, information gathered from the students could provide insight into the knowledge and attitudes on NO-PEP from a wide range of individuals with varying backgrounds, cultures and ethnicities, although participants were limited to only first- and second-year medical students.

Research methods and design

An exploratory cross-sectional descriptive study was performed in August 2013 at the medical campus of Stellenbosch University in Cape Town, South Africa, after obtaining ethics approval from the Stellenbosch University Health Research Ethics Committee (reference S13/06/119). The medical campus is situated at Tygerberg Hospital, a teaching hospital for Stellenbosch University Faculty of Medicine and Health Sciences.[22] Tygerberg Hospital is a tertiary Government-owned facility located in Parow, about 20 km from Cape Town city centre; 'It is the largest hospital in the Western Cape and the second largest hospital in South Africa.'[22]According to Stellenbosch University Faculty of Medicine and Health Sciences: 'The Faculty of Medicine has approximately 3000 full-time undergraduate and postgraduate students, and each year produces an average of 160 doctors, 60 specialists and 180 graduates and diplomates in supplementary health sciences.'[23] Tygerberg campus provides accommodation for about 687 undergraduate students. In 2013 the Faculty had 1522 medical undergraduates (254 in year 1; 298 in year 2; 257 in year 3; 235 in year 4; 174 in year 5; 191 in year 6; 56 in the first-year extended degree programme; and 57 in the second-year extended degree programme).

Participants were included if they were medical undergraduates of Stellenbosch University registered in 2013, attended the lecture in which the questionnaire was administered, and if they agreed to participate in the study. The questionnaire used for this study was adapted from a questionnaire used in a previous study.[2] The researchers modified some of the questions to meet the objectives of the present study. The questionnaire was piloted in a group of Master's in Clinical Epidemiology students before finally being approved by Stellenbosch University Health Research Ethics Committee.

The researchers consulted the timetables for the medical students (year 1 to year 6). Conveners for modules were then requested to allow researchers to administer the questionnaires prior to the start of any lecture on the timetable. Questionnaires were administered on the basis of a convenor agreeing to give some time of their lecture for the researchers to administer the questionnaire. A sample of 197 students was obtained, with 47% in year 1, 40% in year 2, 2.1% in year 3, no fourth year students, 1% in year 5, and 6.7% in year 6.

Students were given information on the study and asked to fill in self-administered questionnaires prior to the start of a class lecture scheduled on their timetables. The questionnaires were handed back to the investigator immediately after completion. Only persons who did not attend the class, those refusing participation, and those with mostly incomplete responses to questions were excluded. Data were carefully captured into an Excel spreadsheet by the primary investigator, and analysed using Microsoft Excel and Stata (version 12.1). Range and consistency checks were used to ensure data quality and minimisation of errors.

Knowledge and attitudes of students towards NO-PEP were assessed by means of frequency tables. Barriers to the use of NO-PEP were also assessed using frequency tables. Associations between self-reported knowledge and selected knowledge questions (objective knowledge) on PEP and NO-PEP were explored using Pearson's chi-square tests for normally distributed data and Fisher's exact tests for non-normally distributed data. Crude odds ratios with 95% confidence intervals were also calculated for the associations between objective and subjective knowledge of PEP and NO-PEP. Persons were excluded from the analysis if either of the questions being evaluated (i.e. subjective or objective knowledge questions) was left blank.

Results

One hundred and ninety seven students participated in the study. Data from the first- and second- year groups (n = 169) were considered representative samples due to low response rates in the other study years (despite efforts to increase participant numbers). Students from third year upwards were busy with clinic rotations and not attending formal lectures at Tygerberg campus. Efforts were made to administer questionnaires to those that had lectures on campus, but these numbers were too low. The researchers tried to administer questionnaires during the students' clinic visits, but it was not possible for students to leave patients unattended to answer the questionnaires. Therefore respondents from third year and above as well as those who submitted questionnaires with the majority of questions incomplete were excluded from the analysis (n = 28).

Just over half of the analysed sample was first-year students (53.8%), whilst 46.2% were in their second-year of study. The mean age of the 169 respondents was 19.7 years (standard deviation 1.9 years) and the range was 17–36 years. There were 40 males and 128 females, with one person not indicating their gender. Students living on campus comprised 53.8% (n = 91) of the sample, and those living off campus 45.6% (n = 77). One person did not indicate where they lived. Forty one per cent of the students were white, 30% Mixed race, 15% African, 11% Indian and 3% did not indicate their race.

Table 1 summarises the responses that were given on HIV transmission and prevention knowledge items. Only 27.8% of the students reported that NO-PEP can be used to prevent HIV infection.

Non-occupational post-exposure prophylaxis

Sixty seven per cent of participants reported that they had heard of NO-PEP from lecturers, whilst 1.4% had heard about it from a partner (Figure 1).

In determining students' attitudes towards NO-PEP, it was found that 66% felt that it is important for people to be given NO-PEP, yet a small proportion (27.8%) reported knowledge thereof. Eighty nine per cent of students felt there were benefits in learning about NO-PEP. Table 2

TABLE 1: Participants' HIV transmission and prevention knowledge.

Participants knowledge	Sources	Yes		No		Unsure		Excluded	
		n	%	*n*	%	*n*	%	*n*	%
Knowledge on how HIV can be transmitted	Sexual contact	162	95.9	7	4.1	0	0.0	0	0.0
	Mother to child	160	94.1	8	4.7	1	0.6	0	0.0
	Blood transfusion	161	95.3	5	3.0	3	1.8	0	0.0
	Skin cuts	155	91.7	11	6.5	3	1.8	0	0.0
	Needle sharing	163	96.4	6	3.6	0	0.0	0	0.0
	Kissing	9	5.3	148	87.6	10	5.9	2	1.2
Knowledge on how HIV can be prevented	Abstinence	166	98.2	1	0.6	1	0.6	1	0.6
	Being faithful to one partner	151	89.3	11	6.5	4	2.4	3	1.8
	Condom use	151	89.3	10	5.9	7	4.1	1	0.6
	Showering after sex	5	3.0	161	95.3	1	0.6	2	1.2
	ART prophylaxis	125	74.0	12	7.1	26	15.4	6	3.6
Specific knowledge items	Know occupational PEP is used to prevent HIV infection	129	76.3	30	17.8	4	2.4	6	3.6
	Know NO-PEP is used to prevent infection	47	27.8	91	53.8	22	13.0	9	5.3

TABLE 2: Attitudes towards non-occupational post-exposure prophylaxis.

Attitudes	Item	Yes		No		Unsure		Excluded	
		n	%	*n*	%	*n*	%	*n*	%
Would take ART if they thought they were exposed to HIV	-	144	85.2	6	3.6	7	4.1	12	7.1
Students' reported attitudes regarding making NO-PEP available under the following circumstances	Rape	156	92.3	2	1.2	2	1.2	9	5.3
	Sharing razors	74	43.8	58	34.3	28	16.6	9	5.3
	Sharing piercing objects	110	65.1	36	21.3	14	8.3	9	5.3
	Sharing needles	125	74.0	28	16.6	7	4.1	9	5.3
	Having unprotected sex	111	65.7	38	22.5	11	6.5	9	5.3
Students' reported attitudes regarding benefits of learning about NO-PEP	Learning about NO-PEP is beneficial	151	89.3	10	5.9	2	1.2	6	3.6
Reported benefits of learning about NO-PEP	To prevent HIV infection	120	71.0	15	8.9	18	10.7	16	9.5
	To seek early medical help	131	77.5	4	2.4	15	8.9	19	11.2
	To protect partner	133	78.7	6	3.6	13	7.7	17	10.1
	To protect unborn baby	133	78.7	7	4.1	12	7.1	17	10.1
	Proxy diagnosis of partner	76	45.0	16	9.5	57	33.7	20	11.9

NO-PEP, non-occupational post-exposure prophylaxis; ART, antiretroviral therapy.

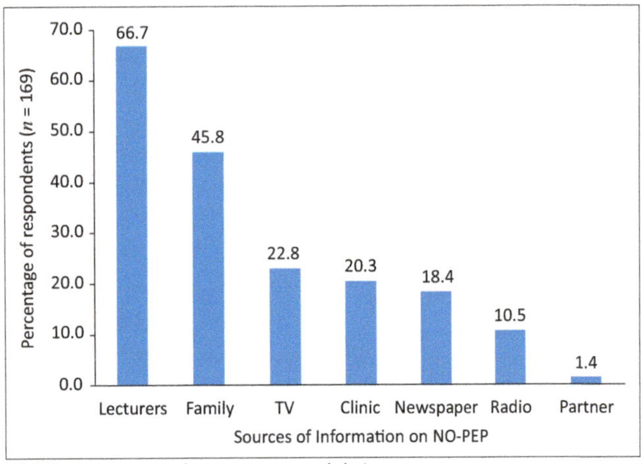

NO-PEP, non-occupational post-exposure prophylaxis.

FIGURE 1: Sources of information on NO-PEP.

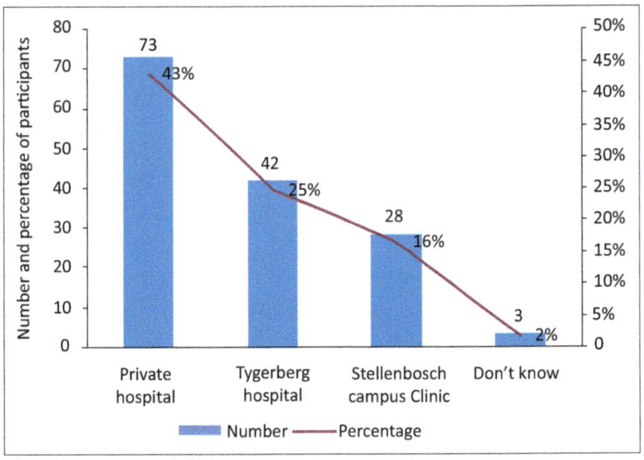

PEP, post-exposure prophylaxis.

FIGURE 2: Where students would go to access PEP services.

highlights circumstances under which students thought NO-PEP should be given and those under which NO-PEP is beneficial.

In assessing barriers to accessing NO-PEP, although students chose more than one option a large proportion reported that they would access NO-PEP services from a private hospital or doctor, whilst a few did not know where such services could be accessed (Figure 2).

Students also identified barriers to the use of and access to PEP (Table 3).

There was a high non-response rate for questions relating to knowledge on medication to be taken for NO-PEP and precautions to be taken whilst on the medicines. For those who answered these questions, when comparing objective (assessed via specific knowledge questions) and subjective (self-reported) knowledge about NO-PEP, the associations

TABLE 3: Barriers to use of and access to non-occupational post-exposure prophylaxis.

Item	Yes		No		Unsure		Excluded	
	n	%	*n*	%	*n*	%	*n*	%
Rejection by family.	80	47.3	52	30.8	30	17.8	7	4.1
Being neglected by partner.	108	63.9	32	18.9	22	13.0	7	4.1
Being neglected by friends.	102	60.4	36	21.3	24	14.2	7	4.1
Discrimination by healthcare workers.	91	53.8	50	29.6	21	12.4	7	4.1
Discrimination by friends.	121	71.6	23	13.6	18	10.7	7	4.1
Discrimination by colleagues.	115	68.0	29	17.2	18	10.7	7	4.1
Discrimination by employers.	115	68.0	26	15.4	21	12.4	7	4.1
Discrimination by family.	112	66.3	29	17.2	20	11.8	8	4.7
Accessibility of PEP services.	84	49.7	28	16.5	47	27.8	10	5.9
Ashamed to discuss condom use.	10	5.9	148	87.6	5	3.0	6	3.6
Ashamed to discuss not sharing needles.	4	2.4	157	92.9	2	1.2	6	3.6
Ashamed to discuss not doing drugs.	3	1.8	158	93.5	2	1.2	6	3.6
Ashamed to discuss going for HIV test.	11	6.5	147	87.0	5	3.0	6	3.6

PEP, post-exposure prophylaxis.

TABLE 4: Associations between subjective and objective knowledge of non-occupational post-exposure prophylaxis.

Item	*n*	%	OR 95%	CI	*p*-value	Excluded†	
						n	%
Know HIV can be prevented with medication.	55	35.3	1.9	0.9–3.8	0.079	60	35.3
Know how PEP should be taken.	91	71.7	2.1	0.8–5.4	0.105	81	47.6
Know how long PEP should be taken.	46	37.1	1.7	0.8–3.7	0.183	83	48.8
Know what to do in case of a forgotten dose.	38	31.1	2.4	1.1–5.4	0.029	86	50.6
Know to practice safe sex.	116	93.5	3.3	0.4–27.6	0.433	84	49.4
Know to refrain from blood donations.	102	82.3	1.2	0.4–3.4	0.705	84	
Know not to share razors, toothbrushes, needles.	115	92.7	3.8	0.5–31.5	0.273	84	49.4
Know to avoid pregnancy.	80	64.5	2.2	0.9–5.2	0.068	84	49.4
Know to stop breastfeeding.	85	68.5	1	0.4–2.3	0.984	84	49.4

†, Participants who did not answer both of the questions.

PEP, post-exposure prophylaxis; NO-PEP, non-occupational post-exposure prophylaxis.

shown in Table 4 were observed. Respondents who knew the correct procedure to take when a dose is forgotten were 2.4 times more likely to report knowledge of NO-PEP than those who did not know what to do when a dose is forgotten ($p = 0.029$). No other associations were statistically significant.

Discussion

This exploratory study was conducted amongst first- and second-year students at Stellenbosch University to determine knowledge and attitudes towards NO-PEP. The results indicate low reported levels of knowledge of NO-PEP in this population. This is possibly because the topic is not given enough attention in schools and communities, but this assumption needs to be explored further. Although NO-PEP knowledge was low, students reported good knowledge on HIV transmission and the modes of preventing transmission. This shows the need to increase awareness through the clinic (via increased educational campaigns) and mass media (especially radio, TV, and newspapers, as people listen to, watch and read these). This lack of knowledge on NO-PEP is in line with the findings of other studies.[12,13,18,19,20,21]

Most students reported that they would take ART if they thought they had been exposed to HIV infection, showing a positive attitude towards the use of NO-PEP. High numbers reported that it should be used for rape cases and in cases where piercing objects and needles are shared. A high number of students felt that NO-PEP should be given for consensual unprotected sex. This could mean that the students engage in risky sexual behaviour, and warrants further investigation. Investigations also need to be done to explore why most students felt NO-PEP should not be given for people sharing razors.

Two-thirds of the students thought that it is important to use NO-PEP, yet only 28% reported knowledge of NO-PEP. Further studies need to be done to explore why students think NO-PEP is important whilst they do not know what NO-PEP is, and why some students consider NO-PEP to be unimportant. A large number of students felt that it was beneficial to learn about NO-PEP. Preventing HIV infection, seeking early medical help, protecting a partner, and protecting an unborn baby were stated as benefits to learning about NO-PEP. However, substantial numbers did not think it beneficial to learn about NO-PEP. Inappropriately, a large number of students thought that testing for HIV and being on NO-PEP are beneficial to act as proxy diagnosis for a partner.

In identifying barriers to access to NO-PEP, most students knew where it can be accessed. It was noted that most students reported that they would get NO-PEP from private hospitals as opposed to getting it from the campus clinic. This could implicate fear of discrimination from their friends on campus and healthcare workers, as these were specifically mentioned as barriers. Further investigations need to be done to verify this assumption. Students reported discrimination (by friends, colleagues, employers, family and healthcare workers), being neglected by partner and friends, rejection by family and poor accessibility to PEP services as barriers to the access to and use of NO-PEP. These perceived barriers, as anticipated, are probably related to stigmatisation around HIV-related issues. These barriers could be addressed if efforts were made to reduce stigmatisation, and this is beyond the scope of this study. Students felt that discussing the following were not barriers to the use of NO-PEP: condom use, not sharing needles, not doing drugs, and going for HIV testing.

There was a low response rate on questions relating to knowledge of medication used for NO-PEP and precautions to be taken whilst on treatment. This could be due to these students being in their preclinical years and not having been taught on such. The lack of knowledge in this sample of students could, however, mean that knowledge on NO-PEP in the general population is low. Further investigations are needed for clarification. When measuring associations between self-reported and objective knowledge on medication used for PEP, students only knew what needs to be done if a person on NO-PEP forgets a dose. However, some trends were observed indicating that self-reporting may be an appropriate tool to measure knowledge; this should be confirmed in further studies. On precautions to be taken whilst on NO-PEP, the high non-response rate is worrying, as one would expect this group to know. Even amongst those who responded, there were substantial numbers that did not know. This high non-response rate needs to be explored in more detail.

Strengths and limitations

This study is the first of its kind at this campus involving medical undergraduates, and thus provides valuable information. However, the sample comprised mostly first- and second-year students, as the numbers of students from third to final year that participated were not representative of the years and were excluded from analyses. For this reason these findings cannot be generalised to all medical students. There also could have been measurement biases, whereby we over-report on students' knowledge. This is because the questionnaire had answer options displayed below each question which participants had to choose from, i.e. the questions were not open-ended. It is thus unclear whether participants actually had this knowledge on NO-PEP or whether recognition of the options artificially increased the reported knowledge levels. The questionnaire used for the study was developed from one used by another author and modified to meet the objectives of this study, and this could have resulted in unclear questions.

Conclusion and recommendations

This was an exploratory study to obtain some information on knowledge and attitudes towards NO-PEP in this particular population, in order to get some baseline information on this topic and to evaluate simple associations existing in the dataset. Findings from this study show that knowledge of HIV infection prevention and transmission is good amongst this group of students, although there are still concerns on the numbers that lack knowledge. Knowledge on NO-PEP is poor and this shows the need to improve educational programmes in life sciences in schools, in healthcare facilities, in communities and the media to increase awareness.

Findings from this study also show that there is stigmatisation around the use of NO-PEP, as shown by the barriers identified by the students. Increasing awareness through the above-mentioned measures could potentially reduce this stigmatisation and ultimately reduce new HIV infections. Information gathered from this study could provide insight on whether medical students are being equipped with the necessary information pertaining to NO-PEP. Hence this study could potentially influence policy regarding teaching practices on HIV infection treatment and prevention. Further studies should investigate issues as highlighted in the discussion. Investigations should also be done to assess whether the level of knowledge is different between the various years of study.

Acknowledgements

Competing interests

The authors declare that they have no financial or personal relationship(s) that may have inappropriately influenced them in writing this article.

Authors' contributions

N.B.Q.N. (Stellenbosch University) completed this project as part of the MScMedSc (Clinical Epidemiology) degree. L.C. (Stellenbosch University) supervised the project from conceptualising, writing the proposal, and obtaining ethics clearance. W.A.J.M. (Stellenbosch University) supervised data collection and analysis. Both supervisors were involved in the write-up and preparation of the manuscript.

References

1. World Health Organization Media Centre.HIV/AIDS. WHO/HIV/AIDS [homepage on the Internet]. No date [cited 2012 Nov 15]. Available from: http://www.who.org
2. Orisakwe EE, Ross AJ, Ocholla PO. Correlation between knowledge of HIV, attitudes and perceptions of HIV and a willingness to test for HIV at a regional hospital in KwaZulu-Natal, South Africa. Afr J Prm Hlth Care Fam Med. 2012;4(1):8.
3. Dube NM, Summers R, Tint KS, Mayayise G. A pharmacologivilance study of adults on highly active antiretroviral therapy, South Africa: 2007–2011. Pan Afr Med J. 2012;11:39.
4. Hamers RL, Sigaloff KC, Wensing AM, Wallis CL, Kityo C, Siwale M, Mandaliya K, Ive P, Botes ME, Wellington M, Osibogun A, Stevens WS, Rinke de Wit TF, Schuurman R. PharmAccess African Studies to Evaluate Resistance (PASER). Patterns of HIV-1drug resistance after first-line antiretroviral therapy (ART) failure in 6 sub-Saharan African countries: implications for second-line ART strategies. Clin Infect Dis. 2012;54(11):1660–1669. http://dx.doi.org/10.1093/cid/cis254
5. World Health Organization Department of HIV/AIDS. Prevention and treatment of HIV and other sexually transmitted infections for sex workers in low- and middle-income countries. Recommendations for a public health approach [homepage on the Internet]. No date [cited 2012 Oct 1]. Available from: http://www.who.int/hiv/pub/guidelines/en/
6. Kathmandu, T. National anti-retroviral therapy guidelines [homepage on the Internet]. 2009 [cited 2012 Nov 30]. Available from: http://www.who.int/search?q=hiv+firstaid+pep
7. World Health Organization. HIV post exposure prophylaxis for occupational and non-occupational exposure to HIV [homepage on the Internet]. No date [cited 2012 Dec 2]. Available from: http://www.who.int/hiv/topics/prophylaxis/meeting/en/index.html

8. Minas B, Laing S, Jordan H, Mak DB. Improved awareness and appropriate use of non-occupational post-exposure prophylaxis (nPEP) for HIV prevention following a multi-modal communication strategy. BMC Public Health. 2012;12:906. http://dx.doi.org/10.1186/1471-2458-12-906

9. Western Cape Provincial Department of Health. Treatment guidelines for the use of post-exposure prophylaxis (PEP) for the prevention of the transmission of human immunodeficiency virus (HIV) in males and females who have been raped or sexually assaulted [homepage on the Internet]. 2002 [cited 2012 Nov 30]. Available from: http://www.doh.gov.za/aids/docs/rape-protocol.html

10. Kim JC, Martin LJ, Denny L. Rape and HIV post-exposure prophylaxis: Addressing the dual epidemics in South Africa. Reprod Health Matters. 2003;11(22):101–112. http://dx.doi.org/10.1016/S0968-8080(03)02285-7

11. Laporte A, Jourdan N, Bouvet E, Lamontagne F, Pillonel J, Desenclos J. Post-exposure prophylaxis after non-occupational HIV exposure: Impact of recommendations on physicians' experiences and attitudes. AIDS. 2002; 16(3):397–405. http://dx.doi.org/10.1097/00002030-200202150-00011

12. Rey D, Bouhnik AD, Peretti-Watel P, Obadia Y, Spire B. Awareness of non-occupational HIV postexposure prophylaxis among French people living with HIV: The need for better targeting. AIDS. 2007; 21:S71–S76. http://dx.doi.org/10.1097/01.aids.0000255088.44297.26

13. Mehta SA, Silvera R, Bernstein K, Holzman RS, Aberg JA, Daskalakis DC. Awareness of post-exposure HIV prophylaxis in high-risk men who have sex with men in New York City. Sex Transm Infect. 2011; 87(4):344–348. http://dx.doi.org/10.1136/sti.2010.046284

14. Hayter M. Knowledge and attitudes of nurses working in sexual health clinics in the united kingdom toward post-sexual exposure prophylaxis for HIV infection. Public Health Nursing. 2004; 21(1):66–72. http://dx.doi.org/10.1111/j.1525-1446.2004.21109.x

15. Giele C, Maw R, Carne C, Evans B. Post-exposure prophylaxis for non-occupational exposure to HIV: Current clinical practice and opinions in the UK. Sex Transm Infect. 2002; 78(2):130–132. http://dx.doi.org/10.1136/sti.78.2.130

16. Roland ME, Myer L, Martin LJ, et al. Preventing human immunodeficiency virus infection among sexual assault survivors in Cape Town, South Africa: An observational study. AIDS Behav. 2012; 16(4):990–998. http://dx.doi.org/10.1007/s10461-011-9892-3

17. Kim JC, Askew I, Muvhango L, et al. Comprehensive care and HIV prophylaxis after sexual assault in rural South Africa: The Refentse intervention study. BMJ 2009;338:b515. http://dx.doi.org/10.1136/bmj.b515

18. Levy I. Post exposure prophylaxis (PEP) to prevent HIV after sexual exposure in Israel. Harefuah. 2005;144(4):252–254.

19. Chogle NL, Chogle MN, Divatia JV, Dasgupta D. Awareness of post-exposure prophylaxis guidelines against occupational exposure to HIV in a Mumbai hospital. Natl Med J India. 2002; 15(2):69–72.

20. Fadeyi A, Fowotade A, Abiodun MO, Jimoh AK, Nwabuisi C, Desalu OO. Awareness and practice of safety precautions among healthcare workers in the laboratories of two public health facilities in Nigeria. Niger Postgrad Med J. 2011; 18(2):141–146.

21. Liu AY, Kittredge PV, Vittinghoff E, et al. Limited knowledge and use of HIV post- and pre-exposure prophylaxis among gay and bisexual men. J Acquir Immune Defic Syndr. 2008; 47(2):241–247. http://dx.doi.org/10.1097/QAI.0b013e31815e4041

22. Western Cape Provincial Department of Health. Tygerberg Hospital: Overview [homepage on the Internet]. April 2014 [cited 2014 May 29]. Available from: www.westerncape.gov.za/your_gov/153

23. Stellenbosch University Faculty of Medicine and Health Sciences. 2013 Health Sciences Yearbook. 2013 [cited 2014 May 29]. Available from: http://sun.ac.za/english/Documents/Yearbooks/2013/2013_WEB_Medicine_and_Health%20Sciences_25Jan2013.pdf

Management of cryptococcal meningitis in a district hospital in KwaZulu-Natal: A clinical audit

Authors:
Benjamin O. Adeyemi[1]
Andrew Ross[2]

Affiliations:
[1]Department of Family Medicine, Pietermaritzburg Hospitals Complex and University of KwaZulu-Natal, South Africa

[2]Department of Family Medicine, University of KwaZulu-Natal, South Africa

Correspondence to:
Benjamin Adeyemi

Email:
ben_adeyemi@yahoo.com

Postal address:
PO Box 8786, Cumberwood 3235, South Africa

Background: Despite the development of context-specific guidelines, cryptococcal meningitis (CCM) remains a leading cause of death amongst HIV-infected patients. Results from clinical audits in routine practice have shown critical gaps in clinicians' adherence to recommendations regarding the management of CCM.

Aim: The aim of this study was to review the acute management of CCM at an urban district hospital in KwaZulu-Natal, South Africa with a view to making recommendations for improving care.

Setting: An urban district hospital in KwaZulu-Natal, South Africa.

Methods: A retrospective audit was performed on clinical records of all patients (age > 13 years) admitted to the hospital with a diagnosis of CCM between June 2011 and December 2012.

Results: Measurement of cerebrospinal fluid opening pressure at initial lumbar puncture (LP) was done rarely and only 23.4% of patients had therapeutic LPs. The majority of patients (117/127; 92.1%) received amphotericin B, however, only 19 of the 117 patients (16.2%) completed the 14-day treatment target. Amphotericin B-toxicity monitoring and prevention was suboptimal; however, in-patient referral for HIV counselling and testing was excellent.

Conclusions: The quality of care of CCM based on selected process criteria showed gaps in routine care at the hospital despite the availability of context-specific guidelines. An action plan for improving care was developed based on stakeholders' feedback. A repeat audit should be conducted in the future in order to evaluate the impact of this plan and to ensure that improvements are sustained.

Gestion de la méningite cryptococcique dans un hôpital régional au KwaZulu-Natal: une vérification Clinique.

Historique: Malgré le développement de directives spécifiques au contexte, la méningite cryptococcique (CCM) reste une des causes principales de décès parmi les patients infectés du VIH. Les résultats des vérifications cliniques dans la pratique courante ont montré des lacunes critiques dans l'adhésion des cliniciens aux recommandations sur la gestion du CCM.

Objectif: Le but de cette étude était de revoir la gestion active du CCM dans un hôpital régional urbain du KwaZulu-Natal, en Afrique du Sud afin de faire des recommandations pour améliorer les soins de santé.

Lieu: un hôpital régional urbain au KwaZulu-Natal, en Afrique du Sud.

Méthodes: Les dossiers cliniques de tous les patients (âgés de plus de 13ans) admis à l'hôpital avec un diagnostique de CCM de juin 2011 à décembre 2012 ont été vérifiés rétrospectivement.

Résultats: La mesure de la pression d'ouverture du CSF à la ponction lombaire initiale (PL) a rarement été effectuée et seuls 23.4% des patients ont subi des PL thérapeutiques. La majorité des patients (117/127; 92.1%) ont reçu de l'amphotéricine B. Cependant, seuls 19 sur 117 patients (16.2%) ont atteint l'objectif de traitement de 14 jours. L'identification et la prévention de la toxicité de l'Amphotéricine B laissaient à désirer. Cependant, l'admission des patients en consultation interne pour le conseil et dépistage du VIH était excellente.

Conclusions: La qualité des soins de la CCM basés sur des processus de sélection des critères a révélé des lacunes dans les soins courants à l'hôpital malgré la disponibilité des lignes directrices particulières au contexte. Un plan d'action pour améliorer les soins a été développé basé sur les feed-back des parties prenantes. Il faudra faire dans le futur une vérification de contrôle pour évaluer l'impact de ce plan et assurer que les améliorations sont maintenues.

Introduction

Cryptococcal meningitis (CCM) has emerged as one of the leading causes of death amongst HIV-infected patients worldwide.[1,2] Recent epidemiological shifts and an explosion of the HIV pandemic have resulted in the emergence of CCM as a major public health problem and a leading cause of community-acquired meningitis in sub-Saharan Africa.[3,4] Estimates from sub-Saharan Africa in 2009 suggested that CCM killed more people than tuberculosis – with more than half-a-million deaths recorded per annum.[1,5,6]

HIV-associated CCM is a life-threatening disease with a 100% case fatality rate in the absence of treatment.[7] Effective management of CCM requires rapid fungicidal induction therapy with amphotericin B and flucytocine, followed by suppressive therapy with fluconazole, as well as aggressive management of raised intracranial pressure (ICP) and appropriate management of immune reconstitution inflammatory syndrome (IRIS).[4,6,8] Raised ICP, which often complicates CCM,[4,9] is a common cause of severe headache, neurological deficit and death.[9]

Despite restricted access to flucytocine, there are effective guidelines for the management of HIV-associated CCM in South Africa.[10] The South African treatment guidelines for the management of CCM comply substantially with best practices[11] by emphasising the use of amphotericin B for induction, advocating the aggressive management of raised ICP as well as the use of secondary prophylaxis with oral fluconazole in order to prevent recurrence of CCM.[10,12] The guidelines also provide recommendations for the prevention and management of amphotericin B-related nephrotoxicity through provision of routine pre-hydration and electrolyte supplementation for patients on amphotericin B.[10,11,12] In line with the recognition of the association between improved survival outcomes and timely introduction of antiretroviral therapy (ART),[4,10,13] clinicians are also enjoined to ensure that patients with AIDS-related CCM are initiated on lifelong ART.[10,12,14]

Cryptococcal meningitis is a common AIDS-defining illness seen at the hospital where this audit was conducted. An exploratory clinical audit carried out in 2006 on the management of CCM at the hospital highlighted concerns about the management of patients with CCM and drew attention to the unavailability of clearly-defined, local clinical guidelines at that time.[15] Context-specific, comprehensive and evidence-based guidelines for the management of HIV-associated CCM in South Africa were introduced at the hospital in 2007 following the aforementioned audit.[10,12] Other studies have shown that despite the availability of national guidelines there is no evidence to suggest that the availability of these guidelines has been associated with significant corresponding improvements in care of and outcomes for HIV-infected patients with CCM in South Africa.[16,17] Critical gaps in routine management of CCM were also highlighted by a clinical audit conducted in the United States.[18]

The aim of this study was to conduct a clinical audit of clinicians' level of adherence to published context-specific guidelines on the management of CCM with a view to making recommendations for the improvement of care. Whilst some have argued that the evidence for the usefulness of clinical audit on improving professional practice is not particularly strong,[19] a Cochrane Systematic Review[20] on the effects of clinical audit and feedback on professional practice and clinical outcomes concluded that audit is an effective tool for improving practice. In fact, the positive effects of clinical audit may be magnified greatly when the feedback emanating from the audit is given in an intense manner,[20] especially in settings where the initial baseline adherence to practice guidelines is low.

Research method and design

This was a clinical audit conducted at an urban district hospital in KwaZulu-Natal, South Africa using a retrospective descriptive study design. The hospital has a full package of district-level services.

The clinical audit topic was selected based on routine observation of the high mortality seen amongst patients with CCM at the hospital and the recognition of the possible impact of improved quality of care on mortality outcomes. An audit team, supported by a broader team of healthcare workers, was formed. The study method comprised the four essential steps of a quality improvement cycle: agreeing on criteria and setting target standards; collecting data on current practice; comparing current practice with target standards; and, finally, planning care and implementing changes.[21]

Based on the prevailing published guidelines over the study period,[10,11,12] criteria were developed around key issues regarding the diagnosis and management of HIV-associated CCM. The key issues selected for audit were: baseline cerebrospinal fluid (CSF) manometry and management of raised ICP; amphotericin B treatment and prevention and/or management of its toxicity; as well as patients' linkage with antiretroviral services. Target standards were set based on published literature[15,16,17,18] and with due consideration for the complexity and constraints of the study setting.[21]

The clinical records of all patients aged 13 years and older who were admitted to the hospital with a diagnosis of CCM between 01 June 2011 and 31 December 2012 were reviewed retrospectively in order to extract information regarding clinical data and patient management. A diagnosis of CCM based on a positive India ink, positive cryptococcal latex agglutination test or a positive culture of *Cryptococcus neoformans* was essential for inclusion in this study. Patient records were identified using the hospital's admission, transfer and discharge registers. Further review of clinical records, mortality records and laboratory data (accessed from the National Health Laboratory Service [NHLS] database) was done in order to extract information on the patients' demographic data and parameters relevant to the audit criteria. A data extraction tool was developed to collect the information and the data were captured onto a Microsoft® Excel spreadsheet. Simple frequencies and percentages were generated for agreed criteria and these were compared to target standards.

The results of the clinical audit were presented at an audit feedback meeting at the hospital in November 2013. The meeting was attended by senior management staff, NHLS laboratory staff representatives, pharmacy representatives, stores department staff, medical doctors, nursing staff and other members of the healthcare team involved in caring for medical patients. The gathering reflected on the findings and the implications of the identified practice gaps. An action plan aimed at improving the quality of acute management of HIV-associated CCM was agreed upon following extensive discussions amongst the stakeholders present at the meeting.

Ethical considerations

Ethical approval was obtained from the University of KwaZulu-Natal Biomedical Research Ethics Committee (REF: BE086/12) and the management of the hospital.

Results

The demographic and clinical profiles of the patients included in the study are presented in Table 1.

Table 2 shows the criteria selected for audit and the level of performance compared to target standards for each criterion. Of the 95 patients who had no therapeutic lumbar puncture (LP), there was no evidence in the notes that the procedure was offered to 82 (86.3%) of the patients; and it was declined by 2 (2.1%) patients and contraindicated in one (1.1%) patient who needed further assessment for new-onset blindness. In 8 cases (8.4%), the patients died before the LP was performed, even though the clinician(s) had made a decision to do a therapeutic LP. There was one instance (n = 1; 1.1%) where the clinical record showed that there was no manometer and another where many LP attempts were recorded as 'unsuccessful' (n = 1; 1.1%).

Out of the 127 patients, analgesics (prescribed separately and in fixed-dose formulations) were employed for the management of headaches associated with CCM in 104 (81.9%) of the patients in this study. Seventy-seven (60.6%) patients had paracetamol; 58 (45.7%) had a paracetamol-codeine fixed-dose combination analgesic; 27 (21.3%) had non-steroidal anti-inflammatory drugs whilst 15 (11.8%) had other opiates such as tramadol and morphine.

Assessment of the pattern of amphotericin B prescription showed that the most frequently-prescribed daily dose was 50 mg. Evidence of determination of actual dose using patients' weight was found for only 23/127 (18.1%) patients. The median duration of induction therapy with amphotericin B was 8 days (interquartile range [IQR] 3–5 days). Only 19/127 (15.4%) patients completed 14 days of amphotericin B. The reasons why patients did not complete 14 days of amphotericin B were as shown in Table 3.

Discussion

Results of this clinical audit from routine practice in a district hospital provide evidence of important gaps in

TABLE 1: Demographic and clinical profiles of patients admitted with cryptocccal meningitis.

Variable	Male	Female
No. of patients (%)	65 (51.2)	62 (48.8)
Age (yrs) median (IQR)	37 (31–42)	33 (27–42)
CD4 cell count (cells/mm^3)† - Median (IQR)	36 (19–80)	56 (23–137)
CCM Case definition - New	49	53
Symptomatic relapse	16	9

IQR, interquartile range; †, CD4 count results available for 74 patients only; CCM, cryptococcal meningitis.

TABLE 3: Reasons for amphotericin B induction therapy < 14 days.

Reason	Frequency (n = 104)	%
Died	61	58.7
Improved	23	22.1
Toxicity	10	9.6
Not prescribed	4	3.9
Renal failure at diagnosis	3	2.9
Refusal of hospital treatment	2	1.9
Out of stock (amphotericin B)	1	1.0

TABLE 2: Comparison of performance and target standards.

Criteria	Target standard (%)	Number of patients (n)	Performance standard n (%)	Target met (yes/no)
CSF manometry at initial LP	80	127	2 (1.7)	No
ICP monitoring and therapeutic LP	100	124†	29 (23.4)	No
Weight-based correct dosing of amphotericin B	80	117‡	23 (19.7)	No
Complete 14-day amphotericin B	80	117‡	19 (16.2)	No
Saline loading	100	117‡	68 (58.1)	No
Prophylactic magnesium supplementation	100	117‡	5 (4.3)	No
Prophylactic potassium supplementation (unless contraindicated)	100	117‡	31 (26.5)	No
Adequate renal function monitoring (3x/ week U&E, Mg)	100	80†	26 (32.5)	No
Weekly haemoglobin monitoring	100	72†	14 (19.4)	No
Referral for HIV counselling and testing when admission HIV status was unknown and/or negative	100	31†	31 (100)	Yes
Incidence of renal impairment	< 40%	88†	32 (36.4)	Yes
Two-week mortality	< 40%	127	71 (55.9)	No

CSF, cerebrospinal fluid; LP, lumbar puncture; ICP, intracranial pressure; U&E, urea and electrolytes; Mg, magnesium; †, Total number of patients < 127 because of missing data and early mortality making evaluation of adequacy of monitoring for toxicity impossible; ‡, Only 117 patients received amphotericin B.

the clinical management of CCM. Similar to findings from a clinical audit conducted in Washington D.C. amongst patients treated for CCM,[18] failure to measure CSF opening pressure at initial LP was the most common deviation from clinical guidelines in our setting. The percentage of patients who had their CSF opening pressure measured at baseline in this audit was 10 times lower than figures (1.7% versus 17%) reported amongst patients seen at the district hospital level in the Western Cape.[17] Clinicians' failure to perform routine measurement of CSF opening pressure at baseline has been attributed to non-availability of spinal manometers;[17] clinicians' limited awareness of the epidemiological significance of *C. neoformans* as one of the leading causes of community-acquired meningitis; and inadequate knowledge of important role of ICP management in the treatment of CCM.[18] The consensus from discussions at the audit feedback meeting was that spinal manometers were generally available in the hospital. This assertion was supported by the fact that there was only one instance where the clinical record showed that the CSF opening pressure was not measured because of the non-availability of a spinal manometer. However the reasons for non-adherence were not explored in this study but are likely to be similar to the findings of other studies.[18]

Only 23.4% of the patients admitted with CCM had ICP monitoring and therapeutic LPs. Although this adherence level is considerably lower than our target of 80%, it is higher than the compliance level of 14.9% reported from a study in a rural district hospital from KwaZulu-Natal in 2011.[16] A review of our patients' clinical records showed that clinicians preferentially prescribed analgesics for persistent headaches in patients with CCM rather than performing therapeutic LPs. However, such practices have been associated with worse neurological outcomes[18] and there are concerns that the use of non-steroidal anti-inflammatory drugs (NSAIDS) could potentially increase the risk of amphotericin B-related nephrotoxicity.[22] In fact, NSAIDS were prescribed as analgesics for 21.3% (27/127) of the patients during the induction phase with amphotericin B. Whilst therapeutic LPs remain '... the best form of "analgesia" for headaches associated with raised intracranial pressure ...'[22] (p. 18), the perceived onerous effort required for the consistent performance of serial LPs has been found to constitute a major factor limiting clinicians' compliance with clinical guidelines on therapeutic LPs.[18]

Despite existing evidence on the dose-dependent nephrotoxic potential of amphotericin B,[23] analysis of the pattern of amphotericin B prescription in this study showed limited evidence of weight-based dosing. In this study, in 43.6% of the cases, clinicians prescribed a 50 mg daily dose of amphotericin B. This may be because amphotericin B comes in standard preparations of 50 mg/vial in South Africa and this may thus represent a convenient dosing schedule for both doctors and nurses. Another possible factor limiting accurate weight-based dosing that was raised by those at the audit feedback meeting was the fact that some of the patients with CCM were too ill to get on a standard weighing scale. The reasons for this practice need to be explored in a further study. The retrospective nature of this study made it impossible to determine the impact of this practice on CSF sterilisation rate or the risk of amphotericin B-related nephrotoxicity.

Whilst amphotericin B remains the preferred and most effective drug for the treatment of serious systemic fungal infections such as CCM,[23,24] universal access to amphotericin B remains a challenge in developing countries.[8,25] In a retrospective case review series at a rural hospital in northern KwaZulu-Natal, only 35% of patients diagnosed with CCM received amphotericin B and only 8.1% completed the recommended 14 days of induction therapy.[16] Apart from amphotericin B stock-outs, early mortality and renal impairment were the other major reasons why patients did not complete 14 days of induction therapy with amphotericin B in an audit in the Western Cape.[17] In the study setting, drug stock-out did not appear to be a major problem; 92.1% of the patients received amphotericin B with only one case where the drug was not available. Deviations from the 14-day induction target were mainly a result of early mortality; clinicians' decision to discontinue amphotericin B on account of improvement in the clinical status of the patient; and amphotericin B-related toxicity. Given the finding from a prospective study in India that even the standard 14-day amphotericin B monotherapy might be suboptimal for one third of patients,[26] clinicians' decision to discontinue amphotericin B before 14 days on the premise of clinical improvement remains a concern. It is pertinent to mention that the South African National Department of Health (NDOH) conceded that completing the 14-day course of amphotericin B might not always be 'feasible' given the high demands for hospital beds and thus recommended that '... an earlier switch to oral fluconazole may be considered ... [*by the clinician*] ... if there has been a good clinical response'[12] (p. 169). The impact of this practice on CCM recurrence rates, CCM-related IRIS and survival outcomes warrants further study.

The prevailing guidelines during the study period (from the Southern African HIV Clinicians Society [SAHIVSOC] and the NDOH) included recommendations on the prevention, monitoring and management of amphotericin B-related toxicities.[10,12] The guidelines recommend pre-emptive saline loading and electrolyte (potassium and magnesium) supplementation; weekly haemoglobin monitoring; monitoring of potassium and creatinine levels; and management of ensuing electrolyte(s) and creatinine derangements.[10,11,12] Similar to a clinical audit report from the Western Cape,[17] clinicians' adherence to these recommendations was suboptimal in the study setting. This was particularly poor with respect to prophylactic magnesium supplementation. These gaps have been attributed to inadequate awareness amongst clinicians regarding toxicity monitoring and prevention recommendations.[17] Despite these gaps, the incidence of renal impairment was within the clinical audit target.

Optimal in-patient linkage to ART counselling services of patients diagnosed with CCM has been attributed to the integrated nature of district level services.[17] All the patients whose HIV status was unknown or negative at admission for CCM were referred for counselling and testing. However, 22.5% (7/31) of the patients could not be counselled and/or tested mainly due to early mortality.

Similar to other reports from routine care in sub-Saharan Africa,[1,16,17,27] acute CCM survival outcomes were poor. The two-week in-patient mortality outcome of 55.9% (71/127) was worse than the preset audit target of 40%. Concerns about the persistently-high burden of CCM and the poor mortality outcome in routine care have led to calls for screening and treatment of early cryptococcal disease amongst patients with no prior CCM but with advanced immunodeficiency whenever they present for ART initiation.[22,28] This pre-emptive strategy, specifically targeting ART-naïve HIV-infected patients with a CD4 cell count < 100 cells/mm^3, has been started in some provinces in South Africa.[29] In 2013, the SAHIVSOC published an updated guideline that reflects recent recommendations for the prevention, diagnosis and management of CCM amongst HIV-infected patients.[22]

Strengths and limitations

Given the retrospective nature of this clinical audit, it was impossible to standardise the quality of information documented in the patients' folders and there were instances of missing or incomplete clinical records. These limitations notwithstanding, the clinical audit and the subsequent feedback session provided a forum for stakeholders to learn and also discuss their concerns with regard to CCM management in the hospital. It also ensured that the reasons for the identified practice gaps and the ensuing recommendations were based on collective feedback and agreement.

Conclusion

This audit of the quality of acute management of CCM in routine care showed gaps in the management of this life-threatening illness, despite the availability of context-specific guidelines. The low adherence to practice guidelines represents an opportunity to improve care through feedback of the audit results coupled with implementation of a comprehensive action plan based on stakeholders' recommendations. Thus, in conjunction with the Quality Improvement Manager at the hospital, the audit team has developed an action plan aimed at improving the management of CCM at the facility. A repeat audit will be conducted six months after the implementation of the plan in order to evaluate its impact and to ensure that improvements are sustained.

Acknowledgements

We wish to thank the laboratory and administrative staff at the hospital for their help in gathering data for this study. B.O.A. gratefully acknowledges the European AIDS Clinical Society (EACS) for clinical research training.

Competing interests

The authors declare that they have no financial or personal relationship(s) which may have inappropriately influenced them in writing this article.

Authors' contributions

B.O.A. (Pietermaritzburg Hospitals Complex and University of KwaZulu-Natal) was responsible for all the work done in this study, including the study design, data collection and analysis. A.R. (University of KwaZulu-Natal) was involved with the initial conceptualisation of the study and assisted with the development and editing of the final manuscript.

References

1. US Centers for Disease Control and Prevention. Fighting a deadly fungus: A new strategy to reduce deaths due to cryptococcus [document on the Internet]. c2011 [cited 2013 Sep 11]. Available from: http://www.cdc.gov/ncezid/dfwed/PDFs/FACTSHEET_Cryptococcus_remediated.pdf
2. US Centers for Disease Control and Prevention. Cryptococcal meningitis: a deadly fungal disease among people living with HIV/AIDS [document on the Internet]. c2012 [cited 2013 Sep 11]. Available from: www.cdc.gov/fungal/pdf/at-a-glance-508c.pdf
3. Jarvis JN, Meintjes G, Williams A, et al. Adult meningitis in a setting of high HIV and TB prevalence: Findings from 4961 suspected cases. BMC Infect Dis. 2010;10:67. http://dx.doi.org/10.1186/1471-2334-10-67
4. Bicanic T, Harrison TS. Cryptococcal meningitis. Br Med Bull. 2004;72:99–118. http://dx.doi.org/10.1093/bmb/ldh043
5. Park BJ, Wannemuehler KA, Marston BJ, et al. Estimation of the current global burden of cryptococcal meningitis among persons living with HIV/AIDS. AIDS. 2009;23(4):525–530. http://dx.doi.org/10.1097/QAD.0b013e328322ffac
6. Perfect JR, Dismukes WE, Dromer F, et al. Clinical practice guidelines for the management of cryptococcal disease: 2010 update by the Infectious Diseases Society of America. Clin Infect Dis. 2010;50(3):291–322. http://dx.doi.org/10.1086/649858
7. Mwaba P, Mwansa J, Chintu C, et al. Clinical presentation, natural history, and cumulative death rates of 230 adults with primary cryptococcal meningitis in Zambian AIDS patients treated under local conditions. Postgrad Med J. 2001;77(914):769–773. http://dx.doi.org/10.1136/pmj.77.914.769
8. Sorrell TC, Chen SC. Recent advances in management of cryptococcal meningitis: Commentary. F1000 Med Rep. 2010;2:82.
9. Gallant JE, Pham PA, editors. Johns Hopkins HIV guide: Management of HIV infection and its complications. Burlington, MA: Jones & Bartlett Learning, 2012.
10. McCarthy K, Meintjes G, Arthington-Skaggs B, et al. Guideline for the prevention, diagnosis and management of cryptococcal meningitis and disseminated cryptococcosis in HIV-infected patients. S Afr J HIV Med. 2008;8(3):25.
11. World Health Organization. Rapid advice: diagnosis, prevention and management of cryptococcal disease in HIV-infected adults, adolescents and children [document on the Internet]. c2011 [cited 2012 Feb 11]. Available from: http://whqlibdoc.who.int/publications/2011/9789241502979_eng.pdf
12. National Department of Health. Ch 10 – HIV and AIDS. Standard Treatment Guidelines and Essential Drug List. 2nd ed. Pretoria, South Africa: National Department of Health, 2006; p. 168–169.
13. Lortholary O, Poizat G, Zeller V, et al. Long-term outcome of AIDS-associated cryptococcosis in the era of combination antiretroviral therapy. AIDS. 2006;20(17):2183–2191. http://dx.doi.org/10.1097/01.aids.0000252060.80704.68
14. Sloan D, Dlamini S, Paul N, et al. Treatment of acute cryptococcal meningitis in HIV infected adults, with an emphasis on resource-limited settings. Cochrane Database Syst Rev. 2008;4:CD005647.
15. Sirkar S. Quality improvement process/cycle: action orientated audit 2006 [presentation on the Internet]. c2006 [cited 2012 Dec 17]. Available from: http://www.kznhealth.gov.za/family/pres6.pdf
16. Lessells RJ, Mutevedzi PC, Heller T, et al. Poor long-term outcomes for cryptococcal meningitis in rural South Africa. S Afr Med J. 2011;101(4):251–252.
17. Von Pressentin KB, Conradie HH, Mash B. A medical audit of the management of cryptococcal meningitis in HIV-positive patients in the Cape Winelands (East) district, Western Cape. S Afr Fam Pract. 2012;54(4):339–346. http://dx.doi.org/10.1080/20786204.2012.10874246
18. Shoham S, Cover C, Donegan N, et al. Cryptococcus neoformans meningitis at 2 hospitals in Washington, D.C.: Adherence of health care providers to published practice guidelines for the management of cryptococcal disease. Clin Infect Dis. 2005;40(3):477–479. http://dx.doi.org/10.1086/427213
19. Benjamin A. Audit: How to do it in practice. BMJ. 2008;336(7655):1241–1245. http://dx.doi.org/10.1136/bmj.39527.628322.AD

20. Jamtvedt G, Young JM, Kristoffersen DT, et al. Audit and feedback: Effects on professional practice and health care outcomes. Cochrane Database Syst Rev. 2003;3:CD000259.

21. Mash B. Ch 151 – How to audit or improve the quality of your service. In: Mash B, Blitz-Lindeque J, editors. South African Family Practice Manual. Pretoria, South Africa: Van Schaik, 2006; p. 402–403.

22. Govender NP, Meintjes G, Bicanic T, et al. Guideline for the prevention, diagnosis and management of cryptococcal meningitis among HIV-infected persons: 2013 update. S Afr J HIV Med. 2013;14(2):76–86. http://dx.doi.org/10.7196/sajhivmed.930

23. Laniado-Laborín R, Cabrales-Vargas MN. Amphotericin B: Side effects and toxicity. Rev Iberoam Micol. 2009;26(4):223–227. http://dx.doi.org/10.1016/j.riam.2009.06.003

24. Deray G. Amphotericin B nephrotoxicity. J Antimicrob Chemother. 2002;49 (Suppl 1):37–41. http://dx.doi.org/10.1093/jac/49.suppl_1.37

25. Nussbaum JC, Jackson A, Namarika D, et al. Combination flucytosine and high-dose fluconazole compared with fluconazole monotherapy for the treatment of cryptococcal meningitis: a randomized trial in Malawi. Clin Infect Dis. 2010;50(3):338–344. http://dx.doi.org/10.1086/649861

26. Patel AK, Patel KK, Ranjan R, et al. Management of cryptococcal meningitis in HIV-infected patients: Experience from western India. Indian J Sex Transm Dis. 2010;31(1):22–26. http://dx.doi.org/10.4103/0253-7184.68996

27. Jarvis JN, Meintjes G, Harrison TS. Outcomes of cryptococcal meningitis in antiretroviral naïve and experienced patients in South Africa. J Infect. 2010;60(6):496–498. http://dx.doi.org/10.1016/j.jinf.2010.03.007

28. Jarvis JN, Lawn SD, Vogt M, et al. Screening for cryptococcal antigenemia in patients accessing an antiretroviral treatment program in South Africa. Clin Infect Dis. 2009;48(7):856–862. http://dx.doi.org/10.1086/597262

29. Govender NP, Chetty V, Roy M, et al. Phased implementation of screening for cryptococcal disease in South Africa. S Afr Med J. 2012;102(12):914–917. http://dx.doi.org/10.7196/samj.6228

Working in rural areas – the experiences of Umthombo Youth Development Foundation graduates

Author:
Andrew J. Ross[1]

Affiliation:
[1]Department of Family Medicine, University of KwaZulu-Natal, South Africa

Correspondence to:
Andrew Ross

Email:
rossa@ukzn.ac.za

Postal address:
24 Jupiter Road, Westville
3629, South Africa

Background: Recruiting and retaining healthcare professionals (HCPs) for rural areas is challenging throughout the world. Although rural origin HCPs have been identified as being the most likely to work in rural areas, only a small number of rural-origin South African scholars are trained as HCPs each year and many do not return to work in rural areas.

Aim: The aim of this article was to present the experiences of rural-origin HCPs who returned to work in a rural area after graduation.

Setting: Umthombo Youth Development Foundation has been running an innovating rurally-based scholarship scheme since 1999. By December 2013, 184 students supported by the scheme had graduated and all had returned to work in a rural area for a period of time.

Methods: This was a qualitative study using a life history methodology to explore the educational experience of six rural-origin HCPs working in rural areas.

Results: The four themes that emerged from the data were: (1) contribution to service delivery; (2) professional development (3) the challenges and frustrations of working in rural hospitals; and (4) the impact of working as an HCP.

Conclusion: Rural-origin HCPs are willing to return and work in rural areas. However, context and content factors need to be addressed if a work-back scholarship scheme is to be a long-term strategy for the recruitment and retention of HCPs.

Travail dans les zones rurales – les expériences des Diplômés de la Fondation Uthombo pour le Développement de la Jeunesse.

Contexte: Le recrutement et la rétention des Professionnels de la Santé (HCP) pour les zones rurales est un problème mondial. Bien qu'on considère que les HCP d'origine rurale seront probablement ceux qui accepteront de travailler dans les régions rurales, un très petit nombre d'étudiants sud-africains d'origine rurale reçoivent une formation de HCP chaque année et beaucoup d'entre eux ne retournent pas travailler dans les zones rurales.

Objectif: Cette étude a pour objectif de décrire les expériences des HCP d'origine rurale qui sont retournés travailler dans les régions rurales après leurs études.

Cadre: la Fondation Umthombo du Développement de la Jeunesse dirige un système de bourses innovant en région rurale depuis 1999. En décembre 2013, 184 étudiants boursiers avaient reçu leur diplôme et tous étaient retournés travailler un certain temps dans une zone rurale.

Méthode: Cette étude qualitative a utilisé la méthode de l'histoire de vie pour étudier 'expérience éducationnelle de six HCP d'origine rurale travaillant dans les zones rurales.

Résultats: Trois thèmes ont émergé des données: (1) la contribution à la prestation de services; (2) Les défis et frustrations de travailler dans des hôpitaux ruraux; et (3) l'impact de travailler comme HCP.

Conclusion: Les HCP d'origine rurale veulent bien retourner travailler en zone rurale. Cependant, il faudra examiner le contexte et le contenu si l'on veut que le système de bourses à rembourser par le travail devienne une stratégie de recrutement et de rétention à long terme des HCP.

Introduction

Without sufficient numbers of well-trained professional staff, key health outcomes will never be realised.[1] Many rural areas in South Africa have a high burden of infectious diseases, high under-five mortality and reduced life expectancy at birth. The 10 districts with the highest deprivation index in South Africa in 2008 were all rural.[2] There are major inequalities between staffing levels at hospitals in rural and urban areas which contribute to poor health outcomes.[2,3] These disparities remain, despite the commitment of the National Department of Health to 'Health for All'[4] and the prioritisation of recruitment of healthcare professionals (HCPs) for rural areas.[5] Maternal, child and infant mortality rates increase as the number of healthcare workers (HCWs) decreases, whilst increasing the number of HCWs has been shown to improve health outcomes in underserved areas.[6]

Rural-origin healthcare professionals (HCPs) have been identified as being the most likely to work in rural areas after qualification and to contribute to improving health outcomes in these areas.[7] However, only a small number of rural-origin South African scholars are trained each year as HCPs[8] and finding staff for rural hospitals is an ongoing challenge. Absent role models, dysfunctional families, poorly-performing schools and limited financial support all make it challenging for rural-origin students to gain access to tertiary institutions in order to train as HCPs.[9,10,11,12,13,14] Compounding the issue of staffing for rural institutions is the fact that only a small percentage of rural-origin HCPs actually choose to work in rural institutions.[15]

The Friends of Mosvold scholarship scheme (now the Umthombo Youth Development Foundation Scholarship Scheme [UYDF SS]), an innovative rural scholarship scheme, was started in 1999. It was based on international research which showed that the training of rural scholars was potentially a long-term solution to the chronic staff shortages in rural and remote areas. Although there are a number of definitions of 'rural' (based on distance from urban areas, resources available, geographic location, economic activity, etc,),[16] by any definition students supported by UYDF SS would be considered to be of rural origin. By November 2013, 184 HCPs supported by the scheme had graduated. All graduates have returned to work at a rural district hospital near where they live to fulfil their work-back obligation. Less than 10% of graduates have bought themselves out of a portion of their work-back obligation and more than 60% have continued to work in a rural area after their work-back obligations were complete.[17]

The willingness of these graduates to return and work in rural hospitals stimulated this research project which is part of a PhD dissertation looking at the educational journeys of rural-origin healthcare professionals working in rural areas. The aim of this article was to present the experiences of these rural-origin HCPs who returned to work in rural areas after graduation. It is hoped that this article will contribute to the discussion regarding the selection and support of rural-origin scholars and strategies for the staffing of rural health care institutions.

Research methods and design

Study design

This was a qualitative study using a life history methodology to explore the educational experience of rural-origin HCPs.

Selection of participants

Six rural origin HCPs were selected purposively from UYDF SS graduates. The criteria for selection of graduates were: (1) their willingness to participate; (2) the ability to articulate their thoughts and express themselves clearly; and (3) whether they were working in a rural context.[18] A variety of HCPs from different disciplines were included in this study in order to ensure that the voices of several members of the healthcare team were heard, many of whom play a significant role in service delivery in rural areas.[19] In addition, women's experiences may be substantially different from those of men – particularly the experiences of rural women – and it was important that the voices of women should also be heard.

The six graduates who were selected (details provided in Table 1) are referred to throughout the rest of this article by their initials only.

Data collection

Data were collected by the author using two unstructured interviews where participants were asked the question, 'tell me about your educational experiences from rural scholar to healthcare professional and what it means to work in a rural setting'. Interviews were supplemented by photographs and artifacts from different stages of

TABLE 1: List of those healthcare professionals who participated in the study.

Name	Current position	Professional qualification	Professional experience	Years of professional experience	Age	Gender	Originally from
DG	Student mentor coordinator based in Mtubatuba	BSc Physiotherapy UKZN 2003	2004–2008 Physiotherapist 2008 – current mentor coordinator	11 years	37 years	M	Ingwavuma
FN	Sub-Saharan coordinator Brian Holden Eye Institute	BSc Optometry UKZN 2003	2004–2009 Optometrist – Mosvold, Pelopele train 2010 – current Brian Holden Eye Institute	11 years	34 years	M	Ingwavuma
SM	Psychologist at Hlabisa Hospital	MSc Clinical psychology UJ 2009	Clinical psychologist Hlabisa Hospital 2010 – current	4 years	29 years	M	Ingwavuma
TM	Physiotherapist at Emmaus Hospital	BSc Physiotherapy Wits 2004	Physiotherapist 2005 – current	6 years	33 years	M	Ingwavuma
NM	Pharmacist Military research post in Mtubatuba	BSc Pharmacy Wits 2004	Pharmacist 2005 – current	10 years	35 years	F	Ingwavuma
LH	Medical officer Mseleni Hospital	MBChB UKZN 2006	Intern / community service officer / Medical officer 2007 – current	9 years	30 years	F	Ubombo

F, Female; M, Male; UKZN, University of KwaZulu Natal; UJ, University of Johannesburg; Wits, University of Witwatersrand.

their educational experiences and by the construction of a collage of a day in their lives (see Figure 1). Participants were asked to describe the photographs and/or artifacts and/or pictures chosen for the collage and how they were connected to their educational experiences. All interviews and discussions were recorded on a voice recorder and transcribed verbatim.

Data analysis

A reconstructed story was written from the transcripts[20] and was sent to the participants for content validity. The stories were read and re-read, codes and categories identified, patterns and relationships between categories reviewed and themes developed.[18]

Ethical consideration

Ethical approval was obtained from the Social Science Ethics Committee of the University of KwaZulu Natal (HSS/1205/012D). Written informed consent, including possible identification, was obtained from all of the participants after the aims of the study were explained to them.

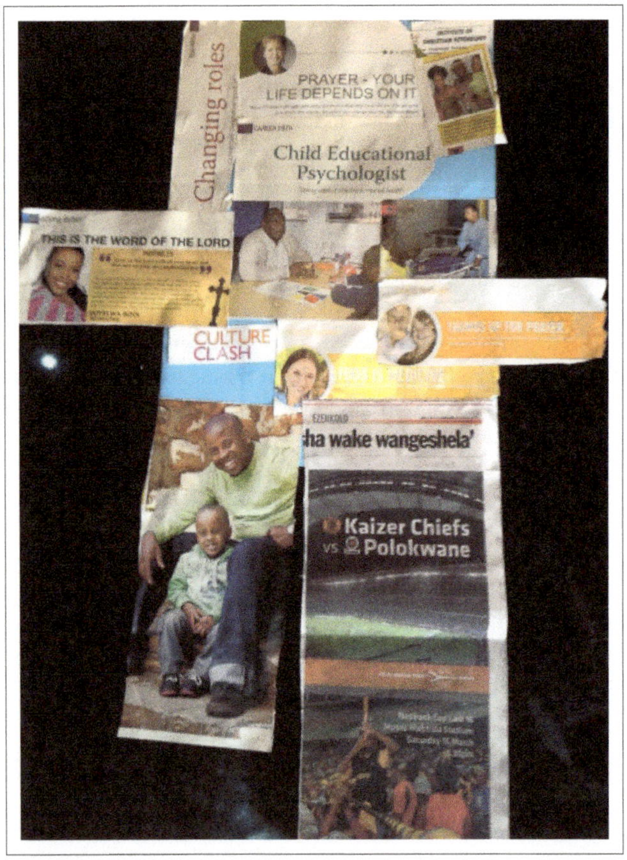

Source: Photo taken by Andrew Ross

FIGURE 1: Collage development [SM].

BOX 1: Discussion of collage in Figure 1.

> In the discussion following the construction of the collage, SM highlighted the importance of his job as a clinical psychologist and the important role that he was playing in the community. He also mentioned the contribution that he was making as a clinical psychologist and as a graduate in the community. He also talked about his changing role within his family, the importance of family and the fact that he was looking forward to having a family of his own. The importance of his religious beliefs, along with how these had impacted upon his choice to return to work at the local district hospital, were also discussed, as well as his love for soccer.

Results

These UYDF SS graduates were chosen to participate in this study because they have continued to work in rural areas. They all had a year-for-year work-back obligation to UYDF to return to the area they came from. Although this was important, because '... I wanted to fulfill my contract with Friends of Mosvold' [DG], fulfilling a contractual obligation was not the primary reason for returning to the hospitals.

SM had a 'great offer to run an employee wellness programme from one of the mining houses'. He could have bought himself out of the contract and remained in Johannesburg, but because of his personal commitment he chose '... to come back for the community. Not returning would have been cheating. I had this moral obligation to my mum and the community'. There were also community expectations that students, who had been chosen by a committee made up of hospital and community members, would return to work on the area after graduating. Graduates were motivated to return because:

> '... [*p*]eople kept on asking me "when are you coming back?". So that kind of put pressure on me ... they must see me coming back now.' [DG]

Working at the local district hospital enabled some of these graduates to stay at home. Even those who had accommodation at the hospital found it easy to visit and provide support to their families. An additional advantage of living in a rural area was that it was cheaper than staying in an urban area because less money was spent on transport as home was close to work and there were less things to spend money on:

> '... [*M*]oney-wise, you don't really spend as much as you would be spending in the urban areas. If you really want to save, you can, and that this [*sic*] was an important advantage of working at a rural district hospital.' [NM]

The following themes were identified from the data:

- Contributing to service delivery.
- Professional development.
- The challenges and frustrations of working in rural hospitals.
- Personal, family and community impact of working as a healthcare professional.

Theme one: Contributing to service delivery

These professional graduates were able to contribute toward service delivery:

> '... [*W*]e worked hard seeing patients in the wards and in OPD [*the outpatient department*] and visiting the clinics.' [DG]

Having grown up in rural areas, they understood what life was like for the majority of the population and this influenced their work ethic and attitude to work. SM recognised that:

'... [*i*]f I don't go to a certain clinic, there's a person there who is waiting for me, who has only that option, to go to that clinic, and nothing else.'

Graduates were able to extend the services provided:

'I saw the therapy department grow from one therapy assistant visiting 16 out of the 34 clinics on her own ... to four physios, two OTs [*occupational therapists*], two audiologists and two speech therapists.' [DG]

Using contacts established through UYDF, they were also able to raise money for equipment needed to support these services.

They brought new skills to the hospitals:

'... I made it my responsibility to make eye services a priority in the whole district ... because of my rural origin I am passionate about making sure that quality healthcare is delivered to people.' [DG]

These graduates were proactive in motivating for posts to be created, staff to be recruited and equipment to be purchased:

'... [*T*]hings never happen by chance ... I always had a plan for the eye clinic.' [FN]

Meaningful contributions were made both to patient care and to the training and support of other HCPs:

'... [*W*]hen I started, the TB [*tuberculosis*] cure rate was below 40%; by the end of the first year, we managed to get it up to 60%, then we got it up again to 75%.' [LH]

'... I orientate [*sic*] them about the HIV and TB programmes.' [LH]

Theme two: Professional development

These HCPs found the work to be interesting, varied and stimulating, with DG commenting that:

'... I remember seeing conditions that you would never see at university – I used to phone the lecturers and say "I'm seeing this, what is it?" Seeing those kind of conditions helped me to say, "[*L*]et me learn more."'

They were also able to take advantage of opportunities for professional development. LH was involved in 'a research project on multiple drug resistant TB' and is '... currently working on modifying the new antiretroviral guidelines'.

SM has had the opportunity to develop professionally as he learnt more about community psychology and culture-bound psychology.

There were also opportunities for promotion which happened more quickly than would have happened in urban hospitals and at some hospitals they felt valued and appreciated by the management, other staff members, patients and members of their community. For most, working in a rural district hospital:

'... [*h*]as been a wonderful journey and I'm loving what I'm doing ... I'm developing caring, supportive relationships and working as a healer and comforter. I see my work as somebody who brings hope to the sick.' [LH]

Theme three: Challenges and frustrations

Graduates, however, found that there were significant challenges and frustrations when working at rural district hospitals. These graduates were chosen by a local selection committee which included community members and management based on a prioritisation of services needed. As students they had returned to the hospital for work-based experience every year and management were aware of their graduation date. Despite this:

'... [*t*]here were no [*optometry*] posts [*when I graduated in December*] ... I eventually started work on the 5th of April in an oral hygienist post; there was no job description and the necessary equipment was not available to function [*sic*].' [FN]

Keeping graduates and making them feel that they were valued and important members of the hospital staff did not appear to be a priority for hospital management at some hospitals. At these hospitals, management was not perceived to be proactive in the creation and filling of posts or in the provision of basic facilities such as suitable accommodation:

'I was willing to fulfill my five year contract but the hospital could only offer me accommodation in a dorm in the Nurses Home with the student nurses although the hospital offered houses to other professional staff.' [DG]

Although management had high expectations of them, graduates often did not feel supported or appreciated:

'... I was left alone to do the job of three [pharmacists] ... [*T*]hey told us that we could not close at four but needed to work until five pm but there was no money for overtime. They offered us the opportunity to take time back but it wasn't easy to take time off when I was the only pharmacist.' [NM]

All of the graduates experienced many frustrations whilst working at the hospitals. LH remembered the following regarding working as a newly-qualified doctor:

'... [*D*]uring a particularly difficult and stressful operation ... I called one doctor. He told me "I'm not on call today. You are a doctor, just see how you can handle it."'

She concluded with:

'... [*T*]hat's how rural medicine is like. Everyone always said rural medicine was horrible and I experienced that first hand.'

She had planned to work at a rural hospital for a number of years, but after that experience she decided:

'... I couldn't stay in rural medicine; the only option was just to quit and go do fashion designing. So I waited for the end of the year and in December when my contracted ended I packed everything and said, "I'm leaving medicine" and I stayed at home without a job until I was approached by Dr F who asked me to work at Mseleni hospital.'

Opting out and leaving rural medicine was an understandable consideration for some of these HCPs when working in an unsupportive environment and faced with overwhelming challenges. However, the HCPs who participated in this study remained and continue to work in rural areas. Some of them (LH, DG, NM, TM) moved to other rural, more supportive institutions whilst others found perspective and were able to continue to work in the same hospital (FN, SM). However even when moving to another hospital, perspective was important as there are challenges in every environment:

'... I realised that there are problems wherever you go ... [I]f you can make a difference here, you can make a difference anywhere. You just need to find a solution to whatever challenges you are facing.' [DG].

Theme four: Personal, family and community impact

For these rural-origin scholars, graduation brought status and respect to them and to their families and has changed their lives forever:

'Graduating changed me and changed the way people relate to me and my family. Graduation brought a belief that I could do things.' [FN]

Working as an HCP meant that they had material resources which they used to build houses for their families, provide water and electricity at home and make sure that other members of their family had opportunities to further their education:

'... Since finishing "varsity", I have helped my eldest sister. After matric she spent two years at home without doing anything as she couldn't continue because of the money. I supported her to go college.' [TM]

These graduates were looked to for health advice as:

'... I can diagnose and give information to improve their condition.' [DG]

They are seen as role models in the community, helping to inspire others to undertake their own educational journey:

'When I speak at schools I start off telling them where I come from and a lot of them get surprised ... [W]hen I tell them, "this is what has happened to me – you can make it", that's when they start relating to the message. I start at the beginning and then go on to tell them about the options.' [SM]

However, perhaps even more profound than being a role model to scholars in the area, was the impact they had on the wider community. Returning to work in the areas and sharing their educational experience with others has changed the communities' perspective regarding the value of higher education:

'... [T]hrough seeing us, through us talking to them they then got encouraged and now maybe 20% of people in that rural area are taking their kids to places of higher learning. When we started, no-one was sending their kids to university. But now, people in the community sell their cows to send their kids to university because they are able to see what education can do for other kids. That's why quite a lot of kids have gone to university from that side – not only kids from good families, but from poor families as well. Parents are putting in their last pennies for their kids to go to university because they can see it does change the family structure, the economics and all that. It's massive. From what I see now. It's massive.' [FN]

Discussion

Using a life history methodology enabled these rural-origin HCPs to tell their life story within the context in which they worked. The stories provided a window to understand the meanings that they attached to their experiences and how they made sense of their world as they worked as an HCP at a rural hospital. Interviews tend to be linear and limited by words whilst the use of arts-based techniques allowed these HCPs to move away from linear thought. Photographs, artifacts and pictures selected for the collages have meaning and memory associated with the experience that the photograph, artifact or picture represents. Using these techniques broadened and deepened my understanding of their experiences as they recalled experiences and explained the meaning relative to the photo or the artifact or the pictures chosen.[21] The use of these tools in this research project was innovative and provided insight and a better understanding of their experiences of working as an HCP in a rural context.[22,23]

A number of recruitment and retention strategies have been proposed with regard to staffing rural hospitals. These include: educational interventions (rural recruitment, early exposure to rural sites, rural campuses); coercion (compulsory service, regulatory requirements); incentives (increased pay, more holidays); and the creation of an enabling environment (increased support, community appreciation). The UYDF SS, as a rurally-based scholarship scheme, could be considered both a recruitment tool in getting graduates to rural areas and a retention tool in the year-for-year work-back obligation imposed on the graduates. The success of the scheme in encouraging graduates to return and fulfil their work-back obligations supports the evidence from international observational studies that the recruitment and training of rural-origin students is an effective strategy for the long-term staffing of rural facilities.[7,24] Studies from Australia have shown that that rural origin students are twice as likely to work in rural areas than graduates from urban areas.[25] Studies from Canada suggest that rural doctors are five times more likely to have originated from rural areas than from urban areas.[26]

In keeping with other studies, reasons given by these graduates for choosing to return to work in a rural district hospital included being able to make a contribution to their communities and to their families, as well as the opportunity to live close to home.[27,28] It was interesting to note that it was not predominately their contractual obligation which motivated them to return but rather a personal commitment to themselves and their community.

A World Health Organization report published in 2013 reiterated the critical role that HCWs play in improving healthcare, stating that governments must prioritise the training, recruitment and retention of HCWs as there can be 'no health without a workforce'.[29] Having and retaining these rural origin HCPs at a district hospital meant that health services could be provided and extended and important services such as optometry and psychology could be introduced. The graduates' intimate knowledge of the community fueled their passion to both improve and extend the healthcare service. Having graduates who understand the local conditions and who appreciate the value and the need for their services is an important asset which should contribute toward the provision of a service of excellence. These graduates found their work to be both interesting and challenging. Opportunities were provided for professional development, they had opportunities for promotion and they felt valued and appreciated by the community. These experiences are similar to the reasons given for remaining at a district hospital by community service officers who were already working in rural district hospitals in South Africa. HCPs who feel valued and appreciated by management, their patients and community members and who feel that they are providing a worthwhile service have been shown to be more likely to choose to remain in a rural setting.[27] Purohit has identified these as being the content factors and/or intrinsic motivators which contribute to HCW motivation, quality of work, job satisfaction and a willingness to remain in rural areas.[30]

However, whilst working at rural district hospitals, many of these graduates experienced multiple frustrations and challenges – often with regard to issues such as a lack of posts, lack of policies (no job description), lack of equipment, inadequate accommodation and poor supervision. Purohit has identified these as context or hygiene factors, which are things that should be in place for the smooth running of a healthcare institution. If they are absent, they can lead to high levels of frustration and dissatisfaction. Context and content factors are complementary and not opposites and both need to be addressed if HCPs are to be retained at rural district hospitals.[30] For example, dealing with accommodation issues may reduce frustration but does not necessarily increase motivation. Doing interesting and worthwhile work which is valued by the community may be motivating but could be undermined by high levels of frustration and plans to leave if, for example, salaries are not paid on time. In this study, four of the six graduates (DG, LH, NM, DG) moved from one district hospital to another, mainly because of context factors. If management wants motivated and productive HCPs who chose to stay and work in rural areas, attention must be given to addressing context factors, in order to reduce and/or eliminate frustrations, as well as to content factors that both motivate and provide a sense of purpose because of doing something that is worthwhile.

The graduates who participated in this study are contributing to service delivery and, in turn, are having a profound influence on their families and on their communities. However the main long-term impact that these graduates have may not be on the health services that they provide but rather on their ability to inspire others to study and to see the potential in education. Ray (2006) has commented that, in relation to aspirations to achieve a better life for oneself and one's family, 'there is no experience quite as compelling as the experience of your immediate family and more broadly those in your socioeconomic and spatial neighbourhood'.[31] The experiences of these rural-origin HCPs echo the words of Nelson Mandela:[32]

> Education is the great engine of personal development. It is through education that the daughter of a peasant can become a doctor, that the son of a mineworker can become the head of the mine, that a child of farm workers can become the president of a great nation ...

Strengths and limitations

The strength of this study lies in the fact that it gives voice to rural-origin HCPs, enabling them to share their experiences. The small number of participants and the qualitative nature of the study mean that the findings cannot be generalised to other settings. However, it is hoped that those reading this study will be able to identify with the participants and apply what has been learnt to their own context.

Conclusion

This study has shown that the recruitment and training of rural scholars is a worthwhile, viable, long-term strategy for the staffing of rural institutions in a developing country such as South Africa and that a scholarship scheme can be a successful strategy for both recruitment and retention. These graduates found their work to be both satisfying and enjoyable and were able to provide and extend healthcare services. They gained status and respect within the community and were role models to scholars in the area. Access to resources improved conditions at home and changed the trajectory of the lives of their family members. However, if such a scheme is to be an effective long-term strategy for the recruitment and retention of HCPs for other rural areas, managers needs to invest in the effort of finding and supporting such rural origin scholars. They also need to give attention to addressing context factors (which lead to frustration) and content factors (that promote motivation) in the workplace.

Acknowledgements

I wish to thank my parents for their assistance in the reviewing of the many drafts of this manuscript. Funding for the research was provided by Discovery Foundation as part of a grant for research into improving rural healthcare delivery. Six months' sabbatical was given by the University of KwaZulu-Natal for data collection as part of the PhD of which this article forms a part.

Competing interests

The author was the founder of the Friends of Mosvold Scholarship scheme (now the UYDF scholarship scheme). He was intimately involved in running the scheme until 2007 and knew all of the participants since they were supported by the scheme. However, since 2007 he has no longer had an active involvement in the selection or financial support of any student and serves only as a trustee of the scheme and a local mentor at the University of KwaZulu Natal. None of those who participated in the research have any financial or other obligation to the author or any personal relationship with the author.

Author's contributions

The author was responsible for the conceptualisation of the research project, the collection and analysis of the data and the writing of this manuscript.

References

1. World Health Organization. Models and tools for health workforce planning and projections. Human Resources for Health Observer – Issue No 3. Geneva: World Health Organization, 2010.
2. Health Systems Trust. The district health barometer 2008/09 [page on the Internet]. c2009 [cited 2012 Feb 08]. Available from: http://www.hst.org.za/publications/district-health-barometer-200809
3. The Rural Health Advocacy Project [homepage on the Internet]. n.d. [cited 2011 Apr 15]. Available from: http://www.rhap.org.za/
4. Declaration of Alma-Ata. International conference on primary health care, Alma-Ata, USSR, 6–12 September, 1978 [document on the Internet]. c1978 [cited 2014 Sep 07]. Available from: http://www.who.int/publications/almaata_declaration_en.pdf
5. Department of Health (South Africa). Human resources for health for South Africa 2030 (Draft) [document on the Internet]. c2011 [cited 2014 Sep 07]. Available from: http://www.hst.org.za/publications/human-resources-health-south-africa-2030
6. World Health Organization. Increasing access to health workers in remote and rural areas through improved retention [document on the Internet]. c2009 [cited 2014 Sep 07]. Available from: http://www.who.int/hrh/migration/background_paper_draft.pdf
7. Wilson NW, Couper ID, De Vries E, et al. A critical review of interventions to redress the inequitable distribution of healthcare professionals to rural and remote areas. Rural Remote Health. 2009;9(2):1060.
8. Tumbo JM, Couper ID, Hugo JF. Rural-origin health science students at South African universities. S Afr Med J. 2009;99(1):54–56.
9. Soudien C. The 'A' factor: Coming to terms with the question of legacy in South African education. Int J Educ Dev. 2007;27(2):182–193. http://dx.doi.org/10.1016/j.ijedudev.2006.07.006
10. Gilmour D, Soudien C. Learning and equitable access in the Western Cape, South Africa. Comp Educ. 2009;45(2):281–295. http://dx.doi.org/10.1080/03050060902920989
11. Letseka M, Cosser M, Breier M, et al. Student retention & graduate destination: Higher education & labour market access & success. Cape Town: HSRC Press; 2009.
12. Adam F, Backhouse J, Baloyi H, et al. Access and throughput in South African Higher Education: Three case studies. Council on Higher Education; 2010.
13. Department of Basic Education. Educational statistics in South Africa 2009 document on the Internet]. c2010 [cited 2014 Sep 07]. Available from: http://www.education.gov.za/LinkClick.aspx?fileticket=8RQsvgahSgA%3d&tabid=462&mid=1326
14. Chisholm L, Morrow S, Wa Kivilu M, et al. Emerging voices. A report on education in South African rural communities. Cape Town: HSRC Press; 2005.
15. Mateen FJ. Future practice location and satisfaction with rural medical education: Survey of medical students. Can Fam Physician. 2006;52(9):1106–1107.
16. Couper ID. Rural hospital focus: Defining rural. Rural Remote Health. 2003;3(2):205.
17. MacGregor RG. Umthombo Youth Development Foundation Annual report 2012–13 [document on the Internet]. c2013 [cited 2014 Sep 07]. Available from: https://www.givengain.com/cause_data/images/1781/UYDF_Annual_Report_2013_e.pdf
18. Terre Blanche MJ, Durrheim K, Painter D, editors. Research in practice: Applied methods for the social sciences. Cape Town: University of Cape Town; 2006.
19. Naidu C, Irlam J, Diab PN. Career and practice intentions of health science students at three South African health science faculties. AJHPE. 2013;5(2):68–71. http://dx.doi.org/10.7196/ajhpe.202
20. Clandinin DJ. Narrative inquiry: A methodology for studying lived experience. RSME. 2006;27(1):44–54.
21. Northcutt N, McCoy D. Interactive qualitative analysis: A systems method for qualitative research. California: Sage Publications; 2004.
22. Butler-Kisber L, Poldma T. The power of visual approaches in qualitative inquiry: The use of collage making and concept mapping in experiential research. Journal of Research Practice. 2010;6(2):1–16.
23. Samaras AP. Explorations in using arts-based self-study methods. Int J Qual Stud Educ. 2010;23(6):719–736. http://dx.doi.org/10.1080/09518390903426212
24. Versteeg M, Couper ID. Position paper: Rural health – key to a healthy nation. Johannesburg: Rural Health Advocacy Project; 2011.
25. Laven G, Wilkinson D. Rural doctors and rural backgrounds: How strong is the evidence? A systematic review. Aust J Rural Health. 2003;11(6):277–284. http://dx.doi.org/10.1111/j.1440-1584.2003.00534.x
26. Rourke J, Dewar D, Harris K, et al. Strategies to increase the enrollment of students of rural origin in medical school: Recommendations from the Society of Rural Physicians of Canada. CMAJ. 2005;172(1):62–65. http://dx.doi.org/10.1503/cmaj.1040879
27. Ross A, Reid SJ. The retention of community service officers for an additional year at district hospitals in KwaZulu-Natal and the Eastern Cape and Limpopo Provinces. SA Fam Pract. 2009;51(3):249–253. http://dx.doi.org/10.1080/20786204.2009.10873856
28. Manafa O, McAuliffe E, Maseko F, et al. Retention of health workers in Malawi: Perspectives of health workers and district management. Hum Resour Health. 2009;7:65. http://dx.doi.org/10.1186/1478-4491-7-65
29. Global Health Workforce Alliance and World Health Organization. A universal truth: No health without a workforce. Geneva: World Health Organization; 2013.
30. Purohit B, Bandyopadhyay T. Beyond job security and money: Driving factors of motivation for government doctors in India. Hum Resour Health. 2014;12:12. http://dx.doi.org/10.1186/1478-4491-12-12
31. Ray D. Ch 28: Aspirations, poverty, and economic change. In: Abhijit V, Mookherjee D, Banerjee RB, editors. Understanding poverty [ebook]. Oxford: Oxford University Press, 2006. http://dx.doi.org/10.1093/0195305191.003.0028
32. Anonymous. Nelson Mandela quotes [document on the Internet]. n.d. [cited 2014 Sep 08]/ Available from: http://www.education.gov.za/LinkClick.aspx?fileticket=8d6cPhef/L8%3D

29

The effect of formal, neonatal communication-intervention training on mothers in kangaroo care

Authors:
Alta Kritzinger[1]
Elise van Rooyen[2]

Affiliations:
[1]Clinic for High-Risk Babies (CHRIB), Department of Speech-Language Pathology and Audiology, University of Pretoria, South Africa

[2]Kangaroo Mother Care Unit, Department of Paediatrics, Kalafong Hospital, University of Pretoria, South Africa

Correspondence to:
Alta Kritzinger

Email:
alta.kritzinger@up.ac.za

Postal address:
Private Bag X20, Hatfield 0028, South Africa

Background: Due to low-birth-weight, preterm birth, HIV and/or AIDS and poverty-related factors, South Africa presents with an increased prevalence of infants at risk of language delay. A Kangaroo Mother Care (KMC) unit offers unique opportunities for training.

Aim: The aim of the present study was to determine if formal, neonatal communication-intervention training had an effect on mothers' knowledge and communication interaction with their high-risk infants.

Methods: Three groups of mothers participated: Group 1 was trained whilst practicing KMC; Group 2 was not trained but practiced KMC; and Group 3 was also not trained but practiced sporadic KMC. Ten mothers per group were matched for age, education level and birth order of their infants. The individual training was based on graded sensory stimulation and responsive mother-infant communication interaction, which emphasised talking and singing by the mother.

Results: Significant differences were found in mother-infant communication interaction between all three groups, which indicated a positive effect on Group 1 with training. Group 2, KMC without training, also had a positive effect on interaction. However, Group 1 mothers with training demonstrated better knowledge of their infants and were more responsive during interaction than the other two groups.

Conclusion: The present study suggests that neonatal communication-intervention training adds value to a KMC programme.

Les effets de la formation formelle d'intervention et de communication néonatales chez les mères ayant recours à la méthode kangourou.

Contexte: En raison d'un poids de naissance trop faible, de la prématurité, de facteurs tels que le VIH et/ou le SIDA et de la pauvreté, les risques de retard de langage chez les enfants sont plus prévalents en Afrique du Sud. Le service des soins maternels de type kangourou (KMC) offre une opportunité unique de formation.

Objectif: L'objet de cette étude est de déterminer si la formation formelle d'intervention et de communication néonatales avait un effet sur le savoir et l'interaction communicative des mères avec leurs enfants à haut risque.

Méthodes: Trois groupes de mères y ont participé: le Groupe 1 a été entrainé en pratiquant le KMC; le Groupe 2 n'a pas été entrainé mais a pratiqué le KMC; et le Groupe 3 n'a pas non plus été entrainé mais a pratiqué sporadiquement le KMC. On a réuni dix mères par groupe selon l'âge, le niveau d'éducation et l'ordre de naissance de leurs enfants. On a basé l'entrainement individuel sur la stimulation sensorielle et l'interaction communicative mère-enfant, où la mère parle et chante à l'enfant.

Résultats: On a remarqué des différences importantes dans l'interaction communicative mère-enfant parmi les trois groupes, ce qui a montré un effet positif sur le Groupe 1 entrainé. Le Groupe 2, avec le KMC sans entrainement, a aussi eu un effet positif sur l'interaction. Cependant, les mères du Groupe 1 entrainées ont fait preuve d'une meilleure connaissance de leur enfant et réagissaient mieux au cours de l'interaction que les deux autres groupes.

Conclusion: Cette étude montre que la formation d'intervention communicative néonatale ajoute de la valeur au programme KMC.

Introduction

Kangaroo mother care (KMC) has a strong impact and focus on mother-infant communication interaction.[1,2] Therefore, speech-language therapists should support and utilise this method to develop neonatal communication-intervention programmes for high-risk infants and their caregivers. In KMC, a neonate is securely carried in an upright position, skin-to-skin, between the mother's breasts. This evolutionary, reclaimed care pattern offers benefits to the infant, the parents and family, healthcare systems, and to speech-language therapy practice.

Kangaroo mother care stabilises a neonate's physiological functions,[1] improves behavioural and state of alertness regulation and may enhance brain organisation and neuromaturation in preterm infants, as sleep patterns are better organised and cyclical.[3] Cyclical sleep during the foetal period, and when interrupted by preterm birth, is important for early sensory development.[4,5] The benefits of KMC to the mother include: increased oxytocin levels in herself and her infant, resulting in enhanced lactation and bonding to her new-born infant; and reduced stress, anxiety and postnatal depression.[1] Family members, especially fathers and grandmothers, can also participate in kangaroo care.[1] Since the neonate is discharged earlier from hospital than with conventional incubator care,[6] and the mother is already skilled in caring for the very small baby at home, the family rather than the hospital is central to the infant's caregiving. Research indicates that mothers and families from different cultures worldwide respond spontaneously and favourably to KMC when trained to apply the procedure.[7] Although the physical implementation of KMC is only applicable during the first weeks or months of an infant's life, the benefits of the intervention are far reaching.

All the benefits of KMC converge at a point where the ideal opportunity arises for speech-language therapists to intervene early and ameliorate threats to typical language development in high-risk infants. Recent studies have clearly shown that those children born preterm, even those born late preterm, are at risk of language and academic difficulties.[8] As described by ASHA,[9] KMC endorses some of the most important principles of early communication-intervention. Similar to early-intervention principles, KMC: is family centred, culturally responsive and developmentally supportive; represents a natural environment of care and prolonged breastfeeding; is team based; starts as early as possible in a child's life; and is supported by high-quality evidence.

There is also an additional rationale as to why speech-language therapists should be involved in a KMC unit or a neonatal intensive care unit (NICU) where the intervention procedure is promoted. When mothers and their high-risk neonates are discharged from a KMC unit they disperse to areas where follow-up early intervention services may not be accessible to them. Since the average lodging of a mother and infant in the KMC unit, where the research was conducted, is 13 days,[6] the unit offers a short period of unique access to mothers and their high-risk neonates. The availability of mothers, who already have an increased interest in their infants as they have been primed by KMC, provides a valuable opportunity for speech-language therapists to start an interdisciplinary communication-intervention programme in a KMC unit (see Figure 1). Nurses and doctors train mothers to practice KMC, whilst speech-language therapists can train them at the same time to appropriately facilitate their infants' communication development. The continuous practice of KMC over time allows for strong bonds to develop between mother and neonate.[10] Mother-infant communication interaction results naturally from attachment, and, as stated by Billeaud,[11] attachment forms the basis of mother-infant communication interaction (see Figure 1). Whilst the mother is gradually becoming familiar with her infant through continuous KMC, she also needs information to understand her preterm infant's progress through developmental stages, as described by Gorski, Davidson and Brazelton,[12] and Rossetti.[2] The mother needs to identify the infant's stress signs, its readiness for stimulation, and its subtle cues to communicate. A mother may require training to establish a highly sensitive pattern of successful reciprocal communication interaction with her preterm infant[2] so that the child's auditory system is appropriately stimulated to facilitate language development during the replaced foetal period.

The importance of appropriate auditory system stimulation in preterm infants is recognised in the literature. According to Graven and Browne,[4] the period from 25 weeks gestation to 5–6 months postnatal age is most sensitive to the neurosensory development of the auditory system. The developing auditory system requires stimulation by the human voice, language and music during the last 10–12 weeks of foetal life so that the hair cells of the cochlea, the axons of the auditory nerve and the neurons of the auditory cortex are tuned to receive specific frequencies and intensities – a function that can only develop when ambient noise is not louder than 60 dB.[4] The foetus appears to receive an ideal signal-to-noise ratio of auditory input in the womb. The effects of noise exposure on preterm infants were demonstrated by evidence of delayed auditory cortex organisation found in mouse pups when reared in the continuous presence of white noise.[13] Considering the unique potential of the early human auditory system to make language acquisition possible, there appears to be a balance between stimulation provided by the ambient noise of the maternal heartbeat and blood circulation, other internal and external noises, and the consistency of a single maternal voice heard *in utero*. The ideal stimulation of the foetal auditory system during the third trimester of pregnancy, provided by the consistency of the mother's voice against vastly different and diffuse background noises, is interrupted by preterm birth. Logic follows that an appropriate ratio of signal-to-noise auditory compensation

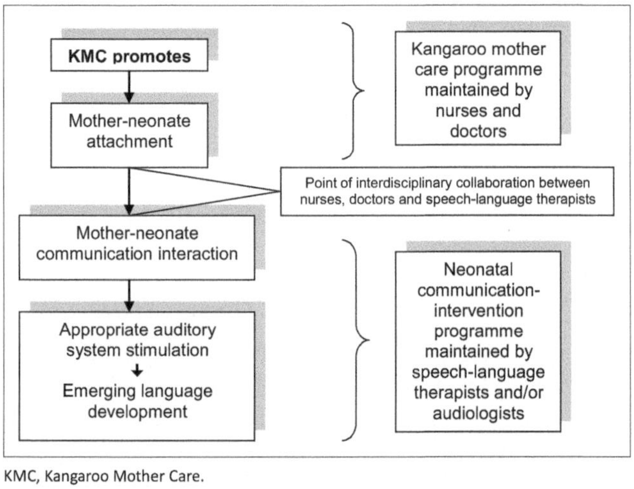

KMC, Kangaroo Mother Care.

FIGURE 1: The interdisciplinary relationship between a KMC programme and a neonatal communication-intervention programme.

must be provided in the caregiving environment during the infant's unplanned perinatal period.

Since the full-term infant is born with a preference for the maternal voice[14] it is clear that complex auditory processing starts before birth and that antenatal auditory system stimulation is required. It is hypothesised that the exclusive maternal-caregiving environment created by continuous KMC provides some form of compensatory auditory system stimulation and possibly an appropriate early language-learning environment for preterm infants (see Figure 1). In the upright KMC position, the infant's ears are in close approximation to the mother's mouth so as to hear her voice. The ambient noise, in contrast to a NICU with much noise created by staff and lifesaving equipment, is typically subdued in a dedicated KMC unit. If a mother is taught to be sensitive to the infant's stress signals, she may provide the appropriate amount and quality of auditory stimulation according to her preterm baby's developmental stage, as described by Gorski et al.[12] and Rossetti.[2]

A further justification to implement a neonatal communication-intervention programme is the high prevalence of at-risk infants born in South Africa, mostly due to low birth weight, preterm birth, HIV and/or AIDS and persistent poverty in many families. If the opportunity to start intervention in the neonatal period is missed in South Africa, case finding may be complicated by a lack of early-intervention services at primary and secondary healthcare facilities. Primary healthcare workers have little capacity to identify infants that require early intervention due to their workload, staff shortages and lack of training.

Since the establishment of the KMC unit at the hospital where the study was conducted, the parent-education programme provided by nurses and doctors has included training and support regarding the KMC method, breastfeeding, and the caring for low-birth-weight infants in the unit and after discharge.[6] As the KMC programme provided limited education to the mothers to enhance the infants' communication development, the opportunity was used to develop a formal communication-based training programme for the mothers, as indicated in Figure 1. The need to contribute to evidence-based neonatal intervention programmes in South Africa provided the stimulus for the research study.

Aim and objectives

The objective of the study was to determine if the short-term knowledge and communication interaction of mothers with their high-risk neonates improved with formal training. To achieve the objective, the participants' language proficiency and confidence had to be determined first in order to establish their readiness for training in English.

Research methods and design

A three-group comparison design was selected to determine whether an experimental group of mothers that received formal communication-intervention training behaved differently with training, as opposed to the two groups who received no training.[15] Group 1 was trained whilst practicing continuous KMC in a well-established KMC unit; Group 2 was not trained, but practiced KMC in the same unit; and Group 3 was also not trained but practiced sporadic KMC at another hospital. The Group 2 was selected after all the mothers of the first group were discharged from the KMC unit. As the KMC unit consisted of one large dormitory, each group's data were collected consecutively to prevent the knowledge of the trained group to influence the first control group, who practiced KMC but did not receive training. The research method is outlined in Table 1.

As seen in Table 1, the interview with the individual mothers was conducted as a pre-test/post-test to determine whether qualitative differences in knowledge of their infants occurred in Group 1 without and with training. Multiple sources of data were utilised to support the mixed methods design of the study. Data were collected from case histories in medical files (quantitative data), interviews with the mothers (text data) and video recordings of mother-infant communication interaction, analysed according to a rating scale.

Ethical considerations

The Research Ethics Committee of the Faculty of Humanities and the Faculty of Health Sciences (Protocol number 40/2004), University of Pretoria and the Provincial Department of Health gave permission to conduct the study. A research assistant informed prospective participants, in English or Setswana, about the aims and procedures of the study. Participant information brochures were available in English and Setswana, the home language of most of the participants. All participants gave written informed consent to participate in the study and to be video recorded. The infants were in stable conditions when their mothers handled them, and when they were video recorded. The researcher handled none of the infants. After the study, a copy of the video recording was given as an incentive to each participant.

TABLE 1: Research design and methods.

Participant groups	Without training	Neonatal communication-interaction training	Post training measurements after two weeks
Kalafong Hospital Continuous KMC	Interview	3 training sessions over two weeks	- Interview - Video recording
Kalafong Hospital Continuous KMC	None	No training	- Interview - Video recording
Another hospital Sporadic KMC	None	No training	- Interview - Video recording

KMC, Kangaroo Mother Care.

Participants and setting

A total of 30 participants, forming three groups of ten mothers in each group, were utilised in the study. The two hospitals were tertiary-level public facilities that received patients from surrounding townships, the inner city or rural towns. The participants of Groups 1 and 2 lodged with their infants in the KMC unit of the first hospital, whilst the participants of Group 3 did not stay in the hospital and had to come in from home to visit their infants in the neonatal unit.

The three groups were matched according to mothers' ages, level of education (either primary or secondary school education), and birth order of their infants. The groups were very similar in composition of factors that could relate to experience of motherhood. Prior experience in motherhood, as measured by the number of children of a participant, was an important variable to equalise between the groups, as parental experience could have given participants an unfair advantage over those with no previous parenting experience.

As further indicated in Table 2, the groups differed in the infants' birth weights, age at the time of the video recordings, number of days in the KMC unit or the neonatal unit, and gender (See Table 2, numbers 4 to 7). The variability of the sample may be a reflection of the diversity that can be expected in the high-risk neonatal population. The differences between the three groups were considered when the results were discussed.

Participant selection

Participants were purposely selected to participate in the study. Criteria for selection included that participants had to be mothers of preterm (born before 37 weeks gestation) and low-birth-weight infants (birth weight < 2 500 g), either in a KMC programme (Groups 1 and 2) or in a neonatal unit (Group 3). Mothers of infants who received oxygen at the time of data collection, infants with congenital disorders, and twins were excluded from the study since these variables were considered to be stressors that could have influenced the mother-infant interaction negatively.

A participant language proficiency and confidence rating scale was designed to rate the participants' language proficiency and perceived confidence, respectively. This was done in order to ensure that the participants were not unfairly judged on their English language skills or intimidated by the researcher. The aim was to recruit participants who scored higher than two points on the rating scale. The 4-point rating scale was used by the research assistant and researcher whilst recruiting the participants, and is presented in Table 3. The research assistant and researcher held informal conversations with prospective participants in English. The research assistant and researcher completed the rating scale separately. A consensus discussion was held when there were differences in the ratings. Mothers who scored lower than two were not included in the study, as they would not have communicated successfully in English.

Group 1 was selected first. Ten participants received three individual training sessions over 14 days whilst they were

TABLE 3: Participant language proficiency and confidence rating scale.

Rating	English language proficiency	Perceived confidence
1	Participant did not understand all questions.	Participant was quiet and did not make eye contact with researcher.
2	Participant understood all questions after rephrasing.	Participant answered questions, but did not volunteer information.
3	Participant understood all questions, but did not elaborate on her answers.	Participant made eye contact and answered all questions.
4	Participant answered questions in full sentences.	Participant initiated conversation with researcher, volunteered information.

TABLE 2: Description of participants (*n* = 30).

Characteristics of mothers and infants	Group 1 (*n* = 10) Continuous KMC and training*	Group 2 (*n* = 10) Continuous KMC, no training	Group 3 (*n* = 10) Sporadic KMC, no training
Dependent variables similar across the three groups			
Mother's age *p*-value: 0.5507	Mean: 27.5 years s.d.: 5.3 Minimum: 20 years Maximum: 36 years	Mean: 29 years s.d.: 6.4 Minimum: 19 years Maximum: 38 years	Mean: 30.3 years s.d.: 5.5 Minimum: 23 years Maximum: 40 years
Educational level	Primary school: 2 Secondary school: 8	Primary school: 2 Secondary school: 8	Primary school: 2 Secondary school: 8
Gravida (number of children, current infant included) *p*-value: 0.9307	Mean: 1.9 children s.d.: 0.7 Minimum: 1 Maximum: 3	Mean: 1.9 children s.d.: 0.8 Minimum: 1 Maximum: 4	Mean: 2.5 children s.d.: 1.9 Minimum: 1 Maximum: 6
Dependent variables not similar across the three groups			
Birth weight of infants (no *p*-values obtained)	Mean: 1613 g Minimum: 1000 g Maximum: 2300 g	Mean: 1335 g Minimum: 978 g Maximum: 1780 g	Mean: 1351 g Minimum: 880g Maximum: 2610 g
Age of infants at video recording *p*-value: 0146**	Mean: 29.5 days s.d.: 13.9 Minimum: 16 days Maximum: 33 days	Mean: 23.5 days s.d.: 8.5 Minimum: 9 days Maximum: 33 days	Mean: 13.6 days s.d.: 13.53 Minimum: 3 days Maximum: 47 days
Number of days in KMC *p*-value: 0.0063**	Mean: 18.4 days s.d.: 10.3 Minimum: 9 days Maximum: 42 days	Mean: 8.8 days s.d.: 3.19 Minimum: 4 days Maximum: 13 days	Mean: 13.6 days in neonatal unit s.d.: 13.5 Minimum: 3 days Maximum: 47 days
Gender of infants	Boys: 9 Girls: 1	Boys: 4 Girls: 6	Boys: 4 Girls: 6

KMC, Kangaroo Mother Care.
Training*, Neonatal communication-interaction training.
*p***, represent significant differences between the three groups on the 0.05% level

practicing KMC. A short interview was conducted with them, before and after their training (see Table 1). Group 2 was selected after all the mothers of the first group had been discharged from the KMC unit. The waiting period was necessary so that Group 1 could not model the trained communication-interaction behaviours with their infants to the group who did not receive training. The participants in Group 2 received no training, but were practicing continuous KMC with their infants in the unit. Group 3 neither practiced continuous KMC, nor did they receive any training to facilitate communication interaction with their infants. As KMC is now widely practiced in South Africa,[16] no state hospital in the area could be found that did not practice KMC at all. The hospital where Group 3 was recruited did not have a KMC unit at the time of data collection, but encouraged mothers to practice KMC when they visited their infants in the neonatal unit. Some mothers in Group 3, therefore, practiced sporadic KMC but did not lodge with their infants in the hospital.

Material and apparatus

Three sets of instruments were used to collect data. The first instrument was a self-designed checklist to record the demographic and biological characteristics of the participants and their infants from the medical files. The second was a self-designed interview schedule to determine participants' knowledge of their infants' communication abilities and development. Five main questions with follow-up questions were posed to the participants during the individual interviews:

1. Do you think your baby can hear?
   - If the response was yes, the following question was asked:
     - How do you know?
   - If no, the following question was asked:
     - When do you think your baby will be able to hear?
2. Do you think your baby can see?
   - If the response was yes, the following question was asked:
     - How do you know?
   - If no, the following question was asked:
     - When do you think your baby will be able to see?
3. Do you know when your baby is tired/needs a break?
   - If yes, the following question was asked:
     - How do you know?
4. Do you know when your baby is happy?
   - If yes, the following question was asked:
     - How do you know?
5. What else can your baby do?

Third, a 4-point scale from Klein and Briggs[17] was used to rate the participants' communication interaction with their infants (see Table 6 later). The participants' interaction with their infants were video recorded and rated as: (1) rarely or never; (2) sometimes; (3) often; and (4) optimally occurring according to the *Observation of Communication Interaction*.[17]

The apparatus included a portable Panasonic VHS-C NV-R33 movie camera, with a hi-fi stereo microphone, a 10 x wide lens and an image stabiliser.

The material also included the neonatal communication-intervention programme. The interdisciplinary parent-training programme is based on three components:

1. The practice of KMC, as explained by Van Rooyen et al.,[6] is taught to the mothers by nurses and doctors. Tactile stimulation is provided to the infants by KMC (i.e. skin-to-skin touching) and vestibular stimulation occurs naturally when the mother is moving.

The researcher, a speech-language therapist, taught the following two components:

2. Graded sensory stimulation[18] is to be provided by the mother according to the three developmental stages of preterm infants: turning in, coming out and reciprocity stages.[12,2.] When the infant is in the turning in and coming out stages, visual stimuli (attempts to make eye contact with the infant) are kept to a minimum. During these stages, the infant may meet attempts at eye contact with gaze aversion. Auditory stimulation is provided by the mother's own voice when she talks and sings softly to the infant during all three developmental stages. During the reciprocity stage, the visual stimulus of eye contact between mother and infant is gradually added. Singing and talking are maintained, provided that the infant is not over stimulated. As indicated by Graven and Browne,[4,] the importance of the mother's voice when she talks and sings to the infant is vital.
3. Responsive interaction between mother and infant[19] is taught. The mother is trained to: identify stress signs in her infant; reduce the infant's stress by decreasing sensory stimuli, such as noise; hold the infant in the KMC position; only initiate interaction once the infant is regulated and calm. The mother is taught to respond to the infant's subtle cues for readiness to communicate and not to provide intrusive stimulation, as cautioned by Klein and Briggs.[17] When the infant is in the reciprocal stage, face-to-face interaction is possible. When stress cues, such as gaze aversion, hiccupping, sneezing, couching, stretching arms and pushing feet are identified, stimulation is reduced and the infant is placed back in the KMC position.

Procedures

A pilot study was conducted with three mothers to test the instruments and procedures, determine the participants' level of understanding English and openness to exchange information with the researcher, who did not share the same culture. The pilot participants were found to be very willing to explain their infants' progress in KMC and wanted new information. The main study proceeded as indicated in Table 1. Participants gave written informed consent. Participants had to be proficient in English to understand the training instructions and interview questions, as the researcher (also the trainer) was not proficient in Setswana. A video recording was made of the interviews and 10–15 min interaction time of the participants with their infants. The participants were asked to play with their infants or perform caregiving tasks whilst the video recording was running and the researcher was studying the medical file. At the beginning of the recording, the researcher assured each mother that her interaction with her infant was appropriate.

The individual communication-interaction training was conducted at each participant's bed by discussing and demonstrating desired behaviours. The researcher identified the infant's developmental stage according to the gestational age and chronological age, and explained it to the mother. Whilst interacting with the infant, the researcher pointed out the infant's hearing responses, eye contact and stress signs to the mother. The mother was gently guided to interact responsively with her infant, whilst encouraging her appropriate behaviours with verbal comments. The training started with the mother's focus of attention, which was usually her infant. The language barriers were managed by adapting vocabulary, following a flexible approach, keeping the conversation interactive, using minimal prompts to encourage the participants and asking open questions instead of questions requiring yes or no answers. With Group 1, after three training sessions over a period of approximately two weeks, a post-training video was recorded. The communication-intervention programme was given to each participant in the form of a handout. Participants of Group 2 and 3 were not trained, but received the handout after their video recordings were made.

Data analysis

Standard deviations (s.d.) were calculated to indicate how far the values deviated from the mean. *P*-values were calculated by means of the Kruskall-Wallis one-way analysis of variance test or Fischer's exact test in order to determine if differences between the groups were statistically significant. The interviews were transcribed from the video recordings and the 'yes', 'no' and 'I don't know' responses were calculated out of ten. The most representative answer to open questions 1 – 4 was selected and reported in Table 5. All of the different themes identified in the answers to question 5 (*What else can your baby do?*) were presented in the results.

Reliability and validity

Evidence of the trustworthiness of the study, expressed as confirmability and internal validity, is as follows: each video recording was analysed three times by the researcher, and 33% of the recordings were analysed by a second rater, for whom the groups were concealed. The average of the ratings was calculated. Data were collected consecutively after Group 1 had been discharged, so that Groups 1 and 2 could not contaminate each other, as participants were selected from the same KMC unit. The objective was dependability, or a refined understanding of the setting. Language and cultural differences were recognised, strategies were applied to be culturally sensitive, to communicate effectively, and to allow trust and spontaneity to develop between the researcher and participants.

Results

The first result describes the participants' language proficiency and confidence, after which the differences in knowledge, mother-infant communication interaction and behaviour types with and without training will be presented.

Participants' language proficiency and confidence

As already determined by the Kruskall-Wallis one-way analysis of variance, the *p*-values indicate no statistical differences between the three groups, for the variables of age, educational level and the number of children (see Table 2). The equivalence between the groups was further determined by the participants' English language proficiency and confidence, as perceived by the researcher and research assistant. A maximum of four points could be obtained. The results are presented in Table 4.

When the decimals points in Table 4 are approximated, the numbers indicate an average value of three for all the groups. The ratings indicate that, on average, the participants understood all the questions asked by the researcher, but did not necessarily elaborate on the answers. The participants were sufficiently confident to answer all questions and made eye contact with the researcher (see rating 3, Table 3). Applying the confidence scale reminded the researcher to be culturally sensitive and to use appropriate interviewing skills when talking to the participants. The ratings of Group 2, who did not receive training, indicated a slight advantage over Groups 1 and 3.

Knowledge of infants

According to Table 5, and based on the interviews, there was a clear difference in Group 1 before training and after two weeks of training. With training and whilst conducting KMC, Group 1 gave increased descriptions of their infants' behaviours, supplied sophisticated descriptions by using terminology from the training programme (*he shows a stop sign with his hand*), demonstrated an understanding of neonatal listening and visual abilities, and knew about stress signs in their infants, as opposed to before the training.

Group 2 gave similar accounts of their infants to Group 1 without training, as both groups were conducting KMC without additional training at that stage. Without training, both groups were mostly sure that their infants could hear, were ambivalent about their infants' vision and stress cues, and were mostly certain when their infants were content. Groups 1 and 2 practiced continuous KMC and gave better

TABLE 4: Results of participant language proficiency and perceived confidence.

Variables	Group 1	Group 2	Group 3
Language proficiency of participants in averages (maximum 4).	2.7	3.4	2.6
Perceived confidence of participants in averages (maximum 4).	3.0	3.4	2.9

answers during the interview than Group 3. Participants in Group 3, who practiced sporadic KMC, could hardly describe their infants' sensory abilities, cues and behaviours. The difference in knowledge of the infants between the two groups practicing continuous KMC, and the third group conducting KMC only sporadically, may indicate the positive effect of KMC on the first two groups with regards to understanding their infants' behaviour. The fact that Groups 1 and 3 knew their infants longer than Group 2 (see Table 2, number 6), appeared not to have made a difference in the knowledge of their infants, which they displayed during the interviews. Group 1 and 2 were equally unsure about their infants' abilities to hear and see, and whether their infants were tired or happy. Participants in Group 3 were least sure about these aspects of their infants' behaviour.

Mother-infant communication interaction

The results obtained through observation of mother-infant communication interaction, as presented in Table 6, show that all *p*-values indicate statistically significant differences between the three groups on the 0.05% level according to Fischer's exact test. Participants in Group 1 showed significantly higher scores on the mother-infant communication-interaction scale with training and KMC, as opposed to Groups 2 and 3 who did not receive training. The ten items of the communication-interaction scale included general interaction behaviours, assessing a mother's sensitivity to respond to her infant's immediate behaviour or withhold stimulation, and communication-specific behaviours. The general interaction behaviours included: holding and rocking (Item 1), displaying pleasure (Items 2 and 5), and responding contingently to the infant (Items 3, 8 and 9). The participants in Group 1 almost always positioned themselves so that the infant was able to make eye contact, talked 'motherese' to the infant by varying the pitch and tone of their voices, and encouraged conversation with the infant. Again, Group 1 and 2 showed better scores than Group 3. The age difference in the infants and the longer time spent with their infants in KMC could have advantaged Group 1 (see Table 2). Participants in Group 1 could have known their infants better than participants in Group 2 or 3. Participants in Group 3 did not know their infants well, as they had to come in from home to see their infants every day and did not spend sufficient time with their infants. Since the groups were matched for age, education level, gravida and birth weight, it may indicate that both KMC and the training programme had an effect on the participants' communication interaction with their infants. None of the groups displayed optimal behaviours on Item 10, which may be too advanced for neonatal communication skills.

Further differences between the groups were observed. The different behaviours that the participants displayed whilst

TABLE 5: Results of the interviews (n = 30).

Question	Group 1 Continuous KMC without training	Group 1 Continuous KMC with training	Group 2 Continuous KMC alone	Group 3 Sporadic KMC Neonatal unit
1. Do you think your baby can hear?	Yes: 10 Don't know: 0 No: 0	Yes: 10 Don't know: 0 No: 0	Yes: 9 Don't know: 1 No: 0	Yes: 6 Don't know: 2 No: 2
How do you know? Example	'Cannot say.'	'He turns his head when you talk.'	'When I touch him he becomes quiet.'	'He jerks if you bang the incubator.'
2. Do you think your baby can see?	Yes: 5 Don't know: 5 No: 0	Yes: 10 Don't know: 0 No: 0	Yes: 4 Don't know: 3 No: 3	Yes: 6 Don't know: 3 No: 1
How do you know? Example	'He sleeps.'	'He follows my hand if I move it.'	'Difficult to tell, she is so small.'	'She has eyes.'
If no, when will your baby be able to hear and see? Examples	'After one or two months.'	N/a	'Maybe after two weeks.'	'Maybe next month.'
3. Do you know when your baby is tired?	Yes: 5 No: 5	Yes: 10 No: 0	Yes: 7 No: 3	Yes: 4 No: 6
How do you know? Examples	'I can see when he is tired.'	'He shows the stop sign with his hand.'	'When he sleeps.'	'When he stretches.'
4. Do you know when your baby is happy?	Yes: 9 Don't know: 1 No: 0	Yes: 10 Don't know: 0 No: 0	Yes: 9 Don't know: 1 No: 0	Yes: 6 Don't know: 0 No: 4
How do you know? Examples	'He smiles.'	'He smiles when he is sleeping.'	'He is happy in KMC.'	'When he feeds.'
5. What else can your baby do? All themes of verbatim responses:	'Nothing.' 'Cries when hungry.' 'She likes moving.' 'Opens her eyes.' 'He looks, but he sees nothing.' 'He can sleep.' 'He likes to play.' 'Stretches.' 'He can suck now.'	'He drinks well.' 'He cries, sleeps.' 'Moves more.' 'Opens her eyes.' 'Cries for her food.' 'More responsive when she is awake.' 'She would stare at me for a long time.' 'She recognises my voice.' 'Drinks and stops, drinks and stops.' 'Sucks his thumb.' 'He can see better.' 'Sleeps at night, but (also) awake at night.' 'He follows me when I go away.' 'Smiles more.' 'Can do more things now.' 'Still sleeps too much.'	'Nothing.' 'Cries a lot.' 'Moves his legs and arms.' 'When I put him down he moves.' 'Pushes herself forwards.' 'She likes playing.' 'Responds when I talk to him.'	'Nothing.' 'Stretches his body.' 'Kicks.' 'I don't know' 'Moves.' 'Smiles.' 'Opens his eyes.' 'Cries sometimes.'

KMC, Kangaroo Mother Care.

interacting with their infants were counted when the video recordings were analysed. The results are displayed in Table 7.

Behaviour types during mother-infant communication interaction

Statistically significant differences were found between the groups: Group 1 displayed the most behaviours, followed by Group 2, and then Group 3. The results confirm the findings of the mother-infant communication-interaction scale, where Group 1 mostly displayed optimal behaviours. The different types of behaviours displayed by the participants clearly show that their first interest was with their infants. A summary of the different caregiving behaviour types demonstrated by the three groups of participants is as follows: holds infant on her lap; touches infant's head, mouth, face, hands, feet; adjusts infant's position; puts infant down next to her; rocks infant; holds infant close, but not skin-to-skin; holds infant on her chest, skin-to-skin (KMC position); looks at infant; smiles at infant; kisses infant; wipes infant's mouth; changes nappy; feeds infant; talks to infant; strokes infant; covers infant with blanket; caresses infant; tickles infant; picks fluff from infant's blanket; adjusts blanket; adjusts infant's nasogastric tube; opens infant's blanket; pats infant gently.

As can be seen from these observations, the participants demonstrated a wide range of natural and spontaneous behaviours with their infants whilst the videos were recorded. It appeared that the participants were not inhibited by the unnatural communication-interaction context created by a video recording. The participants who talked to their infants demonstrated the typical features of 'motherese', as described by Gleitman, Newport and Gleitman,[20] although it was not explicitly taught to them. One of the mothers in Group 1 softly sang a praise song, a traditional chant of ancestral names, to her infant.

Discussion

On three different measures (interview, mother-infant communication interaction and types of behaviours), Group 1 (who practiced continuous KMC and received training in communication interaction with their infants) showed consistently better results with training. On average, the participants in Group 1 showed a high prevalence of communication-facilitating behaviours whilst interacting with their infants. It appears that, despite language and cultural differences between participants and trainer, the training had a direct, positive effect on the participants.

The significant differences on all measures between Group 2 and 3 (who did not receive training) may indicate that KMC without any explicit communication-interaction training may also have a positive effect on the participants' knowledge, mother-infant communication interaction and types of behaviours. The finding is supported by numerous studies indicating the positive effect of KMC on mother-infant communication interaction during the neonatal period and beyond.[1,21]

It appears that the formal neonatal communication-intervention training made a difference to the participants' knowledge of their infants. The lack of knowledge amongst all participants (Group 1 without training, Groups 2 and 3) points to a crisis of information about their children's development, as stated by Guralnick[22] and experienced by mothers.

The results are interpreted with caution, since a small sample of 30 participants was utilised. It was also not possible to randomly allocate the participants to different groups, as trainee participants could not be removed from those who were untrained. The 20-bed KMC unit where the research was conducted is in the form of a dormitory, with mothers continuously in close contact with one another. Therefore, the participants who were untrained would have observed the training and could have copied behaviours seen in the trained participants. The results indicate only the short-term effects of the interdisciplinary neonatal communication-intervention programme on the mothers and not their infants' development, and no long-term outcomes can be deduced.

TABLE 7: Number of behaviour types displayed by participants whilst interacting with infants (n = 30).

Group	Mean	Median	s.d.	Minimum	Maximum
1	7.10 types	7	1.19	6	9
2	5.70 types	6	1.16	3	7
3	3.20 types	3	1.14	2	5

Note: P-value < 0.0001, indicating a significant difference between the 3 groups
s.d, standard deviation.

TABLE 6: Comparison of mother-infant communication interaction between the three groups (n = 30).

Test items adapted from Klein and Briggs[17] (The mother ...)	Group 1† (%)	Group 2 (%)	Group 3 (%)	P-values
1. Provides appropriate tactile and kinesthetic stimulation	90	60	30	0.0291
2. Displays pleasure whilst interacting with infant	100	90	30	0.0013
3. Responds to infant's distress	100	60	33.33	0.0482
4. Positions self and infant for eye-to-eye contact	90	40	20	0.0089
5. Smiles contingently at infant	80	28.57	0	0.0001
6. Varies prosodic features of speech when talking to infant	90	20	0	0.0001
7. Encourages conversation	80	30	0	0.0001
8. Responds contingently to infant's behaviour	80	40	20	0.0366
9. Modifies interaction in response to negative cues from infant	83.33	33.33	22.22	0.0985
10. Uses communication to teach language and concepts	30	0	0	0.0887

†, Post training results.

Confounding factors could include that the groups were not matched for the infants' ages, or the number of days in KMC or in the neonatal unit. The participants in Group 1 knew the researcher well due to the three training sessions, and the familiarity with the context could have given this group an unfair advantage over the other groups who only met the researcher once. The results could have been more robust if a fourth group of participants had been included in the hospital that did not routinely practice KMC. The fourth group should have received training without conducting KMC, thereby isolating the impact of the training programme. As only mothers who could communicate well in English were selected for the study, the transferability of the results is limited.

The positive results of Group 1 with training may indicate that the neonatal communication-interaction programme adds value to the evidence-based practice of KMC in the hospital where the training was conducted, and should become part of the routine KMC programme. The challenge ahead is to implement the training programme on a sustainable basis. Further research should determine the long-term effects of the training programme and determine the effects on both the mother-infant communication interaction and infant auditory, speech and language development.

Acknowledgements

The authors wish to thank Prof. R.C. Pattinson, Head of Department Obstetrics and Gynecology, Kalafong Hospital and Head of the Medical Research Unit for Maternal and Infant Health Care Strategies, University of Pretoria, and Dr A.P. Bergh, senior researcher at the same unit, for their valuable input in planning the research project. The authors also wish to thank Dr W. Lubbe of the School of Nursing Science, North-West University for reviewing the manuscript and providing valuable recommendations.

Competing interests

The authors declare that they have no financial or personal relationship(s) that may have inappropriately influenced them in writing this article.

Author' contributions

A.K. (University of Pretoria) conducted the research. A.K. (University of Pretoria) and E.v.R. (University of Pretoria) planned the research and wrote the article.

References

1. Feldman R. Mother-infant skin-to-skin contact (kangaroo care). Theoretical, clinical and empirical aspects. Infants and Young Children. 2004; 17(2):145–161. http://dx.doi.org/10.1097/00001163-200404000-00006
2. Rossetti LM. Communication Intervention. Birth to Three. 2nd ed. Australia: Singular Thomson Learning; 2001.
3. Ludington-Hoe SM, Johnson MW, Morgan K, Lewis T, Gutman J, Wilson PD, Scher MS. Neurophysiologic assessment of neonatal sleep organization: Preliminary results of a randomized, controlled trial of skin contact with preterm infants. Pediatrics. 2008; 117:e909–e923. http://dx.doi.org/10.1542/peds.2004-1422
4. Graven SN, Browne JV. Auditory development in the fetus and infant. Newborn Infant and Nursing Reviews. 2008; 8(4):187–192. http://dx.doi.org/10.1053/j.nainr.2008.10.010
5. Peirano P, Algarı´n C, Uauy R. Sleep-wake states and their regulatory mechanisms throughout early human development. Journal of Pediatrics. 2003; 143:S70–S79. http://dx.doi.org/10.1067/S0022-3476(03)00404-9
6. Van Rooyen E, Pullen AE, Pattinson RC, Delport SD. The value of the kangaroo mother care unit at Kalafong hospital. Geneeskunde. The Medicine Journal. 2002; April:06–10.
7. Ruis-Peláez JG, Charpak N, Cuervo LG. Kangaroo mother care, an example to follow from developing countries. British Medical Journal. 2004;329:1179–1181. http://dx.doi.org/10.1136/bmj.329.7475.1179
8. Lee EL, Yeatman JD, Luna B, Feldman HM. Specific language and reading skills in school-aged children and adolescents are associated with prematurity after controlling for IQ. Neuropsychologia. 2011;49:906–913. http://dx.doi.org/10.1016/j.neuropsychologia.2010.12.038
9. American Speech-Language-Hearing Association. Roles and responsibilities of speech-language pathologists in early intervention: Guidelines. [Homepage on the Internet]. 2008. Available from: http://www.asha.org/policy/PS2008-00291/#sthash.s7ccQ9LN.dpuf
10. Ludington-Hoe SM. Thirty years of kangaroo care. Science and practice. Neonatal Network: The Journal of Neonatal Nursing. 2011;30(5):357–362.
11. Billeaud FP. Communication disorders in infants and toddlers: Assessment and intervention. 3rd ed. Boston: Butterworth-Heinemann; 2003.
12. Gorski PA, Davidson MF, Brazelton TB. Stages of behavioural organization in the high-risk neonate: Theoretical and clinical considerations. Seminars in Perinatology. 1979;3(1):61–72.
13. Chang EF, Merzenich MM. Environmental noise retards auditory cortical development. Science, 2003;300(5618):498–502. http://dx.doi.org/10.1126/science.1082163
14. Owens RE. Language development. An introduction. 8th ed. New Jersey: Allyn & Bacon; 2012.
15. Leedy PD, Ormrod JE. Practical research. 8th ed. New Jersey: Pearson Education International; 2005.
16. Pattinson RC, Bergh A-M, Malan AF, Prinsloo R. Does kangaroo mother care save lives? Journal of Tropical Pediatrics. 2006;52(6):438–441. http://dx.doi.org/10.1093/tropej/fml032
17. Klein MD, Briggs MH. Observation of communication interaction. Journal of Childhood Communication Disorders. 1987;10(2):95–106.
18. Gottlieb G. Ontogenesis of sensory function in birds and mammals. In: Tobach E, Aronson LR, Shaw E, editors. The biopsychology of development. New York: Academic Press; 1971.
19. Pepper J, Weitzman E. It takes two to talk. A practical guide for parents and children with language delays. Toronto: The Hanen Centre; 2004.
20. Gleitman LR, Newport EL, Gleitman H. The current status of the motherese hypothesis. Journal of Child Language. 1984;11:43–79. http://dx.doi.org/10.1017/S0305000900005584
21. Tallandini MA, Scalembra C. Kangaroo mother care and mother-premature infant dyadic interaction. Infant Mental Health Journal. 2006;27(3):251–275. http://dx.doi.org/10.1002/imhj.20091
22. Guralnick MJ. The effectiveness of early intervention. Baltimore: Paul. H. Brookes Publishing Company; 1997.

African Primary Care Research: Participatory action research

Author:
Bob Mash[1]

Affiliation:
[1]Family Medicine and Primary Care, Stellenbosch University, South Africa

Correspondence to:
Bob Mash

Email:
rm@sun.ac.za

Postal address:
PO Box 19063, Tygerberg 7505, South Africa

This article is part of the series on African primary care research and focuses on participatory action research. The article gives an overview of the emancipatory-critical research paradigm, the key characteristics and different types of participatory action research. Following this it describes in detail the methodological issues involved in professional participatory action research and running a cooperative inquiry group. The article is intended to help students with writing their research proposal.

La recherche sur les soins de santé primaire en Afrique: la recherche sur l'action participative. Cet article fait partie de la série consacrée à la recherche sur les soins de santé primaire en Afrique et traite essentiellement de la recherche sur l'action participative. L'article donne un aperçu du paradigme de recherche émancipatoire-critique, les caractéristiques fondamentales et les différents types d'études sur l'action participative. Elle poursuit en décrivant dans le détail les problèmes méthodologiques qu'implique la recherche professionnelle sur l'action participative et l'organisation de groupes de discussion de manière coopérative. Cet article est destiné à aider les étudiants à rédiger leur proposition de recherche.

Introduction

Participatory action research (PAR) is particularly suited to the primary care context, not only because of its tradition of working with communities, but also because of its ability to improve clinical practice.[1,2] Primary care services, by their nature, are close to the communities that they serve and questions often arise regarding how to work with community groups in order to address the underlying determinants of ill health. Likewise, questions often arise about how to improve clinical practice or the performance and organisation of the health system. Participatory action research is well suited to bridging the gap between evidence and practice, where evidence produced in clinical trials or expressed in national guidelines must be implemented in and adapted to a particular context. This article will describe the essential characteristics of PAR with the intention of helping the reader to develop a research proposal using this study design. The general approach to writing a research proposal has been described in the first article in the series and the structure used in that article is adopted here.[3]

The emancipatory-critical paradigm

Before getting to the more practical details of study design it is important to recognise that PAR requires the reader to embrace a different research paradigm, with different values and assumptions to the more orthodox empirical-analytical paradigm of most medical research.[4] PAR as a methodology is embedded within this emancipatory-critical paradigm (ECP). Table 1 compares the essential characteristics of these different research paradigms. At heart, the ECP is about creating new knowledge by transforming or changing the world in which the research is embedded and reflecting critically on what is learnt in the process. People in the ECP are neither objects to be measured, nor subjects to be understood, but are rather participants in both action and research. Contrary to conventional research, the researcher himself is also a participant in and not an observer of the research process. New knowledge in the ECP is generated as a consensus of the participant's learning and participants may use both quantitative and qualitative techniques in this process. In the ECP, research usually starts with a question regarding how a particular problem can be solved and the participants will align themselves with solving this problem. In doing this, they may generate additional research questions and in some cases even redefine the nature of the problem as the process unfolds. The ECP closes the gap between evidence and practice as learning is immediately put into practice as part of the process. The knowledge that is generated by the research process is highly contextualised and cannot be generalised automatically to other contexts. The concept of transferability applies in that readers of research articles in this paradigm must decide on which findings can be transferred to their own context. The complexity

TABLE 1: The emancipatory-critical paradigm.

Paradigm	Empirical-analytical	Interpretative-hermeneutic	Emancipatory-critical
Relationship of researcher to 'reality'	Testing and measuring	Exploring and interpreting	Changing and transforming
View of the researched person	Object to be measured	Subject to be understood	Participant in the process
View of truth	Correspondence to the facts	Coherence within the data	Consensus of each person's learning
Research process	Predominantly quantitative measurements	Predominantly qualitative measurements	Participatory using both quantitative and qualitative techniques
Research question	Fixed hypothesis Set by the researcher	Open-ended question Set by the researcher	Open-ended question Negotiated with group and can evolve
Implementation of results	Recommendations made for action by other people Generalisable	Insights offered for use by other people Transferable	Findings implemented as part of the research Transferable

of the specific community or health system in which the research is embedded makes it difficult to assume that the application of what has been learnt will work automatically in another context.

For medical practitioners to embrace this paradigm fully it usually requires them to undergo a journey in which they unlearn many of the positivist values and assumptions and become comfortable with trusting the participatory process. Many of these lessons are learnt by being willing to attempt research with the help of a competent mentor.

Key characteristics of participatory action research

Participatory action research can be considered as one methodological approach within this emancipatory-critical paradigm. As the name implies, PAR is an iterative process between action and research.[5,6,7] On the one hand, action requires one to put one's learning into practice, whilst research requires one to reflect and clarify what one has learnt from this experience and to develop new theory and propositional knowledge that is then incorporated into new action. It is participatory and always involves working *with* rather than *on* people. This requires attention to issues of power and hierarchy so that there is a genuinely respectful, open and democratic group process. At its core, PAR believes that people can change their reality and create new knowledge through engaging both consciously and systematically with the steps of the learning cycle as shown in Figure 1.[8] In this cycle, the participants engage with a process of observing and reflecting on their own concrete experience, agreeing on what has been learnt in the form of new propositional knowledge or abstract concepts and then planning to experiment actively with this new knowledge in another cycle of action and reflection.

Although most academic institutions and scientific journals are most interested in the propositional knowledge that is generated by PAR, it is clear that other types of knowledge will also be created. For example, by changing their practice participants will develop new skills and competencies, which can be seen as practical knowledge and will inevitably also engage with personal growth and change, which can be seen as experiential knowledge.

Types of participatory action research

PAR is not a homogenous field and there are different traditions within it. Three broad traditions have been identified.[5]

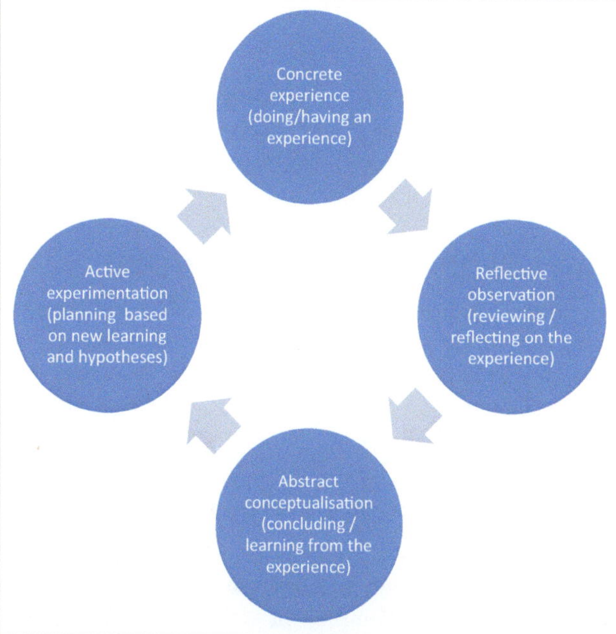

Source: Kolb (1984)[8]

FIGURE 1: Action-reflection learning cycle.

Empowering PAR works with communities to liberate, emancipate and empower them. Proponents of empowering PAR would include people such as Paulo Freire who spoke of the need to develop critical consciousness amongst oppressed communities and to assist them with transforming their reality.[9] His iconic book, 'Pedagogy of the Oppressed',[9] speaks to this perspective and has also had an influence on the development of adult learning theory. In the context of African primary care research, it is easy to see how empowering PAR may have application within community-oriented primary care and in engaging communities in solving their own health problems.[1] One example of empowering PAR in the South African context is a group of community members and health workers who looked at how to prevent mortality and morbidity from traditional circumcision in the Eastern Cape.[10]

Organisational PAR has developed in the context of business, industry and the corporate sector so as to solve organisational problems in a more participatory way.

Professional PAR works with professionals who want to change their practice and has been embraced by both the educational and health sectors. Examples of this within the health sector include a group of general practitioners adapting a World Health Organization programme on mental disorders to their South African context,[11] the leadership of a community health centre trying to develop continuity of care within practice teams,[12] a group of nurse counsellors adapting a protocol on the recognition and management of intimate partner violence to the South African primary care setting,[13] or chronic care teams within community health centres trying to improve the annual review of people with diabetes.[14]

The main principles of professional PAR have been summarised in the CRASP model:[15]

Critical collaborative inquiry by
Reflective practitioners being
Accountable and making the results of their inquiry public
Self-evaluating their practice and engaged in
Participative problem solving and continuing professional development

The cooperative inquiry group

The rest of this article will use the example of a cooperative inquiry group (CIG) to illustrate the key issues that should be covered when writing a PAR proposal.[16] The CIG is one specific method that has been used to conduct professional PAR in the healthcare sector.[11,12,13,14]

Research question, aim and objectives

One should define the problem to be solved or the broad question that the group will address. This is often a 'How to …' question, for example, 'How to improve the annual review of people with diabetes in community health centres?' The research question often arises out of an awareness of the problems encountered in clinical practice – for example, why so many patients with diabetes are controlled poorly.

Study design

The key characteristics of the research paradigm and PAR study design have been described above and illustrated in Figure 1. In the proposal, after stating the type of study design (e.g. a CIG), the steps of the action-research cycle can be described and illustrated in a figure.

Selection of participants

A cooperative inquiry group, as with any small group, functions best with 10–15 people. The research proposal must describe the criteria to be used to invite people to join the group and how this process will be facilitated. Sometimes the initiating researcher will make a presentation to the people that might be interested and invite them to come forward, whilst key people may also be invited specifically. The facilitator of the group is usually the initiating researcher who will also function as a group member and participate in the action-reflection process. Members of the group must be able to engage with relevant action and be interested in the topic of the inquiry. In selecting group members, attention should be given to issues of power and hierarchy within the group and how these will be handled, for example, will doctors, nurses and reception staff be able to engage each other in a collaborative and equitable manner. If the group is too heterogeneous it may struggle to function effectively and yet the facilitator can anticipate these issues and plan ways to overcome them. For example, the venue chosen for the group, the names that people use to refer to each other and the way in which contributions are elicited can all help to establish a spirit of respect, equality and openness. Participants will need to give informed consent.

Cooperative inquiry group process (the intervention)

At the start of the CIG, the researcher must describe how they will go about forming the group and explain the PAR process. Specific training may be needed in order to develop reflectivity in group members. It will be necessary to reach agreement on the research question to be addressed and to be open to modify the question with the group. The group will need to agree on how they will start the inquiry, which often involves developing initial plans for changing practice based on their prior experience and additional information.

In PAR it is not known beforehand what actions the group will engage with or what they will learn. Only the process to be followed can be described in detail. The fundamental process is a cyclical one with continuous cycles of action, observation, reflection and planning in an ongoing spiral format (see also Figure 1). These group members go through these steps in a structured manner:

- *Action*: Putting into action the plans that have been generated from reflection on one's previous experience and understanding of the context.
- *Observation*: Being aware of one's experience and documenting what happened or what has changed; this may include awareness of one's thoughts, feelings and reactions.
- *Reflection*: Reflecting in a structured way on one's observed experience and conceptualising in more abstract forms what one has learnt.
- *Planning*: Incorporating what one has learnt into well-formulated plans for new action at the start of the next cycle.

It should be possible to decide how long the research will last and how many such cycles you anticipate having. All of the steps can be completed as an individual, but reflection and planning should involve the group meeting together to share observations and reflect and plan collectively.

Documentation of the group process (data collection)

It is important to describe how you will document each part of the process. At an individual level people should keep a personal journal in which they regularly record what they have done, what happened and their thoughts, feelings and reactions. People may also reflect at an individual level and record new concepts or ideas to share with the group.

When the group meets at the beginning and end of each cycle, the group's feedback, reflections and planning should be recorded. This can be done using an audio tape, newsprint and/or field notes. It is often helpful for the facilitator to write a summary of the meeting and circulate this soon afterwards.

Sometimes the group's actions generate their own data, for example, if the group decides to perform interviews or administer a questionnaire. Data will need to be analysed and presented for reflection in the group meeting. The researcher should ensure that the data are captured and stored and the results are documented.

Building a consensus of the group's learning (data analysis)

At the end of the inquiry process, the group should build a consensus of what they have learnt in a participatory process. This may involve looking back over the whole inquiry process and the various summary documents. Each person should contribute in terms of what they have learnt. Such a consensus does not imply that the group should just summarise everything that they agree on. The consensus can include learning that appears seemingly contradictory. This is possible because it may not yet be apparent how these ideas fit together to make sense of their experience and the group should not reject aspects of their learning for this reason. Consensus can be built through group discussion, but sometimes more formal techniques such as the nominal group technique can be used to ensure a fair and democratic final process. How you plan to facilitate this process should be described.

In the event that the researcher must also write up the CIG for their thesis it is not unusual for the researcher to perform a further analysis on all the qualitative and quantitative data collected once the group has finished meeting. However, their final interpretation of the group's findings should be checked explicitly with the whole group so as to ensure that they remain a valid representation of the group's learning.

Quality in cooperative inquiry

Orthodox approaches to the appraisal of quality cannot be used in cooperative inquiry because concepts such as bias, confounding and chance do not apply. Concepts used in qualitative research such as triangulation, respondent validation, thick description, reflexivity and deviant case analysis may not be sufficient, although some of them can be relevant to the CIG. For example, it is possible to triangulate the findings from the CIG with evidence from other sources, such as the results of the audit of clinical practice confirming that change has taken place. The following criteria have been proposed for the appraisal of cooperative inquiry:[16]

- *Alignment with purpose*: Alignment of the group members with the purpose of the research both drives the process and acts as the contract between the members. Aligning oneself with a particular outcome or personal intention, rather than the purpose of the research, may lead to a lack of openness in the inquiry.
- *Ownership of the inquiry process*: Ownership of the research by members of the group is crucial to the quality of the inquiry. The initiating researcher will need to transfer power, knowledge of the research methodology, ownership of the research questions and process so that after the group is established he or she does not dominate the inquiry.
- *Development of reflectivity*: As the members of the group are both the researchers and the researched, the quality of the inquiry will depend on their ability to witness themselves. This requires a reflective stance that is characterised by heightened awareness, open-mindedness, critical questioning and commitment to dialogue.
- *Democratic and collaborative group dynamics and facilitation*: The facilitator must strive for a genuine collaborative and democratic group process. The level of trust will be related to telling the truth without judgement and staying within the common purpose. Breaking this contract with each other leads to a loss of trust and commitment and the facilitator must guard against this.
- *Commitment to practical action and experience*: The group must be committed to a balance of both action and reflection. Some groups may find it easy to take action, but difficult to pause for adequate documentation and reflection. Others may be good at planning and reflecting, but short on actually engaging with the practical action.
- *Documentation of the process*: The following three aspects must be documented: (1) the individual experience and action, (2) the group process and dynamics and (3) the developing reflections, learning and final consensus. When writing an account of the CIG it will be necessary to give a 'thick description' of the research process and the way in which the final consensus was reached. How these different aspects will be documented should be described in the research proposal. In terms of publications, the scientific journals are more interested in the final consensus (the findings of the study), but the description of the process will be needed to establish its quality and trustworthiness. Making the results available to the public and being accountable as professionals is emphasised in the CRASP model of professional PAR.
- *Transferability*: Transferability is another aspect of quality whereby the group's findings and context should be sufficiently clearly described to enable readers to understand what aspects of the inquiry can be appropriated to their own context. The reporting of this research should therefore describe the context in some detail so that readers can judge to what extent their own context is similar to or different from the study context.
- *Construction of new knowledge*: The purpose of cooperative inquiry is to construct new knowledge through cycles of action and reflection. One way of judging the quality of the research is in the practical usefulness of this new knowledge. It should be clear that this knowledge is derived from the actions of the group and has been

implemented practically. The way in which the final consensus of learning is constructed will also reflect on the quality of the inquiry.

Ethical considerations

All of the usual ethical considerations apply,[3] but there are some specific issues that arise in cooperative inquiry.[17] Although members of the CIG will have given their consent to participate, the activities of the group will inevitably impinge on other people in the practice environment. Consent must, therefore, also be obtained before group members make observations of others or examine documents that were produced for another purpose. Confidentiality of all involved should be maintained.

Often the group is facilitated by a researcher who is also intending to write up the work for a thesis and publication. This intention must be made clear to the group members at the beginning and ownership of the findings and authorship explicitly discussed. Because of its participatory nature, the 'development of the work must remain visible and open to suggestions from others'.[17]

Conclusion

This article has described the key characteristics and types of participatory action research. It has then described in detail the methods of the cooperative inquiry group within the tradition of professional PAR. It is hoped that this will enable researchers to develop better research proposals using PAR as a study design.

Acknowledgements

The authors gratefully acknowledge funding received from the U.S. President's Emergency Plan for AIDS Relief (PEPFAR), through HRSA under the terms of T84HA21652., and via the Stellenbosch University Rural Medical Education Partnership Initiative (SURMEPI).

Competing interests

The author declares that he has no financial or personal relationship(s) which may have inappropriately influenced him in writing this article.

References

1. Minkler M, Wallerstein N. Community-based participatory research for health. 2nd ed. New York: Jossey-Bass; 2008. PMCid:PMC2444051
2. Malterud K. Action research – a strategy for evaluation of medical interventions. Fam Pract. 1995;12(4):476–481. http://dx.doi.org/10.1093/fampra/12.4.476, PMid:8826069
3. Mash R. African primary care research: choosing a topic and developing a proposal. Afr J Prm Health Care Fam Med. 2013. In Press.
4. Habermas J. Knowledge and human interests (paperback). USA: Beacon Press; 1972.
5. Meyer J. Using qualitative methods in health related action research. BMJ 2000; 320(7228):178–181. http://dx.doi.org/10.1136/bmj.320.7228.178, PMid:10634744
6. Cornwall A, Jewkes R. What is participatory research? Soc Sci Med. 1995;41(12): 1667–1676. http://dx.doi.org/10.1016/0277-9536(95)00127-S
7. Baum F, MacDougall C, Smith D. Participatory action research. J Epidemiol Community Health. 2006;60(10):854–857. http://dx.doi.org/10.1136/jech.2004.028662, PMid:16973531, PMCid:PMC2566051
8. Kolb DA. Experiential learning: experience as the source of learning and development. Englewood Cliffs, NJ: Prentice-Hall; 1984.
9. Freire P. Pedagogy of the oppressed. New York: Continuum International Publishing Group; 2000.
10. Nwanze O, Mash R. Evaluation of a project to reduce morbidity and mortality from traditional male circumcision in Umlamli, Eastern Cape, South Africa: outcome mapping. SA Fam Pract. 2012;54(3):237–243.
11. Mash B. How to design education on mental disorders for general practitioners in South Africa. SA Fam Pract. 2002;25(5):4–10.
12. Mash B, Mayers P, Conradie H, et al. How to manage organisational change and create practice teams: experiences of a South African primary care health centre. Educ Health. 2008;21(2):132.
13. Joyner K, Mash B. A comprehensive model for intimate partner violence in South African primary care: action research. BMC Health Services Research. 2012;12(1):1–10. http://dx.doi.org/10.1186/1472-6963-12-399, PMid:23151248, PMCid:PMC3534545
14. Mash R, Levitt NS, Van Vuuren U, et al. Improving the annual review of diabetic patients in primary care: an appreciative inquiry in the Cape Town District Health Services. SA Fam Pract. 2008;50(5):50.
15. Zuber-Skerritt O. Action research in higher education: examples and reflections. London: Kogan Page; 1992.
16. Mash RJ, Meulenberg-Buskens I. "Holding it lightly": the co-operative inquiry group as a method for developing educational materials. Med Educ. 2001;35(12):1108–1114. http://dx.doi.org/10.1046/j.1365-2923.2001.01057.x, PMid:11895234
17. Denscombe M. Action research. In: M Denscombe, editor. The good research guide: for small-scale social research projects. 4th ed. Maidenhead: Open University Press; 2010. p. 125–135.

Knowledge of HIV and benefits of male medical circumcision amongst clients in an urban area

Author:
Abidemi Faleye[1]

Affiliation:
[1]Department of Family Medicine, University of KwaZulu-Natal, Durban, South Africa

Correspondence to:
Abidemi Faleye

Email:
abidemi.faleye@gmail.com

Postal address:
PO Box 33093, Montclair 4061, South Africa

Background: Male medical circumcision (MMC) has been shown to reduce the risk of HIV transmission in circumcised men by up to 60%. Following recommendations from the World Health Organization, South Africa adopted MMC as a preventative strategy against HIV in 2010 and set up circumcision camps across the country. Concerns have been raised about condom avoidance following MMC because of a mistaken belief about the benefits of MMC.

Aim and setting: The aim of this study was to describe the profile and knowledge about HIV and circumcision amongst men presenting for MMC in an urban area in KwaZulu-Natal.

Methods: This was a cross-sectional descriptive study of 394 clients over the age of 18 years who presented to two MMC sites in Durban between November 2012 and March 2013. A validated questionnaire was used to collect data.

Results: The mean age of clients presenting for MMC was 28 years. Most clients were black, single, unemployed and sexually active. The majority presented for MMC because they believed that MMC would reduce their risk of acquiring HIV infection. Knowledge about HIV transmission was very good and 86.3% of clients were aware that risky sexual behaviour such as condom avoidance could reverse the benefits of MMC.

Conclusion: The knowledge of HIV and benefits of MMC was very good amongst those presenting for MMC. However as MMC is primarily a preventative strategy, innovative methods to promote MMC prior to first sexual encounter need to be explored. Further research is needed to determine whether the benefits of MMC on the reduction of HIV transmission are sustained in routine practice.

La connaissance du VIH et les bienfaits de la circoncision médicale masculine chez les clients qui se présentent pour la circoncision dans les zones urbaines.

Contexte: Il a été démontré que la circoncision médicale masculine (MMC) réduit de 60% les risques de transmission du VIH chez les hommes circoncis. A la suite des recommandations de l'Organisation mondiale de la Santé, l'Afrique du Sud a adopté en 2010 la MMC comme stratégie de prévention contre le VIH et établi des camps de circoncision dans tout le pays. On a montré de l'inquiétude sur la non utilisation de préservatifs suite à la MMC due aux idées fausses sur les bienfaits de la MMC.

Objectif et cadre: Cette étude avait pour but de décrire le profil et les connaissances sur le VIH et la circoncision chez les homes qui se présentent pour la MMC dans une zone urbaine du Kwa Zulu Natal.

Méthodes: Ceci était une étude transversale descriptive de 394 clients de plus de 18 ans qui se sont présentés à deux services de la MMC à Durban de novembre 2012 à mars 2013. On s'est servi d'un questionnaire validé pour collecter les données.

Résultats: L'âge moyen des clients se présentant pour la MMC était 28 ans. La plupart des clients étaient noirs, célibataires, chômeurs et actifs sexuellement. La majorité se présentaient pour la MMC parce qu'ils croyaient que la MMC réduirait le risque d'être infecté par le VIH. Ils étaient bien au courant de la transmission du VIH et 86.3% des clients savaient que les comportement sexuels risqués tel que la non utilisation des préservatifs pouvaient annuler les bienfaits de la MMC.

Conclusion: Les hommes qui se présentaient pour la MMC avaient une bonne connaissance du VIH et des bienfaits de la MMC. Cependant, étant donné que la MMC est en premier lieu une stratégie de prévention, il faut trouver des méthodes innovatrices pour promouvoir la MMC avant la première relation sexuelle. Il faut faire des recherches supplémentaires pour déterminer si les bienfaits de la MMC sur la réduction de la transmission du VIH sont durables dans la pratique quotidienne.

Introduction

Currently, 2.3 million new HIV infections occur each year and 35.3 million people worldwide are living with HIV.[1] With such large numbers of people infected with HIV, prevention and treatment of HIV are an international priority. New prevention strategies such as male medical circumcision (MMC), use of vaginal microbicides, pre-exposure prophylaxis with anti-retroviral agents, herpes suppressive therapy, cervical barrier methods, HIV vaccines and early initiation of antiretroviral therapy are all being promoted as potential methods for the reduction of HIV transmission.[2]

Male medical circumcision (MMC) is the surgical removal of the prepuce from the glans of a flaccid penis. Epidemiological studies have shown a geographical correlation between male circumcision and HIV prevalence, with countries that traditionally practise male circumcision having lower rates of HIV prevalence than countries that do not.[3,4] Three randomised controlled trials done in South Africa (SA), Kenya and Uganda in 2005 and 2007 showed that MMC reduced HIV transmission in circumcised men by 60%, 53% and 51%, respectively.[5,6,7] This reduction in HIV transmission results from the removal of the prepuce which contains a large number of Langerhans cells. These cells are immunological in nature and are rich in CD4 cells, making them a target for HIV entry and replication.[3] In addition, MMC has been shown to protect circumcised men from ulcerative sexually-transmitted infections (STIs)[6,7] such as Herpes simplex virus type 2 (HSV-2), which predisposes one to HIV infection, as well as against human papilloma virus (HPV) infections.[8] The reduced incidence of HPV infection in circumcised men has resulted in the reduction of penile carcinoma amongst circumcised men and indirectly protects women against cervical cancer.[9,10,11] MMC has also been noted to lead to a reduced risk of prostate carcinoma, less inflammation and infection of the skin of the penis and better genital hygiene.[12] A number of African studies have shown MMC to be an acceptable intervention with high levels of uptake.[3,5]

In 2007, based on the evidence of these studies, an expert consultative forum of the WHO/UNAIDS (World Health Organization/Joint United Nations Programme on HIV/AIDS) recommended that MMC be introduced in countries with a high prevalence of HIV and a low prevalence of male circumcision as part of the comprehensive HIV prevention package offered in these countries.[2] As SA meets these criteria, MMC was adapted in 2010 as part of the national strategy for reducing HIV transmission. Since then, a large number of circumcision camps have been set up across SA in order to provide MMC services to males willing to be circumcised, with a target of circumcising 80% of uncircumcised men over a period of five years.[13]

However, concerns have been raised regarding the adaptation of the WHO recommendation and taking this strategy to scale in the South African context. Ncayiyane argues that the scientific evidence for large-scale roll out of MMC is insufficient to justify the energy, money and resources which have been devoted to the roll out of circumcision services. He further posits that the potential increase in risky behaviour based on the belief that circumcision prevents transmission of HIV, termed risk compensation, could nullify any gains from circumcision.[14,15] This concern was supported by data from a 2003 study in the Westonaria district of SA which showed that 30% of circumcised men believed that they could safely have sex with many women without using condoms because they believed that circumcision prevented the transmission of HIV.[15] However, in a study conducted in Johannesburg in 2010, Bridges showed that even though a section of the population found condom avoidance attractive post-circumcision, this risk was overstated in the 2003 study by Lagarde.[16] In fact, a study done in Kenya in 2006, which examined attitude, beliefs and behaviour regarding HIV and MMC, showed that condom use went up in both circumcised and uncircumcised groups (i.e., control and experimental groups) following an intensive circumcision drive and this was linked to the counseling provided to men considering circumcision.[17]

Despite the concerns about condom avoidance in circumcised men, MMC is an important preventative intervention, as men who engage in risky sexual behaviour do not consistently use condoms and circumcision has been shown to lead to a significant reduction in the risk of HIV transmission in men.[18] There is, however, a lack of information on the profile of men who access the MMC services in KwaZulu-Natal as well as their knowledge of HIV, their understanding of the benefits of MMC and their understanding of the importance of condom use post-MMC. This study aimed to address this gap and to make recommendations to the Department of Health regarding its circumcision campaign.

Research methods and design

Study design and setting

This was a cross-sectional descriptive study carried out at Wentworth and St Aidan's Hospitals in Durban, KwaZulu-Natal. Since March 2010, as part of the MMC roll-out programme, MatCH (Maternal Adolescent and Child Health) has been providing a free circumcision service to the population of Durban at Wentworth Hospital, St Aidan's Hospital and KwaMashu Polyclinic. Since the inception of the project, MatCH has run MMC educational programmes and recruitment drives in the townships around Durban and has provided free transport to the most convenient circumcision site. To date over 10 000 clients have been circumcised at these sites.

Study population and sampling strategy

With up to 1000 clients presenting per month for MMC at Wentworth Hospital (WWH) in 2011, a sample of 400 clients representing 40% of those presenting in a month was considered sufficient for an observational descriptive study.[19] Inclusion criteria were males 18 years or older presenting for MMC who agreed to participate in the study. There were no exclusion criteria. All clients who presented for MMC on the days that the research assistant was available were asked to participate in the study. No one who was approached refused to participate in the study. Prior to enrolment, patients were given an information sheet and informed consent was obtained by the research assistant. Data were collected prior to the MMC procedure using a questionnaire adapted from a validated questionnaire previously used by MatCH.[20] Clients were asked to complete the questionnaire on their own and were assisted by the research assistant when necessary.

In October 2012, as a result of transport challenges associated with getting clients to WWH, the number of men presenting at the hospital for MMC dwindled significantly. As MatCH is also responsible for the MMC programme based at St Aidan's Hospital, where more than 50 clients per day were presenting for MMC, permission was requested from the ethics committee, the KwaZulu-Natal Department of Health and the hospital management to switch the study site from WWH and to gather data from St Aidan's from January 2013. Data were collected at WWH from November to December 2012 and from St Aidan's from January to March 2013.

Data analysis

Data were captured onto a Microsoft® Excel spreadsheet and analysed using the Statistical Package for Social Sciences (SPSS) version 21 (IBM Corp., Armonk, NY, 2012).

Ethical considerations

Approval for the study was given by the Biomedical Ethics Committee of the University of KwaZulu-Natal (reference number BE001/12), the hospital management and the KwaZulu-Natal Department of Health.

Results

Three hundred and ninety-four clients completed the questionnaires. Seventy-eight (19.8%) were from WWH and 316 (80.2%) from St Aidan's hospital. The mean age of clients was 28 years (standard deviation 8.67). The demographic profile of the participants is shown in Table 1.

The majority (n = 210, 53.3%) of the clients came from local urban townships, with a few presenting from other districts. The majority had attended high school; over 60% (n = 324) were unemployed, most were single and sexually active.

The majority of clients presented for MMC because it offered partial protection against HIV with only 30 (7.6%) having a circumcision because of social and/or religious reasons. Knowledge of transmission of HIV was excellent. Almost all of the clients had been counselled and tested for HIV and 85% (n = 337) were HIV negative.

Most of the clients had a good understanding of the effects of MMC and the risk of acquisition of HIV and

TABLE 1: Demographic profile of clients (N = 394).

Variable	Frequency	Percentage
Race		
Black people	356	90.4
White people	0	0.0
Indian	21	5.3
Mixed race	12	3.5
Missing	5	0.8
Age		
18–30	285	72.3
31–43	79	20.1
44–56	23	5.8
> 56	7	1.8
Highest level of education		
Never attended school	8	2.0
Attended primary school (Grade 1–Grade 7)	62	15.7
Attended high school (Grade 8–Grade 12)	145	36.8
Passed Matric	60	15.2
Post Matric training (either at college or university)	119	30.2
Sexually active		
Yes	392	99.5
No	2	0.5
Marital status		
Single	361	91.6
Married	30	7.6
Widowed	2	0.5
Divorced	0	0.0
Missing	1	0.3
Job status		
Unemployed	240	61.1
Employed	153	38.9
Missing	1	0.3
Area/Address		
Urban	154	39.9
Urban townships	210	53.3
Urban informal	19	4.8
Rural	11	3.0

understood that MMC is just part of the preventative package against HIV.

Discussion

The majority of those who participated in this study were in the 18–30 year age group (72.3%), with an average age of 28 years as seen in Table 1. These figures may have been distorted by the exclusion for ethical reasons of clients less than 18 years of age (109 clients were aged less than 18 years). However, these figures are consistent with a study by Connolly in 2005 which reported a similar age distribution in a national survey of MMC.[21]

Almost all of those who participated in this study (99.5%) were sexually active. As MMC is intended to prevent HIV transmission it would be preferable to circumcise men prior to initiation of sexual relationships, especially in a society with a high prevalence of HIV. Pre-pubertal circumcision has been associated with the greatest reduction in the risk of HIV acquisition.[22] Although the age of circumcision varies with race, tribe and religion,[14,15] local studies are needed in order to determine the ideal age for MMC and to assess the acceptability of neonatal circumcision as a strategy for the prevention of HIV in SA.

The majority of those who participated in this study cited partial protection against HIV and personal hygiene as their reasons for seeking circumcision, as depicted in Table 2. Surprisingly, social and/or religious and cultural reasons accounted for less than 8% of the participants. This was unexpected, as in 2007 King Zwelithini stated that circumcision was a well-established Zulu cultural practice and that all young men should be circumcised.[23]

In keeping with a Namibian study done in 2010,[24] most clients had excellent knowledge of HIV, its transmission and benefits of circumcision. These men were aware that MMC provides only partial protection, that condoms are still needed to prevent HIV and that the benefits of MMC could be reversed if other protective lifestyle choices such as condom use are not adhered to (Tables 2 and 3). This is encouraging, as it suggests that HIV-related knowledge and the benefits of circumcision are reaching the target population. Recent findings have shown a significant drop in HIV prevalence in SA, which may suggest that not only is knowledge better but that HIV prevention messages are having an effect on sexual practices.[25]

MMC has been shown to reduce the risk of HIV transmission from men to women. Although most of those who participated in this study believed that circumcision does not protect women from being infected with HIV (Table 3), Alsallaq found that by reducing the pool of HIV-positive men, circumcision can indirectly protect women from HIV infection.[26] This information appears to be lacking and could be used as another reason for men to consider circumcision.

Just over 13.2% of those who participated in this study were HIV-positive (Table 2). Initial Department of Health guidelines recommended MMC only for men who were HIV negative. However, the WHO currently recommends MMC for HIV-positive men for medical indications and because of the possible reduction in risk of transmitting HIV in those already infected with HIV.[2] HIV-positive men also benefit from the reduced risk of ulcerative STIs which is associated with MMC.[7] In 2012, the Department of Health updated its guidelines and currently recommends MMC in HIV-positive men if their CD4 is above 350 cells/mm^3, as studies have shown good wound healing at such CD4 levels.[7] Currently, most of the HIV treatment programmes across SA have more women than men on treatment.[27,28] This may be because women tend to access healthcare services more often than men and have more opportunities for testing than men (during antenatal care, when presenting at a clinic with a sick child, etc.).[27,28] There is a need to find innovative ways to encourage men to test for HIV and for those who are positive to participate in treatment programmes. With the ambitious target of reaching 80% of uncircumcised men, the MMC programme may present such an opportunity for testing and for channelling men who are HIV-positive into HIV treatment programmes.

TABLE 2: Knowledge of male medical circumcision, HIV infection and reason for seeking male medical circumcision amongst clients.

Variable	Frequency	Percentage
Reasons for seeking MMC		
Partial protection against HIV	338	85.8
Social and/or Religious reasons	30	7.6
Personal hygiene	329	83.5
Others	0	0.0
Benefits and advantages of MMC		
Improved sexual performance	8	2.0
Prevention of HIV transmission	315	79.9
Reduce risk of STIs	350	88.8
Cultural acceptability	17	4.3
Knowledge about HIV		
Yes	390	98.5
No	4	1.0
Knowledge about HIV		
Sexual intercourse	383	97.2
Blood transfusion	358	90.9
Mother to child	353	89.6
Sharing needles	356	90.0
Hugging and kissing	7	1.8
Others	2	0.5
Previous VCT		
Yes	388	98.5
No	4	1.0
Missing	2	0.5
HIV status		
Positive	56	13.2
Negative	337	85.0
Missing	1	0.3
Duration of MMC healing		
1 day	7	1.8
1 week	4	1.0
2 weeks	8	2.0
> 2 weeks	374	94.9
Missing	1	0.3
Having sex whilst circumcision heals		
Yes	11	2.8
No	381	96.7
Unsure	1	0.3

MMC, male medical circumcision; VCT, voluntary counselling and testing; HIV, Human Immunodefiency Virus; STI, sexually-transmitted infections.

TABLE 3: Effect of male medical circumcision and the risk of acquisition of HIV (N = 394).

Variable	Frequency	Percentage
Effect of MMC on the risk of acquiring HIV		
No effect	11	2.8
It increases the risk of acquiring HIV	6	1.5
It reduces the risk of acquiring HIV	375	95.2
Other	1	0.3
Missing	1	0.3
Whether risky sexual behaviour can remove the benefits of male circumcision		
Yes	340	86.3
No	35	8.9
Unsure	18	4.6
Missing	1	0.3
Whether male circumcision protects women from being infected with HIV		
Yes	34	8.7
No	347	94.9
Unsure	11	11.0
Missing	2	0.5

MMC, male medical mircumcision; HIV, Human Immunodefiency Virus.

Limitations

This was a small study conducted at two sites in KwaZulu-Natal. Because of the convenient nature of the sampling method, the results of this study may not be representative of the study population and may not be generalisable to other settings. The exclusion of clients younger than 18 years of age was a limiting factor as their experience and knowledge may be different from older clients.

Recommendations

More local studies are needed to gain a better understanding of the effect of MMC on sexual behaviour and to measure the impact of MMC on HIV transmission when it is incorporated into routine practice. There is also a need for research to be done amongst those under 18 years of age in order to determine their reasons for presenting for MMC and their knowledge of the benefits of MMC.

Conclusion

This study found that the average man presenting for MMC at these MatCH sites is young, lives in an urban township and is black, single and sexually active. Those presenting for MMC have excellent knowledge of the effects of circumcision on the transmission of HIV, were aware that MMC provides only partial protection, that condoms are still needed to prevent HIV and that the benefits of MMC can be reversed if condom use is not adhered to. Although the concerns about risk compensation are legitimate, most of the men in this study understood that condom use is still necessary post-circumcision. Circumcision presents an opportunity to educate young men about HIV prevention and to channel those who are positive into HIV treatment programmes.

Acknowledgements

Competing interests

The author declares that he has no financial or personal relationship(s) that may have inappropriately influenced him in writing this article.

References

1. UNAIDS. Global report: UNAIDS report on the global AIDS epidemic 2013 [document on the Internet]. c2013 [cited 2014 Jan 15]. Available from: http://www.unaids.org/en/media/unaids/contentasset/document/epidemiology/2013/gr2013/UNAIDS_Global_Report_2013_en.pdf
2. UNAIDS. New data on male circumcision and HIV prevention: policy and programme implications [document on the Internet]. c2007 [cited 2014 Nov 02]. Available from: http://www.who.int/hiv/pub/malecircumcision/research_implications/en/
3. Bailey RC, Plummer FA, Moses S. Male circumcision and HIV prevention: Current knowledge and future research directions. Lancet Infect Dis. 2001;1(4):223–231. http://dx.doi.org/10.1016/S1473-3099(01)00117-7
4. Peters F, Marcus TS. Circumcision weeks: Making circumcision part of routine training and service delivery at district-level hospitals in South Africa. S Afr Fam Pract. 2011;53(3):262–266. http://dx.doi.org/10.1080/20786204.2011.10874096
5. Auvert B, Taljaard D, Lagarde E, et al. Randomized, controlled intervention trial of male circumcision for reduction of HIV infection risk: The ANRS 1265 Trial. PLoS Med. 2005;3(5):e226. http://dx.doi.org/10.1371/journal.pmed.0030226
6. Bailey RC, Moses S, Parker CB, et al. Male circumcision for HIV prevention in young men in Kisumu, Kenya: A randomised controlled trial. Lancet. 2007;369(9562):643–656. http://dx.doi.org/10.1016/S0140-6736(07)60312-2
7. Gray RH, Kigozi G, Serwadda D, et al. Male circumcision for HIV prevention in men in Rakai, Uganda: A randomised trial. Lancet. 2007;369(9562):657–666. http://dx.doi.org/10.1016/S0140-6736(07)60313-4
8. Tobian AA, Serwadda D, Quinn TC, et al. Male circumcision for the prevention of HSV-2 and HPV infections and syphilis. N Engl J Med. 2009;360(13):1298–1309. http://dx.doi.org/10.1056/NEJMoa0802556
9. Auvert B, Sobngwi-Tambekou J, Cutler E, et al. Effect of male circumcision on the prevalence of high-risk human papilloma virus in young men: Results of a randomized controlled trial conducted in Orange Farm, South Africa. J Infect Dis. 2009;199(1):14–19. http://dx.doi.org/10.1086/595566
10. Castellsaqué X, Bosch FX, Muñoz N, et al. Male circumcision, penile human papillomavirus infection, and cervical cancer in female partners. N Engl J Med. 2002;346(15):1105–1112. http://dx.doi.org/10.1056/NEJMoa011688
11. Ewings P, Bowie C. A case-control study of cancer of the prostate in Somerset and east Devon. Br J Cancer. 1996;74(4):661–666. http://dx.doi.org/10.1038/bjc.1996.418
12. Morris B. Male circumcision guide for doctors, parents, adults & teens [page on the Internet]. c2010 [cited 2014 May 12]. Available from: http://www.circinfo.net
13. Bateman C. Millions of snips will bolster our Health system. S Afr Med J. 2009;99(12);840–844.
14. Ncayiyana DJ. The illusive promise of circumcision to prevent female-to-male HIV infection – not the way to go for South Africa. S Afr Med J. 2011;101(11):775–776.
15. Lagarde E, Dirk T, Puren A, et al. Acceptability of male circumcision as a tool for preventing HIV infection in a highly infected community in South Africa. AIDS. 2003;17(1):89–95. http://dx.doi.org/10.1097/00002030-200301030-00012
16. Bridges JF, Selck FW, Gray GE, et al. Condom avoidance and determinants of demand for male circumcision in Johannesburg, South Africa. Health Policy Plan. 2011;26(4):298–306. http://dx.doi.org/10.1093/heapol/czq064
17. Westercamp M, Bailey RC, Bukusi EA, et al. Male circumcision in the general population of Kisumu, Kenya: Beliefs about protection, risk behaviors, HIV, and STIs. PLoS One. 2010;5(12):e15552. http://dx.doi.org/10.1371/journal.pone.0015552
18. Goldstuck ND. Adult circumcision in the prevention of HIV/AIDS. S Afr Med J. 2014;104(1):17. http://dx.doi.org/10.7196/samj.7216
19. Terre Blanche M, Durrheim K, Painter D, editors. Research in practice: Applied methods for the social sciences. Cape Town: University of Cape Town; 2006.
20. Maternal, Adolescent and Child Health (MatCH). Male circumcision: Medical Case report form. Version 4.4 [document on the Internet]. n.d. [cited 2014 Aug 04]. Accessed from: www.match.org.za/publication [no longer available on site].
21. Connolly C, Simbayi LC, Shunmugam R, et al. Male circumcision and its relationship to HIV infection in South Africa: Results of a national survey in 2002. SAfr Med J. 2008;98(10):789–794.
22. Kelly R, Kiwanuka N, Wawer MJ, et al. Age of male circumcision and risk of prevalent HIV infection in rural Uganda. AIDS. 1999;13(3):399–405. http://dx.doi.org/10.1097/00002030-199902250-00013
23. IRIN. South Africa: Zulu king revives male circumcision [article on the Internet]. c2009 [cited 2013 Dec 01]. Available from: http://www.plusnews.org/report/87441/South Africa [updated 2014 Sep 28; available from: http://www.irinnews.org/report/87441/south-africa-zulu-king-revives-male-circumcision]
24. Ngodji TK. Knowledge, attitudes and practices of male circumcision for HIV prevention among voluntary counseling and testing clients in Onandjokwe District Hospital, Namibia [Master's thesis on the Internet; School of Public Health, Faculty of Community and Health Sciences, University of the Western Cape]. c2010 [cited 2014 Sep 28]. Available from: http://etd.uwc.ac.za/bitstream/handle/11394/2576/Ngodji_MPH_2010.pdf?sequence=1
25. UNAIDS. New HIV report finds big drop in new HIV infections in South Africa [article on the Internet]. c2014 [cited 2014 Jan 30]. Available from: http://www.unaids.org/en/resources/presscentre/featurestories/2014/january/20140117southafrica/
26. Alsallaq RA, Cash B, Weiss HA, et al. Quantitative assessment of the role of male circumcision in HIV epidemiology at the population level. Epidemics. 2009;1(3):139–152. http://dx.doi.org/10.1016/j.epidem.2009.08.001
27. Nteta TP, Mokgatle-Nthabu M, Oquntibeju OO. Utilization of the primary health care services in the Tshwane region of Gauteng province, South Africa. PLoS One. 2010;5(11):e13909. http://dx.doi.org/10.1371/journal.pone.0013909
28. Statistics South Africa. Mid-year population estimates 2010 [document on the Internet]. c2010 [cited 2013 Aug 20]. Available from: http://www.statssa.gov.za/publications/P0302/P03022010.PDF

Assessment of the impact of family physicians in the district health system of the Western Cape, South Africa

Authors:
Meyer Swanepoel[1]
Bob Mash[1]
Tracey Naledi[2]

Affiliations:
[1]Division of Family Medicine and Primary Care, Stellenbosch University, South Africa

[2]Health Programmes, Department of Health, Western Cape Government, South Africa

Correspondence to:
Meyer Swanepoel

Email:
meyer.esme@gmail.com

Postal address:
Private Bag X2, Somerset West 7129, South Africa

Background: In 2007, South Africa made family medicine a new speciality. Family physicians that have trained for this new speciality have been employed in the district health system since 2011. The aim of the present study was to explore the perceptions of district managers on the impact of family physicians on clinical processes, health system performance and health outcomes in the district health system (DHS) of the Western Cape.

Methods: Nine in-depth interviews were performed: seven with district managers and two with the chief directors of the metropolitan and rural DHS. Interviews were recorded, transcribed and analysed using the ATLAS-ti and the framework method.

Results: There was a positive impact on clinical processes for HIV/AIDS, TB, trauma, non-communicable chronic diseases, mental health, maternal and child health. Health system performance was positively impacted in terms of access, coordination, comprehensiveness and efficiency. An impact on health outcomes was anticipated. The impact was not uniform throughout the province due to different numbers of family physicians and different abilities to function optimally. There was also a perception that the positive impact attributed to family physicians was in the early stages of development. Unanticipated effects included concerns with their roles in management and training of students, as well as tensions with career medical officers.

Conclusion: Early feedback from district managers suggests that where family physicians are employed and able to function optimally, they are making a significant impact on health system performance and the quality of clinical processes. In the longer term, this is likely to impact on health outcomes.

Evaluation de l'impact des médecins de famille dans le système de santé du district du Western Cape, en Afrique du Sud.

Contexte: En 2007, l'Afrique du Sud a institué une nouvelle spécialité, la médecine de famille. Les médecins de famille qui se sont spécialisés dans cette nouvelle discipline sont employés dans le système de santé de district depuis 2011. L'objet de cette étude était d'étudier les perceptions des gestionnaires de district sur l'impact que les des médecins de famille avaient sur les processus cliniques, la performance du système de santé et les résultats des systèmes de santé des districts (DHS) du Western Cape.

Méthodes: On a effectué neuf entrevues approfondies: sept avec les gestionnaires de district et deux avec les directeurs principaux du DHS rural et métropolitain. On a enregistré, transcrit et analysé les entrevues en utilisant ATLAS-ti et la méthode de structure.

Résultats: Il y a eu un effet positif sur les processus cliniques du VIH et/ou du SIDA, la Tuberculose, le traumatisme, les maladies chroniques non-contagieuses, la santé mentale, et la santé de la mère et de l'enfant. La performance du système de santé a été positivement affectée en termes d'accès, coordination, exhaustivité et efficacité. On s'attendait à un impact sur les résultats en matière de santé. L'impact n'était pas uniforme dans toute la province en raison du nombre différent de médecins de famille et des différentes capacités à fonctionner de manière optimale. On avait aussi l'impression que l'impact positif des médecins de famille en était aux premiers stades de développement. Les effets inattendus comprenaient leurs inquiétudes d'avoir à gérer et à former les étudiants, ainsi que les tensions avec les médecins de carrière.

Conclusion: Les premiers commentaires des directeurs de district indiquent que quand on emploie des médecins de famille qui ont la possibilité de fonctionner d'une manière optimale, ils ont un impact important sur la performance du système de santé et la qualité du processus clinique. Cela aura probablement un impact sur la santé, à long terme.

Introduction

South Africa is following an international movement towards strengthening primary healthcare (PHC) services. This is being done in an attempt to improve the health of the citizens and reduce the cost of healthcare delivery.[1,2,3] In South Africa, strategies for improving PHC and district health systems are being explored.[4,5] The current national health insurance (NHI) roll-out has set the re-engineering of PHC as a priority.[6]

In 2007, the discipline of family medicine was recognised as a new speciality in South Africa, and as a result the eight South African medical schools changed their existing degree programmes to Master of Medicine (MMed). The Department of Health created full-time registrar training posts with family physician supervisors. The first Mmed-qualified family physicians graduated in 2011. In the Western Cape, 21 family physicians were employed in 2011, 32 in 2012 and 42 in 2014. It is expected that this number may increase to 60–80 over the next 5 years.

Nationally, there are 52 health districts, of which 6 are located in the Western Cape. The Cape Town metropolitan district is further sub-divided into 4 sub-structures. In the Western Cape, the Department of Health committed to establishing family physicians in a central role in the DHS, particularly at the district hospital, in order to improve patient outcomes. They do not provide first-contact care, but capacitate and support PHC teams in a clinical and mentorship capacity. They are custodians of clinical governance, provide leadership, and are catalysts in implementing community-orientated primary healthcare.[7,8] The roles rest on the foundation of academic and clinical knowledge acquired within the new family medicine curriculum.

Overall, the perception is that the current family physicians in the Western Cape are making a difference, although no formal research has yet been conducted in a South African or African context.[7] In the United States, Barbara Starfield showed that family physicians impact positively on health outcomes.[9] Both Australia and the United Kingdom have established the central role of the trained family physician in the PHC system.[10] In Brazil, the family healthcare teams, composed of one family physician, one nurse, one auxiliary nurse and 4–6 community health workers, serve 600–1000 families. They aim to provide first-contact care, as well as integrate care with acute level facilities.[11] In Nepal, trained family physicians are making a significant difference to utilisation and provision of services at district hospitals.[12]

In the PHC re-engineering, apart from the roles described above, family physicians will also support community-based PHC teams. These teams will consist of community health workers and nurses, who will take responsibility for visiting a specific group of households. Family physicians will also form part of the district clinical specialist teams (DCSTs), which will, in addition, consist of an obstetrician, paediatrician, midwife, paediatric and PHC nurse. These specialist teams are meant to focus on improving maternal and child health services.[6]

BOX 1: Definition of terms in study objectives.

Health system performance includes the following primary health care characteristics: (14)
• Access (availability of services, geographic access, organisation of access, affordability, acceptability and satisfaction, utilization, equality of access). • Co-ordination (referrals, gate keeping, teamwork, skills-mix, integration of services between different levels and with community orientated primary care activities). • Comprehensiveness (range of equipment, range of first contact care, range of diagnoses dealt with, range of preventive services, range of procedures, range of promotive services). • Efficiency (Allocative or productive (e.g. waiting times, cost-effectiveness); technical (use of resources/laboratory tests); work force (referral rates, number consultations, duration of consultations, frequency of prescriptions).
Clinical processes refer to the care pathways and quality of care for key conditions across the burden of disease, and include: HIV, TB, child health, maternal health, trauma and emergency services, non-communicable diseases and mental health.
Health outcomes refer to measures of morbidity and mortality.

In the Western Cape, such support is being offered in an alternative model by placing the family physicians at posts within the district and supporting them by outreach from the other specialists at the regional hospital. Therefore, no DCSTs, as envisaged by the national DoH, currently exist in the Western Cape. The new information from the present study, which is part of a larger study with the same title, will be useful to the Western Cape Department of Health in evaluating their strategy for the large-scale deployment of family physicians.[7] This data will also be relevant in the broader South African context, considering the phased implementation of NHI.[6] The Primafamed network (a network of departments of family medicine in Sub-Saharan Africa) will also be interested in the results of the research and the implications for their own countries.[5,13] Sub-Saharan African policymakers may also find the results of the present study useful when uncertainty exists regarding their future commitment to the discipline of family medicine.

Aim and objectives

The aim of the present study was to explore the perceptions of district managers on the impact of family physicians in the Western Cape. Specific objectives were to: (refer to Box 1 for greater detail):

1. Explore the perceived effect of family physicians on health system performance.
2. Explore the perceived effect of family physicians on clinical processes.
3. Explore the perceived effect of family physicians on health outcomes.

Methods

Study design

This was a qualitative study using in-depth interviews.

Setting

The present study was conducted in the public sector of the DHS of the Western Cape. The Western Cape DHS consists of four metropolitan sub-structures and five rural districts. Each of these entities has an overall manager, except the Central Karoo District, which is currently managed by the

Eden district manager as the Eden/Central Karoo geographic service area. The four metropolitan sub-structures fall under a Chief Director of the Metro DHS and the five rural districts fall under a Chief Director of the Rural DHS. The Western Cape public health sector has aligned its Comprehensive Service Plan with the model of having a family physician at each district hospital (> 50 beds) and each community health centre (> 30 000 people served).

The researcher was a registrar in family medicine at the time of the research. Due to previous work as a clinical manager, he had an interest in health systems. He was interested to explore the effect of the appointment of well-positioned senior clinicians in the Western Cape DHS.

Selection of participants

The managers of each of the rural districts and urban sub-structures in the Western Cape were selected for participation in the study, based on their broad scope of knowledge of the functioning of the DHS and overview of the impact that family physicians have made. In addition, the chief directors of the metropole (four sub-structures) and rural areas (five districts) were also selected.

Data collection

In-depth interviews were performed face-to-face in the interviewee's office using an interview guide, and ranged from 60–80 mins. Interviews were performed in either English or Afrikaans by the researcher and were audiotaped. Interviews took the form of an open process of exploration that made use of open questions, reflective listening, summaries and clarification. The interview guide reflected the objectives of the study and ensured that all relevant points were explored. The audiotape of the first interview was reviewed by the first two authors to ensure that the guide was constructed appropriately and the interviewer demonstrated the necessary skills.

Data analysis

Interviews performed in Afrikaans were translated into English prior to transcription and analysis. All interviews were transcribed and checked against the audiotapes by the researcher. Data were analysed using ATLAS-ti and the framework method. This involved the steps of: familiarisation with raw data; identifying an index of all the codes and categories to be used from the raw data; applying the index to all the raw data by annotating transcripts with the codes; charting all the raw data from the same code in a single document; and interpreting themes from the charts in terms of the range and strength of opinions, as well as any associations or relationships between themes.[15] Quotations from these interviews are used in the present article to illustrate key points.

Results

The study population consisted of nine interviewees, as described above. Three of them were male and 6 were female. All were middle aged (> 40 years) and had at least 5 years of experience in healthcare management. Two managers were very new in their positions, having served as facility managers for a number of years. One of the chief directors was also very new in the position, having served as a district manager for several years. One manager could not be reached for an interview; it is anticipated that this one interview would not have introduced new themes because no new issues emerged during the final interviews that were performed.

General benefits

Respondents reported that overall family physicians had impacted the DHS positively, although benefits were perceived to be in the early stages of development. Those family physicians who impacted positively on the DHS earned the respect of colleagues. This respect was manifested in the number of applications received for family medicine training posts at these facilities:

> 'You can actually see the places where family medicine is respected and where it's not by the number of applications we receive from the juniors.'

Graduates from the new training programme were considered to be well-trained and balanced clinicians, with a comprehensive skills set due to rotations through the 10 clinical domains. Senior registrars, during their third and fourth years of training, also benefitted the DHS in terms of their clinical impact:

> 'You could already start seeing the impact that the registrars have in the senior years.'

Roles of the family physician

The family physicians were perceived to have raised the clinical levels of functioning in the DHS, in terms of management of clinical emergencies, consultations on difficult cases and guidance to juniors to work more efficiently in terms of time and resources. They have taught juniors how to do ward rounds quicker and they have run specialist family physician clinics. Their seniority has given them the necessary authority to communicate directly with other consultants and senior managers:

> 'You know it is just that seniority, that clinical knowledge, the more kind of decisiveness about what it is to be done.'

Clinical proficiency is the foundation for effective clinical governance, and family physicians were seen to be well suited for this function in the DHS, based on their comprehensive clinical training and the ensuing higher level of clinical reasoning. Regular morbidity and mortality meetings were held and recorded. Clinical audits to improve quality of care were done by means of folder reviews:

> 'As a family physician she brings in the clinical governance oversight. So it's very much on clinical proficiency and whether you're making the right decisions.'

The role of family physicians appears to have evolved to that of a district family physician in some districts. Clinical governance in the sub-district still resided with the sub-district family physician, but one of these senior family physicians provided guidance to the sub-district family physicians in developing a clinical governance framework for their sub districts. The two senior family physicians had quarterly forums with the sub-district family physicians where they focused on clinical issues and lessons learned.

Clinical processes

Family physicians were perceived to provide leadership for the campaign against diarrhoeal disease and helped co-ordinate activities. They identified the desired clinical outcomes and the appropriate course of action for each category of sick child in the diarrhoeal care pathway:

> 'So there's a system that's put in place, but there's also that senior clinical decision making that's there and I think the diarrheal seasons is a great example of that.'

Respondents felt that the Integrated Management of Childhood Illness (IMCI) programme was impacted by family physicians, but the impact was limited. Those family physicians that had a clear understanding of the IMCI programme provided support and in-service training to nursing staff in order to attain better outcomes. Family physicians were perceived to impact the DHS positively in terms of mental health. One family physician was doing a situational analysis of the psychiatric services for the drainage area of their district hospital. He was working with the outreach psychiatrist and they were busy integrating the mental health services within the community, PHC facilities and the district hospital; as well as providing training and support for nursing staff. Some interviewees were of the opinion that the current DHS psychiatric care model is insufficient and it would be unfair towards the family physician to expect them to have a positive impact. However, some felt that even with the short comings of the current model that there are positive contributions that family physicians could make. Family physicians impacted positively on chronic disease management through clinical leadership and direct patient contact. They tended to think more holistically in terms of patient care. A particular family physician developed a risk stratification tool that was implemented in one district and used in the day-to-day care of non-communicable chronic diseases. This tool enabled trained healthcare providers to easily stratify these patients as either stable, at risk or decompensated according to appropriate clinical criteria applicable to each condition, and respond accordingly. These patients would then either continue with routine chronic disease care, or intensified chronic disease care, as characterised by more regular visits and special investigations, or by transfer to the casualty for possible admission to the hospital. This tool was later commissioned by the Western Cape Department of Health and piloted by several districts during their chronic disease drive. Many family physicians then implemented this risk stratification tool in their own sub-districts. They also impacted on chronic disease management by means of quality improvement cycles and staff training. Their inputs helped to integrate systems across a range of chronic diseases, rather than focusing on specific diseases:

> 'I think the success is that we took a clinical governance perspective and not a programmatic perspective in implementing the chronic disease management plan. That to me it is really a strength and I think the family physician involvement there made a huge impact.'

Family physicians also had a significant impact on the care of patients with HIV and TB. They were seen as chipping away at the vertical nature of the HIV care model and providing a more holistic approach to patient care:

> 'When she approaches chronic diseases she approaches it systemically. From where she's sitting that all chronic disease has got something in common and the systems that you put in place for good outcomes for the client is a uniform way of doing things.'

One family physician conducted a quarterly anti-retroviral (ARV) morbidity and mortality meeting and used this to capacitate nursing staff and doctors. She also communicated with the district office about routine ARV data, identifying the need for resources allocation and training gaps.

Maternal care in the metropolitan sub-structures was almost exclusively run by obstetricians, but in the rural districts maternal care was the domain of the generalist. Quality of clinical care at family physician managed facilities in the metropolitan areas was seen as on a par with other facilities of the metropolitan area. One family physician was tasked with improving prevention of mother-to-child transmission (PMTCT) rates. Good ante-natal care practices were implemented and PMTCT rates dropped:

> 'So it's had a massive impact which I don't think we are capturing fully in that there's a story to be told about the impact of family medicine on the Midwife Obstetric Units, because I think it has been positive.'

It is recognised that the majority of patients with trauma and medical emergencies in the metropolitan area presented to the 24-hour community healthcare centres. The clinical governance and leadership that family physicians provided to medical officers in the emergency centres impacted indirectly on emergency care on a large-scale:

> 'You know the family physicians take pride in the fact that they've actually with the full-time doctors, with the cosmos, with the general medical officers that work there – they have systematically improved the outcomes and the clinical decision making and the impact.'

Health system performance

Respondents agreed that access to healthcare services was impacted positively by family physicians in different ways. This particularly included improved access to primary healthcare services via the clinical governance function of the family physician, which improved the quality and acceptability of care:

> 'Look, I think access is probably the one area where family medicine has played a huge, huge impact. Because in our system ninety per cent of our contacts are on the primary health care platform.'

Access was also improved by expanding the clinical services offered by the DHS. This included the establishment of outreach services to new service points, as well as strengthening of existing outreach services from district hospitals to their feeding clinics by both qualified family physicians and registrars. This had the advantage of providing additional service delivery to the respective communities, whilst also training future family physicians within the context in which they will be expected to function in future. Consequently, a more seamless service and functional interface is created between the primary care services and the district level hospital. For example, one family physician analysed the referral and prescription patterns in the sub-district and introduced weekly outreach sessions by a family physician and nurse. This led to improved clinical care and adherence by the patients, and a reduction in emergency referrals.

Organisational access was positively impacted by family physicians. One family physician implemented a stratified approach to consultations, whereby the patient first consulted a clinical nurse practitioner (CNP). The consultation level was then escalated to the junior doctor, senior doctor and, eventually, the family physician as the need arose. This layered approach improved the quality of clinical decision making in their facility since there was a method of dealing with difficult cases:

> 'When she got there three, four years ago, it was chaotic. The doctors there revolved and they didn't want to return to the place. So in four years she turned the place around.'

Patient satisfaction was affected directly by the intervention of family physicians. Respondents reported that family physicians were perceived by both staff and patients to be knowledgeable, senior and empathetic:

> 'The child died at birth or just a few minutes after birth but the way in which the family physician and the staff supported that family was very positive. So it actually prevented the department from, you know from a legal case.'

Coordination of healthcare services in the district was also positively impacted by the family physician in many aspects:

> 'I think the most important thing for me is really the person placing themselves at the centre of a team. And you know it's being at the centre of the team with a purpose. Being patient centred with a population outcome in mind.'

Family physicians impacted the referral system by means of appropriate improvements, such as training nursing staff at the clinic level to perform appropriate patient work-up prior to the referral. These family physicians were also perceived to be good at referring patients themselves as they know the referral routes and have more authority as a specialist. They were also perceived to have easier access to clinical management protocols. As the family physician in the sub-district they are more aware of all the problem cases and they also create awareness of referral problems at the geographic service area meetings where these issues may be solved. The range of procedures being done in the DHS was impacted significantly by family physicians. Training in surgical procedures was perceived to be appropriate and more of these procedures were being performed in the DHS. Equipment was being improved as a result:

> 'I do think there's been a gradual introduction based on patient needs, of a wider range of services. And I think family physician has been at the centre of it.'

Family physicians were actively and routinely involved in curbing the cost of healthcare in the DHS. They considered the burden of disease profile and developed protocols for the cost-effective use of X-rays, laboratory services and medicines.

Unanticipated effects

Family physicians were involved in meetings related to clinical governance but, in addition, they were unexpectedly drawn into more general district management meetings as well. This consumed the time of the family physician with management tasks they were not intended to perform:

> 'What we didn't anticipate was that once we put family physicians on board everybody will call them into meetings'

Some family physicians also had joint appointments with the university, where they were responsible for certain academic responsibilities. It is perceived in some districts that the lack of description of standardised university and management tasks leads to a lessened impact as it removes the family physician from the DHS platform for a significant amount of time and becomes a source of misunderstanding and role uncertainty.

One district had no district manager and had also not appointed any family physicians, whilst it was reported that another had multiple district managers over a period of 4 years. This lack of consistent leadership may have undermined the potential contribution of family physicians who were working more like medical officers in this district. In another district, the introduction of the first family physicians created tension with the long-serving clinical managers and medical officers. The clinical managers were performing clinical governance functions and the medical officers at the district hospitals were perceived to be already sufficiently competent in their specific disciplinary areas. The need for family physicians was, therefore, not clear since the skills-mix they offered at the district hospital was already present and functioning well:

> 'I think the fact that there are a lot of career medical officers and that there are medical managers together with the clinical managers, the family physicians are actually functioning as pure clinicians.'

Some districts commented on the financial implications of appointing family physicians. Creating a family physician post implied taking the budget away from a medical officer and nursing post, as there was no additional money. As the family physician does not just perform clinical care, this may be perceived as a loss of capacity at the coal-face.

Outcomes

The general consensus was that family physicians definitely impact positively on health outcomes, although this perception needs further statistical verification:

> 'Obviously that's anecdotal, so I would just say that my perception is, my indication is that it's probably better but that's only, that's only the impression.'

Discussion

The findings suggest that family physicians are important contributors to improving the quality of primary and district

BOX 2: Summary of key findings.

Key findings
• An overall positive impact on health system performance and clinical processes.
• Positive impact is in the early stages of development.
• Positive impact is centred around individuals and not found uniformly throughout the district health services.
• The expected roles of the family physician have been largely fulfilled.
• FP have brought more clinical seniority into the district health services.

hospital care. Refer to Box 2 for a summary of the health benefits of family physicians. The findings also underscore their value in contributing to the performance of the district healthcare system. Family physicians should, therefore, be important contributors to the implementation of local and national policy in the Western Cape. The findings resonate with the goals of the Healthcare 2030 policy in the Western Cape, which emphasises the need to build patient-centred quality of care and to improve district health services. The study findings also resonate with the goals of the national Negotiated Service Delivery Agreement, which emphasises the need to decrease maternal and child mortality rates, combat HIV/AIDS and TB as well as strengthen the health system.[16,17]

The findings are also congruent with the internationally recognised contribution of family physicians to strengthening health systems,[1] and the resolution of the World Health Assembly on the importance of family physicians as part of a multi-disciplinary team in PHC (along with community health workers, primary health care nurses, midwives, and allied health professionals). The findings support the recommendations of the 2008 World Health Report that physicians with a specialisation in family medicine are needed to avoid a restrictive and watered-down approach to PHC in low-resource settings.[18]

Despite the mainly positive findings, the impact of these family physicians is still at an early stage and they have yet to fully evolve into their place within the developing DHS. In some areas, long-serving competent medical officers function as well as, and sometimes better than, newly qualified family physicians. Lower grade medical officer posts are not as expensive as family physicians and managers may wonder what the advantages are of employing family physicians. However, previous research has revealed significant clinical skills gaps in the district health services, due in part to variation in competencies between medical officers.[20]

Training programmes for family physicians aim to ensure a consistent set of competencies that are appropriate to the district health services, and an attractive career pathway for generalist doctors. In addition, family physicians are trained in a broader scope of practice that goes beyond clinical care to mentoring, capacity building, leadership, clinical governance and community-orientated primary care.[20] In the future, it may be desirable for all doctors pursuing a long-term career in the district health services to be trained as family physicians. In the short to medium term, the picture will inevitably involve a mix of family physicians and medical officers working together to deliver the service.

The role of the family physician in terms of leadership, management and administration is variable, and respondents were worried that, as well-trained clinicians, they spent too much time in meetings. As a new speciality, the number of family physicians to support a wide range of management and planning processes in the sub-district and district is relatively small, which places a significant demand on each individual. The district health services expect the family physicians to make an impact on the continuum of care and clinical governance, which also requires their participation in a number of meetings.[16] Most of the family physicians would be regarded as newly qualified and, usually, such junior consultants would focus more on clinical work and leadership within the immediate clinical team; however, the absence of senior colleagues forces many of them to take on significant leadership roles from the beginning – for example, being the first family physician in a newly opened district hospital. The intention is for family physicians to be expert generalists, working clinically, but with an important contribution to make to clinical leadership of the facility and DHS, rather than taking on the role of manager. More extensive management roles have been taken on by the few more-senior family physicians in the DHS.

Whilst there is an expectation that all family physicians would mentor and build capacity through training of the clinical teams where they work, some family physicians take on more-specific roles in relationship to teaching of undergraduate and postgraduate students.[7] This teaching role and academic involvement at universities, at times, removed family physicians from the DHS platform (for example, teaching in the afternoon at the skills lab or involvement in clinical examinations). This remains a contentious issue between the universities and Department of Health and is currently the focus of new contractual agreements.[21] These contracts will regulate access to the service platform for teaching, and also who will be regarded as joint staff with the university and have a more-specific academic role. Such joint staff would have job descriptions that indicate an academic component and would be allowed to attend specific training to capacitate them for this role.

In the 1990s, the introduction of training for doctors on the district health services platform was welcomed as a sign that medical schools were becoming more relevant, community-orientated and socially responsible. However, as the number of students and length of exposure has grown there is a valid concern that this is taking too much time away from service delivery and scarce resources, especially when this occasionally means teaching at the university campus. The district health services have no tradition of postgraduate training and the collaboration between service and academia, as exists in the tertiary hospitals. There is, thus, a need for both parties to better understand each other's perspectives and work towards developing a mutually beneficial culture of learning that leverages academic and service perspectives.[22] Nevertheless, the need to increase the supply of doctors and family physicians is a national priority.[23] Ultimately, the district health services are dependent on a supply of well and appropriately trained generalists, the universities are dependent on access to the district health services to provide this training, and both institutions must work together to fulfil their shared goal of improving health and the quality of health services.

Limitations of the study methods

Senior healthcare managers do not work directly alongside family physicians and their perception might, thus, represent the opinion of others. Nevertheless, respondents were found to know family physicians by name and the impacts of individual family physicians were attributed specifically to individuals rather than generically. Respondents for the present study did not perform clinical work, and in some instances, respondents were not doctors, but had trained in another aspect of the health sciences such as nursing. Thus, their opinion on the impact of family physicians was not based on direct physical observation, but was a function of their managerial role and perspective within the DHS. They, therefore, represented an important overview of the district and were not necessarily biased towards a positive view of family physicians.

Interviewees may have been reluctant to express positive and negative perceptions about the impact of family physicians, due to the fact that the primary researcher was a family medicine registrar. This limitation was attenuated by explicitly exploring lack of impact or negative impact during the in-depth interviews.

A further limitation of this study was that it was set in the first year of appointment of newly graduated family physicians, with few other family physicians appointed in the DHS; their impact might not yet be fully developed.

Implications or recommendations of the study for policy makers or future researchers

The proposed increase in the number of family physicians in the Western Cape DHS is supported by the present study's findings. It is anticipated that their positive impact will translate to improved outcomes and tangible improvements for staff and patients. The strengthening of the DHS through the deployment of family physicians should be considered by other South African provinces.

Family physicians that completed the new training curriculum were trained for the African context; however, the Western Cape is a different context to many African countries. Nevertheless, the findings of the present study could be transferable to other resource-constrained settings in Africa, and could add weight to the argument for the deployment of family physicians.

As part of a larger study, it is intended to interview managers on an annual basis for three years. This will allow researchers to qualitatively monitor changes in perceived impact over time. The findings from the present study can also be triangulated with findings from the larger study, which will provide quantitative evidence for the impact of family physicians.

Conclusion

The appointment of family physicians in the DHS, who are trained within the new speciality training programmes, is in the early stages of development. They have impacted the DHS positively in terms of health system performance and clinical processes. It is anticipated that this will lead to a positive impact on health outcomes. The positive impact was centred on individual family physicians and was not found uniformly throughout the DHS. This refers to the fact that some districts did not have family physicians, and in other districts, family physicians were not able to function as intended due to a lack of other clinical staff. A few appeared to be under-performing because they had not yet grasped their leadership role and clinical governance function. The appointment and development of family physicians is a work in progress. The functioning of the DHS needs adjustment in some districts in order to better accommodate family physicians and enable them to have the impact that they are trained for.

Acknowledgements

The two chief directors, four rural district managers and three urban substructure managers of the Western Cape DHS are acknowledged with gratefulness for their time offered and quality information provided. This work is based on research supported by the National Research Foundation.

Competing interests

The authors declare that they have no financial or personal relationship(s) that may have inappropriately influenced them in writing this article.

Authors' contributions

M.S. (Stellenbosch University) was the primary researcher. He designed this study, conducted the interviews, performed data analysis and wrote the article up in publishable format. B.M. (Stellenbosch University) was the study leader. He designed the over-arching bigger study, of which this research work forms a part. He provided appropriate and valuable guidance towards the completion of this work. T.N. (Department of Health, Western Cape Government) was a secondary author and contributed towards the initial design of the study. She also reviewed the complete manuscript and provided an invaluable contribution towards the final work.

References

1. De Maeseneer J, Haq C, Markuns J, et al. The Contribution of Family Medicine to Improving Health Systems: A guidebook from the World Organization of Family Doctors. 2nd Ed. Singapore: Wonca; 2013.
2. Van Driel M, De Sutter A, Christiaens T, De Maeseneer J. Quality of care: The need for medical, contextual and policy evidence in primary care. J Eval Clin Pract 2005;11(5):417–429. http://dx.doi.org/10.1111/j.1365-2753.2005.00549.x
3. Mash B, Blitz-Lindeque J. Clinical skills for future family physicians. SA Fam Pract 2006;48(10):3. http://dx.doi.org/10.1080/20786204.2006.10873471
4. Department of Health. Healthcare 2020 - Western Cape Government [Homepage on the internet] c2011 [updated 2011, Nov; cited 2012, Feb 16]. Available from: http://www.westerncape.gov.za/other/2011/12/healthcare_2020_-_9_december_2020.pdf
5. Chopra M, Lawn J, Sanders D, et al. Health in South Africa 6: Achieving the Millenium Development goals for South Africa: challenges and priorities. The Lancet 374. 9694 (Sep 19–Sep 25):1023–31.

6. Department of Health. National health insurance: The first eighteen months. [Homepage on the internet] Pretoria; No date [cited 2013, Jun 8]. Available from: http://www.sarrahsouthafrica.org/LinkClick.aspx?fileticket=wgMmGElMkRk%3D&tabid=2311

7. Nathan R, Rautenbach P. Risks identified in implementation of district clinical specialist teams. South African Medical Journal, [S.l.], 2013;103(3):144–146.

8. Mash B. Reflections on the development of family medicine in the Western Cape, South Africa: A 15 year review. SA Fam Pract 2011;53(6):557–562. http://dx.doi.org/10.1080/20786204.2011.10874152

9. Mash B, Reid S. Statement of consensus on Family Medicine in Africa. Afr J Prm Health Care Fam Med. 2010;2(1),Art.#151, 4 pages.

10. Macinko J, Starfield B, Shi L. Quantifying the health benefits of primary care physician supply in the United States. International Journal of Health Services 2007;37(1):111-126. http://dx.doi.org/10.2190/3431-G6T7-37M8-P224

11. Nicholson C, Jackson C, Marley J, Wells R. The Australian Experiment: How Primary Health Care Organizations Supported the Evolution of a Primary Health Care System. JABFM 2012;25: Supplement S18–26.

12. Paim J, Travassos C, Almeida C, Bahia L, Macinko J. The Brazilian health system: History, advances, and challenges. The Lancet.

13. Nick Simons Institute [Homepage on the internet] Nepal; No date [cited 2013, Jun 11]. Available from: http://www.nsi.edu.np

14. De Maeseneer J, Flinkenflögel M. Primary health care in Africa: do family physicians fit in? Br J Fam Med 2010;60:286–292.

15. Kringos DS, Boerma WG, Hutchinson A, Van der Zee J, Groenewegen PP. The breadth of primary care: a systematic literature review of its core dimensions. BMC health services research 2010;10:65. http://dx.doi.org/10.1186/1472-6963-10-65

16. Pope C, Ziebland S, Mays N. Qualitative research in health care: Analysing qualitative data. BMJ 2000;320:114–6. http://dx.doi.org/10.1136/bmj.320.7227.114

17. Department of Health. Healthcare 2030. Cape Town: Western Cape Government; 2013. [cited 2014, Mar 28]. Available from: http://www.capegateway.gov.za/health

18. Office of the Presidency. Negotiated Service Delivery Agreement. For outcome 2: A Long and Healthy Life for All South Africans [Online] [cited 2014, Mar 28]; Available from: http://www.thepresidency.gov.za/MediaLib/Downloads/Home/Ministries/DepartmentofPerformanceMonitoringandEvaluation3/TheOutcomesApproach/Health%20Sector%20NSDA.pdf

19. World Health Organisation. World Health Report. Primary Health Care: Now More Than Ever [Homepage on the internet] c2014 [cited 2013, Jun 11]; Available from: http://www.who.int/whr/2008/en

20. De Villiers MR, De Villiers PJT, Kent AP. The maintenance of competence of rural district hospital medical practitioners. SA Family Practice 2006;48(3):18. http://dx.doi.org/10.1080/20786204.2006.10873353

21. Couper I, Mash B, Smith S, Schweitzer B. Outcomes for family medicine postgraduate training in South Africa. SA Fam Pract 2012;54(6):501–506. http://dx.doi.org/10.1080/20786204.2012.10874283

22. Western Cape Government. Western Cape Government Signs Multilateral Agreement for Health Professionals [Homepage on the internet] c2012 [upated 2012, May 28; cited 2014, Mar 31]. Available from: http://www.westerncape.gov.za/news/western-cape-government-signs-multilateral-agreement-health-professionals

23. Jenkins L, Mash B, Derese A. The national portfolio of learning for postgraduate family medicine training in South Africa: experiences of registrars and supervisors in clinical practice. BMC Medical Education 2013; 13:149. http://dx.doi.org/10.1186/1472-6920-13-149

24. National Department of Health. Human Resources for Health, South Africa. Pretoria: Department of Health; 2011.

The roles of community health workers in management of non-communicable diseases in an urban township

Authors:
Lungiswa P. Tsolekile[1]
Thandi Puoane[1]
Helen Schneider[1]
Naomi S. Levitt[2]
Krisela Steyn[2]

Affiliations:
[1]School of Public Health, University of the Western Cape, South Africa

[2]Faculty of Health Sciences, Department of Medicine, University of Cape Town, South Africa

Correspondence to:
Lungiswa Tsolekile

Email:
tsolekile@uwc.ac.za

Postal address:
Private Bag X17, Bellville 7535, South Africa

Background: Community health workers (CHWs) are increasingly being recognised as a crucial part of the health workforce in South Africa and other parts of the world. CHWs have taken on a variety of roles, including community empowerment, provision of services and linking communities with health facilities. Their roles are better understood in the areas of maternal and child health and infectious diseases (HIV infection, malaria and tuberculosis).

Aim: This study seeks to explore the current roles of CHWs working with non-communicable diseases (NCDs).

Setting: The study was conducted in an urban township in Cape Town, South Africa.

Method: A qualitative naturalistic research design utilising observations and in-depth interviews with CHWs and their supervisors working in Khayelitsha was used.

Results: CHWs have multiple roles in the care of NCDs. They act as health educators, advisors, rehabilitation workers and support group facilitators. They further screen for complications of illness and assist community members to navigate the health system. These roles are shaped both by expectations of the health system and in response to community needs.

Conclusion: This study indicates the complexities of the roles of CHWs working with NCDs. Understanding the actual roles of CHWs provides insights into not only the competencies required to enable them to fulfil their daily functions, but also the type of training required to fill the present gaps.

Le rôle des agents de santé communautaires dans la gestion des maladies non-contagieuses dans un township urbain.

Contexte: Les agents de santé communautaires (CHW) sont de plus en plus considérés comme un élément capital du personnel de santé en Afrique du Sud et dans d'autres parties du monde. Les CHW assument divers rôles, tels que l'autonomisation des communautés, la prestation de services et le lien entre les communautés et les services de santé. Leurs rôles sont mieux compris dans les domaines de la santé maternelle et infantile et les maladies infectieuses (infection par le VIH, le paludisme et la tuberculose).

Objectif: Cette étude examine les rôles actuels des CHW s'occupant des maladies non contagieuses (NCD).

Cadre: L'étude a été menée dans un township urbain du Cap, en Afrique du Sud.

Méthode: On s'est servi d'une méthode de recherche qualitative et naturaliste qui utilise des observations et des entretiens approfondis avec les CHW et leurs superviseurs travaillant à Khayelitsha.

Résultats: Les CHW ont des rôles multiples pour soigner les NCD. Ils sont éducateurs sanitaires, conseillers, personnel de rééducation et animateurs de groupes de soutien. Ils décèlent les complications de la maladie et aident les membres de la communauté à mieux naviguer dans le système de santé. Ces rôles sont déterminés selon les attentes du système de santé et les réponses aux besoins de la communauté.

Conclusion: Cette étude indique les complexités des rôles des CHW travaillant avec les NCD. La compréhension des rôles des CHW donne une idée non seulement des compétences requises pour leur permettre de s'acquitter de leurs tâches quotidiennes, mais aussi du type de formation requis pour combler les lacunes actuelles.

Introduction

Community health workers (CHWs) are increasingly being recognised as a crucial part of the health workforce.[1] In South Africa and worldwide, CHWs have provided health care to communities for many decades and have assumed a variety of roles, including community empowerment, provision of services and linking communities with health facilities. Their roles are better understood in the areas of maternal and child health.[2] For the purposes of this article CHWs are defined as health workers with informal job-related training and no professional or paraprofessional tertiary training, and limited in-service training to contribute to patient management at community level. They may receive a stipend or work voluntarily[3] and work in communities in which they reside.

CHWs' tasks over the years have evolved from mainly focusing on prevention and promotion to more supportive roles that are associated with the increased burden of chronic lifelong conditions. South Africa, like many countries in transition, has experienced an increase in the burden of chronic lifelong conditions associated with the HIV infection epidemic and the parallel emergence of non-communicable diseases (NCDs). This burden of disease has led to increased workloads, overcrowding at health facilities and poor quality of care,[4] and has exerted a tremendous strain on human resources in the healthcare system, especially those working at primary healthcare (PHC) level.[5] The use of CHWs as part of a solution to the human resources crisis in health settings has been suggested.[6,7]

The South African Government has made significant strides in providing free PHC for all, meaning that people with chronic diseases such as NCDs are provided with long-term treatment at no cost and will further need ongoing support to assist them to adhere to treatment. As part of disease management, patients diagnosed with NCDs and placed on treatment are typically advised to attend support groups run or facilitated by professional nurses at the health facilities.[6] Despite the efforts made at health facilities in managing NCDs, these conditions continue to be managed poorly[8] and a need for extended and continued care at community level therefore exists.

Given the fact that not all patients utilise health facilities for routine check-ups and that NCDs' symptoms are not recognised until the late stages when complications are apparent, employing CHWs to increase awareness about prevention and control of diseases in communities is crucial. CHWs could strengthen the link between health services and the community, increasing access to services, especially in underserved communities.[9]

In South Africa CHWs have been largely utilised in programmes that target infectious conditions such as HIV/AIDS and tuberculosis (TB) as well as maternal and child health. Their roles in such programmes are clearly defined and have an established base of evidence illustrating the benefits.[2] The focus of programmes has been propelled by the need to achieve the Millennium Development Goals, resulting in less attention being given to other conditions such as NCDs.[10]

Numerous interventions for NCDs have been described that utilise the CHW model in disadvantaged communities.[11,12] Studies from developed countries highlight varied roles and relevance or importance of CHWs in the management of NCDs. These roles include patient education,[13,14] care and support,[13,15,16] provision of social support and acting as a liaison with the healthcare system.[3] For example, in a diabetes intervention CHWs assisted in monitoring blood glucose, blood pressure and potential complications, and provided social support to patients as well as their families.[15] Despite general support of the CHW model in the management of diseases, there is a need to further understand the roles of CHWs in the prevention and management of NCDs, especially in resource-poor settings.

Recent policy reforms in South Africa prioritise the revitalisation of PHC and stronger community-based services.[17] On the eve of the re-engineering of PHC and the implementation of PHC outreach teams in South Africa it becomes imperative to understand the roles of CHWs, particularly in caring for conditions previously not included in their work. According to the policy statements on re-engineering of PHC, the work of CHWs has been conceptualised to be comprehensive and to cover household and community level.[18] With respect to NCDs, at household level their roles will include health promotion, that is education on diet, exercise and lifestyle, and screening for those at high overall cardiovascular disease risk and in particular for diabetes and hypertension, foot care and an integrated approach to adherence support. At community level the focus will be on campaigns, support groups and promoting action on risk factors related to diet and exercise.

Objectives

In the light of these broadly stipulated roles of CHWs, this study therefore explored CHWs' current roles in NCDs care with a view to identifying existing challenges. The information gathered will assist in informing a training curriculum that relates to CHWs' daily activities and can support a meaningful response to NCDs.

Contribution to field

Understanding the CHWs' current roles, especially on the eve of re-engineering of PHC, is important for adapting current roles to what will be expected in their new roles in PHC outreach teams. This is especially true as re-engineering of PHC may require an expansion of skills as well as new knowledge. Providing an understanding about current roles will give insight into how CHWs organise their work, the type of activities related to NCDs that they engage in, as well as coping strategies employed in order to address deficiencies in their own work. The results will provide information about the key challenges of managing NCDs at community level, and also highlight possible models that could be used when training opportunities are limited.

Research methods and design

Study design

A qualitative naturalistic research design utilising observations and in-depth and unstructured interviews to investigate the actual daily activities of CHWs working with NCD patients was adopted. A naturalistic observation assumes that the roles of CHWs are socially organised and involve examining[18] the CHWs in their natural environment whilst carrying out their everyday tasks as they would normally do.[19] The use of naturalistic observations facilitated an understanding of the complex realities of CHWs working in resource-limited settings with clients with NCDs as well as various influences affecting their work.

Setting

The non-governmental organisation (NGO) studied was located in Khayelitsha, an urban township in Cape Town, South Africa. Khayelitsha is an economically disadvantaged community with predominantly informal dwellings. According to Census data, Khayelitsha subdistrict has an estimated population of 406 779;[20] however, this number is expected to have increased to over half a million because of an increased influx of people from rural to urban areas over the past few years.[21] More than half of the population (67%) is unemployed.[22]

The CHWs who work in this area are employed by an NGO operating in Khayelitsha and receiving funding from the Government. Some of the CHWs within the NGO are also involved in TB programmes, where they act as directly observed TB therapy (short course) supporters. In addition, CHWs also work as home-based carers. At the time of the study there were no ward-based teams operating in the area as is the case in other parts of South Africa.

CHWs within this NGO are supervised by professional nurses and coordinators who oversee their daily activities, including administration. However, the ratio of CHWs to supervisors varies amongst organisations. The daily clinic nurse workload in the subdistrict is above the national average, as each nurse provides community-based care for about 33 people per day.[23] Such findings highlight the importance of community-based services as well as the need for CHWs. Compared to other subdistricts in the Western Cape, Khayelitsha has the highest burden of HIV/AIDS, chronic NCDs and injuries.[24] This makes it an appropriate setting for encouraging preventive and promotive community health services.

Study population and sampling strategy

Community health workers employed by the NGO were included in the study. Purposive sampling was used in the selection of one NGO, which was chosen on the basis of location as well as its involvement in the management of clients with NCDs. This NGO had 126 employees at the time of the study.

Data collection

A total of 10 CHWs were observed. Data were collected during August 2011 over a period of four weeks through observations and unstructured interviews. During observations which occurred during a working day (4.5 hours), the researcher collected data through note taking. Unstructured interviews with CHWs were conducted to stimulate discussions related to roles, issues pertaining to training and understanding of the relations and links with the health facility. These were introduced at the end of each observation when there were questions that stemmed from the observations. Data collected from informal conversations during observation were recorded in the form of notes. This was complemented by the researcher further reflecting on and summarising the proceedings of the day. In order for the researcher to have a clearer understanding of some of the CHW activities and practices observed in the field, in-depth interviews were conducted with two coordinators who supervise CHWs' daily activities.

In preparation for data collection the researcher spent a week with the CHWs, accompanying them in whatever activities they were carrying out. This served three purposes, namely to familiarise the researcher with the day-to-day activities of the NGO, to gain trust and to establish rapport with the CHWs. In addition, the researcher participated in some of the activities undertaken by the CHWs, such as morning prayers and debriefing sessions. Building trust was an important element in the data collection process and assisted in gaining insider status.

Data analysis

Data from field notes obtained from observations and in-depth interviews were analysed through thematic content analysis. The data analysis process started with identification of units of meaning, which were then categorised. Central themes were identified after the data were categorised.

Ethical considerations

Permission to conduct the study was obtained from the Research and Ethics Committee at the University of the Western Cape, the Department of Health and the NGO which employed the CHWs. Voluntary informed consent was requested from the CHWs in order for them to participate in the study.

Results

Analysis of the field notes revealed several primary themes. Principally, the CHWs had multiple roles and these could be summarised into six broad themes: advisor; provision of direct services; monitoring of clients; linking clients with the health system; capacity building; and administration.

The scenario shown in Box 1 indicates some of the roles and realities of CHWs working in the area of NCDs.

BOX 1: Observation of community health workers' conducting their daily work.

Scenario

The day started at the NGO base and I was assigned to accompany a pair of CHWs. We walked for about 20 minutes before reaching a newly formed support group in a more formal settlement. The group was organised and had a chairperson and a secretary who took minutes. The support group opened with a prayer and CHWs commenced with the support group activities. I was introduced to the members as a colleague visiting the club to see the work that CHWs do.

One of the CHWs started taking out the instruments that were going to be used to measure blood pressure, weight and blood glucose. There were about 15 members on this day and I watched them getting ready to be measured. The majority of the members were women and many of them were overweight. A bathroom scale was used to measure weights and an automated blood pressure monitoring machine was used to measure blood pressure.

One CHW conducted weight and blood pressure measurement, whilst the other was responsible for measuring blood glucose. The same cuff size was used on all members. The cuff could not fit one of the women's arms and it was put around the wrist and a measurement was recorded. All the measurements were recorded in a book. Members whose weights were above the scale's threshold could not be measured. One of the members had an elevated blood pressure reading and another one had an above-normal glucose reading. The client with an elevated blood pressure reading was instructed to relax whilst the one with a high blood glucose reading was given water; both clients sat for a about 30 minutes before a second reading was taken. The CHW then wrote a note in her booklet and told both clients that the supervisor, a nurse, would come to observe them the next day.

After measurements were completed an education session was delivered by one CHW who spoke about diabetes and hypertension. The lecture focused on explaining what the conditions are and how they can be prevented, and finished with a lecture on diet. This lecture took about 20 minutes.

Lastly an exercise session was conducted for about 15 minutes. All members of the group participated, including the male participant with elevated blood pressure. After the exercise session CHWs recorded dates for collecting medication from the clinic cards. Thereafter we left the support group.

We walked to another area and found that the support group we were visiting did not convene on that day, as there was a death in the area and all the members went to support the bereaved family. We then proceeded to several households where we delivered medication packets to clients. Once at the household the person who received the medication had to sign in the CHWs' booklet. Once the CHWs were done we then proceeded to the office to deliver the equipment that was used. This is how the day ended.

NGO, non-governmental organisation; CHW, community health workers.

Advisor

CHWs offered advice to clients, which ranged from health advice to social issues that concerned participants. The following field notes recorded during a support group session demonstrate CHWs' advisory role which extends beyond the health domain:

> After the health education session at the support group, the CHW opened the session for questions. One of the elderly participants enquired about the registration process for the Child Support Grant. The CHW could not offer concrete advice but promised to ask relevant people that may have appropriate answers. (Field notes, support group, day 2)

The advisory role was also confirmed by the coordinators during an in-depth interview and one commented as follows: 'Community health workers are there to advise clients on number of issues such as what they should eat and where to go in order to get help' (Co-ordinator, day 8).

Provision of direct services

It was evident from the observations that CHWs provided direct services to their clients which included facilitation of support groups, health education, distribution of medication as well as rehabilitation exercises.

Facilitation of support groups

Facilitation of support groups consisting of clients with diabetes and/or hypertension was one of the roles identified. As facilitators, CHWs assumed a leadership position:

> On arrival at the support group the participants were already sitting and waiting for the CHW. She introduced herself and then explained how the session will be structured. Thereafter she started with the day's activities. (Field notes, support group, day 1)

This was also observed in three other support groups that were facilitated by CHWs, where CHWs led support group sessions.

Health education

At the support groups and within households, CHWs work as educators. Education sessions offered by CHWs varied and included matters pertaining to nutrition in the management of NCDs as well as explaining about risk factors, symptoms and prevention measures for diabetes and hypertension. In certain instances CHWs explained healthy eating as consuming plenty of fruit and vegetables. The observation highlights gaps in knowledge on diet and nutrition:

> I attended an education session delivered by a CHW at a support group. She started the session by describing hypertension; she further explained the risk factors for hypertension and how conditions such as hypertension can be prevented. She completed the session with a lecture on nutrition and how nutrition can prevent diabetes and hypertension. The CHW emphasised the importance of a 'healthy diet' and explained that this diet should consist of vegetables and fruit. The information provided to the participants was in the form of a didactic lecture with no illustrations or educational materials to assist the participants in their learning and the CHW in her teaching. (Field notes, support group, day 3)

In addition, health education also occurred during home visits; however, the health education at homes was not of the same depth as within support groups. Health education provided during home visits was in response to questions posed by a particular client rather than routine practice as done in support groups.

Distribution of medication

Chronic medication for selected clients assigned to CHWs was distributed in households and at the designated support groups. The delivery of medication to clients by CHWs is a way of improving access to treatment and serves a dual purpose for both the clients and the health facility, by not only ensuring that clients receive medication timeously, but also enabling them to bypass the long queues and long waiting times usually encountered at health facilities and the transport costs involved:

> After recording the medication in the record book, we went to deliver the medication to clients. We first visited a client that was bedridden to deliver her medication; we then visited a support group where we delivered the bulk of the medication. All the clients collected their medication and were then reminded about their next doctor's appointment. (Field notes, support group, day 6)

In certain instances CHWs did emphasise the importance of taking medication as prescribed; however, this was not a common practice and was mostly communicated during household visits.

Although education about medication was not included in the sessions with clients, CHWs still assisted with medication-related issues and communicated these to the health facility or nurse supervisor. This is highlighted in the scenario and conversation about what CHWs do when confronted with issues relating to medication:

> When CHWs delivered medication at a client's house, the client could not recognise some of the medication that was included in the package and relayed his concern to the CHW. (Field notes, home visit, day 8)

The CHW resolved this issue through a verification process:

> 'I look at the boxes, write down the substances, the milligrams [*dosage*] and the drug name that is written in the box. I then go to the book where we record the medication to see if what is given corresponds with what is in the book. If I'm not sure, I ask the nurse supervisor or pharmacist at the clinic. After getting a response I then tell the client what I have been told.' (Conversation with a CHW, support group, day 6)

Rehabilitation services

A single CHW was observed providing exercises to a client with hemiplegia resulting from a stroke. The CHW was assisted by another CHW to handle the client. Whilst conducting the exercises the CHW kept communicating with the client, who seemed pleased with the service provided. The CHW then encouraged the client to visit the local health facility in order to access further rehabilitation services. Interestingly, no clients from the other support groups were observed receiving rehabilitation exercises. The lack of CHWs assisting clients with rehabilitation exercises in other support groups was explained by the co-ordinator:

> 'A few years ago we received funding to train CHWs to work with community members that could not readily access physiotherapy services. Our CHWs were then trained in rehabilitation exercise; however, when the funding ended we could not continue with the work we were doing. Currently we only have two CHWs who were part of that training and others have retired.' (Co-ordinator, day 7)

Monitoring of clients

CHWs assisted support group members with information that would enable them to better manage their conditions. Whilst conducting support groups, the CHWs collected anthropometric measurements, namely blood pressure, blood glucose and weights of all the participants. Blood pressure was measured using only one cuff size, despite varying mid-upper arm circumferences. Notably, in cases where the cuff was too small to fit the size of upper arm, CHWs placed the cuff on a client's wrist. Finger-prick blood glucose was measured using a new lancet for each person, and clients' readings were recorded. Weights were measured using a dial bathroom scale and put on surfaces that were sometimes uneven. During weight measurements at no point was the scale calibrated. Calculations of body mass index were not performed. In all the observations, individuals with abnormal blood pressure and/or blood glucose readings were informed of their results and referred to the facility. The appreciation on the faces of the support group members was clearly evident during the taking of measurements. During home visits no CHWs were observed taking any client measurements.

Linking clients with the health system

At the support groups CHWs referred people who were identified with elevated blood glucose levels as well as raised blood pressure to the nurse supervisor, who then referred the clients to the nearest health facilities. Referred clients were given a referral letter by the nurse to present to the health facility. Although clients reported being attended to at the health facility, no letters were sent back to the nurse supervisor or CHW. When clients were followed up by CHWs through home visits, CHWs could only rely on the clients' recollection of their clinic attendance and by inspecting the clinic card to ensure that the client did indeed visit the health facility as instructed.

Capacity building

Peer educator

CHWs assisted other CHWs with 'on-the-job' experience. It was evident from one of the field observations that CHWs also acted as peer educators by assisting peers with the skills required to fulfil daily tasks:

> On one of the visits I noticed that CHWs were working as a trio and one CHW would constantly be observing what was happening. When I enquired about this, I was told that the third CHW was newly recruited and therefore did not have experience in doing the work, thus they had to teach her what is usually done. (Field notes, support group, day 9)

According to the coordinators, this was a way of infusing knowledge about field work to new recruits and to assist them in gaining on-the-job experience. One of the coordinators commented as follows:

> 'We have team leaders that we use in the field; they are the ones that we use to partner with a newly recruited CHW. [...] the team leaders are CHWs who have been working for the organisation for a long time and they really know the work.' (Co-ordinator, day 7)

Administration

CHWs completed forms with information relating to the clients on a daily basis. The information recorded includes patients' medication, and particulars of the clients to be visited on that day. In addition, CHWs completed daily statistic sheets for clients (clients seen the day before or planned to be seen). The completion of forms was a daily activity done at the beginning of the day, whilst some of the forms that involved updating patient information were completed after home visits and submitted to the coordinators on the next day. CHWs were also responsible for collected signatures of clients when they receive medication, so as to keep a record of the clients who have collected their medication.

Discussion

The findings of this study show that CHWs fulfil a variety of roles in the management of NCDs. As such they have a crucial role in community level NCD public health care in South Africa. It is evident that the varied roles fulfilled by CHWs seem to be in response to clients' needs. Consequently a degree of flexibility in the way they approach their work may be necessary so as to allow them to react to the community's needs.

In a society where community needs vary, acting as an advisor may be one of the crucial roles played by CHWs. However, as demonstrated in this study, their knowledge and available support material may need to extend beyond health-related issues, especially in communities with social problems. Other studies have shown that CHWs trained in health-related issues such as diabetes management were often confronted with issues unrelated to diabetes, and therefore suggested the need to prepare them for unanticipated non-diabetes issues.[11] Such expectations pose a challenge to CHWs' scope of practice and what can be realistically expected of them. In addition, this illustrates the need to form meaningful networks with other community structures such as social development. These findings further support the broader debate that CHWs need to be integrated into Government programmes and be incorporated into professional teams[1] who can offer support. Furthermore, communication with other team members whilst in the field can provide more streamlined services for the clients.

Playing the role of a health educator meant that CHWs are expected to act as sources of information, creating an expectation that CHWs possess current and relevant information related to NCDs. The study also highlighted the shortfalls in CHWs' knowledge, in that information provided was not always accurate. Inability to clarify certain nutrition concepts emphasises the need for training and continuous education that is tailored to the context that addresses the everyday realities of CHWs, as well as the need for teaching aids to further enforce and standardise the health information given to clients. Indeed it has been suggested that the community's perception of CHW knowledge, skills and ability to assist communities with their health needs is crucial in inspiring respect and acceptance of CHW services.[9]

As lay workers based in communities, CHWs play a fundamental role in community-based support groups, and as demonstrated in this study, within such groups their roles could vary. As facilitators, CHWs require a diverse range of skills which includes communication skills, as part of facilitation includes communicating with the audience. CHWs set the subject or topics for discussion and have the potential to influence the focus of the group, and as such require leadership skills. This leadership role presents its own challenges and expectations, as it would imply that CHWs are expected to know how to guide and support group members. In addition, increased demands to support and provide information may rise to a point where expectations on the leader may exceed their capabilities.[25] Thus it is necessary to structure facilitation of support groups in such a way that forges partnerships, and co-ownership between participants and facilitators.

The distribution of medication to clients on chronic medication serves several purposes that benefit the clients as well as the health facility. Distribution of medication in the community may assist in improving access to treatment, ensure that medication is received timeously and reduce long waiting times in pharmacies at the health facilities. Clearly delivering medication in such settings is helpful, as it minimises the number of trips to the health facility and also reduces overcrowding at health facilities. This benefit could be enhanced considerably if CHWs were to advise on improving adherence and provide education relating to medication for the management of conditions. Our findings highlight the lack of adherence support given to clients with NCDs, in stark contrast to the extensive support provided by CHWs to patients on HIV infection and TB treatment.

As CHWs in this study mainly worked with individuals already known to have a chronic disease, it is crucial that they possess skills in physical rehabilitation of clients. This is particularly pertinent because of the increase in risk factors for cardiovascular disease; an increase in the aging population suggests a similar increase in the burden of cardiovascular disease in sub-Saharan Africa and elsewhere in the developing world. In the absence of appropriate interventions, stroke and heart disease-related deaths are expected to increase from 3 million in 1998 to 5 million in 2020 in developing regions as outlined by the World Health Organization.[26,27] Such statistics suggest that there will be a need for community-based services such as CHWs with specialised skills to deal with the burden of increased numbers of people with physical disabilities caused by strokes and those who suffer from ischaemic heart disease. This will then extend services to clients in areas where there is a scarcity of rehabilitation workers or where people may have limited access to these services.

The role of CHWs in measuring vital parameters in children has been shown to be feasible (reliable) in numerous studies on children.[28] This role could be extended to NCDs, for the detection of abnormal readings and thus the facilitation of referral. In instances when such measurements are incorrectly conducted, this may lead to CHWs' work being devalued. Furthermore, such inadequacies in practice highlight insufficiencies in training and supervision. Thus adequate training, supervision and regular evaluation of tasks are essential in ensuring good practice.

One of the major roles for CHWs has been to connect or link community members to the health facility.[7] In this study this role was fulfilled in numerous ways, such as the delivery of medication and referral of clients identified in the community to a health facility. In communities where health-seeking behaviour is poor and people only visit health facilities when they have serious symptoms, CHWs can play a crucial role in identifying problem cases early enough for health professionals to intervene timeously. However, it is evident that the relationship or communication between health facilities and CHWs has its challenges. Improved communication between health facilities and CHWs could assist in increasing CHWs' legitimacy in the eyes of the community.

The role of CHWs as peer educators is an illustration of innovative thinking by their NGO in order to deal with a lack of appropriate formal training services, although innovative peer education needs to be supervised and better formalised to ensure that the knowledge transferred is appropriate and accurate. Peer education in this context shows how an organisation tailors practices to meet the needs of those they serve.

This article shows some of the limitations and challenges to the roles and responsibilities of CHWs in an NCDs programme. For example, home visits were not utilised maximally, as these could serve as places where health education is delivered. In addition, the work of CHWs concentrated on people with NCDs, thus excluding the population at risk which could benefit from their services. In a place where there is an increase in NCDs there is a need for primary prevention, and CHWs can be used in communities to identify those at risk.

Limitations of the study

The study is limited by the methodology utilised. Although observations are an accepted qualitative research method, they have several constraints, one being that observations are context-specific. A second constraint is that study subjects may alter behaviour when observed by an outsider. Furthermore, observations were based on data collected from one NGO. It is thus important to remember that different organisations may organise work differently. Therefore the findings of this study indicate the issues relating to roles in managing NCDs rather than being generalisable.

Recommendations

On the basis of the findings of this study, the following recommendations are made:

1. CHWs should be empowered with resources as well as forging links with non-health organisations so that they can better refer clients with non-health problems.
2. The main issue of this study is the role of CHWs relating to NCDs. On the one hand there are factors that may inhibit their roles, which may undermine their value in society; on the other hand, the varied roles add value to their work. There is therefore a need to develop the capacity of CHWs in a sustained manner and to create on-going education that is organised and relevant to the context in which they work. In addition, it will be crucial to explore the concept of peer education and how the process can be formalised and supported.
3. It is important to look at community-to-facility referral pathways, as this is important in linking clients to formal health services as well as in the continuity of care, especially for chronic conditions.

Conclusion

This study shows the complexities of the work done by CHWs working with NCD-related conditions. Thus, understanding the actual roles of CHWs provides insights not only into the competencies required to enable them to fulfil their daily functions, but also into the type of training required to fill the present gaps.

Acknowledgements

We would like to acknowledge the Chronic Diseases Initiative for Africa for the funding support. We would like to thank the participants and the NGO concerned for their time and valuable contributions during the study.

Competing interests

The authors declare that they have no financial or personal relationship(s) that may have inappropriately influenced them in writing this article.

Authors' contributions

L.P.T. (University of the Western Cape) initiated the study and was responsible for the data collection, data analysis and writing of the manuscript. T.P. (UWC) contributed in conceptualisation of the study design, preparation of the manuscript and critical revision of the article. H.S. (UWC) assisted in conceptualisation of the study design, preparation of the manuscript and critical revision of the article. N.L. (University of Cape Town and Chronic Disease Initiative for Africa) contributed in conceptualisation of the study, drafting the manuscript and critical revision of the article. K.S. (Chronic Disease Initiative for Africa) contributed in conceptualisation of the study, drafting the manuscript and critical revision of the article.

References

1. Lehmann U, Sanders D. Community health workers: What do we know about them? The state of the evidence on programmes, activities, costs and impact on health outcomes of using community health workers. Geneva: World Health Organization; 2007, pp. 1–42.
2. Lewin S, Munabi-Babigumira S, Glenton C, Daniels K, Bosch-Capblanch X, Van Wyk BE, Odgaard-Jensen J, Johansen M, Aja GN, Zwarenstein M, Scheel IB. Lay health workers in primary and community health care for maternal and child health and the management of infectious diseases. Cochrane Database Syst Rev. 2010 Mar 17;(3):CD004015.
3. Lewin SA, Babigumira SM, Bosch-Capblanch, et al. Lay health workers in primary and community health care: A systematic review of trials. Geneva: World Health Organization [homepage on the Internet] c2006 [cited 2014 Jan 11]. Available from: www.who.int/rpc/meetings/LHW_review2.pdf
4. Mayosi BM, Flisher AJ, Lalloo UG, Sitas F, Tollman SM, Bradshaw D. The burden of non-communicable diseases in South Africa. Lancet 2009; 374(9693):934–947. http://dx.doi.org/10.1016/S0140-6736(09)61087-4

5. Tollman SM, Kahn K, Sartorius B, Collinson MA, Clark SJ, Garenne ML. Implications of mortality transition for primary health care in rural South Africa: A population-based surveillance study. Lancet 2008; 372(9642):893–901. http://dx.doi.org/10.1016/S0140-6736(08)61399-9

6. Steyn K, Levitt NS. Health services research in South Africa for chronic diseases of lifestyle. In: Steyn K, Fourie J, Temple N, editors. Chronic diseases of lifestyle in South Africa: 1995–2005, Technical report. Cape Town: South African Medical Research Council; 2006, pp. 226–248.

7. Singh P. One million community health workers: technical task force report [homepage on the Internet] c2011 [cited 2014 January 11]. Available from: http://1millionhealthworkers.org/files/2013/01/1mCHW_TechnicalTaskForceReport.pdf

8. Steyn K, Levitt D, Patel M, et al. Hypertension and diabetes: Poor care for patients at community health centres. S Afr Med J. 2008;98(8):618–622.

9. Jaskiewicz W, Tulenko K. Increasing community health worker productivity and effectiveness: A review of the influence of the work environment. Hum Resour Health 2012;10(1):38. http://dx.doi.org/10.1186/1478-4491-10-38

10. Perry H, Zuliger R. How effective are community health workers? An overview of current evidence with recommendations for strengthening community health worker programs to accelerate progress in achieving the health-related Millennium Development Goals [homepage on the Internet] c 2012 [cited 2014 Jan 15]. Available from: http://www.coregroup.org/storage/Program_Learning/Community_Health_Workers/review%20of%20chw%20effectiveness%20for%20mdgs-sept2012-condensedversion.pdf

11. Puoane T, Tsolekile L, Sanders D, Parker W. Chronic Non-communicable diseases. In: Barron P, Roma-Reardon J, editors. South African Health Review 2008. Durban: Health Systems Trust, 2008; pp. 73–87.

12. Wadler BM, Judge CM, Prout M, Allen JD, Geller AC. Improving breast cancer control via the use of community health workers in South Africa: A critical review. J Oncol. 2011; Article ID 150423, 8 pages.

13. Gary TL, Bone LR, Hill MN, Levine DM, McGuire M, Saudek C, Brancati FL. Randomized controlled trial of the effects of nurse case manager and community health worker interventions on risk factors for diabetes-related complications in urban African Americans. Prev Med. 2003;37(1):23–32. http://dx.doi.org/10.1016/S0091-7435(03)00040-9

14. Cherrington A, Ayala GX, Amick H, Allison J, Corbie-Smith G, Scarinci I. Implementing the community health worker model within diabetes management challenges and lessons learned from programs across the United States. Diabetes Educator. 2008;34(5):824–833. http://dx.doi.org/10.1177/0145721708323643

15. Fedder DO, Chang RJ, Curry S, Nichols, G. The effectiveness of a community health worker outreach program on healthcare utilization of west Baltimore City Medicaid patients with diabetes, with or without hypertension. Ethn Dis. 2003;13(1):146.

16. McDermott R, Tulip F, Schmidt B, Sinha A. Sustaining better diabetes care in remote indigenous Australian communities. BMJ 2003;327(7412):428. http://dx.doi.org/10.1136/bmj.327.7412.428

17. Naledi T, Barron P, Schneider H. Primary health care in SA since 1994 and implications of the new vision for PHC re-engineering. In: Padarath A, English R, editors. South African health review. Durban: Health Systems Trust, 2011; pp. 17–28.

18. Bolster D, Manias E. Person-centred interactions between nurses and patients during medication activities in an acute hospital setting: Qualitative observation and interview study. Int J Nurs Stud 2010;47(2),154–165. http://dx.doi.org/10.1016/j.ijnurstu.2009.05.021

19. Pillay Y, Barron P. The implementation of PHC re-engineering in South Africa. Public Health Association of South Africa [homepage on the Internet] c2011 [cited 2013 July 20]. Available from: http://www.phasa.org.za/articles/the-implementationof-phc-re-engineering-in-south-africa.html

20. Department of Social Services and Poverty Alleviation. The population register update: Khayelitsha [homepage on the Internet] c2006, p. 72 [cited 2013 July 20]. Available from: http://www.capegateway.gov.za/other/2007/10/kprufinal_2005_october_2007_publish_date.pdf

21. Provincial and Local Government. Nodal economic profiling project: Khayelitsha Western Cape. Republic of South Africa [homepage on the Internet] c2011, p. 8 [cited 2013 July 20]. Available from: http://www.btrust.org.za/library/assets/uploads/documents/3_CIPPN_Khayelitsha%20profile.pdf

22. Department of Social Services. Department of Social Development nodal baseline survey: Khayelitsha results [homepage on the Internet] c2010 [cited 2013 July 20]. Available from: http://www.sarpn.org/documents/d0003004/

23. Day C, Monticelli F, Barron P, Haynes R, Smith J, Sello E, editors. The District Health Barometer 2008/09. Durban: Health Systems Trust; 2010.

24. Groenewald P, Bradshaw D, Daniels J, et al. Local-level mortality surveillance in resource-limited settings: A case study of Cape Town highlights disparities in health. Bull WHO 2010; 88(6): 444–451. http://dx.doi.org/10.2471/BLT.09.069435

25. Keene A. Complexity theory: The changing role of leadership. Ind Comm Training 2000;32(1):15–18. http://dx.doi.org/10.1108/00197850010311121

26. Leeder S, Raymond S, Greenberg H, Liu H, Esson K. A race against time: The challenge of cardiovascular disease in developing countries. New York: Centre for Global Health and Economic Development, Columbia University; 2004.

27. World Health Organization. Report of the Commission on Macroeconomics and Health: Investing in health for economic development. Geneva: World Health Organization; 2001.

28. Amarchandi R, Sharmaii H, Krishnaniii A. Community health workers can be trained to measure blood pressure: Experience from India. Regional Health Forum. 2013;17(1):26–31.

Mental healthcare in Kenya: Exploring optimal conditions for capacity building

Authors:
Elijah Marangu[1]
Natisha Sands[1]
John Rolley[1]
David Ndetei[2]
Fethi Mansouri[3]

Affiliations:
[1]School of Nursing and Midwifery, Deakin University, Australia

[2]Africa Mental Health Foundation and University of Nairobi, Kenya

[3]Centre for Citizenship and Globalization, Deakin University, Australia

Correspondence to:
Elijah Marangu

Email:
elijah.marangu@deakin.edu.au

Postal address:
Deakin University, School of Nursing and Midwifery, Geelong Waterfront Campus, Locked Bag 20000, Victoria 3220, Australia.

The global burden of disease related to mental disorders is on the increase, with the World Health Organization (WHO) estimating that over 450 million people are affected worldwide. The Mental Health Global Action Program (mhGAP) was launched by the WHO in 2002 in order to address the widening gap in access to mental healthcare in low-income countries. Despite these efforts, access to mental healthcare in low-income countries remains poor and is often described as inadequate, inefficient and inequitable, with an 85% estimated treatment gap in low-income countries, as compared with 35% to 50% in high-income countries.In this article, the authors argue that integrating mental health services into primary healthcare settings through capacity building is vital with regard to achieving mhGAP goals. The article explores the challenges to and potential enablers for the improvement of the delivery of broad-based mental healthcare services in Kenya. The authors propose the integration of the conceptual dimensions of both the cosmopolitanism and capabilities approaches as a combined strategy for dealing with capacity building in heterogeneous settings such as Kenya.

Introduction

The World Health Organization (WHO) estimates that 450 million[1] people worldwide experience a mental disorder, which accounts for nearly 12%[1] of the total global burden of disease. High- and low-income countries experience a similar prevalence for mental disorders,[2,3,4] yet large discrepancies exist between resources dedicated to mental health services in low-income countries compared with high-income countries.[2] Kenya, a country in East Africa with a population of approximately 43 million, has less than 500 mental health professionals. Furthermore, inadequate funding and underdeveloped policy frameworks add to the challenge of delivering broad population-based mental healthcare.

This article explores the challenges facing Kenya with regard to improving the delivery of broad-based mental healthcare, including potential barriers and enablers. Both the Cosmopolitanism[5] and Capabilities Approach[6] as theoretical frameworks for improving mental healthcare delivery will be discussed in terms of engaging in capacity-building strategies in primary health settings.

Mental healthcare in Kenya

Mental illness is common in Kenya, with prevalence rates of 4%[7] for major mental disorders, which is comparable with the prevalence rates reported in high-income countries.[8,9] Poverty, unemployment, internal conflict, displacement and HIV[7] add to the mental health burden. Mental health services in Kenya are mainly government funded, with very few privately-funded programmes and facilities.[10] Based in Nairobi, Mathari Hospital is the largest psychiatric hospital, providing inpatient services for the whole of Kenya.[9]

Epidemiologic transition in Kenya and its impact on mental healthcare delivery

Omran's[11] theory of epidemiological transitions is useful when accounting for recent changes in disease patterns in sub-Saharan Africa and Kenya. His theory outlines three 'ages' of relevance to epidemiology and argues that these affect all societies. These ages are: (1) the age of pestilence and famine, characterised by high mortality rates and a life expectancy of about 30 years; (2) the age of receding pandemics and an increase in life expectancy up to 50 years; and (3) the age of degenerative diseases and fluctuating life expectancy.[11] Regarding mental health, the burden of mental disorders is expected to increase in low- and middle-income countries such as Kenya as a result of the epidemiologic transition occurring within these countries, characterised by a marked increase in non-communicable diseases such as diabetes, cardiac disease and mental disorders.[12]

In recognition of these trends, the WHO launched the Mental Health Global Action Program (mhGAP) in 2002 in order to help address the disparity in mental healthcare between high- and low-income countries.[13] The WHO-mhGAP package includes human resources development, increased financing and effective budgeting, advocacy, information system development and monitoring and evaluation.[13]

Prioritising mental health in the face of other complex health issues

Since attaining independence from Britain in 1963, Kenya has engaged in a number of health reforms as a means toward strengthening health services, eradicating communicable diseases and improving health access for the whole population.[14] Whilst there have been improvements with regard to child and maternal mortality and a reduction in morbidity and mortality rates related to communicable diseases, access to healthcare is still hampered by poverty, political instability, corruption and rapid population increase.[14,15] Mental healthcare has received little attention in Kenyan health reform and it remains a low policy and budget priority.[10]

Prioritising resource allocation for mental health services in a country the likes of Kenya is often a challenge because of competing health priorities, including infectious diseases such as HIV, malnutrition, unsafe drinking water, malaria and increasing rates of chronic disease such as diabetes, cardiac disease and renal failure.[16]

Policy and stigma

Mental Health Policy is integral to setting the agenda for planning and delivering mental health services.[2] At present, Kenya has no formal, ratified mental health policy, which severely limits the mental health reform agenda.[17] Jenkins argues that health administrators need to play a role in influencing politicians to take a more active role in advocating for mental healthcare, observing that integration of mental healthcare into the national health sector strategic plan at every level (community to tertiary) is likely to lead to better, more sustainable changes and positive health outcomes.[18]

Studies undertaken in Australia[19] have concluded that stigmatising attitudes toward people with mental illness impact on service delivery and recovery from mental illness.[19] Stigma and discrimination against people with mental illness (and the healthcare staff who work in mental health settings) is a significant challenge for capacity-building efforts in Kenya.[20] and this may explain why very few health professionals choose to work in mental health services.[10] Capacity-building efforts in Kenya must commence by, firstly, addressing the endemic issues of stigma and lack of mental health literacy in the health workforce and, secondly, addressing the society on a broader scale.[21] Public education through social marketing is an effective way of achieving a reduction in stigma and educating the public about mental health and illness. The success of social marketing approaches in addressing HIV prevention and public education in Kenya, Ghana and Uganda[22] confirms the power of social marketing for health promotion and capacity-building; these same approaches could be applied to mental health capacity building.

The limitations of a traditional mental health workforce

A major challenge for mental healthcare in Kenya is the severe shortage or, in some regions, total lack of a specialist mental health workforce.[10] The WHO[1] reports the global median mental health workforce to population ratio as 10.7 staff per 100 000, which is in stark contrast to current resourcing to mental health in Africa, reported as being 1.7 mental health staff per 100 000. Kenya has 54 psychiatrists, 418 trained psychiatric nurses, 10 medical social workers and very few psychologists[10] to cater to a population of about 43 million,[23] 4%[7] of whom are likely to suffer from a major mental disorder. The low levels of mental health literacy amongst health workers at all levels of the Kenyan healthcare system compounds the problem of lack of access to mental healthcare resulting from mental health workforce shortages.[20]

Compounding the workforce issues, a 'brain drain', or the trend of losing trained health workers from low- to high-income countries has had a significant impact on healthcare in sub-Saharan Africa.[24] Of the 74 psychiatrists who have been trained in Kenya since 1980, only 54 have remained to practise in Kenya.[25] There are 418 trained psychiatric nurses in Kenya, but only 250 are currently working in mental health services; others have either emigrated or are working in non-governmental organisations.[10] Attracting and retaining a specialist mental health workforce remains a significant challenge in Kenya.[9]

The problem

Kenya faces a set of complex challenges if it is to realise its goal of improved mental healthcare. The devolving healthcare system away from a Nairobi-centric model to the Counties[26] is an important indicator. However, the persisting lack of investment in real terms, insistence on maintaining traditional approaches in training a professional mental health workforce and the pervading stigma of mental illness continue to hamper the best of intentions.[20]

Improving mental healthcare delivery for the broadest base of the population will require a different approach from that taken in the past. Central to the WHO's mhGAP initiative[13] is for countries to have a robust and efficient mental health workforce at the primary healthcare level.[27] Thornicroft and Tansella, similarly, recommend low-income countries to focus resources on primary healthcare with specialist back-up and the gradual increase of specialist mental health component services as more resources become available.[28] Thornicroft and Tansella's model can be achieved in Kenya by training and by the task shifting of basic mental health assessment, diagnostic and treatment functions from tertiary level institutions to primary healthcare settings through education, training and other knowledge dissemination strategies. In this approach, the existing network of public and non-governmental organisations, including faith-based health facilities at the primary healthcare level, would be used as a vital component of the educational capacity-building strategy. Adopting a primary healthcare focus optimises the potential for a more sustainable and broad-based reach to basic mental healthcare in Kenya.

Theoretical approaches

Two theoretical frameworks are relevant with regard to guiding capacity building: Cosmopolitanism and the Capabilities Approach. The former provides a philosophical foundation that locates the Kenyan context within a broader humanitarian imperative,[6] whilst the Capabilities Approach, an economic model for developing capacity, would provide an operational framework[29] consistent with the goals of Cosmopolitanism.

Cosmopolitanism: Understanding the Kenyan historical, social and political context

Whilst cosmopolitanism, as a philosophical construct, has been around for centuries and has often indicated an outward orientation, along with a capacity to exhibit care and empathy toward strangers and the less-fortunate members of society, some scholars, including Delanty[30] suggest that cosmopolitanism can best be represented as a 'transformative condition' concerned with possibilities in the present. It is a 'condition' of openness to the world that involves social transformation in light of encounters with the 'other'.[30] As such, cosmopolitanism has been applied successfully to studies involving complex political, economic and social settings.[5,31] Kenya has been described similarly as a multi-cultural and multi-linguistic society blending African, Arabic and European elements.[32] Strand (2010) suggests that cosmopolitanism is a conceptual approach rather than a prescriptive theoretical framework; it is a way of seeing the world, on the one hand, as an evolving and complex social reality and, on the other, as a paradigm of political and social analysis;[33] as such, is an appropriate lens through which to understand and then analyse the Kenyan health context. Kenya is a post-colonial, emerging economy, with many political and social challenges that impact on health resourcing and planning. With multiple government and non-governmental organisations involved in healthcare delivery, as well as having a rich cultural heritage and diverse ethnic population, Kenya is 'cosmopolitan' in the truest sense of the word. Cosmopolitanism, in this context, capitalises on these unique contextual factors with regard to both planning and delivering capacity-building strategies and provides a standpoint from which to examine 'who' the actors are and 'what' their agendas may be;[33] this information is critical with regard to planning effective and sustainable mental healthcare capacity-building strategies for Kenya.

Capabilities Approach: Mental health capacity building in Kenya

Sen's Capabilities Approach (CA)[34] is a prominent framework that could be employed for the design and development of a mental health capacity-building model for Kenya. The CA is essentially an economic model that challenges the welfare approach and considers the different *Commodities* and *Capabilities* within the society that can enable its *Abilities* (development). Kenya is currently in a state of political stability, giving rise to positive developments in a number of sectors, including health.[35] According to the current (2013) World Bank forecast,[35] the Kenyan economy is set to grow by at least 6% in the next few years and inflation will be less than 10%.[35] Using Sen's approach, an appraisal of the current strengths in the Kenyan economy and healthcare system can be achieved; this is an important step in developing mental health programmes that are sustainable into the future, with less dependence on foreign funding. Political stability and economic prosperity in Kenya are factors that optimise the likelihood of reform in the health sector,[24] including mental healthcare.

Building primary healthcare capabilities

Despite many political, economic and social challenges that have impeded mental health services improvements and reform, Kenya has many strengths that can be harnessed in order to enable further development of its mental healthcare system.

The stakeholders

Kenya has a wide network of non-governmental organisations, charitable organisations and development partners such as the United Nations International Development Agency (USAID).[26] These stakeholders have been vital to healthcare delivery in Kenya for many years[32] and in involving them in collaborative mental health capacity building is likely to add significant value to strategies developed by the Kenyan Ministry of Health. The African Mental Health Foundation and Basic Needs (UK) are examples of stakeholders currently involved in advocacy, planning and delivery of mental healthcare in Kenya.[8] The activities of these groups include engagement with mental health consumers, public education, engaging in research on psychotrauma which has been common during times of political instability and offering mental health outreach services in rural and remote areas of Kenya.[7] Strengthening these existing collaborative partnerships through educational exchange, training, pooling of resources and collaborative research would be a logical way forward when planning future mental health reform and capacity building in Kenya.

Mental health literacy

Jorm et al. define mental health literacy as 'knowledge and beliefs about mental disorders which aid their recognition, management and prevention'.[36] Mental health literacy is important for both the general public and health professionals for the early identification, treatment of and ongoing support for people with mental disorders.[37] The ability to read and write is key with regard to getting information about mental disorders to the public or primary healthcare workers. Literacy levels in Kenya are estimated to be over 85%[35] and there has been an increase in the number of higher education institutions in recent years.[15] The high levels of literacy and increasing availability of educational opportunities in Kenya are positive attributes that will present opportunities for capacity building through mental health literacy. Incorporating mental health literacy programmes[38] into education programmes in schools and universities and through social marketing-based mental health promotion campaigns, will be an important step in increasing awareness of mental disorders and fighting the associated stigma.

Traditional and faith healers

Kenya has a parallel healthcare system, which works alongside the Western-based system and includes indigenous 'traditional' and faith healers;[3] yet the role of traditional healers in the Kenyan healthcare system is neither officially recognised nor remunerated.[9] A study undertaken amongst people with mental illness in Nairobi by Ndetei et al.[39] found that the majority of patients who participated in the study consulted both Western medical practitioners as well as traditional and faith healers; the authors thus concluded that there was a need for linkages between Western medical practitioners and traditional healers because their roles were complementary.[39] Traditional and faith healers are increasingly involved in delivery of healthcare in rural and remote settings in Kenya; examples include traditional birth attendants and tuberculosis programmes.[14] Mental health capacity-building initiatives implemented in Kenya should include faith and traditional healers. An important first step would be to recognise their role and then to offer training in basic mental healthcare and to clarify referral pathways for the more difficult cases that they are not able to deal with. This approach would acknowledge the cultural importance[40] of this dimension of healthcare in Kenya and recognise the capacity-building potential of strengthening and working collaboratively with existing healthcare workers with formal medical or traditional backgrounds.[39] This inclusive approach is also consistent with the core values of cosmopolitanism.

Technology and capacity building

In recent years there has been a marked increase in the use of mobile technologies in Kenya; and it is estimated that up to 70%[23] of the adult population in Kenya use their mobile phone for mobile banking.[23] Similarly, mobile phones in Kenya are now increasingly used by farmers, pastoralists and business people in order to monitor market conditions.[41] Trials using mobile technology to improve antenatal care and tuberculosis programmes in Kenya have shown positive results.[26] The increasing use of technology in Kenya presents opportunities to use this technology for mental healthcare capacity-building strategies, for example, in training health workers in rural and remote areas and as a potential platform for public mental health promotion through a variety of social networking platforms accessible via phones and other mobile technologies. Mobile technologies are also useful with regard to extending the reach of clinical care, for example, to provide follow-up for consumers with mental illness and to enhance monitoring and communication about mental disorders within and across health facilities.

Devolution

In the past, Kenya has had a highly-centralised health system whereby the vast majority of health resources were concentrated in the capital city, Nairobi,[32] which made access to healthcare difficult for people living in rural and remote areas. The recent devolution and decentralisation of government functions to the county level[35] has potential to lead to more equitable use of available health resources if implemented. There is already evidence emerging[35,42] to suggest that counties within Kenya are reassessing the needs of their jurisdictions and planning service development targeting areas of healthcare neglected in the previous system;[35] this, in turn, could present opportunities for mental health capacity building in the primary health sector.

Conclusion

Whilst Kenya is not unique in the prevalence of mental illness, it does, as with other low-income countries, experience an overwhelming gap in basic mental healthcare delivery to the majority of the population. The growing political stability and burgeoning economic prosperity bode well for the improvement of healthcare in general, yet substantial investment in building capacity for effective mental healthcare is still vital. Whilst, philosophically, cosmopolitanism is not a new idea, its application in the context of improving mental healthcare in Kenya is innovative. The transformative nature of cosmopolitanism with its emphasis on the possibilities of the present can aid in developing sustainable solutions that recognise the critical importance of local stakeholders and which capitalise on Kenya's unique cultural context.

The other deeply complementary framework discussed in this article, namely, the Capabilities Approach, looks to the strengths inherent in the context from which to build capacity for better mental healthcare. These strengths include existing literacy levels, the level of population connectivity through technology and alternative healthcare models such as traditional healers who can complement the efforts of Western-trained healthcare workers. In keeping with WHO recommendations, focusing on capacity building at the primary healthcare level may provide a sustainable way of improving access to basic mental healthcare.

Acknowledgements

The authors thank and acknowledge their anonymous reviewers; their comments and feedback were invaluable in improving this article.

Competing interests

The authors declare that they have no financial or personal relationship(s) which may have inappropriately influenced them in writing this article.

Authors' contributions

E.M. (School of Nursing and Midwifery, Deakin University), a PhD candidate and the first author, was involved in the conceptualisation, design, preparation and submission of the manuscript. N.S. (School of Nursing and Midwifery, Deakin University) was the principal supervisor to E.M and was involved in the conceptualisation, design and review of the manuscript. J.R. (School of Nursing and Midwifery, Deakin University) and F.M. (Centre for Citizenship and Globalization, Deakin University) were E.M.'s co-supervisors and were involved in the conceptualisation, design and review of the manuscript. D.N. (Africa Mental Health Foundation) was E.M.'s co-supervisor and was involved in the conceptualisation and review of the manuscript.

References

1. World Health Organization. Mental health atlas 2011. Geneva: World Health Organization; 2011.
2. World Health Organization. Improving health systems and services for mental health. Geneva: World Health Organization; 2009.
3. World Health Organization. Mental health systems in selected low- and middle-income countries: a WHO-AIMS cross-national analysis. Geneva: World Health Organization; 2009.
4. Goldberg D, Mubbashar M, Mubbashar S. Development in mental health services – a world view. Int Rev Psychiatry. 2000;12(3):240–248. http://dx.doi.org/10.1080/713673748
5. Axtmann R. Cosmopolitanism and globality; Kant, Arendt, and Beck on the global condition. German Politics & Society. 2011;29(3):20–37. http://dx.doi.org/10.3167/gps.2011.290302
6. Clark DA. The Capability Approach: its development, critiques and recent advances [document on the Internet]. c2005 [cited 2014 Aug 31]. Available from: http://www.gprg.org/pubs/workingpapers/pdfs/gprg-wps-032.pdf
7. Ndetei D, Khasakhala L, Kuria MW, et al. The prevalence of mental disorders in adults in different level general medical facilities in Kenya: A cross-sectional study. Ann Gen Psychiatry. 2009;8:1. http://dx.doi.org/10.1186/1744-859X-8-1
8. Kiima D, Jenkins R. Mental health policy in Kenya – an integrated approach to scaling up equitable care for poor populations. Int J Ment Health Syst. 2010;4:19. http://dx.doi.org/10.1186/1752-4458-4-19
9. Ndetei D, Khasakhala L, Omolo JO. Incentives for health worker retention in Kenya: An assessment of current practice. EQUINET discussion paper 62 [document on the Internet]. c2008 [cited 2014 Aug 31]. Available from: http://www.equinetafrica.org/bibl/docs/DIS62HRndetei.pdf
10. Ndetei D, Ongecha F, Mutiso V, et al. The challenges of human resources in mental health in Kenya. S Afr Psychiatry Rev. 2007;10:33–36.
11. Omran AR. The epidemiologic transition theory. A preliminary update. J Trop Paediatr. 1983;29(6): 305–316. http://dx.doi.org/10.1093/tropej/29.6.305
12. Patel V, Thornicroft G. Packages of care for mental, neurological, and substance use disorders in low-and middle-income countries: PLoS Medicine Series. PLoS Med. 2009;6(10):e1000160. http://dx.doi.org/10.1371/journal.pmed.1000160
13. World Health Organization. mhGAP Mental Health Gap Action Programme: Scaling up care for mental, neurological, and substance use disorders. Geneva: World Health Organization; 2008.
14. Oyaya CO, Rifkin SB. Health sector reforms in Kenya: An examination of district level planning. Health Policy. 2003;64(1):113–127. http://dx.doi.org/10.1016/S0168-8510(02)00164-1
15. Rakuom C. Nursing human resources in Kenya: Case study. Geneva: International Centre for Human Resources in Nursing; 2010.
16. Luoma M, Doherty J, Muchiri S, et al. Kenya health systems assessment 2010. Bethesda, MD: Health Systems 20/20 Project, 2010.
17. Jenkins R, Kiima D, Njenga F, et al. Integration of mental health into primary care in Kenya. World Psychiatry. 2010;9(2):118–120.
18. Jenkins R. How to convince politicians that mental health is a priority. World Psychiatry. 2013;12(3):266–268. http://dx.doi.org/10.1002/wps.20073
19. Reavley NJ, Jorm AF. Stigmatising attitudes towards people with mental disorders: Changes in Australia over 8 years. Psychiatry Res. 2012;197(3):302–306. http://dx.doi.org/10.1016/j.psychres.2012.01.011
20. Muga FA, Jenkins R. Training, attitudes and practice of district health workers in Kenya. Soc Psychiatry Psychiatr Epidemiol. 2008;43(6):477–482. http://dx.doi.org/10.1007/s00127-008-0327-z
21. Ndetei D. Early intervention in psychosis: Concepts, evidence and perspectives. World Psychiatry. 2008;7(3):164–165.
22. England R. Head to Head: Are we spending too much on HIV? BMJ. 2007;334(7589):344. http://dx.doi.org/10.1136/bmj.39113.402361.94
23. World Bank. Kenya at a glance [document on the Internet]. c2012 [cited 2014 Aug 31]. Available from: http://devdata.worldbank.org/AAG/ken_aag.pdf
24. Davies S. Global politics of health. Cambridge, UK: Polity Press; 2010.
25. Jenkins R, Baingana F, Ahmad R, et al. International and national policy challenges in mental health. Ment Health Fam Med. 2011;8(2):101–114.
26. Republic of Kenya. Kenya health sector strategic and investment plan (KHSSP) July 2013 – June 2017 [document on the Internet]. c2012 [cited 2014 Aug 31]. Available from: http://www.who.int/pmnch/media/events/2013/kenya_hssp.pdf
27. Saxena S, Thornicroft G, Knapp M, et al. Resources for mental health: Scarcity, inequity, and inefficiency. Lancet. 2007;370(9590):878–889. http://dx.doi.org/10.1016/S0140-6736(07)61239-2
28. Thornicroft G, Tansella M. Components of a modern mental health service: A pragmatic balance of community and hospital care: Overview of systematic evidence. Br J Psychiatry. 2004;185(4):283–290. http://dx.doi.org/10.1192/bjp.185.4.283
29. Goerne A. The capability approach in social policy analysis – yet another concept? REC-WP Working Papers on the Reconciliation of Work and Welfare in Europe (03-2010), 2010.
30. Delanty G. A cosmopolitan approach to the explanation of social change: Social mechanisms, processes, modernity. The Sociological Review. 2012;60(2): 333–354. http://dx.doi.org/10.1111/j.1467-954X.2012.02076.x
31. Parekh B. Cosmopolitanism and global citizenship. Review of International Studies. 2003;29(1):3–17. http://dx.doi.org/10.1017/S0260210503000019
32. Muga FA, Jenkins R. Health care models guiding mental health policy in Kenya 1965–1997. Int J Ment Health Syst. 2010;4:9. http://dx.doi.org/10.1186/1752-4458-4-9
33. Strand T. The making of a new cosmopolitanism. Stud Philos Educ. 2010;29(2):229–242. http://dx.doi.org/10.1007/s11217-009-9161-3
34. Sen A. Capability and well-being. In: Nussbaum M, Sen A. The quality of life. Oxford: Oxford University Press, 1993; pp. 30–54. http://dx.doi.org/10.1093/0198287976.003.0003
35. World Bank. Kenya Economic Update: June 2013 [document on the Internet] c2013 [cited 2014 Aug 31]. Available from: http://www.worldbank.org/content/dam/Worldbank/document/Africa/Kenya/kenya-economic-update-june-2013.pdf
36. Jorm AF, Barney LJ, Christensen H, et al. Research on mental health literacy: What we know and what we still need to know. Aust N Z J Psychiatry. 2006;40(1):3–5. http://dx.doi.org/10.1080/j.1440-1614.2006.01734.x
37. Jorm AF. Mental health literacy: Empowering the community to take action for better mental health. Am Psychol. 2012;67(3):231–243. http://dx.doi.org/10.1037/a0025957
38. Ganasen KA, Parker S, Hugo CJ, et al. Mental health literacy: Focus on developing countries. Afr J Psychiatry. 2008;11(1):23–28. http://dx.doi.org/10.4314/ajpsy.v11i1.30251
39. Ndetei D, Khasakhala L, King'ori J, et al. The complementary role of traditional and faith healers and potential laisions with Western-style mental health services in Kenya [document on the Internet]. c2007 [cited 2014 Sep 04]. Available from: https://profiles.uonbi.ac.ke/ndetei/publications/complementary-role-traditional-and-faith-healers-and-potential-liaisons-western-
40. Patel V. Explanatory models of mental illness in sub-Saharan Africa. Soc Sci Med. 1995;40(9):1291–1298. http://dx.doi.org/10.1016/0277-9536(94)00231-H
41. Library of Congress – Federal Research Division. Country profile: Kenya [document on the Internet]. c2007 [cited 2014 Sep 04]. Available from: http://lcweb2.loc.gov/frd/cs/profiles/Kenya.pdf
42. Jenkins R, Njenga F, Okonji M, et al. Prevalence of common mental disorders in a rural district of Kenya, and socio-demographic risk factors. Int J Environ Res Public Health. 2012;9(5):1810–1819. http://dx.doi.org/10.3390/ijerph9051810

African Primary Care Research: Quality improvement cycles

Authors:
Claire van Deventer[1]
Bob Mash[2]

Affiliations:
[1]Department of Family Medicine and Rural Health, University of the Witwatersrand, South Africa

[2]Division of Family Medicine and Primary Care, Stellenbosch University, South Africa

Correspondence to:
Claire van Deventer

Email:
cvandeventer@nwpg.gov.za

Postal address:
PO Box 1197, Potchefstroom 2520, South Africa

Improving the quality of clinical care and translating evidence into clinical practice is commonly a focus of primary care research. This article is part of a series on primary care research and outlines an approach to performing a quality improvement cycle as part of a research assignment at a Masters level. The article aims to help researchers design their quality improvement cycle and write their research project proposal.

La recherche sur les soins de santé primaire en Afrique: les cycles d'amélioration de la qualité. L'amélioration de la qualité de la prise en charge médicale et l'application des données probantes à la pratique clinique font couramment l'objet de l'attention de la recherche portant sur les soins de santé primaire. Cet article fait partie d'une série dédiée à la recherche sur les soins de santé primaire et définit une approche à la réalisation d'un cycle d'amélioration de la qualité, dans le cadre d'un travail de recherche entrepris au niveau du Master. L'objectif de cet article est d'aider les chercheurs à élaborer leur cycle d'amélioration de la qualité et à rédiger leur proposition de projet de recherche.

Introduction

This article outlines the study design for quality improvement (QI) cycles when performed as a research project. QI cycles can be seen as a form of translational research:

> Translational research transforms currently available knowledge into useful measures for everyday clinical and public health practice. Translational research aims to assess implementation of standards of care, understand the barriers to their implementation, and intervene throughout all levels of health care delivery and public health to improve quality of care and health outcomes, including quality of life.[1]

Translational research is important in the context of primary care because there is often more benefit for the population served from ensuring the effective implementation of what is already known than from developing new therapies or technology from basic science. Performing a QI cycle in the discipline of family medicine and primary care is therefore recognised as a legitimate research activity that provides new knowledge on how to improve the quality of care in that context.[2]

One of the roles of family physicians is often that of clinical governance, which at its heart is also an approach to improving the quality of clinical care. Many health services have embedded QI strategies as a routine part of the organisational culture and policy.[3,4] There are publications from South Africa, Scandinavia, the Netherlands, the United States of America and many others, where the long-term advantages of a process of QI in healthcare have been recognised.[4,5,6,7,8,9,10,11] Skills in QI are therefore a necessary competency for family physicians. When performed as part of a research project, however, there must be greater attention to scientific rigour, especially with regard to ensuring sufficient sample size and applying appropriate statistical methods of data collection and analysis or using the best qualitative methods, should this be the preferred route.

There are many reasons to start a QI project:[12]

- Bridging the gap between evidence, policy and practice.
- Improving the patient's experience of care.
- Educating and training health workers in terms of best evidence-based practice.
- Improving teamwork and motivation to improve quality of care.
- Improving management and accountability.
- Improving financial planning and budgeting of healthcare services.
- Identifying further research questions.

Historical background

The earliest examples of quality in health may be seen in Florence Nightingale's interventions in the Crimean war[13] in 1854, the British farming industry in the early 1900s[14] and Donabedian's contribution in the 1960s toward the framework of quality in health that comprises structural, process and outcome elements of quality.[15]

Quality improvement was studied as an industrial process in 1931 by Shewhart.[16] His concepts included identifying customers' needs, reducing variation in processes and minimising unnecessary supervision. Influenced by Shewhart's work, Deming recognised QI as a primary driver for industrial success and subsequently introduced these methods to post-World War II Japanese engineers and executives.[17] Applied strategically, these methods produced considerable growth in the Japanese automobile industry and became recognised worldwide as QI methods.[18]

Based on the above influences, Taiichi Ohno, a Toyota Motor Corporation engineer, revolutionised thinking about process inefficiency or 'waste' in the early 1950s, leading to the creation of the Toyota Production System (TPS).[19] Application of the TPS resulted in the use of the term *lean* in many industries, including healthcare.[20] Lean methodology is driven by the identified needs of the customer and aims to improve processes by removing non-value-added activities.

Non-value-added activities, also referred to as waste, do not add to effectiveness, financial success or the customer's experience; and the customer is often not willing to pay for them. Seven different types of waste have been identified, as shown in Table 1.

Understanding the concept of 'quality' in healthcare

The WONCA Working Party on Quality in Family Medicine defines quality as: 'The best health outcomes that are possible, given available resources, and that are consistent with patient values and preferences'.[21] Quality of care can be defined from different perspectives with different priorities – the patient, the primary care provider, the fund manager or the policy maker. Quality of care can also be evaluated at different levels of the health system, from the individual person, to a whole health centre or clinic, to a subdistrict or district, or even at a national level.

The focus of quality improvement in primary care is often on the quality of clinical care within the consultation for specific conditions such as HIV, diabetes or hypertension. However, there are additional dimensions that should be considered. The performance of the health service as a whole may also be relevant:

- Accessibility:[22] Are patients capable of getting healthcare services when needed, in terms of both geographic and financial barriers? Is care organised in a way that maximises physical access (eg. convenient times, ramps for patients with disabilities) and convenience for patients? Is the clinic able to cope with the volume of patients? Is care equally accessible to all? Is there a financial barrier for certain levels of health (eg. MRI scans for state patients)? Negative attitudes of staff members may also prevent optimal access.
- Acceptability:[23] How satisfied are patients with their care? Are there cultural or spiritual issues that are ignored?
- Continuity:[24] Is care organised in such a way that there is retention of information between visits and over time as well as some longitudinal continuity with at least a team of the same primary care providers?
- Coordination:[22] Is there cooperation between the community and clinic, within the multiprofessional team at the clinic or health centre and between the clinic and the referral hospital?
- Comprehensiveness:[24] Does the facility offer the full range of services needed by this community?
- Effectiveness:[22] 'Doing the right thing' is in many ways addressed directly through the QI cycle in the structural, process and outcome criteria that are set and based on the best available evidence.
- Efficiency:[23] '[*T*]he balance between the level of resources in the system used to treat patients to come to certain outcomes'. From the patient's point of view, allocative or productive efficiency relates to maximising their health outcome whilst minimising the costs and time spent for the patient. Technical efficiency implies that the system cannot reduce its use of resources any further without also eroding its ability to treat patients or deliver on the required outcomes. Performance efficiency may also relate to issues such as the number and duration of consultations, rationale for use of medication or number of new referrals.
- Equity:[23,25] This is '[*t*]he absence of systematic and potentially remediable differences in health status across population groups' and is entrenched in the South African National Core standards as part of the involvement and fairness toward patients when related to issues of quality.

There are a number of confusing concepts regarding QI. Whilst quality assessment (audit) is the process of evaluating the current level of performance, QI is a process of change and improvement that uses the audit as a source of information. Quality assurance requires both these aspects in order to

TABLE 1: Types of organisational waste and examples from healthcare.

Types of waste	Examples for healthcare
Overproduction	Pre-mixing drugs or performing laboratory tests 'just in case' they might be useful.
Wasted inventory	Using beds for patients who are just waiting for test results, getting patients back weekly to see a clinic nurse for tuberculosis (TB) treatment.
Rejects/defects	Mislabelling laboratory specimens, using broken or faulty equipment.
Wasted motion	Having only one emergency trolley between many wards, resulting in having to spend time hunting for equipment to perform a common procedure.
Waiting/delay	Long queues or waiting times, waiting unnecessarily long for medication, results or to see a healthcare worker.
Waste with processing	Time spent on completing irrelevant paperwork, spending time on intravenous treatment when oral is equally effective.
Waste with transport	Transporting patients to a referral hospital for treatment or investigations that should be performed locally, transporting specimens to a laboratory when point-of-care testing would be equally effective.

assure that good standards of care are maintained through repeated cycles of assessment and improvement.[26]

When looking at quality as part of a research project for a Master's degree, it is usually necesssary to go beyond just auditing the current practice (what is happening). At the same time, it is usually impractical to perform continuous quality assurance over several years. Quality improvement is therefore the most usual goal of such a project, implying that a full QI cycle should be completed in which the current quality of care is audited, change to improve the quality of care is implemented and the effect of this intervention is reaudited in order to determine if there has been an improvement.

Choosing a topic

In your research proposal, the argument for the social and scientific value of your chosen topic will be made in the introduction to the proposal. The topic should be of importance to patients' health or wellbeing, be amenable to change, be relatively common with sufficient patient numbers and be practical to study in terms of available time and resources. Topics may be chosen due to the awareness of a gap between evidence and practice, experience of a critical adverse event such as a maternal death, unacceptable variation in practice between people or facilities, or because data is being collected routinely and can be used to identify health priorities as well as to monitor progress. There may be problems that are important for patients, healthcare providers or other partners in healthcare such as policy makers or carers.

Aim and objectives

In QI, the research question is usually a 'How?' question. An example is 'How to improve the quality of care for congestive cardiac failure at a given Community Health Centre?' and the aim, therefore, could be expressed as 'To assess and improve the quality of care for congestive heart failure at a given Community Health Centre'. When writing the objectives one should avoid describing the methodological steps of the QI cycle and rather describe the objectives that you want to achieve as a result of these steps. For example:

- To assess the current quality of care for congestive cardiac failure.
- To plan and implement changes to improve the quality of care.
- To determine if these changes are associated with a measurable improvement in the quality of care.

Methods

Study design

The study design for QI is usually a series of steps that can be conceptualised as a cycle. When writing the research proposal, it may be clearer to describe each of these steps under a number of subheadings (see below), rather than trying to force the description of the design into the traditional subsections of the methods. The overall design of the cycle can be described in the study design section of the proposal and a diagram to illustrate it is often helpful (Figure 1).

Setting

In your research proposal you should describe the clinical setting for the QI cycle with some detail regarding the current service for the topic in question. You should also describe the population served by the facility, in order to provide a context for understanding the topic and for interpreting the data.

Selecting a team

Quality improvement is usually a team effort, as ownership of the problem and process by the people involved is more likely to lead to change in practice than when it is perceived as criticism by an outside researcher or individual. In a study done with a QI team regarding management of diabetic patients in a primary care setting, the following was found:

> Success was more likely in teams in which: the GP or nurse felt personally involved in the audit; they perceived their teamwork as good; they had recognized the need for systematic plans to address obstacles to quality improvement; and their teams had a positive attitude to continued monitoring of care. A positive attitude to audit and a personal interest in the disease were not associated with improvement in care.[27]

Set up a meeting to explain the concept of what QI is, what it is not (policing, criticism), that participation is crucial and explain the process. Involve all the people that could improve the situation and assist in maintaining the long-term outcome. The team will usually consist of key leadership within the facility. Consideration should be given to the involvement of patient advocates. The team should also ensure that they give and receive feedback from the broader healthcare team during the process.

In your research proposal, describe how you will establish your team, what categories of people you intend to be a part thereof and why you have purposefully selected these categories. The team members each need to add value to the project and will influence both the outcome and the sustainability thereof.

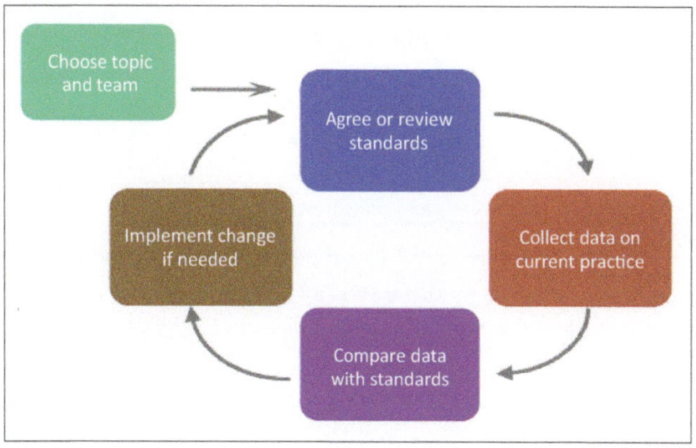

FIGURE 1: The quality improvement cycle.[27]

Agree on or review standards of care

Target standards for QI are usually a combination of a measurable and clearly-defined criteria and a level of desired performance.[22]

Criteria are often aspects of care and are chosen with respect to the structure, process or outcome of care (see Table 2 for examples):

- Structure would include the available physical amenities, human resources, equipment, medication and educational materials.
- Process includes all the healthcare activities that take place during the patient's progress through the facility, including the consultation.
- Outcomes are the end results of the care received, for example the successful treatment of a condition, level of control achieved, or avoidance of complications.

Criteria should be evidence based and derived from a synthesis of the evidence, ideally in the form of a relevant and valid guideline.[22] In the absence of such a guideline, systematic reviews or other types of studies can guide the selection of criteria. The evidence should clearly make the case for why this criterion is linked to the quality of care for this specific condition or topic. Criteria should also be selected that are measurable given available time and resources and should be amenable to change. The number of criteria should also be realistic – not everything needs to be measured. The criteria that best depict the quality of care and which are most sensitive to improvement should be chosen. Criteria should, however, include all the key areas and focus particularly on where the team anticipates the problems with quality to be.

A standard can be agreed upon. This can be based on the results of previous QI cycles or on national or international guidelines or simply agreed to by the project team as a reasonable goal for QI. They should be realistic (for example, levels of 100% are seldom achieved) and yet promote the improvement of quality over time. Table 2 gives examples of criteria for cervical screening. The standard here could possibly be '60% of women qualifying for a papsmear, receive one', based on the national target of 54%.[28]

In your research proposal, you should describe the sources of evidence that you will use with your team and the process that you will follow to set these standards. If this process has not yet happened it may be helpful to at least give some examples of likely standards that may be used.

TABLE 2: Examples of criteria for cervical screening.

Structure	Criteria
All consulting rooms used by professional nurses have specula available in small, medium and large sizes.	Structural criteria
Patients seen have all their details entered into the cervical screening register.	Process criteria
Professional nurses have performed 10 cervical smears per week during the previous month.	Process criteria
Women over 30 years of age have had at least one documented cervical smear in the previous three years.	Outcome criteria

Collect and analyse data on current practice

When performing QI as part of a research project, it is important to ensure a sufficient sample size if you are relying mostly on quantitiave methods. Remember that you intend not only to achieve a representative sample of your target population (e.g. all women over the age of 30 years that require cervical screening or all patients with type 2 diabetes), but also to compare the results at baseline with the results at follow up to determine if there is a statistically-significant improvement in care (this will require sufficient power in your sample size). Sometimes you can demonstrate a statistically-significant improvement even when your standard is not achieved. A suitable sampling strategy must also be used to ensure that you obtain an unbiased sample of your target population. See the article on surveys and questionnaires for help with sample size calculation and sampling strategies.

Common sources of data to measure your criteria in primary care include patients' records, registers (e.g. TB and mental health registers) or routinely-collected statistics on healthcare from the clinic. Data can be collected prospectively, as patients are seen or, more often, retrospectively, from data that has already been collected.[24,25] A data collection tool may be developed and data captured in an Excel spreadsheet for further analysis. See the article on quantitative data analysis elsewhere in this series.

Qualitative data is sometimes also collected to complement the measurement of criteria and to enable a deeper understanding of how to improve quality. For example, in-depth interviews or focus group interviews with patients can provide valuable insights from their perspective. Patient satisfaction and experience can also be measured by means of a questionnaire. This baseline data can then be analysed using descriptive statistics or qualitative data analysis as described in other articles in this series. Make sure that you have analysed your data so as to measure the exact criteria that you defined previously.

In your research proposal, therefore, you need to describe your sample size calculation, sampling strategy, data collection process and analysis of the data.

Compare data with standards

The results of this baseline audit can then be compared to the standards set previously by the team. In essence, this makes the discrepancy between actual and desired practice visible to the team. The researcher should aim to facilitate reflection on these results with the whole team with the goal of reaching a consensus on what has been learnt regarding the strengths and weaknesses of current quality.

In your research proposal you should describe how you will facilitate this process and any specific techniques that you will use. A few useful techniques are described below:

Process mapping

Process mapping is an objective assessment of systems or processes in order to identify road blocks and bottle necks within the processes such as long waiting times in a clinic, or the process from antenatal booking to delivery of a baby.[29] The team can do this as a theoretical exercise where the current situation is analysed. On individual post-it notes, a process is mapped out as shown in Figure 2. Each step is documented starting on the left, with arrows between the post-it notes. At each note, the people involved should be documented. The time taken should be annotated in red if the data point is non-value-added or in green if it is value-added. This leads to objective and constructive discussions relating to bottlenecks, unseen problems, obvious solutions and ongoing monitoring systems. Patient shadowing would require team members to physically accompany a patient through all the processes and note everything that occurs and the time taken.

Fishbone and/or root cause analyses

Process mapping is often used together with other tools such as the fishbone or root cause analyses shown in Figure 3.[29] The fishbone assists in separating and organising the contributing factors towards the root cause of the problem.

The '5 whys' is another way of doing a root cause analysis, by asking the question 'why?' until one reaches a common denominator, as is shown in Figure 4.[29]

Plan and implement change

The reflective and analytical process described above should lead naturally to reflection within the team regarding how to change current practice and improve quality. One should ensure a thorough reflection on the real issues and not jump to conclusions too quickly on what to change. In your research proposal, you should also describe how you will facilitate this process.

As with all planning processes, it should be made very clear what has been agreed to, who is responsible and what the timeframe is for implementation. The plan and the implementation thereof need to be SMART (Specific, Measurable, Achievable, Realistic and Time-framed). Small-scale or individual Plan-Do-Study-Act (PDSA) cycles can be used to pilot suggested changes prior to full-scale implementation within the facility.[30,31] If there is a need for further training in order to implement the plans, this should also be identified and organised. If there is a need for additional resources or input from higher up the organisational ladder, then this should also be identified and a strategy agreed on for engaging with the relevant managers. The results of the audit, interpretation and plans for change should be communicated to the rest of the staff in a way that encourages further feedback, reflection and ownership.

The team should plan the implementation carefully as well as how they will monitor and follow up on progress. Regular meetings are helpful with regard to tracking the progress of the implementation.

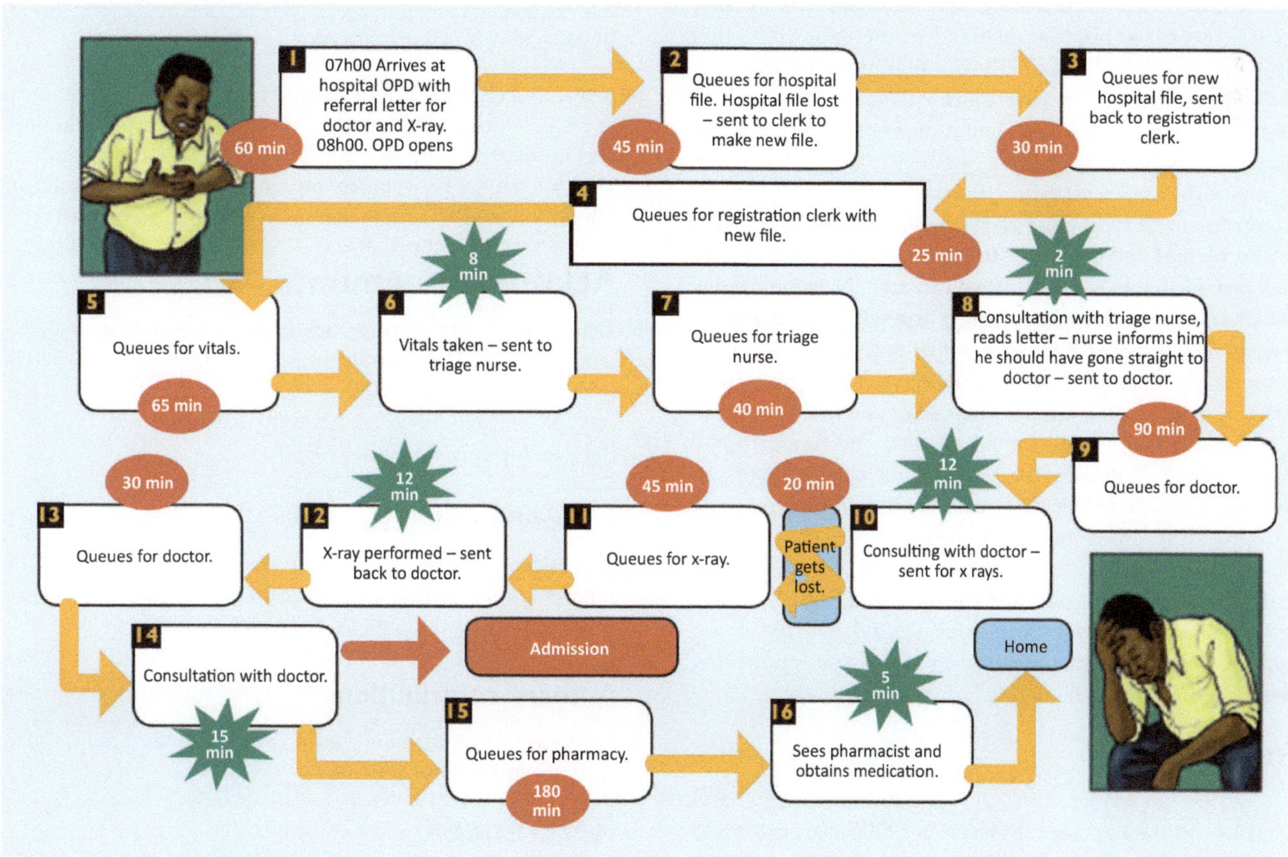

FIGURE 2: Example of process mapping diagram.[27]

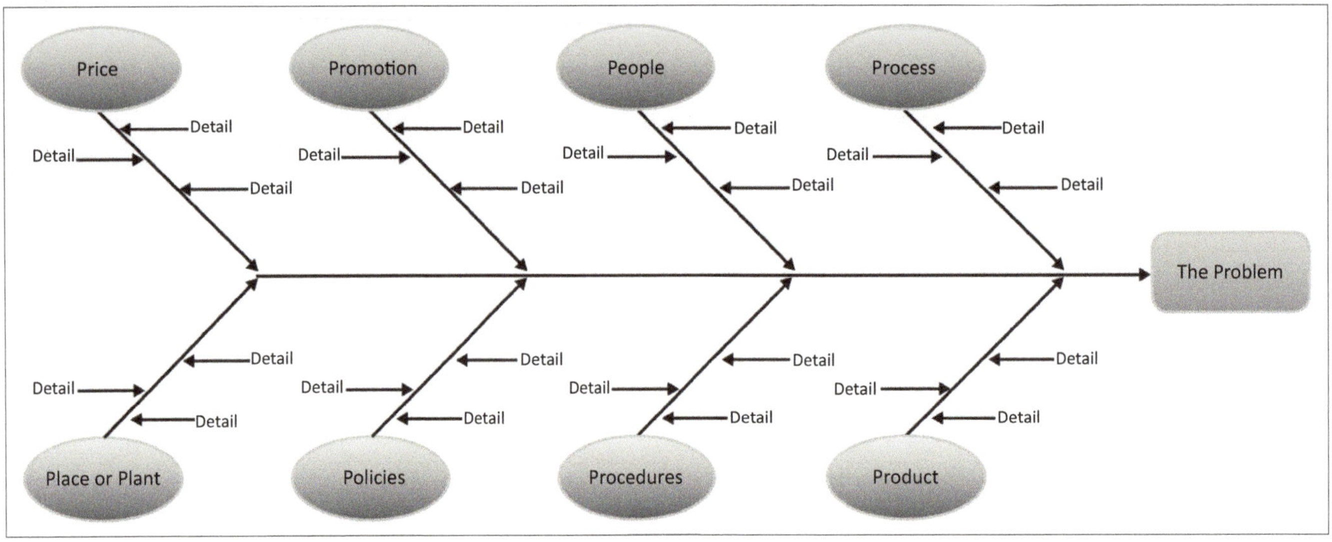

FIGURE 3: Fishbone diagram for root cause analysis.

Your research proposal should describe how you will facilitate this process; how the plans will be implemented, monitored and reinforced over time; and how long you anticipate it will take before they result in a measurable improvement in quality.

Repeat the cycle

After a defined period of time the audit should be repeated to re-measure the criteria. This period is usually six months to one year in order to allow time for the intervention to be effective and this should be anticipated in the timeline for your research proposal. Ideally, the same patients or their medical records should be included in the re-audit so that you are measuring change in the same group of people over time. This makes comparative statistical analysis possible. In your research proposal, you should describe when and how you will re-audit the criteria.

In your final research assignment, it may be useful to report on any further reflections of the team on the final results, what has been achieved and what must be focused on next. You should report on what worked and what did not work in terms of changing clinical practice and how this might be useful to other practitioners. It may also be helpful to reflect on whether the criteria you used need to be modified or adapted in some way for future use. The propositional knowledge generated by the QI cycle includes a report on the quality of care in the study context and on how care can be improved in this context.

Many QI cycles performed for research purposes are once-off projects. Sustaining the change should be considered from the beginning with ongoing QI cycles and monitoring systems built in after the research project has finished.

Conclusion

This article describes the QI programme design and elaborates on the key steps involved in a QI cycle, performed as a translational research study and, in particular, advises on how to write a research proposal for such a study. If a

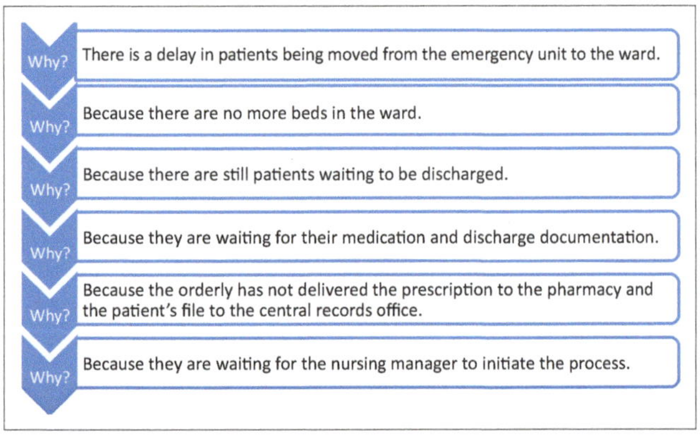

FIGURE 4: The 5 Whys used in root cause analysis.

researcher chooses a relevant and important topic, gathers an appropriate team and has evidence-based target standards and innovative assessment methods, these should result in a SMART plan, which can be implemented and reassessed and which can lead to actual change in clinical practice.

Acknowledgements

The authors gratefully acknowledge funding received from the U.S. President's Emergency Plan for AIDS Relief (PEPFAR), through HRSA under the terms of T84HA21652, and via the Stellenbosch University Rural Medical Education Partnership Initiative (SURMEPI).

Competing interests

The authors declare that they have no financial or personal relationship(s) which may have inappropriately influenced them in writing this article.

Authors' contributions

Both authors contributed to the initial manuscript and made the subsequent revisions.

References

1. Narayan V, Benjamin E, Gregg EW, et al. Diabetes translation research: where are we and where do we want to be? Ann Intern Med. 2004;140(11):958–963.

2. Marincowitz GJO, Fehrsen GS. Caring, learning, improving quality and doing research: different faces of the same process. SA Fam Pract. 2004;46(7):26–29.

3. Gauld R, Mays N. Reforming primary care: are New Zealand's new primary health organisations fit for purpose? BMJ. 2006;333(7580):1216–1218.

4. Bentley J, Fletcher D. Choosing and using: patient choice in 'Choose and Book'. Br J Community Nurs. 2004;12(12):558–562.

5. Stevenson K, Baker R, Farooqi A, et al. Features of primary health care teams associated with successful quality improvement of diabetes care: a qualitative study. Fam Pract. 2003;18(1):21–26.

6. Bradley EH, Holmboe ES Mattera, JA, et al. Data feedback efforts in quality improvement: lessons learned from US hospitals. Qual Saf Health Care 2004;13(1):26–31.

7. Compas C, Hopkins KA, Townsley E. Best practices in implementing and sustaining quality of care: a review of the quality improvement literature. Res Gerontol Nurs. 2008;1(3):209–216.

8. Ferguson L, Calverte J, Davie M, et al. Clinical leadership: using observations of care to focus risk management and quality improvement activities in the clinical setting. Contemp Nurse. 2007;24(2):212–224.

9. Hutchinson J, Armstrong G. Improving standards of care for patients: a pilot project. Nurs Stand. 2009;23(51):43–47.

10. Shojania KG, Grimshaw JM. Evidence-based quality improvement: the state of the science. Health Aff. 2005;24(1):138–150.

11. Wensing M, Wollersheim H, Grol R. Organizational interventions to implement improvements in patient care: a structured review of reviews. Implement Sci. 2006;1:2.

12. Teasdale S. The future of clinical audit: learning to work together [editorial]. BMJ. 1996;313(7057):574.

13. Cook ET. The life of Florence Nightingale: 1862–1910 (Vol 2). London: McMillan; 1914.

14. Liston C. Managing quality and standards. Buckinham: Open University Press; 1999.

15. Donabedian A. Evaluating the quality of medical care. Milbank Q. 2005;83(4):691–721.

16. Shewhart WA. Economic control of quality of manufactured products. New York, NY: D. Van Nostrand Co; 1931.

17. Deming WE. Out of the crisis. Cambridge, MA: MIT Center for Advanced Engineering Study Publishing; 1982.

18. Varkey P, Reller MK, Resar RK. Basics of quality improvement in health care. Mayo Clin Proc. 2007;82(6):735–739.

19. McCarthy M. Can car manufacturing techniques reform health care? Lancet. 2006;367(9507):290–291.

20. Toussant J, Gerard RA, Adams E. On the mend: revolutionizing healthcare to save lives and transform the industry. Cambridge, MA: Lean Enterprise Institute; 2010.

21. Mäkelä M, Booth B, Roberts R. editors. Family doctors' journey to quality. Helsinki, Finland: Stakes; 2001.

22. Armstrong S, editor. Managing quality: tools skills and capacities for health leaders. Cape Town: Pearson; 2012.

23. Kringos DS, Boerma WGW, Hutchinson A, et al. The breadth of primary care: a systematic literature review of its core dimensions. BMC Health Services Research. 2010;10:65.

24. Lawrence M, Schofield T, editors. Medical audit in primary health care. New York: Oxford University Press; 1993.

25. Department of Health. National core standards for health establishments in South Africa. Department of Health; 2011.

26. Grol R, Thomas S, Roberts R. Development and implementation of guidelines for family practice: lessons from the Netherlands. J Fam Pract. 1995;40(5):435–439.

27. Department of Health, IHI, DFID. The five steps to quality improvement: a facility-based guide to improving clinical outcomes. Department of Health; 2012.

28. Massyn N, Day C, Dombo M, et al. District health barometer 2012/2013. Westville: Health Systems Trust; 2013.

29. Moleko W, Marshall C. Quality improvement guide. Quality improvement – the key to providing improved quality of care. Department of Health; 2012.

30. Berwick DM. Developing and testing changes in delivery of care. Ann Intern Med. 1998;128(8):651–656.

31. Langley GJ, Nolan KM, Norman CL, et al. The improvement guide: a practical approach to enhancing organizational performance. San Francisco, CA: Jossey-Bass; 1996.

Human resources for health in Botswana: The results of in-country database and reports analysis

Authors:
Oathokwa Nkomazana[1]
Wim Peersman[2]
Merlin Willcox[3]
Robert Mash[4]
Nthabiseng Phaladze[5]

Affiliations:
[1]Faculty of Medicine, Department of Surgery, University of Botswana, Botswana

[2]Faculty of Medicine and Health Sciences, Department of Family Medicine and Primary Health Care, Ghent University, Belgium

[3]Division of Medical Sciences, Department of Primary Care Health Sciences, University of Oxford, United Kingdom

[4]Division of Family Medicine and Primary Care, Faculty of Medicine and Health Sciences, Stellenbosch University, South Africa

[5]School of Nursing, Faculty of Health Sciences, University of Botswana, Botswana

Correspondence to:
Oathokwa Nkomazana

Email:
nkomazanao@mopipi.ub.bwn

Postal address:
University of Botswana School of Medicine, Private Bag 00713, Gaborone, Botswana

Background: Botswana is a large middle-income country in Southern Africa with a population of just over two million. Shortage of human resources for health is blamed for the inability to provide high quality accessible health services. There is however a lack of integrated, comprehensive and readily-accessible data on the health workforce.

Aim: The aim of this study was to analyse the existing databases on health workforce in Botswana in order to quantify the human resources for health.

Method: The Department of Policy, Planning, Monitoring and Evaluation at the Ministry of Health, Ministry of Education and Skills Development, the Botswana Health Professions Council, the Nursing and Midwifery Council of Botswana and the in-country World Health Organization office provided raw data on human resources for health in Botswana.

Results: The densities of doctors and nurses per 10 000 population were four and 42, respectively; three and 26 for rural districts; and nine and 77 for urban districts. The average vacancy rate in 2007 and 2008 was 5% and 13% in primary and hospital care, respectively, but this is projected to increase to 53% and 43%, respectively, in 2016. Only 21% of the doctors registered with the Botswana Health Professions Council were from Botswana, the rest being mainly from other African countries. Botswana trained 77% of its health workforce locally.

Conclusion: Although the density of health workers is relatively high compared to the region, they are concentrated in urban areas, insufficient to meet the projected requirements and reliant on migrant professionals.

Ressources humaines pour les services de santé au Botswana: les résultats des bases de données et de l'analyse des rapports du pays.

Contexte: Le Botswana est un vaste pays à revenus intermédiaires d'Afrique australe avec un peu plus de 2 millions d'habitants. La pénurie de ressources humaines dans le domaine de la santé est rendue responsable de l'incapacité à fournir des services de santé accessibles et de haute qualité. Cependant, on manque de données accessibles, complètes et intégrées sur les professionnels de la santé.

Objectif: L'objectif de cette étude était d'analyser les bases de données existantes sur les professionnels de la santé au Botswana afin de quantifier les ressources humaines de santé.

Méthode: Le Département de Politique, Planification, Contrôle et Evaluation au Ministère de la Santé, le Ministère de l'Education et du Développement des Compétences, l'Association des Professionnels de la Santé du Botswana, L'Association des Infirmières et Sages-femmes du Botswana et le bureau de l'Organisation mondiale de la Santé dans le pays ont fourni des données brutes sur les Ressources humaines de Santé au Botswana.

Résultats: La densité de docteurs et infirmières par 10 000 habitants était de 4 et 42, respectivement, 3 et 26 dans les zones rurales et 9 et 77 dans les zones urbaines. Le taux moyen de vacance de postes en 2007/2008 était respectivement de 5% et 13% dans les soins primaires et les soins hospitaliers, mais on s'attend à ce qu'ils atteignent respectivement 53% et 43% en 2016. Seuls 21% des docteurs inscrits à l'Association des professionnels de la santé étaient du Botswana, le reste venait surtout d'autres pays africains. Le Botswana a formé localement 77% de ses professionnels de santé.

Conclusion: Bien que la densité des professionnels de santé soit relativement élevée par rapport à la région, ils sont concentrés dans les zones urbaines, et sont insuffisants pour satisfaire les besoins futurs et dépendent des professionnels itinérants.

Introduction

The African region has 3% of the world's health workforce to tackle 24% of the global burden of disease.[1] With only 11% of the world's population, the region accounts for half the world's maternal and child deaths and more than 90% of the world's deaths from malaria and HIV.[2] The United Nation's Millennium Development Goals (MDGs) call for reducing under-five mortality by two-thirds and maternal mortality by three-quarters by 2015. Sub-Saharan Africa is unlikely to achieve those goals without significant increases in skilled human resources for health.[3,4] There is ample evidence that an increase in the number and quality of healthcare workers is associated positively with improved health outcomes.[1] The shortage of human resources for health in sub-Saharan Africa is attributed to a number of complex factors including inadequate numbers trained, inappropriate skill mixes, inequitable distribution and migration.[1] Migration to North America and Western Europe was the major cause of faculty loss in the Sub-Saharan African Medical Schools Survey.[5] The exodus of skilled professionals in the midst of so much unmet health need places Africa at the epicentre of the global health workforce crisis, which contributes to weak health systems.[6]

Botswana and human resources for health

Botswana is a landlocked country in Southern Africa with a landmass of 582 000 km^2 and a population of just over 2 million.[7] It has an annual government and total expenditure on health per capita of $246 and $382, respectively.[3] There are 28 health districts made up of five urban, four rural and 19 rural districts, with one or more urban villages. For the purposes of this paper, urban areas are defined as 'all settlements with a population of 5000 or more persons with at least 75% of labour force in non-agricultural occupations (subsistence farming)[7] and villages are defined as settlements on tribal land, which have tribal administration and some basic services, including a primary care clinic, primary school and a post office. Combining these definitions, 27 villages were designated as 'urban villages' and this then leads to a distinction between districts that are completely rural and districts that are rural with one or more urban villages.[7]

Botswana's health services are mostly public with a small but growing private sector. The healthcare system is based on a primary healthcare model and services are provided through a network of three referral hospitals, seven district hospitals, 14 primary hospitals, three private hospitals, three mine hospitals, two mission hospitals, 265 primary care clinics (101 with maternity beds), a number of specialists and general private outpatient clinics (mostly in towns and some urban villages), 343 health posts and 861 mobile clinic sites. This has brought 95% of the total population (89% of the rural population) within eight kilometres of a healthcare facility. Access to a healthcare facility does not always translate to good health service, as many of the facilities are severely short staffed (MoH, Integrated Health Services Plan [IHSP] 2012, personal communication, Jan 23). Life expectancy at birth is estimated at 61 years.[3] The infant and under-five mortality rates are 36 and 48 per 1000 live births respectively and the maternal mortality ratio (MMR) is 160/100 000 births.[3,8]

The major employer of health workers in Botswana is the government. Prior to 2010, primary healthcare was managed by the Ministry of Local Government, but from April 01 2010, all healthcare was transferred to the Ministry of Health. A shortage of skilled and qualified healthcare workers remains one of the major bottlenecks toward the availability of accessible high quality healthcare in Botswana with 3.4 doctors and 28.4 nurses per 10 000 people.[3] Training of health workers is achieved through a combination of in-country and foreign training institutions. In-country training is done at the eight Institutes of Health Sciences for diploma courses in nursing, midwifery, health education, laboratory, radiography and dental technology. The University of Botswana provides Bachelor's degrees and Master's degree courses in nursing, including specialist nursing, laboratory technology, environmental health and it will graduate its first class of doctors in October 2014. The Institutes of Health Sciences and the University of Botswana are public institutions. There is one private institution which offers training in phlebotomy, plaster, theatre and dental assistance, as well as training for health care auxiliaries.

Botswana has a paucity of readily-accessible, integrated and comprehensive information on human resources for health. A decision was therefore made to collate and analyse the available data from different sources, which are otherwise fragmented and sometimes difficult to access within the Ministry of Health (MoH), Ministry of Local Government and Ministry of Education and Skills Development. Professional regulatory bodies and multiple consultancy reports are also useful sources of information. The Department of Policy, Planning, Monitoring and Evaluation (DPPME) is responsible for human resources planning for the MoH. The Botswana Health Professions Council (BHPC) is the regulatory body for all doctors and allied health professionals, whilst the Nursing and Midwifery Council of Botswana (NMCB) is responsible for the registration and regulation of the practice of nurses and midwives.

The Ministry of Education and Skills Development (MESD) provides scholarships for tertiary education, including health sciences, both inside and outside the country. The Department of Tertiary Education Funding (DTEF) is responsible for administering these scholarships.

For the purposes of this study the following definitions of health cadres are used: 'medical officers' are generalist doctors without specialist training and 'nurses' refers to all nursing cadres including midwives, family nurse practitioners, community health nurses and all other nurses; 'clinical support staff' comprises health workers with minimal to no formal training that assist with patient care including theatre technicians, plaster technicians and nurse auxiliaries. Other health workers' on the other hand refers to healthcare workers with training of up to 18 months, such as lay counsellors, phlebotomists, healthcare auxiliaries and health education assistants. 'Pharmacists' refers to pharmacists and pharmacy technicians (trained at diploma level). 'Medical laboratory scientists' refers to scientists (degree holders) and technicians (diploma holders).

Aim and objectives

The aim of this study was to analyse the existing databases and report on the health workforce in Botswana in order to quantify and describe the situation with regard to the human resources for health. The specific objectives were:

1. To quantify the different types of health workers in Botswana.
2. To determine the vacancy rates for the different health worker categories at primary and higher levels of healthcare.
3. To compare the Botswana Human Resources Strategic Plan for Health (BHRSPH)'s recommended numbers of health workers to baseline levels at primary and higher levels of care.
4. To describe the density and distribution of the different health workers.
5. To describe the country of origin of health workers in Botswana.
6. To determine the number and place of training of Botswana health workers.

Research methods and design

A compilation and analysis of the existing databases on human resources for health was carried out. This entailed face-to-face meetings with the DPPME of the MoH, the DTEF of the MESD, the BHPC, the NMCB and the in-country World Health Organization (WHO) office to explain the purpose of the study. Formal requests for their particular databases were subsequently made to each of the bodies. The data were collected from November 2011 to May 2012 and covered the period from 2007 to 2012.

The DPPME provided raw data on the 2009 head count of all their health workers as well as the 2012 database. The latter database also provided information on the distribution of the health workers in the country and the information on the number of these workers who were Batswana (citizens of Botswana). They also provided a number of consultancy reports, including the National Health Services Situational Analysis (NHSSA) as well as a number of policy and strategy documents including the National Health Policy (NHP), the BHRSPH (2008–2016) and the 10-year IHSP (2010–2020) and the Essential Health Services Package (EHSP). These are sources for some of the information in this study.

The BHPC provided data on the numbers, country of origin and distribution of the healthcare professionals registered with the council. The NMCB provided summary statistics of the nurses and midwives registered with the council, including the total numbers and the countries of origin.

The database on Batswana students, who were funded to study health science courses from 1997 to 2010, was sourced from the DTEF.

The in-country WHO office provided the Botswana Human Resources for Health Country Profile, which is the source of some of the information in this article.

Once the data were collected, attempts were made to improve their quality by seeking clarification on the definition of categories of health workers used by different sources. The databases were created over different time periods, with data collected for different purposes. They therefore had different types of information and none had enough information to answer all the aims of this study. Therefore, each database was used to answer different aspects of the study objectives, based on the relevance and perceived completeness of their information. The data were used to compile the different categories of health workers and calculate summary statistics. There was not enough information to calculate the change in the numbers or types or distribution of health workers over time.

Results

The quantities of health workers

In 2007 and 2008 MoH, Ministry of Local Government had a total staff complement of 6353, which included 2321 health workers (Table 1). The other employees were non-clinical non-technical support staff, administrators and non-clinical managers. The health workers included Bachelor's degree holders such as pharmacists, dentists, laboratory scientists, as well as technicians trained to diploma levels, including dental therapists, pharmacy and laboratory technicians (Tables 1 and 2). Medical Specialists at Primary Health Care level in 2007 and 2008 were Public Health Specialists. The recommended posts (Tables 1 and 2) are the estimated number of healthcare workers that will be required to provide health services in 2016 according to the BHRSPH. The projected 2016 vacancy rate is based on the number of filled positions in 2007 and 2008 (baseline) and the planned 2016 target for posts, assuming that there will be the same number of health workers in 2016 as at baseline.

Prior to 2010, the MoH had a total workforce of 9652 which included 4952 health workers who were employed on the clinical platform in secondary and tertiary health institutions (Table 2). The MoH also employed 220 other health professionals who have been excluded from the analysis as they do not work on the clinical platform, but are teachers at the Institutes of Health Sciences (MoH, BHRSPH 2012, personal communication, Jan. 23)

Vacancies

In 2007 and 2008 there were vacancies in seven of the 13 health worker categories in primary care. The vacancies were highest

TABLE 1: Primary care staff establishment 2007 and 2008 and recommendations for 2016.

Health worker category	Total posts	Filled posts	Current vacancy rate (% total posts)	Recommended posts	Projected 2016 vacancy rate (%) (FP/RP)
Dental therapists	2	2	0	0	-
Dieticians	0	0	0	26	100
Environmental health officers	75	70	7	164	57
Medical laboratory scientists	40	40	0	26	-
Medical officers	69	63	9	79	20
Nurses	1897	1816	4	3089	41
Other allied health workers	23	22	4	26	15
Pharmacists	89	78	12	392	80
Physiotherapists	2	2	0	0	-
Radiographers	4	6	0	0	-
Medical specialists	18	13	28	26	50
Social workers	19	19	0	26	27
Clinical support staff	38	38	0	0	-
Other health workers	45	40	11	868	95
Totals	**2321**	**2209**	**5**	**4722**	**53**

Source: Ministry of Health, Botswana Human Resources Strategic Plan for Health 2012, personal communication, January 23

TABLE 2: Secondary and tertiary hospital staff establishment 2007 and 2008 and recommendations for 2016.

Post category	Total posts	Filled posts	Current vacancy rate (% total posts)	Recommended posts	Projected 2016 vacancy rate (%) (FP/RP)
Dentists	28	21	25	40	48
Dieticians	17	15	12	17	12
Dental therapists	61	79	0	105	25
Environmental health officers	51	0	100	33	100
Medical laboratory technicians	248	254	0	587	57
Medical officers	244	195	20	356	45
Nurses	3552	2898	18	3147	8
Other allied health workers	189	134	29	267	50
Occupational therapists	10	11	0	28	61
Pharmacists	241	245	0	509	52
Physiotherapists	16	16	0	58	72
Psychologists	5	4	20	13	69
Radiographers	48	40	17	104	62
Medical specialists	137	89	35	192	54
Speech therapists	1	0	100	13	100
Social workers	2	38	0	65	42
Clinical support staff	89	233	0	387	40
Other health workers	13	18	0	1671	99
Totals	**4952**	**4290**	**13**	**7592**	**43**

Source: Ministry of Health, Botswana Human Resources Strategic Plan for Health 2012, personal communication, January 23
FP, Filled posts; RP, Recommended posts.

for medical specialists, pharmacists, medical officers and other health workers respectively (Table 1). The number of radiographers employed exceeded the number of established positions. The mean vacancy rate in primary care was 5%. There were very high vacancy rates in 10 of the 18 health worker categories in secondary and tertiary health care, the worst of which was for environmental health officers and speech therapists (Table 2). Dental therapists, social workers, clinical support staff and other health workers (Table 2) exceeded the number of established positions. The mean vacancy rate for secondary and tertiary healthcare services was 13%.

The vacancy rates were much higher in secondary and tertiary healthcare services compared to primary health care (Figure 1), except for pharmacists where there were no vacancies in secondary/tertiary care compared to a 12% vacancy rate in primary care. Other health professionals refer to all other health workers excluding nurses, doctors, dentists and/or dental therapists, and pharmacists and/or pharmacy technicians (Figures 1 and 2).

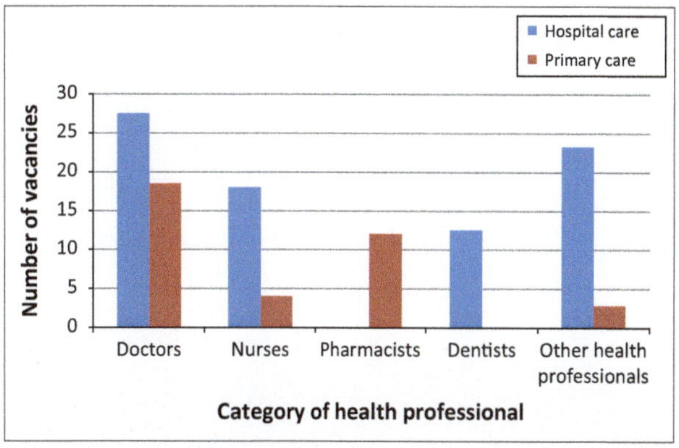

Source: Ministry of Health, Botswana Human Resources Strategic Plan for Health 2012, personal communication, January 23

FIGURE 1: Comparison of vacancy rates in primary care versus secondary and/or tertiary hospital care 2007 and 2008.

Recommended number of health workers for 2016 compared to baseline

To implement the BHRSPH, moderate increases in the numbers of healthcare workers will be required from baseline to the levels planned for 2016 (Tables 1 and 2, Figure 2). The highest increases at all levels of care will be in the 'other health worker' category with a projected 2016 vacancy rate of 95% in primary care and 99% in higher levels of care. Dieticians will be introduced in primary care and pharmacists increased significantly (Table 1). Some types of health workers are to be removed completely from primary care, including dental therapists, radiographers, physiotherapists and clinical support staff (Table 1). The number of nurses in secondary and/or tertiary care is to be reduced whilst those in primary care are to increase significantly (Figure 2). The mean 2016 vacancy rate, based on the 2007 and/or 2008 filled positions and the planned 2016 targets, is 53% in primary care compared to 43% in the secondary or tertiary care levels.

Density and distribution of health workers

The densities of health workers were highest in urban areas and lowest in the rural districts with one or more urban villages (Table 3). In 2012, Gaborone, with 11% of Botswana's population, was home to 250 (34%) doctors and 1113 (17%) nurses whilst Francistown, with 5% of the population, had 100 (13%) doctors and 530 (8%) nurses (MoH 2012, personal communication, Jan. 23). In 2009, the proportion of doctors working in Gaborone and Francistown was 43% and 15% and for nurses, 11% and 4%, respectively (MoH, IHSP 2012, personal communication, Jan. 23).

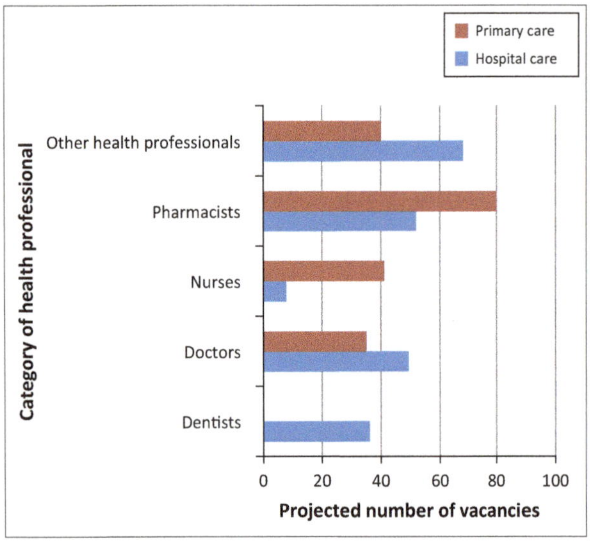

Source: Ministry of Health, Botswana Human Resources Strategic Plan for Health 2012, personal communication, January 23

FIGURE 2: Comparison of projected 2016 vacancy rates for primary care versus secondary and/or tertiary hospital care.

Country of origin of Botswana health workers

In 2012, 13 713 health workers were registered with the BHPC and NMCB. The BHPC had 4416 registrants whilst the NMCB had 9297 (Table 4). There were 1820 doctors registered with the Botswana Health Professions Council. Batswana (native-born and naturalised citizens of Botswana) made up 41% of all health professionals registered with BHPC and 84% of the nurses registered with NMCB (Table 4). Only 21% of the doctors registered with the BHPC were Batswana compared with 84% of nurses (Table 4). Batswana were also in the minority amongst physiotherapists (39%), radiographers (13%) and optometrists (35%) (BHPC 2012, personal communication, May 16).

The major contributors to health professionals registered with the BHPC in 2012 were Botswana, Zimbabwe, Democratic Republic of Congo (DRC) and Zambia (Table 5). Zimbabwe mainly contributed doctors (n = 191), laboratory scientists (n = 127), physiotherapists (n = 34), radiographers (n = 90), pharmacy technicians (n = 49), pharmacists (n = 52) and laboratory technicians (n = 43), whilst Zambia mainly contributed doctors (n = 73), laboratory technicians (n = 28), pharmacy technicians (n = 42), physiotherapists (n = 19) and radiographers (n = 77). The DRC was a significant source of doctors (n = 333) (BHPC 2012, personal communication, May 16).

Training of health workers

Between 1997 and 2010, an estimated 7154 Batswana graduated as health professionals with government financial support (Table 6). Of these, 1665 (23%) graduated from universities in 21 countries in Europe, North America, South America, Australia, Africa and South East Asia. This latter group included doctors (48%), pharmacists (10%), dentists (11%) and nurses (11%), as well as physiotherapists, nutritionists, dieticians, biomedical engineers, optometrists, occupational therapists, radiographers, audiologists and speech therapists and occupational health and safety officers.

Discussion

The density of doctors and nurses per 10 000 population was 4.3 and 41.3, respectively, using the MoH database of 2012. The densities of doctors and nurses in rural districts were significantly lower than urban districts. This is in keeping with the findings in many low- and middle-income countries.[9,10,11] Disparity in the distribution with significant

TABLE 3: Density of health workers (per 10 000 population) in Botswana per district type.

District type	Population	Doctor	Nurses and/or midwives	Pharmacists	Dentists	Healthcare workers
Rural	98 816	3	26	1	0	45
Rural with urban villages	1 515 181	2	22	1	1	35
Urban	424 231	9	77	4	1	115
Total	**2 038 228**	**4**	**42**	**2**	**1**	**65**

Source: Ministry of Health, Department of Policy, Planning, Monitoring and Evaluation 2012, personal communication, April 04

TABLE 4: Health workers who are citizens of Botswana as compared to the total number of health workers in Botswana.

Health workers	Total number	Batswana	
		n	%
Doctors	1820	382	21
Nurses	9297	7845	84
Dentists and/or dental therapists	296	223	75
Pharmacists and/or pharmacy technicians	764	402	53
Other health workers	3645	2226	61
Total	**13 713**	**9635**	**70**

Source: Ministry of Health, Botswana Health Professions Council and Nursing and Midwifery Council of Botswana 2012, personal communication, May 16

TABLE 5: Country of origin of health professionals registered with the Botswana Health Professions Council in 2012.

Country of origin	All healthcare workers (N = 4416)		Doctors (N = 1820)	
	n	%	*n*	%
Botswana	1790	40	382	21
Zimbabwe	630	14	191	10
Democratic Republic of Congo	351	8	333	18
Zambia	266	6	73	4
India	199	4	97	5
Nigeria	174	4	96	5
Republic of South Africa	140	3	101	6
United States of America	110	2.5	70	4
Kenya	109	2.5	37	2
Tanzania	101	2.3	65	4
Ethiopia	72	1.6	69	4
China	59	1.3	55	3
Uganda	56	1.3	40	2
Other African	90	2.0	48	3
Other non-African	269	6.1	163	9

Source: Ministry of Health. Botswana Health Professions Council 2012, personal communication, May 16

TABLE 6: Numbers and place of training of state-supported health professionals graduated between 1997 and 2010.

Health care trained	N	Botswana		Other countries	
		n	%	*n*	%
Dentists[1]	272	89	33	183	67
Pharmacists[1]	350	190	54	160	46
Nurses[1]	5031	4846	96	185	4
Doctors	802	0	0	802	100
Other health workers	699	364	52	335	48
Total	**7154**	**5489**	**77**	**1665**	**23**

Source: Department of Tertiary Education Funding 2012, personal communication, April 06
[1], Bachelors and diploma levels.

skewing favouring urban areas is also well described in many settings.[12,13] The densities are a little higher in purely rural districts because these are very sparsely populated, with some clinics attending to as few as four patients a day (MoH, IHSP 2012, personal communication, Jan 23). The arrangement is necessary to meet the government targets of bringing 95% of the population within eight kilometres of a health facility.[8] The density of doctors and nurses in Botswana was similar to Namibia and higher than many countries in the region such as Zambia and Zimbabwe, but lower than South Africa.[4] A number of African countries are said to have a critical shortage of health workers, with fewer than 2.3 health workers per 10 000 population.[1] Although Botswana is not amongst the countries with a critical shortage of health workers, it still has far fewer numbers than countries with established health systems such as the United Kingdom (UK).[1]

There is evidence that adequate numbers of health workers are associated with positive health outcomes.[1] Botswana's life expectancy at birth as well as maternal and under-five mortalities were similar to Namibia, which had equivalent densities of health workers, but much better than Zimbabwe, Zambia, Uganda, Mali and Sudan, all of which had much lower health worker densities.[4] Surprisingly, Botswana's health indices were better than those of South Africa although the latter had higher health worker densities.[4] Botswana's health indices were much worse than the UK, which was in keeping with the UK's higher densities of health workers.[4] There are, of course, other factors that also contribute to these differences.

The mean vacancy rate in primary healthcare was less than that for secondary and tertiary care. This is different from many low-income countries, which have very high vacancy rates in primary healthcare compared with higher levels of care.[14,15] However, with far fewer posts now than projected for 2016 in primary care compared with secondary and/or tertiary care, the number of health workers required in primary care was grossly underestimated. This shows that the system has been skewed toward recruitment in secondary and/or tertiary care settings since only 34% of filled posts and 32% of total posts were in primary care settings. This is the inverse of what would be needed in a more efficient system based on universal access to good quality primary healthcare.[15]

Since about 2006 and 2007, the government has been rolling out the management of patients with HIV infection to primary care, which may explain the significant projected increases in the numbers of pharmacists, nurses, other health workers and medical specialist, as well as the introduction of dieticians. It is not clear from the data as to which medical specialties were intended for primary care, but according to a more recent strategy document, the EHSP (2010–2020), Family Physicians are to be based in Primary Hospitals and not in primary care clinics (MoH, IHSP 2012, personal communication, Jan. 23). Primary Hospitals are part of secondary-level care with less than 100 in-patient beds and usually do not have specialist doctors. The planned increases in other healthcare workers reflects the intention to shift a number of tasks currently done by nurses and doctors to health workers with shorter training such as health education assistants and lay counsellors as well as an increase in the links between primary care and the community-based services (MoH, EHSP 2012, personal communication, Apr. 06).

Task shifting, when properly implemented and with adequate supervision, can improve significantly the ability of countries to increase their health workforce, improve skill mixes and reduce international migration. The challenges are maintaining the quality of care and patient safety.[16] Removing radiographers, physiotherapists and dental therapists from primary care is likely to have an adverse effect on the ability of the health system to provide equitable and accessible care. The increases in the number of health workers at all levels of the health services mandates significant increases in the training of nurses, other health workers, pharmacists and doctors, including medical specialists. With only 21% of the doctors in the country being Batswana (citizens of Botswana), Botswana is heavily dependent on migrant health workers, mostly from countries such as the DRC, Zimbabwe and Zambia, which are plagued with significant political and/or economic hardships. This overdependence on an expatriate health workforce puts the country at significant risk as these health workers are likely to want to return to their countries as situations improve, or to migrate to higher-income countries.

Local training appears to reduce significantly the dependence on expatriate health workers. The dependence on foreign training institutions for doctors has proven to be ineffective and unsustainable as the majority of the graduates have tended to remain in the host countries on completion of training, which tend to be higher-income countries with better salaries and more career development opportunities (DTEF 2012, personal communication, Apr. 06). Some of the host countries also see the foreign students as a potential solution to their own human resources for health shortages. Australia, for instance is exploring the potential contribution of international medical students in Australian medical schools to the Australian medical workforce.[16] The establishment of a local medical school is intended to reduce the dependence on expatriate doctors. This will need to be monitored closely, however, as many developing countries have continued to experience a reduction in the numbers of doctors despite in-country training, because of migration to higher-income countries.[17]

Limitations

The major limitation of the study was the incompleteness and inaccuracy of the data, which made it difficult to get a reliable estimate of the quantities, densities and distribution of health workers. An unidentifiable number of health professionals on the BHPC register work outside the country. None of the databases had detailed information on health workers in other sectors of the health system such as the private sector and non-governmental organisations. Therefore, an accurate estimation of the total health worker density is not possible. Although the data span from 2007 to 2012, they are not adequate to calculate trends in human resources for health.

None of the databases available had information on the distribution of health workers according to the level of care and the data were not disaggregated to the level of the individual clinic or hospital. The only data on vacancy rates are very old, being from 2007 and 2008.

Recommendations

Botswana has an urgent need to establish a comprehensive human resource information system that will be resourced adequately in order to keep it up-to-date in real-time and accessible to all stakeholders. The information should differentiate between the different levels of healthcare and should also be disaggregated to the level of the healthcare facility. The disparity in the distribution of health workers between the rural and urban districts should be addressed as a matter of priority in order to achieve universal access to healthcare. For an optimally-functioning health system, all levels of care must be resourced both adequately and appropriately. Research is needed so as to find out how health workers can be attracted to and retained in Botswana's rural areas in order to address the disparity.

Training of doctors, including medical specialists, nurses, pharmacists and pharmacy technicians, as well as lay counsellors and health educations assistants, needs to be increased in order to meet the planned EHSP and BHRSPH requirements. All training should be supported by strategies for attraction and retention so as to reduce the heavy dependence of the country on an expatriate health workforce, especially doctors.

Conclusion

The MoH is the sole employer for the public health service. In 2007 and 2008 there were relatively high vacancy rates for different types of health workers, especially in secondary and/or tertiary care. Plans to increase significantly the numbers of health workers at all levels of health care by 2016, if not coupled with a significant injection of new health workers, will exacerbate the vacancy rates. The density of health workers in Botswana is relatively high compared to its neighbours, but this is still too low to enable the country to achieve its MDGs. Similar to many countries, health workers tend to be more densely distributed in urban compared with rural areas. Botswana has a worrisomely high dependence on an expatriate health workforce and, until recently, out-of-country training of doctors and dentists and allied health professionals. Attraction and retention of internationally-trained health workers has been unsuccessful and localisation of training is intended to more effectively meet the country's needs. In order to meet the country's human resources for health needs in a sustainable manner, more health workers will need to be trained, recruited and retained.

Acknowledgements

This work is part of the Human Resources for African Primary Care and is supported through the European Union's FP7 programme; grant agreement no. 265727: http://www.huraprim-project.eu. The researchers acknowledge the facilitation from the MoH, the MESD as well as the BHPC, the NMCB and the in-country WHO office.

Competing interests

The authors declare that they have no financial or personal relationship(s) that may have inappropriately influenced them in writing this article.

Authors' contributions

O.N. (University of Botswana School of Medicine) conceptualised the project, collected and analysed the data and drafted the manuscript. W.P. (Ghent University), M.W. (Oxford University) and R.M. (Stellenbosch University) reviewed the draft manuscript and approved the final version. N.P. (University of Botswana School of Nursing) collected the data, reviewed the manuscript and approved the final version.

References

1. World Health Organization. Working together for health: The world health report 2006. Geneva: World Health Organization; 2006.
2. Chen L, Evans T, Anand S, et al. Human resources for health: Overcoming the crisis. Lancet. 2004;364(9449):1984–1990. http://dx.doi.org/10.1016/S0140-6736(04)17482-5
3. World Health Organization. World health statistics 2012. Geneva: World Health Organization; 2012.
4. African Science Academy Development Initiative. Science in Action: Saving the lives of Africa's mothers, newborns, and children. United States National Academies; 2009.
5. Chen C, Buch E, Wassermann T, et al. A survey of sub-Saharan African medical schools. Hum Resour Health. 2012;10:4. http://dx.doi.org/10.1186/1478-4491-10-4
6. Eastwood JB, Conroy RE, Naicker S, et al. Loss of health professionals from sub-Saharan Africa: the pivotal role of the UK. Lancet. 2005;365(9474):1893–1900. http://dx.doi.org/10.1016/S0140-6736(05)66623-8
7. Botswana Central Statistics Office. 2011 Population and housing census: Preliminary Results Brief [document on the Internet]. c2011 [cited 2014 Oct 28]. Available from: http://ecastats.uneca.org/aicmd/Portals/0/Census%202011%20Preliminary%20%20Brief%20Sept%2029%202011.pdf
8. Ray S, Madzimbamuto F, Ramagola-Masire D, et al. Review of causes of maternal deaths in Botswana in 2010. S Afr Med J. 2013;103(8):537–542. http://dx.doi.org/10.7196/samj.6723
9. Dussault G, Franceschini MC. Not enough there, too many here: understanding geographical imbalances in the distribution of the health workforce. Hum Resour Health. 2006;4:12. http://dx.doi.org/10.1186/1478-4491-4-12
10. Lehmann U, Dieleman M, Martineau T. Staffing remote rural areas in middle-and low-income countries: A literature review of attraction and retention. BMC Health Serv Res. 2008;8:19. http://dx.doi.org/10.1186/1472-6963-8-19
11. Munga MA, Mæstad O. Measuring inequalities in the distribution of health workers: The case of Tanzania. Hum Resour Health. 2009;7:4. http://dx.doi.org/10.1186/1478-4491-7-4
12. Starfield B, Shi L, Macinko, J. Contribution of primary care to health systems and health. Millank Q. 2005;83(3):457–502. http://dx.doi.org/10.1111/j.1468-0009.2005.00409.x
13. Dayrit MM, Dolea C, Dreesch N. Addressing the Human Resources for Health crisis in countries: How far have we gone? What can we expect to achieve by 2015? Rev Peru Med Exp Salud Publica. 2011;28(2):327–336. http://dx.doi.org/10.1590/S1726-46342011000200022
14. Daviaud E, Chopra M. How much is not enough? Human resources requirements for primary health care: A case study from South Africa. Bull World Health Organ. 2008;86(1):46–51. http://dx.doi.org/10.2471/BLT.07.042283
15. Chukwuani CM, Olugboji A, Akuto EE, et al. A baseline survey of the primary healthcare system in south eastern Nigeria. Health Policy. 2006;77(2):182–201. http://dx.doi.org/10.1016/j.healthpol.2005.07.006
16. Hawthorne L, Hamilton J. International medical students and migration: The missing dimension in Australian workforce planning? Med J Aust. 2010;193(5):262–265.
17. Tankwanchi ABS, Özden Ç, Vermund SH. Physician emigration from sub-Saharan Africa to the United States: Analysis of the 2011 AMA physician masterfile. PLoS Med. 2013;10(9):e1001513. http://dx.doi.org/10.1371/journal.pmed.1001513

Management of type 2 diabetes mellitus: Adherence challenges in environments of low socio-economic status

Authors:
Tania Steyl[1]
Julie Phillips[1]

Affiliations:
[1]Department of Physiotherapy, University of the Western Cape, South Africa

Correspondence to:
Tania Steyl

Email:
tsteyl@uwc.ac.za

Postal address:
Private Bag X17, Bellville 7535, Western Cape, South Africa

Background: The efficacy of treatment for clients with diabetes is highly dependent on the individual's ability to manage the disease. Several constraints, such as poverty, illiteracy and insufficient resources (finances and specialised healthcare professionals), especially communities of low socio-economic status, could influence clients' ability to manage their disease.

Aim: The main aim of this study was to outline the obstacles encountered by individuals with type 2 diabetes mellitus from an urban community with regard to management of their disease.

Setting: The study was conducted at a primary health care facility in the Western Cape, South Africa.

Methods: Ethical clearance was obtained from all relevant authorities. Eight (8) conveniently selected clients with type 2 diabetes mellitus per participating community healthcare centre (six approved centres in total) were invited to take part in focus group discussions. Twenty six clients, 15 females and 11 males, with a mean age of 58.92 years (SD = 7.33), agreed to participate. Audiotaped data were transcribed verbatim followed by content analysis and identification of themes.

Results: Themes that emerged were challenges with: a healthy eating plan, physical activity, financial constraints, other people's understanding of the disease, and service received at the community healthcare centre. Verbatim quotes were used to exemplify the themes.

Conclusion: Clients with type 2 diabetes mellitus experienced several challenges in the management of their disease. These challenges should be addressed to assist with better glycaemic control and to curb the emergence of diabetic complications and their attendant cost implications.

Gestion des diabétiques de type 2: les défis d'adhérence dans des environnements à faible socio-économiques.

Contexte: L'efficacité du traitement pour les clients atteints de diabète est très dépendante de la capacité de l'individu à gérer la maladie. Plusieurs contraintes telles que la pauvreté, l'analphabétisme et l'insuffisance des ressources (finances et les professionnels spécialisés de soins de santé), en particulier dans les groupes à faible socio-économique pourraient influencer la capacité des clients à gérer leur maladie.

Objectif: L'objectif principal de cette étude était de décrire les obstacles rencontrés par les personnes atteintes de diabète de type 2 à partir d'une communauté urbaine en ce qui concerne la gestion de leur maladie.

Définition: L'étude a été menée dans un établissement de soins de santé primaires dans le Western Cape, en Afrique du Sud.

Méthodes: jeuéthique a été obtenue à partir de toutes les autorités compétentes. Huit (8) clients modèles ont été sélectionnés avec le diabète de type 2 par participant Centre de santé communautaire (six CSC approuvés au total) ont été invités à prendre part à des discussions de groupe de discussion. Vingt-six (26) clients, 15 femmes et 11 hommes avec un âge moyen de 58 à 92ans (SD = 7.33), ont accepté de participer. Les données enregistrées sur bande audio ont été transcrites intégralement suivies par l'analyse du contenu et l'identification des thèmes.

Résultats: Les thèmes émergents sont les défis avec: un plan d'alimentation saine, l'activité physique, les contraintes financières, la compréhension par les autres personnes de la maladie et le service reçu au CSC. Des citations textuelles ont été utilisées pour illustrer les thèmes.

Conclusion: Les clients avec diabète de type 2 ont connu plusieurs difficultés dans la gestion de leur maladie. Ces défis doivent être relevés pour aider à un meilleur contrôle de la glycémie et à réduire l'apparition de complications diabétiques et les répercussions sur les coûts de celles-ci.

Introduction

Key focus

The benefits of good glycaemic control in patients with diabetes mellitus (DM) have been highlighted in research, as glycaemic control is directly related to development of diabetic complications.[1] The efficacy of treatment for clients with DM is highly dependent on the individual's ability to manage the disease.[2] Several constraints, such as poverty, illiteracy and inadequate resources (finances and specialised healthcare professionals), especially in communities of low socio-economic status, could influence clients' ability to manage their disease.

Background

DM, an international pandemic, is a growing public health concern, and its prevalence is escalating exponentially with a high frequency of morbidity, premature mortality, disability, loss of productivity[3] and socio-economic challenges.[4] Diabetes is a chronic disease with no cure to date, and fewer than 50% of patients with type 2 DM globally meet glycaemic targets, even in developed countries.[5] More disturbingly, less than 10% achieve blood pressure, cholesterol and glycaemic targets, even with multifactorial interventions.[6]

Despite improvement in the management of diabetes in the Western Cape, South Africa, over the past decade, a recent audit revealed that only 48% of patients with DM had an HbA1c test done in the previous year, whilst a mere 35% reached glycaemic control (HbA1c < 7%).[1] This is of great concern as good glycaemic control is the foundation of the prevention of diabetic complications.[5]

Globally the cost implications of the management of DM are exorbitant. Almost 15% of national budgets are spent on the diagnosis and treatment of people with DM in developed countries.[7] The International Diabetes Federation agreed that given its chronic nature, the working adults mostly affected and the resources required to manage the disease, DM is a very costly disease.[8] Financial constraints of affected individuals as well as the healthcare sector could have a negative impact on management of the disease. Clients could not afford transport costs for clinic visits and prescribed healthy food, which was shown to negatively influence the outcome of disease management.[9]

The main focus of short-term management should be on keeping blood glucose levels in a specific range, therefore preventing hypoglycaemia or hyperglycaemia as well as long-term complications due to chronic hyperglycaemia.[10] The long-term aims focus on avoiding hyperglycaemia as well as later complications.[11] The benefits of good glycaemic control were recorded by two major studies, the Diabetic Control and Complication Trial conducted in the United States of America and the United Kingdom Prospective Diabetes study completed in 2003. Both concluded that glycaemic control is directly related to the development of diabetic complications.[5,12]

The Society for Endocrinology, Metabolism and Diabetes of South Africa developed guidelines for the management of patients with diabetes in South Africa, based on the findings of international studies.[5] Specific guidelines for diagnosis and management of type 2 DM for primary health care (PHC) were developed in 2012.[5] These guidelines emphasise the importance of patient education to improve self-management of the disease. Knowledge about the disease as well as management skills is not enough. Effective management of chronic diseases like diabetes calls for an integrated approach with the patient, family and community taking an active supportive role.[13] This is echoed by research which proposed that diabetes education in South Africa should involve people with DM, families, healthcare staff and communities, and should be considered as an integral and significantly important component of DM treatment and management.[14] If DM care is to reach the 'grassroots', then care needs to be focused at PHC level, along with efficient administration and education of PHC staff. As DeCoster and George[15] state: 'Integrating diabetes self-care into daily living demands more than knowledge acquisition and skill mastery; it requires acceptance of the disease, motivation for change, instrumental and emotional support, general problem-solving skills, and control over one's life – empowerment'.

The persistence of inadequate glycaemic control could be attributed to both patients and healthcare providers. Several studies have shown that a key element in the effectiveness of health care is the effective partnership between patients and healthcare providers.[16,17,18] Non-adherence, a characteristic of poor patient self-management, could increase mortality and disability as well as healthcare costs.[19] In addition, patients' attitudes and beliefs, knowledge of the disease, financial resources as well as social and family support have been identified as influencing adherence to management protocols.[16,20]

Social and family support has been shown to be either a barrier or a supporting factor to adherence to a treatment and management programme as well as glycaemic control. Stress, depression, low perceptions of self-efficacy, low levels of family and social support are consistently related to low levels of diabetes self-management.[21] In contrast, Wing and associates[22] reported that participation of spouses in an education programme had a negative effect for obese men with type 2 DM, whilst obese women with type 2 DM adhered to the programme and achieved better results.

Aim

Many factors contributing to adherence to care and management revolve around the patients themselves.[15] Against this background, the main purpose of this article is to outline obstacles encountered by individuals with

DM from an urban community in the Western Cape, South Africa, in management of their disease.

Contribution to field

If the contextual factors contributing to non-adherence to prescribed treatment and management protocols for DM are unearthed, they should be kept in mind when appropriate health promotion interventions are developed and implemented to mitigate the impact of the disease. This could assist to control the costs of DM management and complications as well as improve patients' experience regarding management of DM in South Africa.

Research methods and design

Study design

The study incorporated a cross-sectional qualitative design.

Setting

The study was conducted in the Cape Metropolitan District of the Western Cape, one of the five district municipalities of the City of Cape Town, Western Cape. The Cape Metropolitan District covers an area of 2460 km^2, has a population of 3 740 026 million people,[23] and is divided into four substructures with 39 community health centres (CHCs), of which 22 provide diabetes care and management. Of the individuals diagnosed with type 2 DM in the Western Cape, 55% are from the Cape Metropolitan District.

Study population and sampling strategy

Eight conveniently selected clients with type 2 DM per participating CHC (6 approved CHCs in total) were invited to take part in the focus group discussions (FGDs). Of the total of 48 invited clients, 26 agreed to participate, resulting in a response rate of 54.2%. The decision was made to conduct six FGDs, and if saturation was not reached more participants would be recruited. A total of six FGDs was conducted.

Data collection

The FGDs were conducted at a venue organised by the respective CHCs on a day convenient for the consenting clients. The procedure was explained to the participants and each consenting participant completed an FGD binding form. Participants were asked to reflect on the challenges they experience in the management of their disease. They were encouraged to talk freely and participate fully in the discussions. The facilitator guided the discussions to permit and encourage participation from everyone in the language used by the majority of the participants (English). The decision about language medium was made by the group. The sessions were concluded when each participant said they could not think of anything else to add. Each session lasted between 45 minutes to an hour. The responses were audiotaped and recorded on paper.

Data analysis

Data from the audiotape recordings was transcribed verbatim by an independent person with experience in transcription to produce a manuscript. A comparison was made between notes taken during the discussions to verify accuracy. Content analysis was done by extracting meaningful ideas from the participants' opinions (coding into themes). Thereafter the transcripts were read several times by the authors to look for emerging themes. The themes identified by the authors were compared to the themes identified by an independent researcher. Grouping of the themes into broader categories was done in order to fit small categories together.

Data storage

All tapes were destroyed once they had been transcribed and documented according to themes. The transcribed data were stored in a locked and safe place.

Ethical considerations

Ethical approval was obtained from the relevant university authority of the University of the Western Cape, South Africa (clearance number 11/4/2), the Western Cape Department of Health (six of the seven randomly selected CHCs) and the facility managers of the six approved CHCs.

The purpose of the study was clearly explained to all consenting participants using an information sheet. Signed, written informed consent was obtained from 26 of the clients with DM prior to the FGDs. The consent form, information sheet and questionnaire were available in English, Afrikaans and isiXhosa. Participation in the study was voluntary. The participants were informed of their right to withdraw from the study at any time without any consequences. Identification codes using numbers were employed on data forms to ensure anonymity. Only the researcher and research assistant had the details of the participants. Information obtained from the informal discussions was handled with confidentiality. Participants in the discussion signed an FGD binding form in which they undertook not to disclose any information from the discussion.

Minimal perceived risks were expected in the study. However, if participants were affected by the study and experienced questions as traumatic, they would be referred to a counsellor for management. Although the participants will not directly benefit from the study, the results could be used to develop and implement appropriate health promotion strategies at PHC settings in South Africa.

Trustworthiness

Trustworthiness of qualitative data is measured by its credibility, which in qualitative research is determined by the match between assembled realisms of the participants and the data drawn from the participants presented by the researcher.[24] Several steps were considered to build credibility: prolonged engagement and persistent observation; member checks by giving feedback of the data to participants so that they could comment on accuracy of the recordings; responses were transcribed verbatim; and independent researchers were asked to read through the transcripts and generate the themes.

Results

Six FGDs were facilitated by the researcher and research assistant. Twenty six clients, 15 females and 11 males, with a mean age of 58.92 years (SD = 7.33) agreed to participate.

The emerging themes generated from the thematic analysis of the FGDs were as follows, and are outlined below:

> Challenges with a healthy eating plan; Challenges with physical exercise; Financial constraints; Other people's understanding of the disease; and Service received at the CHC.

Verbatim quotes are used to further exemplify the above mentioned themes with regard to challenges experienced in self-management.

Challenges with a healthy eating plan

The majority of participants confided that they found it very difficult to follow a healthy eating plan. Their living circumstances were amongst the reasons mentioned for this:

> 'My wife passed away ... I stay on my own and don't cook for myself. It is so easy to just eat bread with something on it.' (Male, 68 years)

> 'I stay with my daughter and her family. I must eat whatever she cooks.' (Female, 60 years)

> 'I stay with my sister and her husband. She cooks all the food he loves. It is usually unhealthy ... He likes fried foods. I don't have a choice; I must eat what I get.' (Female, 66 years)

> 'I can't cook ... I just eat whatever is in the house ... usually bread and things like pies.' (Male, 57 years)

Working conditions also make it very difficult for some of the participants to follow a healthy meal plan:

> 'I work on a building site. We don't have regular breaks and I am divorced. So I have to pack my own lunch and snacks. It is so much easier just to buy a pie and chips at the shop.' (Male, 57 years)

> 'To say the least, my boss is very strict and does not allow you to eat whilst you work. I work in a factory. Even though I have a letter from the hospital to say that I must eat regular small meals, he insists that I "clock in and out". Now I lose pay!' (Female, 56 years)

Challenges with physical exercise

The clients expressed awareness of the importance of physical activity, although some are not engaging in physical activity. Safety in their neighbourhoods was also of great concern and expressed by the majority of participants in the FGDs. The following quotations illustrate their sentiments:

> 'I wish there was a place in the community where I could go to exercise ... like the church hall or so. And I don't feel safe to exercise around the house.' (Female, 63 years)

> 'I get up early in the morning to go to work and then I get back very late. It is already dark outside. It is really too dangerous to go for a walk then.' (Male, 60 years)

Participants also stated that lack of time hampers their participation in physical activity. This is reflected in the statements below:

> 'I work full-time in an office and when I get home I must do all my housework myself and cook for the family. I really don't have time to exercise during the week.' (Female, 47 years)

> 'I work half-day and then look after my grandchildren in the afternoon. There is no time to do formal exercise.' (Female, 52 years)

Changing a bad habit was also reported to be a challenge when it comes to exercise:

> 'I am very lazy ... I don't even like to walk, I actually hate any form of exercise.' (Male, 69 years)

> 'I am so overweight all the years. I don't have the energy to exercise. I only do some of my housework. Otherwise I sit all day and watch TV.' (Female, 63 years)

There was a sentiment amongst participants that their general feeling of well-being as well as physical disabilities precluded them from exercising:

> 'Some days I am too tired to get out of bed. I also have a heart problem.' (Female, 68 years)

> 'My foot was amputated last year and now I must walk with crutches. My hands get sore and tired when I walk too much.' (Male, 64 years)

Financial constraints

Lack of money was reported to be a key challenge in the management of type 2 DM, as it causes difficulty for the participants in buying healthy food and going to the CHCs for regular check-ups. This is illustrated in the following excerpts:

> 'I get a grant. My two grandchildren stay with us. We don't have money to buy all the right foods like the stuff that you can use in the place of sugar and all the vegetables. The children get a plate of food at school and sometimes we just eat dry bread for days.' (Female, 51 years)

> 'I only have R450 in a month for groceries. So I buy cheap stuff, not the vegetables that are very expensive.' (Female, 59 years)

> 'My daughter takes my grant ... so I can't buy food myself ... I have no money.' (Female, 66 years)

> 'Healthy food is a lot of money ... actually, all foods are expensive. Pap and bread are the cheapest.' (Female, 71 years)

> 'I must take a taxi to go to the clinic every month. It is too far to walk and I sometimes feel too weak to walk. It is very expensive. I only get a grant and have to pay a lot for rent.' (Male, 68 years)

> 'My neighbour charges me a lot to take me to the day hospital and fetch me again. I can't get to the taxi rank; it is too far from my house.' (Female, 63 years)

Other people's understanding of the disease

A few of the participants mentioned that not all people understand what the disease entails. It causes them to struggle with proper self-management of the disease:

> 'It is very difficult at parties or family functions. They [*the family*] look at you in a funny way if you don't eat the food like pies and pastries. So now I just eat it, although I know it will badly affect my sugar. I am tired of explaining why I should not have it.' (Female, 47 years)

> 'I can't help that my clinic appointment is sometimes on the day of deadlines at the work. My boss refuses then that I can go for my appointment. Then I don't always have medication.' (Male, 60 years)

Service received at the CHC

The majority of the participants complained about the service they received at the CHC. The long waiting times to see the doctor or sister and to get their medication at the pharmacy are a major problem:

> 'The long queue at the Pharmacy is very bad. I sometimes wait half a day before I get my medication. And then it is not always the right tablets! I also once did not get enough medication to last me until my next visit.' (Female, 54 years)

> 'The staff is always in a hurry; so they don't have a lot of time to spend with you. I don't get all the information I want as they must help the other people that are waiting outside.' (Male, 68 years)

> 'I sometimes leave without seeing the doctor or sister, because it just gets too much to wait more than three hours in the queue! This also caused me not go to the clinic a few times for my appointments.' (Female, 47 years)

> 'There is not enough staff. They just do the finger-prick test and take your blood pressure, but they don't tell you what it is. If you don't ask them, you will never know if your sugar and blood pressure is high or not. But it is the Government's fault. They should employ more people to work at the clinics.' (Female, 51 years)

Discussion

Outline of the results

The importance of disinterring the perceived circumstantial factors contributing to non-adherence to self-management strategies in clients with DM has been highlighted. This study aimed to assess the challenges experienced by clients with DM in the management of their disease at PHC settings in the Western Cape, South Africa. Recognising the challenges that clients experience in the management of their disease is crucial for development and implementation of health promotion strategies.

Certain challenges with physical exercise were communicated by the participants, barriers to which included safety in the neighbourhood, lack of time, changing a bad habit, and a general feeling of well-being or health-related conditions. These findings replicate those in previous studies that examined exercise preferences and barriers to physical activity in people with type 2 DM in both the developing and developed context.[25,26,27,28] Furthermore, research reported that people's perception of unsafe neighbourhoods resulted in a broad range of negative effects, including physical inactivity[29] that also results in obesity.[30,31] The participants in the current study are from a socio-economically deprived community, hence the lack of access to safe pathways or parks, high levels of crime and low sense of safety in their neighbourhood.

Apart from the environmental factors contributing to physical inactivity, personal factors such as a low motivation to change a bad habit are also a major challenge for some clients. It is very difficult to change a bad habit if you do not have the motivation or if it is not regarded as a priority.[32] The clients' inability to set obtainable goals for themselves and to stick to them could further aggravate their sedentary habits. It is therefore imperative that health promotion strategies for clients with DM should include ways to improve self-efficacy and to set reachable goals. Furthermore, they should take into consideration perceived obstacles to adherence.[33]

As for following a healthy eating plan, the majority of participants reported that they find it very difficult to follow a healthy eating plan. Several reasons were given, i.e. living circumstances, work environment, financial constraints and other people's understanding of the disease. These results are similar to those found in research from other developing countries.[25,26,31] In the present study it was evident that the clients did not have the knowledge to substitute unhealthy food with healthier options of more or less the same price; they were of the opinion that all healthy foods are expensive.

Regarding diabetes care, a number of challenges related to the healthcare services were reported. Almost all of the participants were concerned about the shortage of staff, especially the availability of pharmacists, medical doctors and nursing staff. Some of the participants were unhappy at the short consultation times as well as seldom seeing a medical doctor. The same concerns were reported in a Ghanaian study.[34] The long waiting time in the clinic waiting room – sometimes more than two hours – was also stated to be a problem for the clients. Some of the participants noted that this was a factor in their decision to miss their scheduled appointments, an observation consistent with those of other researchers.[35]

Practical implications

The social environment carries both the potential to underpin poor care and management as well as to ameliorate unhealthy lifestyles and to support adoption of a healthy lifestyle and provision of adequate care and management of the disease. Identification of perceived barriers to self-management and instruction on how to overcome them could considerably enhance adherence to prescribed treatment.

Limitations of the study

Data were analysed cross-sectionally, therefore limiting the ability to make causal inferences.

Recommendations

Although addressing issues such as neighbourhood safety and gang violence seems like a daunting task, collaboration between several national and local government departments and community forums is required to find interim solutions. Tailored physical activity classes in community halls by lay health educators could be seen as a possible solution to increase physical activity participation in this community. This type of intervention will not only provide a safe environment for physical activity but also address social support issues, such as the desire to exercise with others and provide opportunities for socialisation. It is also in line with the *Health Care 2030* document of the Western Cape Department of Health[36] that envisages a more prominent community-based service platform where teams will be assigned with the responsibility of the health of a distinct population. Lastly, the shortage of staff should be addressed at all PHC facilities in South Africa.

Conclusion

The above findings emphasise the challenges that clients with DM experience that negatively influence their self-management strategies. It further points to the fact that clients are disempowered, with seemingly little control over their environment and social interactions. It calls for action to be taken by national and local health departments to empower clients with DM through development and implementation of health promotion strategies that bear the reported challenges in mind. This will assist clients with DM to adopt and maintain a healthy lifestyle.

Acknowledgements

Dr T. Steyl would like to thank the participants and research assistant for their participation, and the study supervisor, Prof. J. Phillips for her guidance and assistance.

Competing interests

The authors declare that they have no financial or personal relationship(s) that may have inappropriately influenced them in writing this article.

Authors' contributions

T.S. (University of the Western Cape) was the principal researcher (PhD study) and J.P. (University of the Western Cape) was the study supervisor. Both authors contributed equally to the writing of this article.

References

1. De Vries E. Integrated chronic disease audit report 2011. Cape Town: Department of Health; Western Cape.
2. Mbanya J, Gill G. Diabetes mellitus. In: E Parry, R Godfrey, D Mabey, G Gill, editors. Principles of Medicine in Africa 3rd ed. Cambridge: Cambridge University Press; 2004.
3. Steyn K. The Heart and Stroke Foundation South Africa: Heart disease in South Africa 2007. Media Data Document, Department of Medicine, University of Cape Town & Chronic Diseases of Lifestyle Unit, Medical Research Council [homepage on the Internet]. No date [cited 2013 Sept 19]. Available from: http://www.mrc.ac.za/chronic/heartandstroke.pdf
4. Mbanya J, Motala A, Sobngwi E, Assah F, Enoru S. Diabetes in sub-Saharan Africa. Lancet. 2010; 375:2254-2266. http://dx.doi.org/10.1016/S0140-6736(10)60550-8
5. Amod A, Ascott-Evans BH, Berg GI, et al. The 2012 SEMDSA Guideline for the management of type 2 diabetes mellitus (Revised). JEMDSA. 2012;17(2)(Supplement 1):S1–S95.
6. Gaebe P, Lund-Andersen H, Paving HH, Pedersen O. Effect of a multifactorial intervention on mortality in type 2 diabetes. N Engl J Med. 2008;358:580–591. http://dx.doi.org/10.1056/NEJMoa0706245
7. Arnoldi A. Functional foods, cardiovascular disease and diabetes. Boca Raton: CRC Press; 2004.
8. International Diabetes Federation. IDF Diabetes Atlas. Brussels: International Diabetes Federation; 2006.
9. Jerant AF, Von Friederichs-Fitzwater MM, Moore M. Patients' perceived barriers to active self-management of chronic conditions. Patient Educ Counsel. 2005; 57:300–307. http://dx.doi.org/10.1016/j.pec.2004.08.004
10. Watkins P, Drury P, Howell S. Diabetes and its management. Oxford: Blackwell Science; 1996.
11. Gerstein C. Mann J, Yi Q, et al. Albuminuria and risk of cardiovascular events, death, and heart failure in diabetic and non-diabetic individuals. JAMA. 2001;286:421–426. http://dx.doi.org/10.1001/jama.286.4.421
12. Genuth S, Eastman R, Kahn R, et al. Implications of the United Kingdom Prospective Diabetes Study. Diabetes Care. 2003; 26(suppl. 1):S28-S32. http://dx.doi.org/10.2337/diacare.26.2007.S28
13. Yach D, Leeder S, Bell J, Kistnasamy, B. Global chronic diseases. Science. 2005;307:317. http://dx.doi.org/10.1126/science.307.5708.317
14. Tshabalala G. Diabetic education in an African setting-focus on South Africa. Diab Int. 2001;11(4):43–44.
15. DeCoster VA, George L. An empowerment approach for elders living with diabetes: A pilot study of a community-based self-help group – the Diabetes Club. Educ Gerontol. 2005;31:699–713. http://dx.doi.org/10.1080/03601270500217787
16. Nam S, Chelsa C, Stotts NA, Kroon L, Janson SL. Barriers to diabetes management: Patient and provider factors. Diabetes Res Clin Pract. 2011;93:1–9. http://dx.doi.org/10.1016/j.diabres.2011.02.002
17. De Belvis AG, Pelone F, Biasco A, Ricciardi W, Volpe M. Can primary care professionals' adherence to evidence based medicine tools improve quality of care in type 2 diabetes mellitus? A systematic review. Diabetes Res Clin Pract. 2009;85:119–131. http://dx.doi.org/10.1016/j.diabres.2009.05.007
18. McGill M, Felton A. New global recommendations: A multidisciplinary approach to improving outcomes in diabetes. Prim Care Diabetes. 2007;1:49–55. http://dx.doi.org/10.1016/j.pcd.2006.07.004
19. Horwitz RI, Horwitz SM. Adherence to treatment and health outcomes. Arch Intern Med. 1993;153(16):1863–1868. http://dx.doi.org/10.1001/archinte.1993.00410160017001
20. Lerman I. Adherence to treatment: A key for avoiding long-term complications of diabetes. Arch Med Res. 2005;36(3):300–306. http://dx.doi.org/10.1016/j.arcmed.2004.12.001
21. Glasgow RE, Toobert DJ, Gillette CD. Psychosocial barriers to diabetes self-management and quality of life. Diabetes Spectrum. 2001;14:33–41. http://dx.doi.org/10.2337/diaspect.14.1.33
22. Wing RR, Marcus MD, Epstein LH, Jawad A. A 'family-based' approach to the treatment of obese type II diabetic patients. J Consult Clin Psychol. 1991;59:156–162. http://dx.doi.org/10.1037/0022-006X.59.1.156
23. Census 2011: Municipal Fact Sheet. Statistics South Africa, 2012 [cited 2013 March 12]. Available from: http://www.statssa.gov.za/Census2011/Products/Census_2011_Municipal_fact_sheet.pdf
24. Lincoln Y, Guba E. Naturalistic Enquiry. Beverley Hills, CA: Sage; 1985.
25. Ganiyu AB, Mabuza LH, Malete NH, Govender I, Ogunbanjo GA. Non-adherence to diet and exercise recommendations amongst patients with type 2 diabetes mellitus attending Extension II Clinic in Botswana. PHCFM. 2013;5(1)..
26. Kahn AR, Al-Adbul Lateef ZN, Al Aithan MA, et al. Factors contributing to non-compliance among diabetics attending primary health centres in the Al Hasa district of Saudi Arabia. J Fam Community Med. 2012;19(1):26–32. http://dx.doi.org/10.4103/2230-8229.94008
27. Nel C, Van Rooijen AJ, Van der Westhuizen, Viljoen I, Steenkamp EM, Mamadi S. Physical activity levels in male and female diabetic patients at the Pretoria Academic Hospital, South Africa. SAJP. 2007;63(3):2–6.
28. Wanko NS, Brazier CW, Young-Rodgers D, et al. Exercise preferences and barriers in urban African Americans with type 2 diabetes. Diabetes Educator. 2004; 30(3):502–513. http://dx.doi.org/10.1177/014572170403000322
29. Foster S, Giles-Corti B. The built environment, neighbourhood crime and constrained physical activity: An exploration of inconsistent findings. Prev Med. 2008; 47:241–251. http://dx.doi.org/10.1016/j.ypmed.2008.03.017
30. Fish JS, Ettner S, Ang A, Brown, AF. Effect of perceived neighborhood safety on body mass index. Am J Publ Health. 2010; 100(11):241–251. http://dx.doi.org/10.2105/AJPH.2009.183293
31. Burdette AM, Hill TD. An examination of processes linking perceived neighborhood disorder and obesity. Soc Sci Med. 2008;67:38–46. http://dx.doi.org/10.1016/j.socscimed.2008.03.029
32. Pender NJ. Health Promotion in Nursing Practice (2nd eds.). Norwalk: Appleton & Lange; 1987.

33. Sarkar U, Fisher L, Schillinger D. Is self-efficacy associated with diabetes self-management across race/ethnicity and health literacy? Diabetes Care. 2006;29:823–829. http://dx.doi.org/10.2337/diacare.29.04.06.dc05-1615

34. De-Graft Aikins, A. Exploring biomedical and ethnomedical representations of diabetes in Ghana and the scope for cross-professional collaboration: A social psychological approach to health policy. Soc Sci Inform. 2002; 41(4):603–630.

35. Al-Malki A. Missed appointment at maternal healthcare clinics in primary health care centres in Riyadh city: Reasons and associated factors. J Hosp Admin. 2014; 3(4):92–100.

36. Western Cape Government Health. Health Care 2030 [cited 2014 July 13]. Available from: http://www.westerncape.gov.za/text/2013/October/health-care-2030-9-oct-2013.pdf

Health sector responses to intimate partner violence: A literature review

Authors:
Kate Rees[1]
Virginia Zweigenthal[1]
Kate Joyner[2]

Affiliations:
[1]Faculty of Health Sciences, School of Public Health and Family Medicine, University of Cape Town, South Africa

[2]Division of Nursing, Faculty of Medicine and Health Sciences, Stellenbosch University, South Africa

Correspondence to:
Kate Rees

Email:
reeskste@gmail.com

Postal address:
Department of Public Health and Family Medicine, Faculty of Health Sciences, University of Cape Town, Anzio Road, Observatory 7925, South Africa

Background: Intimate partner violence (IPV) is a common and serious public health concern, particularly in South Africa, but it is not well managed in primary care.

Aim: This review aims to summarise the current state of knowledge regarding health sector-based interventions for IPV, their integration into health systems and services and the perspectives of service users and healthcare workers on IPV care, focusing on the South African context.

Method: PubMed, CINAHL, PsycINFO and Google Scholar were searched between January 2012 and May 2014. All types of study design were included, critically appraised and summarised.

Results: Exposure to IPV leads to wide-ranging and serious health effects. There is sufficient evidence that intervening in IPV in primary care can improve outcomes. Women who have experienced IPV have described an appropriate response by healthcare providers to be non-judgmental, understanding and empathetic. IPV interventions that are complex, comprehensive and utilise systems-wide approaches have been most effective, but system- and society-level barriers hamper implementation. Gender inequities should not be overlooked when responding to IPV.

Conclusion: Further evaluations of health sector responses to IPV are needed, in order to assist health services to determine the most appropriate models of care, how these can be integrated into current systems and how they can be supported in managing IPV. The need for this research should not prevent health services and healthcare providers from implementing IPV care, but rather should guide the development of rigorous contextually-appropriate evaluations.

Réponses du secteur de la santé à la violence conjugale: Une analyse documentaire.

Contexte: La violence conjugale (IPV) est une grave préoccupation commune de santé publique, particulièrement en Afrique du Sud, mais n'est pas bien gérée au niveau des soins primaires.

Objectif: Ce rapport vise à résumer l'état actuel des connaissances en ce qui concerne les interventions sanitaires contre l'IVP, leur intégration dans le système et les services de santé, et les perspectives des utilisateurs des services et des professionnels de la santé sur les soins pour l'IPV, en mettant l'accent sur le contexte sud-africain.

Méthode: On a fait des recherches en 2012 et 2013 sur PubMed, CINAHL, PsycINFO et Google Scholar. On a inclus tous les types d'études qu'on a évalués et résumés.

Résultats: L'exposition à l'IPV entraine toute une série de graves problèmes de santé. Il y a suffisamment de preuves que l'intervention dans le contexte des soins de santé primaires peut améliorer les résultats. Les femmes ayant été victimes d'IPV ont déclaré qu'une réponse appropriée par les prestataires de soins ne portait pas de jugement et était complète et compréhensive. Les interventions d'IPV qui sont complexes, complètes et utilisent des démarches à l'échelle des systèmes ont été très efficaces, mais les barrières au niveau du système et de la société entravent leur mise en œuvre. Il ne faut pas négliger les injustices liées au genre quand on réagit à l'IPV.

Conclusion: D'autres évaluations de la réaction du secteur de la santé à l'IPV seront nécessaires, pour permettre aux services de santé de déterminer les modes de soins les plus appropriés, comment les intégrer dans les systèmes actuels, et comment on peut les aider à gérer l'IPV. La nécessité de mener cette étude ne doit pas empêcher les services de santé et les prestataires de soins de mettre en œuvre les soins pour l'IPV, mais devrait plutôt guider l'élaboration d'évaluations rigoureuses et appropriées dans ce contexte.

Introduction

Intimate partner violence (IPV) refers to 'behaviour by an intimate partner that causes physical, sexual or psychological harm, including acts of physical aggression, sexual coercion, psychological abuse and controlling behaviours'.[1] The World Health Organization (WHO) estimates that 30% of women globally who have been in a relationship have experienced physical or sexual IPV.[2] In the WHO Africa region, this estimate is as high as 36.6% (95% CI 32.7; 40.5%).[2] These figures do not include emotional violence which is often omitted from prevalence studies, although it appears to be common and has serious mental health implications.[3]

In South Africa, interpersonal violence is the second-highest contributor to years of life lost[4] and, in women, IPV accounts for 62.4% of this high burden.[4] A survey of women in three South African provinces found lifetime levels of physical abuse of between 19% and 28%[5] and, in Cape Town, 42.3% of working men interviewed reported perpetrating physical violence in a relationship in the previous 10 years.[6]

When emotional abuse is measured, the figures are even higher. A survey conducted in Gauteng found that 43.7% of women reported emotional violence, whilst 65.2% of men reported perpetrating it. Emotional violence was experienced more often than any other type of violence.[7]

Despite this notable burden of disease, standardised protocols for IPV care have not been implemented in the South African primary healthcare services, leading to poor identification and inconsistent management.

This review aimed to summarise the current state of knowledge regarding health sector-based interventions for IPV, their integration into health systems and the perspectives of service users and healthcare workers on IPV care, focusing on the South African context.

Methods

Multiple searches of PubMed, CINAHL, PsycINFO and Google Scholar were conducted between January 2012 and May 2014. All types of study design were included. Keywords included intimate partner violence; domestic abuse; violence against women; gender-based violence; South Africa; developing countries; intervention; and health systems. The review was undertaken as part of a larger research project whose protocol was approved by the University of Cape Town's Faculty of Health Sciences' Human Research Ethics Committee (reference 655/2012).

Review findings

Health effects

For women experiencing IPV, the negative effects span all aspects of health and can lead to mortality, morbidity and increased risk factors for poor health outcomes. These effects are mediated through multiple pathways, including physical trauma, psychological trauma and stress, as well as controlling behaviours leading to limited reproductive control and lack of autonomy in healthcare seeking.[2]

Mortality can be caused through homicide, or indirectly through suicide,[8] maternal causes[9] and an association with HIV.[10] Increased morbidity results from increased mental disorders, injuries, increased chronic conditions and physical complaints and reproductive health problems, including HIV and other sexually-transmitted infections.[2,8,11]

Mental disorders that are most prevalent amongst women who have experienced IPV include depression, post-traumatic stress disorder, suicidal tendencies and alcohol and substance abuse.[12] A recent study in South Africa found that of women who obtained protection orders against intimate partners, 66.4% experienced severe depression symptoms and 51.9% experienced symptoms of severe post-traumatic stress disorder.[13] A recent systematic review of longitudinal studies was able to conclude that IPV is associated with incident depression symptoms, adding to evidence of a causal relationship.[14]

Women who have experienced IPV are more likely to report poor overall health and more likely to suffer physical symptoms, including pain.[8] They are also more likely to have gastrointestinal symptoms and diagnosed functional gastrointestinal disorders, gynaecological disorders and many more physical disorders.[11]

IPV is associated with an increased risk of being HIV positive, even after adjusting for risk-taking behaviours.[10] Besides the biological risk resulting from forced sex, male perpetrators are more likely to engage in risky behaviours outside of the relationship and are therefore more likely to transmit HIV.[15] Women who are in controlling or abusive relationships are also less able to negotiate condom use.[2] Risky behaviours associated with IPV include multiple partners, transactional sex and substance abuse.[10]

Pregnancy outcomes are worse for women experiencing IPV, in terms of both maternal and foetal health. Poor maternal health outcomes include increased rates of sexually-transmitted infections, vaginal bleeding and premature rupture of membranes. Poor foetal outcomes include low birth weight and preterm delivery.[9] There is also evidence that IPV can be linked to unintended pregnancy.[16]

Women who have a history of IPV have been shown to have significantly higher levels of healthcare utilisation[17] and the estimated economic burden is significant.[18] In Canada, the annual cost resulting from IPV amongst women who had recently left a violent relationship was estimated to be 6.9 billion Canadian dollars.[19] This emphasises that leaving a relationship does not necessarily mean the end of violence or its impacts.

The high global burden of IPV, its numerous health effects, its impact on efforts to prevent HIV and the opportunity afforded to healthcare providers to inquire about violence, have contributed to growing recognition that IPV is an issue of major public health concern.

Conceptualising intimate partner violence

Many theoretical perspectives and frameworks have been used to explain and guide research on IPV. For example, the feminist perspective highlights patriarchy and male dominance as causes of IPV, whilst the sociological perspective points to prior experiences of violence and unequal resources in relationships.[20] An ecological framework approach attempts to pull together factors that lead to violence on multiple levels, incorporating individual, relationship, societal and structural causes.[21] No one theory fully explains IPV; causes are complex, interrelated and contextual with dynamic, non-linear pathways.[22]

A theoretical model developed by Jewkes[22] describes two community-level factors that operate as necessary causes of IPV. These are gender inequality – or male superiority – and social acceptance of the use of violence to resolve conflict. Both are prevalent features of South African communities.[22]

Poverty interacts with these factors by hampering the ability of women to leave violent relationships; and potentially leading men who are disempowered economically to gain power by exerting dominance over women.[23] Masculine identity is a possible mediator in the relationship between poverty and IPV, with men living in poverty being unable to fulfil their conceptualisation of masculinity, ultimately leading to violence on their part.[22]

On a relationship level, the existence of conflict, negative styles of conflict-management, as well as alcohol abuse (which also acts on an individual level), are important contributors to IPV. Relationship conflict has been hypothesised to be a mediator in the relationship between both poverty[22] and alcohol[23] and IPV, with conflict arising around household finances or one partner's drinking leading to violence. Conflict that is most likely to lead to IPV is related to women contravening accepted gender roles. In South Africa, this often translates to women having multiple partners, women drinking alcohol or conflict about male drinking.[22]

There is evidence that a life course perspective could be useful in understanding IPV risk. Experiences in childhood and early adulthood, such as childhood abuse, earlier age at first sex or forced first sex, have been shown to increase IPV risk in women.[24,25] The WHO multi-country study on women's health and domestic violence found that risk was highest when both the woman and her partner experienced a risk factor,[24] highlighting the importance of prevention approaches that target both men and women.

The response of the health sector to intimate partner violence

Despite growing recognition that IPV is an important public health issue, there has been a relative lack of evidence regarding the most effective health system responses.[26,27,28] A Cochrane review of IPV interventions concluded that there is insufficient evidence to show whether current health sector-based approaches are effective in reducing violence or improving psychological well-being.[28] This points to a need for the development of new health sector responses,[29] as well as more rigorous evaluations of interventions and their integration into health services and systems, particularly in primary care, which is relatively under-represented in the literature.[27,30]

There is, however, sufficient evidence that intervening for IPV in a primary care setting can be beneficial. A recent systematic review of interventions based in primary care found that 76% of 17 included studies showed an improvement in at least one measured outcome, including reductions in IPV, improvement in health-related quality of life and increased safety-promoting behaviours.[31] Included studies were largely of United States origin, with only one study originating in South Africa, one in Peru and one in Hong Kong.

The WHO has recently published clinical and policy guidelines for responding to IPV and sexual violence,[1] synthesising the best available evidence in an attempt to increase the prominence of IPV as a health concern. On a policy level, the guidelines recommend integrating services into existing structures as far as possible, as well as having multiple models of care appropriate for different levels, but prioritising primary care.[1] These recommendations are all based on very low-quality evidence, reflecting the relative lack of quality evaluations of health system responses. The guideline outlines minimum requirements for an appropriate health sector response, including having clear local policies and protocols, ensuring supportive management including financial resources, providing comprehensive care as well as resource materials, working intersectorally, providing appropriate monitoring and evaluation and providing support for carers.[1]

Screening and intervening

In primary care, intervention for IPV usually consists of screening or identification of women experiencing IPV, followed either by on-site intervention or referral to further specialised services.[31] Universal screening for IPV is controversial, although the need to identify cases non-routinely in healthcare settings is widely accepted.[32] Since 2013, the U.S. Preventive Services Task Force has recommended universal screening for IPV in women of childbearing age.[33] However, a more recently-published, well-conducted randomised controlled trial (the WEAVE study) found no difference in primary outcomes between women who were screened routinely for violence and a control group.[34] This trial, in addition to prior evidence,[35,36] has led to the expert conclusion that universal screening for IPV is ineffective in improving health.[29] Although screening is able to identify women experiencing IPV, uptake of interventions is impeded by numerous barriers and is often low and, in the setting of asymptomatic women, current intervention approaches have not been shown to be of benefit.

Inquiring about and discussing violence in specific cases during healthcare encounters (selective screening or case-finding) has been recommended as an alternative approach,[29,37] followed by more complex, individualised interventions.[29] This approach has been demonstrated to be feasible, with a cluster randomised controlled trial showing that training and support can significantly increase the number of women identified and referred to services in the absence of universal screening.[38]

Several trials of IPV interventions in primary care have recently taken place, most of them in developed countries, utilising doctors, nurses and lay providers to deliver interventions either on or off-site.[34,35,38,39] These interventions commonly use empathic approaches and attempt to empower women by helping them to understand their situation, improve their safety and access community resources.[31]

One randomised controlled trial with two levels of intervention (provision of a referral resource card and a protocol administered by a nurse) found both intervention groups experienced significant decreases in violence, suggesting that even the act of disclosure may be an important driver of change for women experiencing IPV.[39]

System-level interventions

Reviews of IPV interventions have emphasised that comprehensive, system-wide approaches have been the most effective.[26,40,41] IPV interventions are complex, requiring more than health care provider training to enable effective programme functioning within a health system. For example, a realist review (focusing on programme mechanisms to understand how and why programmes work) found that providers can be supported by four elements of an IPV programme: institutional support at high levels; effective protocols; ongoing training; and immediate access to support services.[40]

The evidence base informing the scale-up of IPV interventions and their integration into health systems is lacking.[42] However, examples of published investigations that do exist provide lessons of interest to those wishing to institute an appropriate response to IPV. In Malaysia, the national scale-up of One Stop Crisis Centres, an integrated health sector response to IPV, was investigated. Factors relating to health system structure and organisation, as well as external policy constraints, were found to be barriers to implementation.[42] Several system-level factors arising from this case study could be applicable in other contexts. Commitment at policy level was found to be necessary, which could be communicated to service delivery level by incorporating appropriate indicators into routine reporting. Adequate training, as well as adjustments to service delivery, in order to ensure that providers have the necessary time and privacy available to them, were required. Finally, flexibility of the model was important so as to allow for its implementation at different levels of care.

An investigation of the integration of gender-based violence laws into the regional health systems of Spain found institutionalisation to be a challenge.[43] Advancements were often made through the actions of highly-motivated individuals, raising concerns about sustainability. Budget allocation was found to be a key component of sustaining institutional change. It is also noted that since IPV is complex to respond to, protocols, whilst necessary, were insufficient and need to be supported by adequate training.[43]

In South Africa, *Vezimfilho*, a model health sector response to IPV and HIV, was developed and implemented in four districts.[44] Important findings from an evaluation of the implementation process included the need for a systemic response, with political commitment, policies, protocols and effective referral systems being essential.[44] In addition, capacity building needed to include addressing values and attitudes toward IPV and gender norms, as well as interpersonal skills in healthcare providers. Support from managers in the health system and strong relationships between multiple stakeholders were seen as being key to a sustainable approach.[44] System barriers to implementation included insufficient staff and lack of confidence in managerial support, whilst on a societal level, providers' attitudes and perceptions relating to gender hampered implementation.[44] The social barriers relating to gender imply that a comprehensive health sector response requires advocating for wider social change.

This need to engage the wider community to address gender issues has been recognised in recent interventions. A pilot health services-based IPV intervention for pregnant women in Kenya included an explicit focus on community collaboration[45] embedded within an ecological framework.[46] Of note is the pilot's innovative use of 'supported referrals', where community volunteers provide practical assistance for reaching referral services. This pilot was found to be acceptable and feasible and shows promise in intervening for IPV as well as primary prevention.

Primary prevention

Primary prevention of IPV, focusing on underlying causes and risk factors, remains a challenge. Two programmes have been tested in South Africa, attempting to address both IPV and HIV by focusing on the gendered nature of these interlinked epidemics.

The Intervention with Microfinance for AIDS and Gender Equity (IMAGE) study implemented a microfinance intervention combined with participatory training that focused on gender and HIV and encouraged community mobilisation. After two years, women enrolled in the intervention group experienced 55% less IPV in the previous 12 months, compared to the control group (risk ratio 0.45, 95% CI 0.23;0.91).[47] Although it was unable to show a difference in HIV incidence in communities, the trial showed that a structural intervention that empowers households economically can decrease violence.

Stepping Stones is a participatory programme aiming to prevent HIV through improving gender equity in relationships, thereby decreasing sexual risk behaviour. This programme was adapted for the South African context and was both implemented and evaluated through a cluster randomised controlled trial. The trial was unable to show a decrease in HIV incidence, but did demonstrate a decrease in incidence of Herpes simplex virus 2; and men who underwent the intervention reported perpetrating IPV significantly less often after two years of follow-up.[48]

In India, a programme including a process of community mobilisation, aiming to empower the female sex worker community to work together to decrease their risk of HIV, showed a significant reduction in their experiences of violence.[49] The SASA! model,[50] currently being trialled in Uganda, uses community mobilisation in an attempt to alter the community-level factors that increase risk for both HIV and violence. In order to do this, community members and community leaders, as well as professionals such as healthcare workers and police officers, are trained and supported in order to engage with their communities, create networks and share key messages that develop as the empowered group is expanded in the community.

Other instances of IPV-prevention programmes exist, for example the SHARE project in Uganda[51] and a study comparing different combinations of interventions aiming to promote gender equitable behaviour in Brazil.[52] In addition, a recent systematic review of IPV-prevention interventions specifically targeting adolescents, found that half of the included trials were effective.[53] The interventions focused largely on building awareness, with some focusing on social norms and gender inequity. Interventions that reported positive outcomes were conducted in multiple settings (e.g. school and community). A trial of a structured home visitation programme for high-risk pregnant women in the Netherlands showed a decrease in IPV in the intervention group.[54] These examples not only demonstrate that IPV can be prevented through the efforts of the health sector acting in concert with other stakeholders and the community, but also highlight the importance of addressing gender inequity when responding to both IPV and HIV. Approaches that include community empowerment and mobilisation, explicitly recognising that social and structural factors need to be addressed, appear to be particularly successful.

Women's perspectives on intimate partner violence care

The WHO clinical and policy guidelines for responding to IPV and sexual violence against women advocate for woman-centred care.[1] Much literature on the topic of women's experiences and expectations of health services in the context of IPV is available. This includes articles synthesising qualitative research in an attempt to increase evidence availability for policy-making and programme design.[55,56] There are many points of commonality, bearing in mind that the majority of this research was conducted in developed countries.

Consistently, women who have experienced IPV have described an appropriate response by healthcare providers to be non-judgmental, understanding and empathetic.[55,56] Women want their healthcare providers to understand the complexities and consequences of living with violence and the difficulties they face because of it.[56,57] They also want confirmation from their providers that what they are experiencing is abuse; and that it is both unacceptable and wrong.[58,59]

When these features are present, the encounter can be validating and helpful and raising the issue of violence can be viewed as caring.[56] When they are absent, however, particularly when the healthcare provider neglects the psychosocial aspects of care, the encounter can be detrimental[57,60] and can lead to a reluctance to disclose violence in the future.[55]

Another feature women have described as being of central importance is having healthcare providers respect their autonomy.[58] However, one survey found that 71% of women who disclosed IPV reported feeling that their healthcare provider wanted them to leave their relationship, with 37.5% reporting that they had been advised directly to do so.[61] Women have also expressed feeling judged when they did not follow the advice of providers to leave their relationship.[56,59]

Consistent with the need for a non-directive and validating encounter, South African women experiencing IPV reported that counseling was the service they wanted most often (between 36.1% and 45.8% in different provinces).[5]

Common barriers to accessing help through health services include fear of the abuser and fear of having children removed from the home as a consequence of disclosing violence.[55,56] Related to the provider, the fear of judgment and not being believed or understood,[56,57] as well as the fear of loss of confidentiality, are common barriers.[55,56] At a systemic level, the lack of privacy often encountered in healthcare settings, as well as a lack of continuity, can prevent disclosure.[55]

Overall, the appropriateness of the healthcare encounter depends on the empathetic and non-directive attitude of the provider, the attention paid to emotional issues and the maintenance of confidentiality. If these elements are present, having a healthcare provider raise the issue of violence is usually viewed by women experiencing IPV as being both supportive and helpful.[56]

Healthcare provider perspectives

Access to reproductive health services can be affected significantly by the attitudes of healthcare workers.[62] In the case of IPV, perceptions regarding the role of the health system and healthcare workers in intervening for IPV, as well as attitudes regarding the underlying causes of violence, can influence how a patient is managed.[63]

Healthcare workers have dual roles, as care givers and community members, often sharing cultural understandings of violence with their communities. They also experience a similar prevalence of violence to the rest of the community.[64] Ongoing or unresolved experiences of IPV have been found to be an important factor influencing healthcare workers' responses to violence, impeding their capacity to offer effective care.[65] The stigma of seeking help for IPV from colleagues may also make it very difficult for healthcare workers to access care. In a rural South African setting, primary healthcare nurses were found to reflect the dominant culture of normalised violence, viewing IPV as intrinsic to relationships and expressing a preference to deal with abuse within the family structure. Both male and female nurses perceived abuse as an often acceptable form of 'discipline', often elicited by the actions of abused women. A distinction was drawn between 'normal' levels of abuse and abuse resulting in very severe injuries, for which it was considered more acceptable to seek outside help.[64]

Addressing IPV remains a challenge for many healthcare workers, with studies citing numerous barriers to responding appropriately. On a provider level, these include discomfort dealing with emotional issues[66,67] and unrealistic expectations about the outcome of intervention.[63] One survey found that 58% of healthcare workers had unrealistic expectations of IPV interventions.[68] This highlights the need to address how healthcare workers understand the complexities of violence, in particular the realities of why women remain in violent relationships. The same survey found that providers were able to empathise with women who were financially unable to leave their relationships, but were less empathetic toward middle-class or educated women who did not leave their partners.[68]

In medical culture, the view of the healthcare provider as the decision maker in the patient–provider relationship is prominent.[69] This can affect how providers see their IPV encounters, in that a woman choosing not to follow advice to either leave the relationship or seek legal redress, could be interpreted as a failure of the interaction. The provider's inability to provide a solution to the problem may be seen as an inability to intervene effectively.[63]

On a systems level, a lack of time has been cited in many different settings.[66,67,70,71] A Malaysian study found that although providers lacked time within which to deal appropriately with IPV, whether or not this impacted on the provision of care depended on individual providers' varying interest in responding to violence.[63]

A lack of training is also a common barrier,[71,72] with evidence suggesting that those healthcare workers who have had training tend to ask about IPV more often[73] and intervene more.[74] A survey of doctors in South Africa reported that only 9.7% of respondents had received any IPV training.[75] Similarly, a lack of protocols is perceived by providers to inhibit IPV management[66,72] and those who have protocols available report assisting patients more often.[74]

Further systemic barriers include ineffective referral networks[67,71,72] and inadequacies of the healthcare setting in terms of creating a trusting and private environment.[66,70]

There appears to be some disparity between what women experiencing IPV want from health services and what the health system is currently providing. Whilst women feel validated when an understanding of their complex situation is displayed, healthcare providers are undertrained in IPV and may have unrealistic expectations. Whilst women want non-directive counseling and support, healthcare providers may be uncomfortable with psychosocial issues and want to offer assistance in the form of advice, usually to leave the relationship or get legal help. In addition, system-level barriers impact on the ability of providers to offer appropriate care, whilst social and structural barriers impede access. Well-developed intersectoral linkages, with strong support from high-level management, are required to facilitate the provision of IPV care within the health services and in the community.

Limitations

This was not a systematic review, seeking all available literature in order to assess it methodologically and present valid study findings. This was not its intention, as the review was designed to inform considerations in the design of health sector-based IPV interventions, including the perspectives of women and healthcare providers. Nonetheless, there is the possibility that factors such as the authors' opinions and omitted studies have influenced the interpretation of the literature.

Implications and recommendations

Policy makers should ensure that comprehensive policies are in place for responding to IPV in health services and for preventing IPV at a community level. Healthcare providers should be supported in providing appropriate care, taking cognisance of common barriers.

Further evaluations of health sector responses to IPV are needed, both in order to assist health systems to determine the most appropriate models of care and to determine how these can be integrated into current systems in the context of multiple systemic and societal barriers. Further research is needed to explore: how best to support health systems in providing IPV care; how to operationalise intersectoral approaches to IPV in health systems; and how to improve access to, including acceptability of, services.

The need for this research should not prevent health systems from implementing IPV care, but rather should guide the development of rigorous, contextually-appropriate evaluations.

Conclusion

There is sufficient evidence that IPV is a common and serious public health concern and that addressing IPV in health services has the potential to improve outcomes. Furthermore, in countries such as South Africa, addressing IPV and gender inequality should form part of HIV prevention programmes.

The health sector has a responsibility not only to respond to the underlying violence that women seeking health services experience, but also to work together with other stakeholders and communities to try and address the contextual factors that lead to IPV and HIV. This requires the empowerment of healthcare workers, women and communities, as well as adjustments to system-level barriers that impede care. A comprehensive health sector response to IPV has the potential to significantly improve the health of the population.

Acknowledgements

Competing interests

The authors declare that they have no financial or personal relationship(s) that may have inappropriately influenced them in writing this article.

Authors' contributions

K.R. (University of Cape Town) conducted the review. K.J. (Stellenbosch University) and V.Z. (University of Cape Town) made significant intellectual contributions.

References

1. World Health Organization. Responding to intimate partner and sexual violence against women: WHO clinical and policy guidelines. Geneva: World Health Organization; 2013.
2. World Health Organization. Global and regional estimates of violence against women: Prevalence and health effects of intimate partner violence and non-partner sexual violence. Geneva: World Health Organization; 2013.
3. Jina R, Jewkes R, Hoffman S, et al. Adverse mental health outcomes associated with emotional abuse in young rural South African women: A cross-sectional study. J Interpers Violence. 2012;27(5):862–880. http://dx.doi.org/10.1177/0886260511423247
4. Norman R, Bradshaw D, Schneider M, et al. Estimating the burden of disease attributable to interpersonal violence in South Africa in 2000. S Afr Med J. 2007;97(8):653–656.
5. Jewkes R, Penn-Kekana L, Levin J, et al. 'He must give me money, he mustn't beat me'. Violence against women in three South African provinces. Pretoria: CERSA (Women's Health), Medical Research Council; 1999.
6. Abrahams N, Jewkes R, Laubscher R, et al. Intimate partner violence: Prevalence and risk factors for men in Cape Town, South Africa. Violence Vict. 2006;21(2):247–264. http://dx.doi.org/10.1891/vivi.21.2.247
7. Machisa M, Jewkes R, Morna CL, et al. The war at home – GBV indicators project. Johannesburg: Gender Links; 2011.
8. Ellsberg M, Jansen HA, Heise L, et al. Intimate partner violence and women's physical and mental health in the WHO multi-country study on women's health and domestic violence: An observational study. Lancet. 2008;371(9619):1165–1172. http://dx.doi.org/10.1016/S0140-6736(08)60522-X
9. Sharps PW, Laughon K, Giangrande SK. Intimate partner violence and the childbearing year: Maternal and infant health consequences. Trauma Violence Abuse. 2007;8(2):105–116. http://dx.doi.org/10.1177/1524838007302594
10. Dunkle KL, Jewkes RK, Brown HC, et al. Gender-based violence, relationship power, and risk of HIV infection in women attending antenatal clinics in South Africa. Lancet. 2004;363(9419):1415–1421. http://dx.doi.org/10.1016/S0140-6736(04)16098-4
11. Campbell JC. Health consequences of intimate partner violence. Lancet. 2002;359(9314):1331–1336. http://dx.doi.org/10.1016/S0140-6736(02)08336-8
12. Golding JM. Intimate partner violence as a risk factor for mental disorders: A meta-analysis. J Fam Violence. 1999;14(2):99–132. http://dx.doi.org/10.1023/A:1022079418229
13. Peltzer K, Pengpid S, McFarlane J, et al. Mental health consequences of intimate partner violence in Vhembe district, South Africa. Gen Hosp Psychiatry. 2013;35(5):545–550. http://dx.doi.org/10.1016/j.genhosppsych.2013.04.001
14. Devries KM, Mak JY, Bacchus LJ, et al. Intimate partner violence and incident depressive symptoms and suicide attempts: A systematic review of longitudinal studies. PLoS Med. 2013;10(5):e1001439. http://dx.doi.org/10.1371/journal.pmed.1001439
15. Jewkes R, Sikweyiya Y, Morrell R, et al. The relationship between intimate partner violence, rape and HIV amongst South African men: a cross-sectional study. PloS ONE. 2011;6(9):e24256. http://dx.doi.org/10.1371/journal.pone.0024256
16. Pallitto CC, Campbell JC, O'Campo P. Is intimate partner violence associated with unintended pregnancy? A review of the literature. Trauma Violence Abuse. 2005;6(3):217–235. http://dx.doi.org/10.1177/1524838005277441
17. Rivara FP, Anderson ML, Fishman P, et al. Healthcare utilization and costs for women with a history of intimate partner violence. Am J Prev Med. 2007;32(2):89–96. http://dx.doi.org/10.1016/j.amepre.2006.10.001
18. Max W, Rice DP, Finkelstein E, et al. The economic toll of intimate partner violence against women in the United States. Violence Vict 2004;19(3):259–272. http://dx.doi.org/10.1891/vivi.19.3.259.65767
19. Varcoe C, Hankivsky O, Ford-Gilboe M, et al. Attributing selected costs to intimate partner violence in a sample of women who have left abusive partners: A social determinants of health approach. Can Public Policy. 2011;37(3):359–380. http://dx.doi.org/10.3138/cpp.37.3.359
20. Ali PA, Naylor PB. Intimate partner violence: A narrative review of the feminist, social and ecological explanations for its causation. Aggress Violent Behav. 2013;18(6):611–619. http://dx.doi.org/10.1016/j.avb.2013.07.009
21. Heise LL. Violence against women: An integrated, ecological framework. Violence Against Women. 1998;4(3):262–290. http://dx.doi.org/10.1177/1077801298004003002
22. Jewkes R. Intimate partner violence: Causes and prevention. Lancet 2002;359(9315):1423–1429. http://dx.doi.org/10.1016/S0140-6736(02)08357-5
23. Russell M, Cupp PK, Jewkes RK, et al. Intimate partner violence among adolescents in Cape Town, South Africa. Prev Sci. 2014;15(3):283–295. http://dx.doi.org/10.1007/s11121-013-0405-7
24. Abramsky T, Watts CH, Garcia-Moreno C, et al. What factors are associated with recent intimate partner violence? Findings from the WHO multi-country study on women's health and domestic violence. BMC Public Health. 2011;11:109. http://dx.doi.org/10.1186/1471-2458-11-109
25. Kouyoumdjian FG, Calzavara LM, Bondy SJ, et al. Risk factors for intimate partner violence in women in the Rakai Community Cohort Study, Uganda, from 2000 to 2009. BMC Public Health. 2013;13:566. http://dx.doi.org/10.1186/1471-2458-13-566
26. Chibber KK, Krishnan S. Confronting intimate partner violence, a global health priority. Mt Sinai J Med. 2011;78(3):449–457. http://dx.doi.org/10.1002/msj.20259
27. Wathen CN, Macmillan HL. Interventions for violence against women. JAMA. 2003;289(5):589–600. http://dx.doi.org/10.1001/jama.289.5.589
28. Ramsay J, Carter Y, Davidson L, et al. Advocacy interventions to reduce or eliminate violence and promote the physical and psychosocial well-being of women who experience intimate partner abuse. Cochrane Database Syst Rev. 2009;3:CD005043.
29. Jewkes R. Intimate partner violence: The end of routine screening. Lancet. 2013;382(9888):190–191. http://dx.doi.org/10.1016/S0140-6736(13)60584-X
30. Hegarty KL, Gunn JM, O'Doherty LJ, et al. Women's evaluation of abuse and violence care in general practice: A cluster randomised controlled trial (WEAVE). BMC Public Health. 2010;10:2. http://dx.doi.org/10.1186/1471-2458-10-2
31. Bair-Merritt MH, Lewis-O'Connor A, Goel S, et al. Primary care-based interventions for intimate partner violence: A systematic review. Am J Prev Med. 2014;46(2):188–194. http://dx.doi.org/10.1016/j.amepre.2013.10.001
32. Garcia-Moreno C. Dilemmas and opportunities for an appropriate health-service response to violence against women. Lancet. 2002;359(9316):1509–1514. http://dx.doi.org/10.1016/S0140-6736(02)08417-9
33. Moyer VA. Screening for intimate partner violence and abuse of elderly and vulnerable adults: U.S. preventive services task force recommendation statement. Ann Intern Med. 2013;158(6):478–486. http://dx.doi.org/10.7326/0003-4819-158-6-201303190-00588
34. Hegarty K, O'Doherty L, Taft A, et al. Screening and counselling in the primary care setting for women who have experienced intimate partner violence (WEAVE): A cluster randomised controlled trial. Lancet. 2013;382(9888):249–258. http://dx.doi.org/10.1016/S0140-6736(13)60052-5
35. Klevens J, Kee R, Trick W, et al. Effect of screening for partner violence on women's quality of life: A randomized controlled trial. JAMA. 2012;308(7):681–689. http://dx.doi.org/10.1001/jama.2012.6434
36. MacMillan H, Wathen C, Jamieson E, et al. Screening for intimate partner violence in health care settings: A randomized trial. JAMA. 2009;302(5):493–501. http://dx.doi.org/10.1001/jama.2009.1089
37. Joyner K, Mash B. A comprehensive model for intimate partner violence in South African primary care: Action research. BMC Health Serv Res. 2012;12:399. http://dx.doi.org/10.1186/1472-6963-12-399
38. Feder G, Davies RA, Baird K, et al. Identification and Referral to Improve Safety (IRIS) of women experiencing domestic violence with a primary care training and support programme: A cluster randomised controlled trial. Lancet. 2011;378(9805):1788–1795. http://dx.doi.org/10.1016/S0140-6736(11)61179-3
39. McFarlane JM, Groff JY, O'Brien JA, et al. Secondary prevention of intimate partner violence: A randomized controlled trial. Nurs Res. 2006;55(1):52–61. http://dx.doi.org/10.1097/00006199-200601000-00007

40. O'Campo P, Kirst M, Tsamis C, et al. Implementing successful intimate partner violence screening programs in health care settings: Evidence generated from a realist-informed systematic review. Soc Sci Med. 2011;72(6):855–66. http://dx.doi.org/10.1016/j.socscimed.2010.12.019

41. Plichta SB. Interactions between victims of intimate partner violence against women and the health care system: Policy and practice implications. Trauma Violence Abuse. 2007;8(2):226–239. http://dx.doi.org/10.1177/1524838007301220

42. Colombini M, Mayhew SH, Ali SH, et al. An integrated health sector response to violence against women in Malaysia: Lessons for supporting scale up. BMC Public Health. 2012;12:548. http://dx.doi.org/10.1186/1471-2458-12-548

43. Goicolea I, Briones-Vozmediano E, Ohman A, et al. Mapping and exploring health systems' response to intimate partner violence in Spain. BMC Public Health. 2013;13:1162. http://dx.doi.org/10.1186/1471-2458-13-1162

44. Jacobs T, Jewkes R. Vezimfilho : A model for health sector response to gender violence in South Africa. Int J Gynecol Obstet. 2002;78(Suppl 1):S51–S56. http://dx.doi.org/10.1016/S0020-7292(02)00044-9

45. Turan JM, Hatcher AM, Odero M, et al. A community-supported clinic-based program for prevention of violence against pregnant women in rural Kenya. AIDS Res Treat. 2013, Article ID 736926, 10 pages.

46. Latcher AM, Romito P, Odero M, et al. Social context and drivers of intimate partner violence in rural Kenya: Implications for the health of pregnant women. Cult Health Sex. 2013;15(4):404–419. http://dx.doi.org/10.1080/13691058.2012.760205

47. Pronyk PM, Hargreaves JR, Kim JC, et al. Effect of a structural intervention for the prevention of intimate-partner violence and HIV in rural South Africa: A cluster randomised trial. Lancet. 2006;368(9551):1973–1983. http://dx.doi.org/10.1016/S0140-6736(06)69744-4

48. Jewkes R, Nduna M, Levin J, et al. Impact of Stepping Stones on incidence of HIV and HSV-2 and sexual behaviour in rural South Africa : Cluster randomised controlled trial. BMJ. 2008;337:a506. http://dx.doi.org/10.1136/bmj.a506

49. Beattie TS, Mohan HL, Bhattacharjee P, et al. Community mobilization and empowerment of female sex workers in Karnataka State, South India: Associations with HIV and sexually transmitted infection risk. Am J Public Health. 2014;104(8): 1516–1525. http://dx.doi.org/10.2105/AJPH.2014.301911

50. Abramsky T, Devries K, Kiss L, et al. A community mobilisation intervention to prevent violence against women and reduce HIV/AIDS risk in Kampala, Uganda (the SASA! Study): Study protocol for a cluster randomised controlled trial. Trials. 2012;13:96. http://dx.doi.org/10.1186/1745-6215-13-96

51. Wagman JA, Namatovu F, Nalugoda F, et al. A public health approach to intimate partner violence prevention in Uganda: The SHARE Project. Violence Against Women. 2012;18(12):1390–1412. http://dx.doi.org/10.1177/1077801212474874

52. Pulerwitz J, Barker G, Segundo M, et al. Promoting more gender-equitable norms and behaviors among young men as an HIV/AIDS prevention strategy. Washington DC: Population Council; 2006.

53. De Koker P, Mathews C, Zuch M, et al. A systematic review of interventions for preventing adolescent intimate partner violence. J Adolesc Health. 2014;54(1):3–13. http://dx.doi.org/10.1016/j.jadohealth.2013.08.008

54. Mejdoubi J, van den Heijkant SC, van Leerdam FJ, et al. Effect of nurse home visits vs. usual care on reducing intimate partner violence in young high-risk pregnant women: A randomized controlled trial. PloS ONE. 2013;8(10):e78185. http://dx.doi.org/10.1371/journal.pone.0078185

55. Robinson L, Spilsbury K. Systematic review of the perceptions and experiences of accessing health services by adult victims of domestic violence. Health Soc Care Community. 2008;16(1):16–30. http://dx.doi.org/10.1111/j.1365-2524.2007.00721.x

56. Feder GS, Hutson M, Ramsay J, et al. Women exposed to intimate partner violence: Expectations and experiences when they encounter health care professionals: A meta-analysis of qualitative studies. Arch Intern Med. 2006;166(1):22–37. http://dx.doi.org/10.1001/archinte.166.1.22

57. Narula A, Agarwal G, McCarthy L. Intimate partner violence: Patients' experiences and perceptions in family practice. Fam Pract. 2012;29(5):593–600. http://dx.doi.org/10.1093/fampra/cms008

58. Chang JC, Cluss PA, Ranieri L, et al. Health care interventions for intimate partner violence: What women want. Womens Health Issues. 2005;15(1):21–30. http://dx.doi.org/10.1016/j.whi.2004.08.007

59. Reisenhofer S, Seibold C. Emergency healthcare experiences of women living with intimate partner violence. J Clin Nurs. 2013;22(15–16):2253–2263. http://dx.doi.org/10.1111/j.1365-2702.2012.04311.x

60. Stenius VMK, Veysey BM. 'It's the little things': Women, trauma, and strategies for healing. J Interpers Violence. 2005;20(10):1155–1174. http://dx.doi.org/10.1177/0886260505278533

61. Morse DS, Lafleur R, Fogarty CT, et al. 'They told me to leave': How health care providers address intimate partner violence. J Am Board Fam Med. 2012;25(3):333–342. http://dx.doi.org/10.3122/jabfm.2012.03.110193

62. Tavrow P. Promote or discourage: how providers can influence service use. In: S Malarcher, ed. Social Determinants of Sexual and Reproductive Health: Informing Future Research and Programme Implementation. Geneva: World Health Organization, 2010; pp. 15–36.

63. Colombini M, Mayhew S, Ali SH, et al. 'I feel it is not enough...' Health providers' perspectives on services for victims of intimate partner violence in Malaysia. BMC Health Serv Res. 2013;13:65. http://dx.doi.org/10.1186/1472-6963-13-65

64. Kim J, Motsei M. 'Women enjoy punishment': Attitudes and experiences of gender-based violence among PHC nurses in rural South Africa. Soc Sci Med. 2002;54(8):1243–54. http://dx.doi.org/10.1016/S0277-9536(01)00093-4

65. Joyner K. Health care for intimate partner violence: Current standard of care and development of protocol management [doctoral dissertation, Social Science Methods]. Stellenbosch: Department of Sociology and Social Anthropology, Faculty of Arts and Social Sciences, Stellenbosch University [thesis on the Internet]. c2009 [cited 2014 Aug 11]. Available from: http://hdl.handle.net/10019.1/2515

66. Vieira EM, Dos Santos MA, Ford NJ. Seizing an opportunity to help-knowledge and attitudes of doctors and nurses toward women victimized by intimate partner violence in Brazil. Health Care Women Int. 2012;33(3):228–249. http://dx.doi.org/10.1080/07399332.2011.646365

67. Sprague S, Kaloty R, Madden K, et al. Perceptions of intimate partner violence: A cross sectional survey of surgical residents and medical students. J Inj Violence Res. 2011;5(1):1–10.

68. Nicolaidis C, Curry M, Gerrity M. Health care workers' expectations and empathy toward patients in abusive relationships. J Am Board Fam Pract. 2005;18(3):159–165. http://dx.doi.org/10.3122/jabfm.18.3.159

69. Shelton JD. The provider perspective: Human after all. Int Fam Plan Perspect. 2001;27(3):152–161. http://dx.doi.org/10.2307/2673838

70. Laisser RM, Lugina HI, Lindmark G, et al. Striving to make a difference : Health care worker experiences with intimate partner violence clients in Tanzania. Health Care Women Int. 2009;30(1–2):64–78. http://dx.doi.org/10.1080/07399330802523618

71. Zink T, Regan S, Goldenhar L, et al. Intimate partner violence: What are physicians' perceptions? J Am Board Fam Pract. 2004;17(5):332–340. http://dx.doi.org/10.3122/jabfm.17.5.332

72. Djikanovic B, Celik H, Simic S, et al. Health professionals' perceptions of intimate partner violence against women in Serbia: Opportunities and barriers for response improvement. Patient Educ Couns. 2010;80(1):88–93. http://dx.doi.org/10.1016/j.pec.2009.09.028

73. Glowa PT, Frasier PY, Wang L, et al. What happens after we identify intimate partner violence? The family physician's perspective. Fam Med. 2003;35(10):730–736.

74. Leppäkoski T, Paavilainen E. Interventions for women exposed to acute intimate partner violence: emergency professionals' perspective. J Clin Nurs. 2013;22(15–16): 2273–2285. http://dx.doi.org/10.1111/j.1365-2702.2012.04202.x

75. Peltzer K, Mashego TA, Mabeba M. Attitudes and practices of doctors toward domestic violence victims in South Africa. Health Care Women Int. 2003;24(2):149–157. http://dx.doi.org/10.1080/07399330390178431

Health research in the Western Cape province, South Africa: Lessons and challenges

Authors:
Leslie London[1,2]
Tracey Naledi[1]
Sabela Petros[1,2]

Affiliations:
[1]School of Public Health and Family Medicine, Division of Public Health Medicine, University of Cape Town, South Africa

[2]Health Department, Western Cape Government, South Africa

Correspondence to:
Leslie London

Email:
leslie.london@uct.ac.za

Postal address:
School of Public Health and Family Medicine, University of Cape Town Health Sciences Faculty, Anzio Road, Observatory 7925, South Africa

Background: Health research can play a critical role in strengthening health systems. However, little monitoring of health research is conducted in African countries to identify whether research contributes to addressing local health priorities.

Aim/Setting: To review the profile of research on the health service platform in the Western Cape province of South Africa which was approved by the health authorities over the period January 2011 to December 2012.

Methods: Databases held by both the Provincial and City of Cape Town health departments were reviewed. Descriptions of research institution, location of research, topic and funding size and source were analysed.

Results: Of the health research approved in the province, 56% of projects were located on the District Health Services platform and 70% were based in the Cape Metropolitan area. For projects reporting budgetary information, the total funding was US $29.2 million. The primary focus of research was on HIV and tuberculosis (TB), whilst relatively few studies addressed nutrition, mental health or injury and there was little health systems research. Research funding was dominated by very large grants from foreign funders for HIV and/or TB research. South African government sources comprised less than 8% of all health research funding.

Conclusion: There is a partial mismatch of donor funding to local health priorities. Greater focus on neglected areas such as mental health, trauma, nutrition and non-communicable disease, as well as greater investment in health systems research, is needed. Unless governments increase funding for research and a culture of research translation is achieved, health research will have limited impact on both local and national priorities.

Recherches en santé dans la Province du Western Cape, Afrique du Sud: Leçons et Défis.

Contexte: La recherche en santé peut jouer un rôle essentiel dans le renforcement des systèmes de santé. Cependant, il y a peu de suivi sur les recherches en santé dans les pays africains pour déterminer si la recherche contribue à donner suite aux priorités en matière de santé.

Objectif/ Lieu: Revoir la recherche sur la plateforme des services sanitaires dans la province du Western Cape d'Afrique du Sud, approuvée par les autorités sanitaires pour la période allant du mois de janvier 2011 au mois de décembre 2012.

Méthodes: On a révisé les banques de données des départements sanitaires de la Province et de la ville du Cap. On a aussi analysé la description des instituts de recherche, les lieux de recherche, les thèmes et le montant et la source des financements.

Résultats: Parmi la recherche sanitaire approuvée dans la province, 56% des projets des Services de Santé de District, et 70% de ceux-ci se trouvaient dans la zone métropolitaine. Le financement total des informations budgétaires relatives aux projets était de 29.2 millions d'USD. La recherche portait principalement sur le VIH et la tuberculose; alors qu'il y avait relativement peu d'études sur la nutrition, la santé mentale ou les blessures et peu de recherches sur les systèmes de santé. Le financement de la recherche était dominé par les subventions importantes des bailleurs de fonds étrangers pour la recherche sur le VIH/la tuberculose. Les sources provenant du gouvernement sud-africain s'élevaient à moins de 8% de tous les financements de recherche en santé.

Conclusion: Il y a un certain décalage dans le financement des bailleurs de fonds pour les priorités locales en matière de santé. Il conviendrait d'insister d'avantage sur les domaines négligés tels que la santé mentale, le traumatisme, la nutrition et les maladies non contagieuses, et aussi de s'investir plus dans la recherche sur les systèmes de santé. A moins que les gouvernements n'augmentent le financement de la recherche et sa valorisation, la recherche dans le domaine de la santé aura un effet limité sur les priorités locales et nationales.

Introduction

Health research is critical to human development and well-being. Research can contribute to identifying key health problems, the risks for and associations with health states and mustering the evidence for how to address these problems; to assessing health service and health system performance and identifying and evaluating improvement strategies; to informing appropriate policies and programmes; and to building the knowledge base for improved health outcomes. Health research can tell the public, civil society and health managers how their services are doing and what needs improving.[1,2,3] Although the importance of health research for potentially improving health outcomes is undisputed, the extent to which investments in health research deliver desired benefits has been challenged.[4,5,6,7] Concerns have also been expressed regarding whether health research meets local priorities,[6,8] most commonly framed through analysis by Burden of Disease (BoD) categories.[9,10,11,12] Moreover, it has been noted that despite the great potential for enhancing health research in the clinical domain in South Africa, the contribution of clinical research has been severely constrained by lack of funding and undermined by the lack of any monitoring and evaluation systems for health research.[1]

Given the importance of health for development, inequities in the distribution of health research benefits and the role of research in strengthening Primary Health Care, an integrated strategy for health research has been elevated in South Africa to a legislative responsibility of the National Health Council.[13] Accordingly, the *National Health Act* 61 of 2003 provides an institutional and regulatory framework for the undertaking of health research in South Africa, including the establishment of a National Health Research Committee and equivalent provincial structures charged with, amongst other responsibilities, identifying research priorities in the country.[3] Moreover, strengthening of research and development is one of 10 National Ministerial priorities.[14]

In the Western Cape province, the process of oversight and facilitation of health research under the Provincial Health Research Committee involves approval by the Provincial and City of Cape Town (CoCT) health authorities of every research study conducted within their services. In submitting applications to conduct research on the health platform to the authorities, researchers are expected to provide information in their proposals on their projects, to the extent that the services can evaluate whether permission should be given for the research to go ahead. This provides a potential mechanism by which health services can maintain a database of research in the health services, be informed of research findings and make better use of research outputs to inform policy, programmes and practice. Even though the HIV programme in particular has provided very good recent examples of evidence-based policy development,[15] the culture of using evidence more generally to inform decision making in South African health services is weak.[3]

Given calls at the National Health Summit convened to improve the monitoring and evaluation of the performance of the health research system in South Africa, this article presents a review of research by health services in the Western Cape in 2011 and 2012. It aims to describe the location, type and amount of funding for research as well as the institutional affiliation of researchers and funding sources available for health research in the province.

Research methods and design

Databases created and maintained by health authorities in the province for research approval were assembled and reviewed for studies submitted and approved between January 2011 and December 2012. The primary database was that held in the Health Research sub-Directorate of the Health Impact Assessment Directorate in the Department of Health of the Western Cape Government for research conducted on the Provincial District Health Service (DHS) platform. This database captures information through mandatory fields in the application form on study topic and type, funding source, research budget, principal investigator affiliation and location of study (facility, district and subdistrict). The databases of the CoCT Health Department and from four tertiary and psychiatric hospitals (Tygerberg, Groote Schuur, Valkenberg and Stikland hospitals) were also reviewed, but provided data only for the 20 months from January 2011 to August 2012. These databases contained limited information on topic and location but no details about funding or investigator affiliation. At the time of conducting the study, there was no consistent content, structure and field format for the different databases. Moreover, health research conducted outside of provincial and municipal health services was not captured in any health service database.

Based on the study title, the topic was post-coded to a variable that included the main BoD categories (HIV, tuberculosis [TB], injury and/or violence, women's health, child health, non-communicable disease, mental health and nutrition), supplemented by coding for a category 'Other' (which included disease entities not contained in the main BoD categories) and 'General' (which included health system and service issues not specific to a disease or BoD category). The latter included, for example, studies of human resource issues, quality of care and policy studies. Up to three codes for topic were permitted per study. Analysis of study topic included studies conducted in central hospitals as well as on the District and Regional platform for the period January 2011 to August 2012.

For type of study, a descriptor was created for health services research based on the reviewer's assessment of whether the research topic had direct implications for health service development. A second variable was created to code for drug trials.

Investigator affiliation was coded as the South African institution (university or research council) to which the investigator was affiliated or, if the investigator was a

TABLE 1: Coding of funding sources for health research in the Western Cape, 2011–2012.

Category	Includes
SA (South African) Government	All funding from South African government, whether directly through government departments or through research councils such as the Medical Research Council (MRC), Human Sciences Research Council (HSRC) and the National Research Foundation (NRF).
US (United States) Government	Centre for Disease Control (CDC), The U.S. President's Emergency Plan for AIDS Relief (PEPFAR), United States Agency for International Development (USAID), the National Institutes of Health (NIH) and any NIH institute.
Global Agencies	Denotes funding from Foundations (such as AERAS Global TB vaccine foundation, or the Bill & Melinda Gates Foundation) and the Joint United Nations Programme on HIV/AIDS (UNAIDS).
Other International	a. A non-South African university. b. International agencies other than US agencies such as the International Development Research Centre (IDRC), Canadian Institute for Health Research ICIHR), European Union (EU), Wellcome Trust, South African and Netherlands Research Programme on Alternatives in Development (SANPAD), World Health Organisation (WHO), World Dental Federation (FDI) and the European and Developing Countries Clinical Trials Partnership (EDCTP).
Pharma	Private sector pharmaceutical companies.
Foundation	South African Foundations such as the Harry Crossley Foundation.
University	Researchers who indicated their own universities as the source of funding.
Health Services	Researchers who were service providers conducted research funded from within the services.
Self-funded	Researchers who indicated they were unfunded or funded their own research out of their own resources.
Other	a. Local Non-Government Organisations (NGOs): Hospice, ANOVA, Impumelelo, CANSA. b. International NGOs working in South Africa: Médecins Sans Frontierès (MSF), Management Sciences for Health (MSH).

non-national, was coded as 'International'. All investigators based in pharmaceutical companies or private Clinical Research Organisations (CROs) were coded in a single category of 'Pharma'.

Source of funding was coded as listed in Table 1. The main categories were South African (SA) Government, United States (US) Government, Global Agencies, Other International, University, Health Services, Self-funded and Other. Donor grants directed through government were counted as government funding. Those who did not declare their source of funding were reported as 'Unknown'.

Although projects may have received funding from more than one source, only one code was allocated for funding source as the information supplied did not allow for disaggregation of how much funding came from different funders. Where there was any government funding for a study, we coded the funder as 'SA Government', thereby making the code 'SA Government' as the 'trump' code for multiple funders.

Size of budget was based on self-reported budget provided by the researcher in the application documents. Budgets are reported in US$ with a conversion rate from SA currency (ZA Rands) of $1 to ZAR10, the rate prevalent at September 2012. Where researchers failed to report budget or reported budget in unmanageable terms, the data were treated as incomplete.

Results

During the 20-month period January 2011 to August 2012, a total of 615 projects were approved in the province. Just over half (56%) were projects approved on the DHS platform, whilst the rest were projects implemented at specialist or psychiatric hospitals.

Amongst the 341 projects approved on the DHS platform between January 2011 and December 2012, approximately 50% were projects spanning multiple districts: 72% were located in the Cape Metro, with fewer in other districts (23% in the Cape Winelands; 11% in Eden, 8% in the Overberg; 6% on the West Coast and 4% in the Central Karoo). Within the Cape Metro, 18% of projects were not specific to subdistricts or were located in central, regional, TB, rehabilitation and psychiatric hospitals. Across subdistricts, projects were approximately evenly distributed by subdistrict (Eastern and Khayelitsha [30%]; Tygerberg and Northern [33%]; Klipfontein and Mitchells Plain [35%]; and Southern and Western [36%]). Once studies in the central hospitals were included, over 85% of research studies submitted for approval between January 2011 and August 2012 were located in the Cape Metro area. Of these, approximately 23% were co-located in another district.

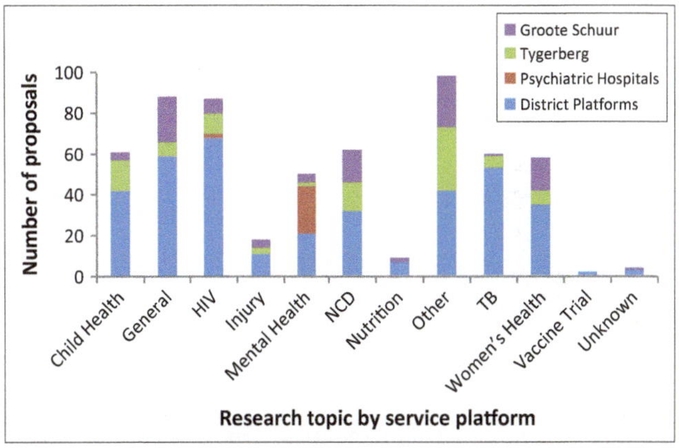

NCD, Non-communicable disease; TB, Tuberculosis.

FIGURE 1: Research topics by service platform, Western Cape, January 2011 to August 2012.

Figure 1 summarises the topics for health research in the province. Combined, HIV (87 projects) and TB (60 projects) comprised the largest single category (28%) for health research in the province. Injury was the topic for only 4% of research projects in the province. Whilst mental health was the topic of 10% of all research in the province, less than half of all mental health projects were located at district level; the majority of studies were in specialised mental health hospitals. A subanalysis at one of the tertiary hospitals

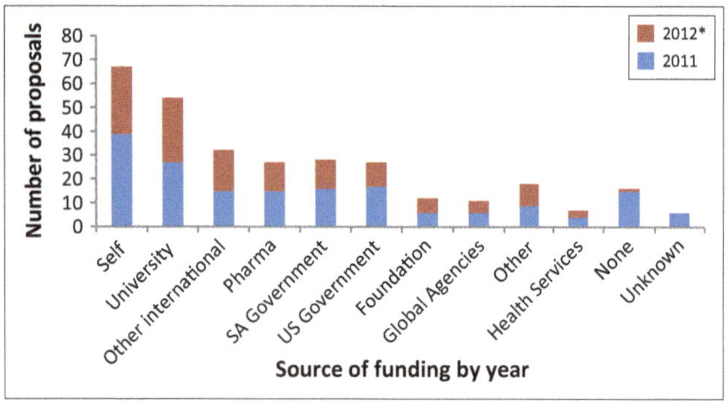

*, Dataset for 2012 comprises eight months only – January to August 2012.

FIGURE 2: Source of funding for health research on the District platform, Western Cape, January 2011 to August 2012.

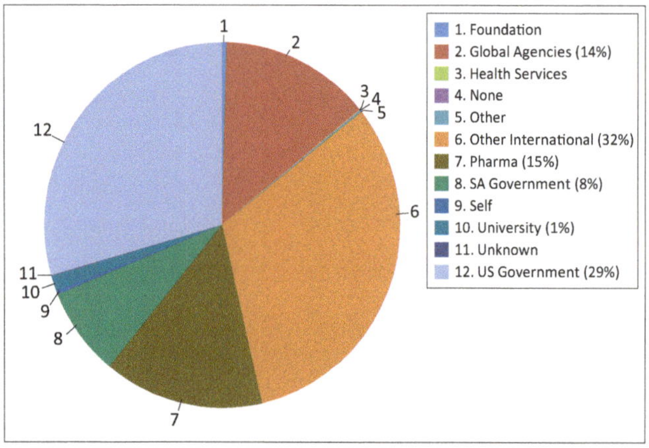

FIGURE 3: Total budget of health research funding on District Health platform, Western Cape, January 2011 to August 2012, by funding source category.

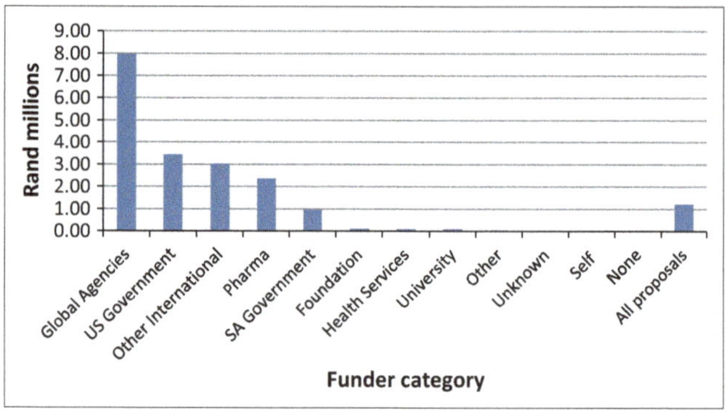

*, Data on budgets missing for ~30% of proposals, including > 50% pharma, global agencies.

FIGURE 4: Average budget in R millions per project*, by funder category.

showed that 29% of studies approved were for drug trials and these were predominantly concentrated in non-communicable disease (NCD) categories (cardiac disease, Chronic Obstructive Pulmonary Disease, seizures, diabetes, cholesterol and oncology trials).

Researcher affiliation reflected local higher education or research institutions, with University of Cape Town (UCT) (36%), University of Stellenbosch (25%) and University of the Western Cape (10%) being the most frequent. A small number of projects (2%) reported an international researcher as principal investigator. The most common category for source of funding was researchers who reported being 'Self-funded' (57 projects or approximately 22%) and 'University-funded' (54 projects or approximately 17%). Projects funded by the pharmaceutical industry, the SA government, the US government and other international sources were all more-or-less equally frequent, comprising about 9% to 11% of projects.

Figures 3 and 4 summarise the size of research funding by funding source. Based on the 72% of projects for which budgetary details were provided, the largest categories of funder were 'other international' (32%) and the 'US Government' (29%), followed by 'Pharma' (15%), 'Global Agencies' (14%) and the 'SA Government' (8%). Of the SA government funding, the bulk came directly from government departments, particularly the Department of Health (88%), with relatively little coming via the two main national Research Councils (National Research Foundation 6% and Medical Research Council 4%). A single contribution from the Department of Health to the *South African National Health and Nutrition Examination Survey* (SANHANES) comprised more than 75% of all government funding. Without this contribution, government funding would have comprised about 2% of all health research funding on the district platform in the province.

In total, of the 72% of projects that reported budgets with sufficient detail to compute, a total of $29.2 million was spent on health research projects on the provincial health department district platform in the province over the 20 months for which budgetary data were available.

Figure 4 shows that funding in projects whose sources were 'US Government' or 'Global Agencies' were very large grants. Average budget per project for Global Agencies was close to $800 000 and that for US government about $340 000. By contrast, the average grant from SA government sources was about $95 000. Grants from the largest funders (Global Agencies, US Government, Other International) tended to focus on TB (37%), HIV (33%) and, less so, on women's health (11%) and child health (18%). Pharmaceutical funding included TB (14%), but was mostly directed at NCDs (30%) and other health conditions (23%). None of the largest funders supported injury-related research and only 4% of grants from these large funders were for mental health.

Discussion

In contrast to developed countries,[16,17,18,19] where health research spending is more-or-less in line with *national* BoD priorities, the findings in the Western Cape suggest a weak correlation with *local* BoD priorities. Whilst HIV and TB are undoubtedly critical contributors to BoD, the dwarfing of other areas of research in the province is striking – about 65% of all funding in the province was for projects related to HIV or TB or both. It is evident that research activities appear to be linked to donor funding availability focused on HIV and TB, rather than specific local priorities. This is a problem reported commonly in developing countries, where donor agendas have set the pattern of research.[8,20,21] The mismatch between BoD and what research is taking place is concerning. For example, whereas the Western Cape suffers a very high burden from trauma, very little funding is directed at research addressing trauma and most of what is done on trauma is supported by SA government sources and smaller funders. Similarly, very little mental health research appears to be supported outside of psychiatric hospitals in the province. The lack of research in the nutrition field and the focus in NCD research on drug trials is another concerning aspect. Good nutrition is a key achievement of MDG goals 1 and 4 and NCDs continue to contribute a huge component of the provincial and national BoD, as well as placing a huge strain on the health services. Equally, the dearth in health systems research is a matter for concern as this denies the country empirical evidence upon which health decision makers can make judgement on how well the system is addressing the BoD, as well as what areas need attention.

This neglect of a certain area is not unique to the Western Cape or South Africa.[8] For example, criticisms have been made regarding the neglect of mental health research in the UK.[22] A review of US funding through the National Institutes of Health found that both mental health (as in depression) and injuries were underfunded areas compared with their US BoD;[23] and both these morbidity categories were also noted as being underfunded in an Australian review of the extent to which health research funding followed the pattern of national with the burden of disease.[17]

Finally, both the quantum and pattern of research funding are potentially problematic. On the one hand, approximately US$30 million was spent on health research in the DHS. If one extrapolated to include studies which did not report funding details and studies in the health services elsewhere on the platform, the true figure may well be in excess of $50 million. This is substantial research expenditure and one may well ask whether the potential from this substantial investment in reduction of the BoD and improvement in quality of care is being realised.[24] At the same time, the very low proportion of research funding in the province sourced from government funding structures is a matter for deep concern. About 8% of all research in the province receives SA government funding, with the bulk of research funding coming from international sources in the north. It is hard to imagine how local and national priorities can be met if 90% of research funding comes from outside sources, even with the best-intentioned forms of international aid. By contrast, there is evidence that Health Ministries in Europe take the lead in shaping and funding public health research in their countries.[18]

Calls have been made in international forums to increase national funding for health research such that at least 2% of the national health budget is allocated to health and development.[8,25,26] Such a step will no doubt enable greater local determination of what kind of research is undertaken. However, it is sobering to think that such an increase would require a five-fold increase in funding in South Africa from the current allocation of 0.38% of the health budget for research.[3] Whether such a massive investment is feasible and whether it will be done in such a way as to enable local priorities to be set and met remains to be seen.

Nonetheless, despite the likely difficulties, it can also been argued that SAs have a right to enjoy the benefits of research, a right which, by implication, imposes on the state an obligation to invest, to the maximum extent possible, in supporting scientific and technological advancement.[27] Indeed, the right to benefit from scientific progress is contained in the International Covenant on Social, Cultural and Economic Rights (ICESCR), a covenant which South Africa signed in 1994 and agreed to ratify in 2012.[28] Increased support and funding for health research, identified as a key action to strengthen the SA health system,[29] would be entirely consistent with the cabinet's commitment to domesticate provisions of the ICESCR and with our Constitution's commitment to advancing the socio-economic rights of all who live in South Africa.

In addition to increased funding, we should also advocate for measures to strengthen the culture of using evidence for decision making, which is generally weak in the health system at present. For research to be of maximum benefit, there needs to be improved feedback of research findings by researchers to the services and to communities, as well as continuous review of research findings by the services in order to identify potential issues for action and translation of evidence into policy and programmes. Current plans to establish a national database of health research in South Africa being steered by the Health Systems Trust (HST) for the Department of Health will contribute to strengthening the health system's capacity to best utilise research findings for implementation.

There are a number of caveats to this study. Firstly, health research occurring off the service platform does not make its way into this database since it does not require health service permission. It is possible that much research in trauma and nutrition might fall into this category and may explain partly the dearth of these topics in the provincial database. Secondly, the database was not complete for all sources, limiting the detailed cross-tabulations regarding size of budget and researcher institution presented here to the Provincial DHS database. Thirdly, information supplied by investigators was often missing or inaccurate, particularly related to financial data and funding source. Lastly, in extrapolating from data provided to reach a minimum figure of $50 million spent on health research in the Western Cape over a 24-month period, there may be a number of variables that make this figure either an under- or over-estimate. The funding profile of projects for which financial data were missing may have been different from those that were reported and there may have been some double counting if the principal investigator applied to more than one authority. Nonetheless, the estimate remains a sizeable figure for health research in the province and points to the need to find mechanisms with which to maximise the added value for the health of the population of the Western Cape from such a large investment of funding.

Conclusion

This audit provides the first provincial report on health research conducted in South Africa. It confirms that considerable resources are invested in research in the province, but that there are key gaps in what is funded. Neglected areas such as mental health, malnutrition and trauma are important contributors to BoD but, presumably because they are not attractive to large donors, do not receive levels of funding commensurate with local need. The National Health Summit in South Africa in 2011 made seven key recommendations regarding the future of health research in this country. The findings of this review echo some of these calls, particularly the need for increased national funding for health research. If South Africa is serious about wanting to shape the portfolio of research for development and evidence-based decision making, the state needs to increase substantially its funding for health research. Otherwise the country's pressing health needs and challenges will not be adequately addressed and research direction will remain determined by the interests of external agencies which may not always be consistent with national and local health priorities. We believe the situation may be even more extreme in other African countries, where national support for health research is even more constrained.

Acknowledgements

The authors wish to acknowledge Charlene Roderick for assistance with management of the provincial research database, as well as the Western Cape Provincial Health Research Committee (WCPHC) for its work managing the process of health research oversight in the Western Cape. Professors Rodney Ehrlich and Deborah Jackson, as Chair and Member of the Committee, respectively, made valuable comments on the manuscript.

Competing interests

The authors declare that they have no financial or personal relationship(s) that may have inappropriately influenced them in writing this article. All the authors were, at the time of writing, employed by the Health Department of the Western Cape Government and involved in the Health Research sub-directorate responsible for managing health research on the provincial platform.

Authors' contributions

L.L. (University of Cape Town; Western Cape Government) was the project leader and led the analysis and writing of the manuscript; T.N. (University of Cape Town) and S.P. (University of Cape Town; Western Cape Government) contributed to the design of the study and made iterative comments on the successive drafts of the manuscript. All authors signed off on the final text.

References

1. Academy of Science of South Africa. Consensus report on revitalising clinical research in South Africa: a study on clinical research and related training in South Africa [document on the Internet]. c2009 [cited 2011 Nov 16]. Available from: http://www.assaf.co.za/wp-content/uploads/2009/09/ASSAf-Clinical-Report-2009.pdf
2. Global Forum for Health Research. The global forum update on research for health, Volume 4: Equitable access: Research challenges for health in developing countries. London: Pro-Brook Publishing; 2007.
3. National Health Research Committee. 2011 National Health Research Summit Report. Strengthening research for health, innovation and development in South Africa. Proceedings and recommendations of the 2011 National Health Research Summit, 26–27 July 2011, OR Tambo Conference Centre [document on the Internet]. c2011 [cited 2014 Nov 18]. Available from: http://www.rmchsa.org/wp-content/uploads/2014/04/National-Health-Research-Summit-Report-2011.pdf
4. Macilwain C. Science economics: What science is really worth? Nature. 2010;465:682–684. http://dx.doi.org/10.1038/465682a
5. FoxNews.com. NIH funds $423,500 study of why men don't like to use condoms. Fox News Politics [newspaper online] 2009 June 19 [cited 2013 Jan 04]. Available from: http://www.foxnews.com/politics/2009/06/19/nih-funds-study-men-dont-like-use-condoms/
6. McCoy D, Sanders D, Baum F, et al. Pushing the international health research agenda towards equity and effectiveness. Lancet. 2004;364(9445):1630–1631. http://dx.doi.org/10.1016/S0140-6736(04)17319-4
7. Moses H 3rd, Dorsey ER, Matheson DH, et al. Financial anatomy of biomedical research. JAMA. 2005;294(11):1333–1342. http://dx.doi.org/10.1001/jama.294.11.1333
8. Ijsselmuiden C, Jacobs M. Health research for development: Making health research work ... for everyone. Scand J Public Health. 2005;33(5):329–333. http://dx.doi.org/10.1080/14034940510032310
9. Lamarre-Cliche M, Castilloux AM, LeLorier J. Association between the burden of disease and research funding by the Medical Research Council of Canada and the National Institutes of Health. A cross-sectional study. Clin Invest Med. 2001;24(2):83–89.
10. Curry CW, De AK, Ikeda RM, et al. Health burden and funding at the Centers for Disease Control and Prevention. Am J Prev Med. 2006;30(3):269–276. http://dx.doi.org/10.1016/j.amepre.2005.10.028
11. Mitchell RJ, McClure RJ, Olivier J, Watson WL. Rational allocation of Australia's research dollars: Does the distribution of NHMRC funding by National Health Priority Area reflect actual disease burden? Med J Aust. 2009;191(11): 648–652.
12. Rubin JB, Paltiel AD, Saltzman WM. Are we studying what matters? Health priorities and NIH-funded biomedical engineering research. Ann Biomed Eng. 2010;38(7):2237–2251. http://dx.doi.org/10.1007/s10439-010-9982-9
13. Republic of South Africa. National Health Act, No 61 of 2003. Pretoria: Government Printers.
14. Health Systems Trust. Kwik Squiz: The 10 point plan, Vol. 2, No. 1 [document on the Internet]. c2010 [cited 2014 Nov 18]. Available from: http://www.healthlink.org.za/uploads/files/ks_1V2_10pointplan.pdf
15. National Department of Health. Policy and guidelines for the implementation of the PMTCT programme. Pretoria: National Department of Health South Africa; 2001.
16. Gross CP, Anderson GF, Powe NR. The relation between funding by the National Institutes of Health and the burden of disease. N Eng J Med. 1998;340(24):1881–1887. http://dx.doi.org/10.1056/NEJM199906173402406
17. Aoun S, Pennebaker D, Pascal R. To what extent is health and medical research funding associated with the burden of disease in Australia? Aust N Z J Public Health. 2004;28(1):80–86. http://dx.doi.org/10.1111/j.1467-842X.2004.tb00637.x
18. Conceição C, Leandro A, McCarthy M. National support to public health research: A survey of European ministries. BMC Public Health. 2009;9:203. http://dx.doi.org/10.1186/1471-2458-9-203
19. Mayor S. Report gives snapshot health research funding in the UK. BMJ. 2006;332(7552):1230. http://dx.doi.org/10.1136/bmj.332.7552.1230-a
20. Sridhar D. Who sets the global health research agenda? The challenge of multi-bi financing. PLoS Med. 2012;9(9):e1001312. http://dx.doi.org/10.1371/journal.pmed.1001312
21. Gonzalez-Block MA. Health policy and systems research agendas in developing countries. Health Res Policy Syst. 2004;2:6. http://dx.doi.org/10.1186/1478-4505-2-6
22. Kingdon D. Health research funding. Mental health research continues to be underfunded. BMJ. 2006;332:1510. http://dx.doi.org/10.1136/bmj.332.7556.1510
23. Gillum LA, Gouveia C, Dorsey ER, et al. NIH disease funding levels and burden of disease. PLoS One. 2011;6(2):e16837. http://dx.doi.org/10.1371/journal.pone.0016837

24. Martin BR, Tang P. The benefits from publicly funded research. SPRU Electronic working paper series. Paper No. 161 [document on the Internet]. c2007 [cited 2014 Jun 20]. Available from: https://www.sussex.ac.uk/webteam/gateway/file.php?name=sewp161&site=25

25. Ministerial Summit on Health Research. The Mexico statement on health research. Knowledge for better health. Strengthening health systems [document on the Internet]. c2004 [cited 2011 Nov 18]. Available from: http://www.who.int/rpc/summit/agenda/en/mexico_statement_on_health_research.pdf

26. Global Ministerial Forum on Research for Health. The Bamako call to action on research for health. Strengthening research for health, development, and equity [document on the Internet]. c2008 [cited 2013 Jun 20]. Available from: http://www.who.int/rpc/news/BAMAKOCALLTOACTIONFinalNov24.pdf

27. Donders Y. The right to enjoy the benefits of scientific progress: In search of state obligations in relation to health. Med Health Care Philos. 2011;14(4):371–381. http://dx.doi.org/10.1007/s11019-011-9327-y

28. South African Human Rights Commission. SAHRC welcomes cabinet's decision to allow for the ratification of the International Covenant on Economic, Social and Cultural Rights (ICESCR) [press release on the Internet]. c2012 [cited 2013 Jun 20]. Available from: http://www.sahrc.org.za/home/index.php?ipkArticleID=141

29. Mayosi BM, Lawn JE, van Niekerk A, et al. Health in South Africa: Changes and challenges since 2009. Lancet. 2012;380(9858):2029–2043. http://dx.doi.org/10.1016/S0140-6736(12)61814-5

Compliance of St Joseph's Hospital Roma, Lesotho with the National Tuberculosis Programme of Lesotho, 2007 and 2008

Authors:
Oladoyinbo O. Samuel[1]
Pierre J.T. de Villiers[1]

Affiliations:
[1]Division of Family Medicine and Primary Care, Stellenbosch University, South Africa

Correspondence to:
Pierre de Villiers

Email:
pierre@aosis.co.za

Postal address:
Private Bag X19, Durbanville 7550, South Africa

Background: In 2009 Lesotho had an estimated TB prevalence of 696 cases/100 000 population – the 4th highest in the world. This epidemic was characterised by high rates of death, treatment failure and unknown treatment outcomes. These adverse outcomes were attributable to a high rate of TB and/or HIV co-infection and weaknesses in the implementation of Lesotho's National Tuberculosis Programme (NTP). This study was conducted in St Joseph's Hospital, Roma (SJHR) to assess the implementation of the NTP.

Method: Records of 993 patients entered into the SJHR TB register between 2007 and 2008 were reviewed. Patients' treatment details were extracted from the register, validated and analysed by STATA 10.0.

Results: Of 993 patients registered: 88% were new patients, 37% were diagnosed on sputum smear microscopy alone, 35% were diagnosed on sputum smear microscopy with chest X-ray, whilst 25% were diagnosed on chest X-ray alone. In addition: 33% were sputum smear positive, 45% were sputum smear negative, and 22% had extra-pulmonary TB. As to treatment outcome: 26% were cured, 51% completed treatment, and 51% converted from sputum smear positive to sputum smear negative over six months, whilst 16% died. Regarding HIV, 77% of patients were tested for HIV and 59% had TB and/or HIV co-infection. Of ten NTP targets only the defaulter and treatment failure rate targets were met.

Conclusion: Whilst only two out of ten NTP targets were met at SJHR in 2007–2008, improvements in TB case management were noted in 2008 which were probably due to the positive effects of audit on staff performance.

Exécution du programme national du Lesotho contre la Tuberculose à l'Hôpital St Joseph de Roma, en 2007 et 2008.

Historique: En 2009 le Lesotho avait une fréquence estimée de Tuberculose de 696 cas pour 100 000 habitants – la 4ème la plus élevée du monde. Cette épidémie était caractérisée par un taux élevé de décès, l'échec des traitements et les résultats des traitements inconnus. Ces résultats négatifs étaient attribués au taux élevé de Tuberculose et/ou à une coïnfection VIH, ainsi qu'à des lacunes dans la mise en œuvre du Programme national du Lesotho contre la Tuberculose (NTP). Cette étude a été réalisée à l'HôpitaL St Joseph de Roma (SJHR) pour évaluer la mise en œuvre du NTP.

Méthode: Les dossiers des 993 patients inscrits dans le Registre de Tuberculose de l'hôpital St Joseph entre 2007 et 2008 ont été révisés. Les informations sur le traitement des patients ont été tirées du registre, validées et analysées par STATA 10.0.

Résultats: sur les 993 patients enregistrés: 88% étaient de nouveaux patients, 37% avaient été diagnostiqués simplement par examen microscopique des expectorations, 35% avaient été diagnostiqués par examen microscopique des expectorations et une radiographie pulmonaire, alors que 25% avaient été diagnostiqués simplement sur radiographie pulmonaire. En outre: 33% des cas avaient un frottis d'expectoration positif, 45% un frottis d'expectoration négatif et 22% avaient une Tuberculose extra-pulmonaire. Quand aux résultats des traitements: 26% des cas étaient guéris, 51% avaient terminé le traitement, et 51% étaient passés du prélèvement d'expectorations positif à un prélèvement négatif en l'espace de 6 mois, alors que 16% étaient décédés. En ce qui concerne le VIH, 77% des malades avaient le VIH et 59% avaient à la fois la Tuberculose et le VIH. Sur les dix objectifs du NTP seuls les objectifs du taux des abandons et du taux d'échec au traitement ont été atteints.

Conclusion: Bien que seulement deux objectifs sur dix du programme NTP aient été réalisés au SJHR de 2007 à 2008, on a remarqué des améliorations en 2008 dans la gestion des cas de Tuberculose, ce qui est

Introduction

Worldwide there were an estimated 9.2 million new cases of tuberculosis (TB) in 2006 of which 4.1 million were TB sputum smear-positive. This TB epidemic is perpetuated by the transmission of the TB bacillus from sputum smear-positive patients to uninfected individuals and will be halted only when 70% of TB smear-positive patients are detected and 85% of those are cured.[1,2]

The member states of the United Nations are determined to halt this epidemic by the application of the World Health Organization (WHO) TB programme through the 12 WHO Regions.[3] This resolve was also evident in 2000 when the United Nations Millennium Declaration was adopted by the 189 member states and detailed eight Millennium Development Goals (MDG). The 6th goal, namely to combat HIV and/or AIDS, malaria and other diseases, included the target to reduce the incidence, prevalence and death rates associated with tuberculosis and to increase the proportion of tuberculosis cases detected and cured under Directly Observed Treatment Short Course (DOTS).[4]

This universal drive was augmented in 2000 by the Stop TB Partnership, which called for action from ministerial delegations from 20 countries with the highest burden of TB. In addition in 2006 the Global Plan to Stop Tuberculosis was launched with the aim of treating 50 million people for TB and enrolling 3 million patients who have both TB and HIV onto antiretroviral therapy (ARV) by 2015. The Plan aims to halve TB prevalence and deaths by 2015 compared with 1990 levels.

National Tuberculosis control programmes

These initiatives are available to assist states to formulate effective National Tuberculosis Programmes (NTPs). States will succeed with their NTPs to the extent that they can find the political will to fund, resource, and drive their NTPs through health care structures capable of effectively delivering TB services. Many of those states that are worst affected by TB lack health care infrastructures capable of delivering TB treatment to infected individuals.[5]

An NTP should be able to detect at least 70% of smear positive pulmonary TB patients and successfully treat or cure 85% of such cases and maintain this level of performance indefinitely. To achieve these goals of high TB case detection and an increased cure rate an NTP must have a permanent presence nationwide and be capable of delivering inexpensive and simplified technologies through its health services. Such NTPs are generally run by a manager based in a central TB unit who is responsible to the minister of health.[6]

The credibility of an NTP is judged by the programme's ability to supply antituberculous drugs to TB patients when they need them – such services are usually provided free. An effective NTP can strengthen a weak health care system in a developing country. Surveillance and standardisation of data recording, collecting and reporting are necessary for successful TB control.[7,8,9]

Conditions necessary for a successful National Tuberculosis Programme

Modern TB treatment hinges on the detection of sputum positive patients, the application of standard treatment protocols and the recording of patient data in records that allow for analysis and comparison of results between different settings. TB case management has been simplified and standardised so that generalists can be trained to diagnose and treat the disease.

TB treatment succeeds where patients complete their treatment, have exit sputa examined, have an accurate account of their treatment recorded in a standard TB register, have drugs available and where DOTS is in place. Treatment succeeds too where TB staff are familiar with TB treatment protocols and where the TB care delivered is patient-centred. Since it was introduced in 1994, DOTS has become a key underpinning element in all successful TB programmes. Since 1994 the global treatment success rate has been high with 8 out of 22 high-burden countries reaching the 85% target rate.

In the four WHO Regions, including the African Region, where TB targets were not met their failure to meet NTP targets were explained by high death rates, treatment failure, and unknown outcomes through default, transfer without follow-up or evaluation. All of these reasons apply in Lesotho. The high HIV infection rate in these countries may explain the high TB death rate seen.

TB services are generally delivered through secondary hospitals in sub-Saharan African (SSA) countries such as Lesotho. TB services need staff who are familiar with WHO TB protocols – these may need adaptation to a particular country's NTP. To ensure that patients comply with TB treatment, staff should relate well to patients and should behave in a patient-centred way. To succeed, an NTP should be fully incorporated into the running of a hospital. Many hospitals in high-burden countries are resource-constrained and obliged to provide TB services to patients from large catchment areas.

Tuberculosis in Lesotho

The Lesotho Department of Health fully subscribes to the WHO TB programme, the MDGs and the Stop TB Partnership target of halving the prevalence and mortality due to TB by 2015, as compared with the 1990 levels. To achieve these goals, Lesotho's NTP will need to be strengthened and allied with the country's HIV and/or AIDS programme – this will require a high level of political commitment to the NTP from the government.

In 2009 the WHO Global TB Report[9] listed Lesotho, as having the fourth highest estimated TB prevalence in the world (696 cases/100 000 population). Lesotho has a high

TB prevalence associated with a high rate of HIV infection. The TB infection rate is rising in SSA countries in contrast with countries in Europe where the TB epidemic has been contained. Lesotho's high TB-HIV burden and the difficulties that Lesotho's health care system experiences are reflected in the poor results it has had in dealing with Lesotho's TB epidemic and meeting TB treatment targets.

St Joseph's Hospital, Roma

St Joseph's Hospital (SJHR) is a 120-bedded district hospital located in Roma, a semi-rural area with a population of 14 000; which is 45 km south of Maseru, the capital of the Kingdom of Lesotho. District hospitals in Lesotho have failed to reach the TB and HIV treatment targets set for them by the national department of health. These hospitals have found it difficult to combine the clinical care of patients with the application of standard TB treatment protocols. The present study was undertaken in SJHR to determine how well the Lesotho NTP was being applied there and to identify areas of weakness and to make recommendations for their rectification.

Methods

This retrospective cohort study was conducted on 993 patients entered into the SJHR TB register for the years 2007 and 2008. The records of seven patients whose records were incomplete or who were started on treatment and then transferred to another facility outside the SJHR catchment area were excluded from the study. A total of 993 patients were therefore included in the study. A baseline evaluation was made, patient records were checked after 2–3 months' intensive treatment, and after 6 months' treatment outcome measurements were made.

TB treatment data was extracted from the TB register for all patients treated at SJHR from 01 January 2007 to 31 December 2008. This register, which was a version adapted from the WHO model, was issued to SJHR by the NTP. The TB patient data was extracted, checked for accuracy, assigned a numerical code to ensure patient anonymity, and entered onto an Excel spreadsheet before analysis by STATA 10.0. Patient confidentiality was maintained by limiting staff access to patient's datasets to the researcher and two assistants. Data checks were performed on all categorical and continuous variables captured for values that were not within plausible range, and cross-checking of variables was also done. Analysis included descriptive statistics, comparison of continuous measurements with a t-test and categorical measurement with a chi-square test. Nine hundred and ninety three (993) patients' records were analysed in 2007 and 2008. Statistical significance level was set at 0.05. TB indicators achieved by St Joseph's hospital were compared with the national targets set by the Lesotho national TB programme.

Results

Demographic and clinical characteristics of the study population

The demographic and clinical characteristics of the study population are shown in Table 1.

Findings of note were that there was no difference in the median age of presentation of TB patients in 2007 and 2008 and that more males attended the TB programme. There was a decrease in sputum bacteriological coverage of patients from 77.2% recorded in 2007 to 65.2% by the end of 2008. The mode of TB presentation showed significant reduction in smear negative PTB (from 59.1% recorded in 2007 to 30.4% by the end of 2008), but an increase in the detection of smear positive patients from 28.9% in 2007 to 36.7% by the end of 2008. There was a significant increase in extra-pulmonary TB from 12.0%, to 32.9% by the end of 2008. There was no change in the pattern of TB presentation in the patients between 2007 and 2008. New TB cases treated in 2007 were 87.6% and 2008 were 88.7%. Sputum conversion showed a marginal increase from 48.8% in 2007 to 53.1% by the end of 2008. Treatment outcome showed a marginal increase in cure rate and treatment success by the end of 2008. There was also a marginal decrease in mortality, treatment failure, defaulters and transferred outcome by the end of 2008. Overall, treatment outcome by the end of 2008 showed improved outcome. HIV collaborative activities showed improved outcome in HIV testing amongst TB patients, cotrimoxazole and antiretroviral uptake amongst TB and/or HIV co-infected patients. There was a decrease in the mean CD4 counts of patients who presented in 2008 (155 cells/Ul) when compared to 2007 (173 cells/Ul).

Comparison of outcome indicators with national TB targets

The comparison of targets achieved by St Joseph's TB programme with the national target set by the Lesotho NTP for 2007 and 2008 are shown in Table 2.

Findings of note were that there was an increase in detection of pulmonary smear positive TB from the baseline value of 28.9% (2007) to 36.7% reported in 2008, though still less than the national target of 50%. An increase from the baseline value of sputum conversion (new smear positive pulmonary TB) from 48.8% to 53.1% was noticed (national target is > 85%). There was an improvement of about 20% in cure rate by the end of 2008 (from 10.9% in 2007 to 29.9% in 2008), though this was still far below the national target of 85%. However, treatment success increased from (74.2% in 2007 to 76.8%) in 2008, 8.2% less than the national target of 85%. There was no significant fluctuations in the defaulter rate between 2007 and 2008, defaulter rates was less than 1% in both years, 0.6% and 0.8% (national target < 5%). There was a 2% reduction in mortality by the end of 2008 from 17.2% in 2007 and 15% in 2008 (national target [< 5%]).

In terms of TB and/or HIV collaboration activities, the proportion of TB patients offered HIV counselling and testing increased from 69.9% in 2007 to 84.7% in 2008 and the proportion of HIV positive TB patients started on cotrimoxazole increased by 7% from 60.3% in 2007 to 67.5% in 2008. An increase of about 60% was seen in the proportion of HIV positive patients eligible for HAART and commenced on it by the end of 2008. In 2007 30.2% of those eligible

TABLE 1: Demographic and clinical characteristics of the study population.

Variables	Clinical characteristics						
	Crude analysis		Stratified analysis 2008		Stratified analysis 2009		*p*-value
	n	%	*n*	%	*n*	%	
Age: mean (s.d.)							
Mean age of presentation	38.4	15.0	38.6	14.8	38.4	15.2	0.7
Sex							
Male	569	57.3	271	53.3	285	61.8	0.008
Female	424	42.7	231	46.7	176	38.2	
Mode of diagnosis							
Smear microscopy only	370	37.3	110	21.7	239	51.8	0.000
Smear microscopy + Chest X-ray	346	34.8	282	55.5	62	13.4	
Smear microscopy + Tissue biopsy	5	0.5	5	0.98	0	0	
Chest X-ray only	251	25.3	109	21.5	142	30.8	
Others (e.g. CSF analysis)	21	2.1	2	0.39	18	3.9	
Mode of TB presentation							
Smear positive PTB	332	33.4	147	-	169	36.7	0.000
Smear negative PTB	447	45.0	300	59.1	140	30.4	
Extrapulmonary TB	214	21.6	61	12.0	152	32.9	
Type of TB cases							
New TB	873	87.9	44	87.6	409	88.7	0.002
Relapse TB	74	7.4	54	10.6	17	3.7	
Transfer in	1	0.1	0	0	1	0.22	
Treatment after default	6	0.6	5	0.9	1	0.22	
Treatment after failure	2	0.2	0	0	2	0.43	
Others	36	3.7	4	0.8	31	0.43	
Sputum conversion: %	51.3	-	48.8	-	53.1	-	0.078
TB treatment outcome							
Cure	253	25.4	101	19.9	138	29.9	0.004
Treatment completed	501	50.5	279	54.9	216	46.9	
Treatment failure		1.0	6	1.2	4	0.87	
Died	162	16.3	87	17.1	72	15.6	
Treatment defaulted	7	0.7	3	0.6	4	0.8	
Transferred out	60	6.0	32	6.3	27	5.9	
TB and/or HIV collaborative activities							
HIV testing uptake	760	76.7	353	69.5	388	84.5	0.000
TB and/or HIV co-infected	592	59.4	280	55.1	297	64.7	
TB and/or HIV co-infected patients on ARVs	388	65.5	97	34.6	277	93.3	
TB and/or HIV co-infected patients on co-trimoxazole	270	45.6	169	60.3	207	69.7	
Mean CD4 counts	163.10	161.43	146.13	173.72	171.20	155.08	0.24

TB, tuberculosis.

for HAART were commenced, and by the end 2008 it had increased to 93.3%. In summary then, of ten TB programme indicators examined in 2007 and 2008 two were met, the defaulter and treatment failure rates.

Discussion

This retrospective cohort study, which essentially amounted to a clinical audit, was undertaken in order to determine where improvements could be made in the delivery of TB and HIV care at SJHR.

Case detection, sputum conversion and treatment outcome

The proportion of patients diagnosed as having TB by means of sputum smear microscopy increased from 29% in 2007 to 37% in 2008, as did the proportion of patients diagnosed by sputum microscopy and chest x-ray (CXR), although these rates still fell far short of the NTP and STOP TB target of 70%.

The low sputum conversion rate (51%) can be attributed to the fact that 30% of patients were started on the secondary phase of TB treatment after an initial 2 months of intensive treatment on the basis of chest x-ray findings alone without sputum examination. In addition 10% of sputum results were not available for evaluation after 2 months and consequently could not be reported either as sputum converted (negative) or as treatment failure (sputum positive). A small but gratifying reduction in deaths was noted from 17% in 2007 to 15% in 2008.

Whilst at 25% the cure rate is far below the requisite 85% this rate did improve from 20% in 2007 to 30% in 2008. The low cure rate is attributable to the low sputum conversion rate during the intensive treatment phase and the high treatment completed rate of 54% without bacteriological confirmation. The high treatment completed rate is reflective of the fact that nearly 60% of the patients attending had TB/HIV co-infection and were either sputum negative or had extra-pulmonary TB and the fact that few patients had end

TABLE 2: Comparison of targets achieved by St Joseph's TB programme with the national target set by the Lesotho National Tuberculosis Programme.

Indicators	National target set by the NTP of Lesotho (2007) (%)	Target achieved by St Joseph's Hospital (2007) (%)	Target met (2007) Yes or No	Target achieved by St Joseph's Hospital (2008) (%)	Target met (2008) Yes or No
Proportion of TB Cases who were smear positive detection	At least 70	28.9	No	36.7	No
Sputum conversion rate at 2 months	> 85	48.8	No	53.1	No
Cure rate	> 85	19.9	No	29.9	No
Treatment success rate	> 85	74.8	No	76.5	No
Defaulter rate	< 5	0.6	Yes	0.8	Yes
Mortality rate	< 5	17.1	No	15.6	No
Treatment failure rate	< 5	1.2	Yes	0.8	Yes
Proportion of TB patients offered HIV testing and counselling	100	69.5	No	84.5	No
Proportion of HIV positive TB patients started on cotrimoxazole	100	60.3	No	69.7	No
Proportion of HIV positive patients eligible for ARVs who are on HAART.	100	34.6	No	93.3	No

TB, tuberculosis.

of treatment sputum examinations that would have allowed cure to be declared.

Most patients over the course of the study were started on treatment without initial sputum microscopy and the course of their illness was tracked by means of chest x-ray alone and they were thus recorded as treatment completed. The STOP TB target for treatment success is 85% consequently at 76% the SJHR success rate is well below this rate due largely to the fact that most SJHR patients were either smear negative or had extra-pulmonary TB.

The audit demonstrated a low cure rate, but relatively high treatment completion rate, which is largely due to the low numbers of patients that had sputum checked at the end of treatment. There was also a practice of advancing the patient to the maintenance phase based on radiological examination, after the initial intensive phase, but without confirmatory sputum conversion. This creates an ideal situation for multiple drug resistant (MDR) TB to go undetected. Data from previous MDR-TB studies done in Lesotho showed that DR-TB and MDR-TB were common amongst patients with treatment failure on the initial regimen. The proportion of MDR-TB was respectively 78% and 28% amongst the treatment failures and suspected failures. Early initiation of empiric second-line anti-tuberculosis treatment, whilst awaiting culture and drug susceptibility testing (DST) results, should be considered for HIV-negative and -positive patients who have failed first-line anti-tuberculosis treatment; and patients suspected to be failing a first-line regimen should undergo DST at the end of the intensive phase. Considering the alarmingly high incidence of MDR-TB in Lesotho, and in the neighbouring country of South Africa, the Lesotho NTP should be addressing this possibility. [10]

The observed failure to follow up seems low for a country with a large number of migrant workers, taking into account a mortality rate of 16% and a transferred out rate of 6% reported in this clinical audit, although the low defaulter rate reported in this audit is in keeping with other previous studies in Lesotho. For example, a study on high risk of DR-TB, when first-line therapy fails in a high HIV prevalence setting in Lesotho, showed that the default rate amongst the study population appeared to be quite low compared to typical default rates of 15% – 20% amongst MDR-TB patients in South Africa.[10] Reasons for these low default rates were not entirely clear.

TB and/or HIV collaborative activities

HIV testing increased from 70% in 2007 to 85% in 2008. Antiretroviral (ARV) provision increased from 34% in 2007 to 93% in 2008. Whilst cotrimoxazole uptake improved from 60% in 2007 to 67% in 2008 it still fell short of the 100% target. Attention to TB/HIV co-infection is fundamental to the lowering of TB/HIV mortality. In SSA 30% of TB and/or HIV patients die within 12 months of treatment, largely from HIV-related infections. The improvements in the management of TB/HIV co-infected patients could explain the decrease in mortality from 2007 to 2008.

Conclusion

This study revealed weaknesses in baseline sputum evaluation, a low cure rate for new sputum smear positive patients, a low sputum conversion rate at 2 and 3 months in new smear positive patients, a high mortality in patients on TB treatment and a low cotrimoxazole uptake. These weaknesses showed how far SJHR has yet to go to meet NTP targets. However, it also revealed the following strengths: a low defaulter rate, an increase in HIV testing amongst TB patients and an improved ARV uptake in HIV co-infected TB patients.

The marginal improvements shown between 2007 and 2008 probably reflect the fact that staff became more familiar with the requirements of the NTP and thus were able to combine the clinical and programmatic aspects of the NTP more closely.

This study constituted a worthwhile clinical audit with the benefits that usually accompany such exercises – the close attention to goals, targets, outcomes and the increase in staff familiarity with NTP protocols as well as the collection and analysis can only have increased their ability to implement the Lesotho's NTP to the benefit of TB patients. Further operational research should be conducted on the application of the NTP to help Lesotho move closer to the MDG goal of halving TB incidence and of achieving a cure rate of 85% in all smear positive patients by 2015. This operational research should align itself with the priorities of the Stop TB Partnership's Global Plan to Stop TB 2011–2015.This research should aim to develop interventions that will result in improved design and better performance of the health system with more efficient methods of service delivery. Suggested areas for priority research should include; access, screening and diagnosis of TB; access to and delivery of treatment for drug-susceptible and M/XDR-TB; and capacity-building of staff for operational research. [11]

Acknowledgements

Competing interests

The authors declare that they have no financial or personal relationship(s) that may have inappropriately influenced them in writing this article.

Authors' contributions

This article is based on a master's thesis submitted to the University of Stellenbosch for the degree M.Med (Fam Med). O.S. (University of Stellenbosch) was the principal researcher and P.deV. (University Stellenbosch) was the study superviser.

References

1. Tuberculosis Coalitions for Technical Assistance. International standards for tuberculosis care. the Netherlands: The Hague TBCTA; 2006.
2. World Health Organization. Global tuberculosis control: Surveillance, planning, financing. WHO Report 2005. Geneva: World Health Organization; 2005.
3. Falzon D, Le Strat Y, Belghiti F, Infuso A. Europe TB correspondents: Exploring the determinants of treatment success for tuberculosis cases in Europe. Int J Tuberculosis Lung Disease. 2005;9:1224–1229.
4. World Health Organization. Global tuberculosis control: Surveillance, planning, financing. Geneva: World Health Organization; 2006.
5. Dye C, Hosseini M, Watt C. Did we meet the 2005 targets for tuberculosis control? Bull World Health Organisation. 2007;85:364–369. http://dx.doi.org/10.2471/BLT.06.037580
6. The international standards for tuberculosis care. Available from: URL: http://www.who.int/tb/publication/2006/istc/en/index.htm.l (no information available)
7. Stylo K, Bumgarner R. Tuberculosis can be controlled with existing evidence Technologies: Evidence. The Hague: Tuberculosis Surveillance Research Unit Progress Report. 1991:60–72.
8. Walley J, Chukwu J. The tuberculosis emergency in Africa: Opportunities and strategies for action. World Hospital Health Serv 1995;31(2):13–16.
9. World Health Organization's (WHO's). Global TB Report; 2009.
10. Satti H, McLaughlin MM, Seung KJ, Becerra MC, Keshavjee S. High risk of drug-resistant tuberculosis when first-line therapy fails in a high HIV prevalence setting. Int J Tuberc Lung Dis. 2013;17(1):100–106. http://dx.doi.org/10.5588/ijtld.12.0344
11. Priorities in Operational Research to improve tuberculosis; care www.stoptb.org/assets/documents/resources/StopTB%20Guide (no information available)

Permissions

All chapters in this book were first published in PHCFM, by AOSIS Publishing; hereby published with permission under the Creative Commons Attribution License or equivalent. Every chapter published in this book has been scrutinized by our experts. Their significance has been extensively debated. The topics covered herein carry significant findings which will fuel the growth of the discipline. They may even be implemented as practical applications or may be referred to as a beginning point for another development.

The contributors of this book come from diverse backgrounds, making this book a truly international effort. This book will bring forth new frontiers with its revolutionizing research information and detailed analysis of the nascent developments around the world.

We would like to thank all the contributing authors for lending their expertise to make the book truly unique. They have played a crucial role in the development of this book. Without their invaluable contributions this book wouldn't have been possible. They have made vital efforts to compile up to date information on the varied aspects of this subject to make this book a valuable addition to the collection of many professionals and students.

This book was conceptualized with the vision of imparting up-to-date information and advanced data in this field. To ensure the same, a matchless editorial board was set up. Every individual on the board went through rigorous rounds of assessment to prove their worth. After which they invested a large part of their time researching and compiling the most relevant data for our readers.

The editorial board has been involved in producing this book since its inception. They have spent rigorous hours researching and exploring the diverse topics which have resulted in the successful publishing of this book. They have passed on their knowledge of decades through this book. To expedite this challenging task, the publisher supported the team at every step. A small team of assistant editors was also appointed to further simplify the editing procedure and attain best results for the readers.

Apart from the editorial board, the designing team has also invested a significant amount of their time in understanding the subject and creating the most relevant covers. They scrutinized every image to scout for the most suitable representation of the subject and create an appropriate cover for the book.

The publishing team has been an ardent support to the editorial, designing and production team. Their endless efforts to recruit the best for this project, has resulted in the accomplishment of this book. They are a veteran in the field of academics and their pool of knowledge is as vast as their experience in printing. Their expertise and guidance has proved useful at every step. Their uncompromising quality standards have made this book an exceptional effort. Their encouragement from time to time has been an inspiration for everyone.

The publisher and the editorial board hope that this book will prove to be a valuable piece of knowledge for researchers, students, practitioners and scholars across the globe.

List of Contributors

Langalibalele H. Mabuza, Indiran Govender and John V. Ndimande
Department of Family Medicine and Primary Health Care, University of Limpopo (Medunsa Campus), South Africa

Olufemi B. Omole
Department of Family Medicine, University of the Witwatersrand, South Africa

Cathy Kande and Robert Mash
Division of Family Medicine and Primary Care, Stellenbosch University, South Africa

Bob Mash
Division of Family Medicine and Primary Care, Stellenbosch University, South Africa

Kangale Izale and Jean-Pierre L. Fina
Department of Family Medicine, Protestant University of Congo, Democratic Republic of Congo

Indiran Govender and John Tumbo
Department of Family Medicine and Primary Health Care, University of the Limpopo, Medunsa Campus, South Africa

Indiran Govender, Langalibalele H. Mabuza and Gboyega A. Ogunbanjo
Department of Family Medicine, University of Limpopo, Medunsa Campus, South Africa

Bob Mash
Division of Family Medicine and Primary Care, Stellenbosch University, South Africa

Brenda S. Mhlanga and Fatima Suleman
Discipline of Pharmaceutical Sciences, School of Health Sciences, University of KwaZulu-Natal, South Africa

Caron L. Jack and Maurice Mars
Department of TeleHealth, Nelson R Mandela School of Medicine, University of KwaZulu-Natal, South Africa

Stephane Tshitenge and Adewale Ganiyu
School of Medicine, University of Botswana, Botswana

Andre Citeya
Mahalapye District Health Management Team, Botswana
Stephane Tshitenge, Adewale Ganiyu and Deogratias Mbuka
Family physicians and lecturers, Department of family medicine, School of Medicine, University of Botswana, Botswana

Joseph M. Shama
Hospital superintendent, Selebi Phikwe Government Hospital, Botswana

Ronette Lategan, Violet L. van den Berg and Corinna M. Walsh
Faculty of Health Sciences, University of the Free State, South Africa

Talitha Crowley and Ethelwynn L. Stellenberg
Division of Nursing, Faculty of Medicine and Health Sciences, Stellenbosch University, South Africa

Violet L. van den Berg and Lisemelo Seheri
Department of Nutrition and Dietetics, University of the Free State, South Africa

Jacques Raubenheimer
Department of Biostatistics, University of the Free State, South Africa

Candice Reardon and Gavin George
Health Economics and HIV and AIDS Research Division (HEARD), University of KwaZulu-Natal, South Africa

Raymond G. Mabaso
Department of Health Studies, University of South Africa, South Africa

Olalekan A. Oduntan
Discipline of Optometry, University of KwaZulu-Natal, South Africa

Ganizani Mlawanda
Faculty of Medicine and Health Sciences, Department of Interdisciplinary Health Sciences, Division of Family Medicine and Primary Care, University of Stellenbosch, Tygerberg, South Africa
Royal Swaziland Sugar Corporation (RSSC) Medical Services, Mhlume, Swaziland

Michael Pather
Faculty of Medicine and Health Sciences, Department of Interdisciplinary Health Sciences, Division of Family Medicine and Primary Care, University of Stellenbosch, Tygerberg, South Africa

Srini Govender
Faculty of Medicine and Health Sciences, Department of Interdisciplinary Health Sciences, Division of Family Medicine and Primary Care, University of Stellenbosch, Tygerberg, South Africa
Khayelitsha Community Health Centre, Khayelitsha, South Africa

Valerie J. Ehlers and Getahun S. Aragaw
Department of Health Studies, University of South Africa, South Africa

Selente Bezuidenhout, Damilola A. Ogunsanwo and Elvera A. Helberg
Department of Pharmacy, University of Limpopo, Medunsa Campus, South Africa

Steve Reid
Primary Health Care Directorate, University of Cape Town, South Africa

Bob Mash
Family Medicine and Primary Care, Stellenbosch University, South Africa

Lilian Dudley
Community Health Division, Faculty of Medicine and Health Sciences, Stellenbosch University, South Africa

Andrew Ross
Department of Family Medicine, Nelson R. Mandela School of Medicine, University of KwaZulu-Natal, South Africa

Bob Mash
Family Medicine and Primary Care, Stellenbosch University, South Africa

Bob Mash
Division of Family Medicine and Primary Care, Stellenbosch University, South Africa

Gboyega A. Ogunbanjo
Department of Family Medicine, University of Limpopo, Medunsa Campus, South Africa

Langalibalele H. Mabuza, Indiran Govender and Gboyega A. Ogunbanjo
Department of Family Medicine, Medunsa Campus, University of Limpopo, South Africa

Bob Mash
Family Medicine and Primary Care, Stellenbosch University, South Africa

Henry I. Okonta and Gboyega A. Ogunbanjo
Department of Family Medicine and Primary Health Care, University of Limpopo, Medunsa Campus, Pretoria

John B. Ikombele
Mamelodi District Hospital, Pretoria

Kayode O. Osungbade
Faculty of Public Health, College of Medicine, University of Ibadan, Ibadan, Nigeria
University College Hospital, Ibadan, Nigeria

Olubunmi O. Ayinde
Oyo State Ministry of Health, Ibadan, Nigeria

Lesley T. Bhebhe and Wilhelm J. Steinberg
Department of Family Medicine, Faculty of Health Sciences, University of the Free State, South Africa

Cornel Van Rooyen
Department of Biostatistics, Faculty of Health Sciences, University of the Frees State, South Africa

Nondumiso B.Q. Ncube
Division of Community Health, Stellenbosch University, South Africa

Willem A.J. Meintjes
Unit for Infection Prevention and Control, Stellenbosch University and Tygerberg Hospital, and Division of Community Health, Stellenbosch University, South Africa

Lumbwe Chola
Health Systems and Services Research, Division of Community Health, Stellenbosch University, South Africa

Benjamin O. Adeyemi
Department of Family Medicine, Pietermaritzburg Hospitals Complex and University of KwaZulu-Natal, South Africa

Andrew Ross
Department of Family Medicine, University of KwaZulu-Natal, South Africa

Alta Kritzinger
Clinic for High-Risk Babies (CHRIB), Department of Speech-Language Pathology and Audiology, University of Pretoria, South Africa

Elise van Rooyen
Kangaroo Mother Care Unit, Department of Paediatrics, Kalafong Hospital, University of Pretoria, South Africa

Bob Mash
Family Medicine and Primary Care, Stellenbosch University, South Africa

Abidemi Faleye
Department of Family Medicine, University of KwaZulu-Natal, Durban, South Africa

Meyer Swanepoel and Bob Mash
Division of Family Medicine and Primary Care, Stellenbosch University, South Africa

Tracey Naledi
Health Programmes, Department of Health, Western Cape Government, South Africa

Lungiswa P. Tsolekile, Thandi Puoane and Helen Schneider
School of Public Health, University of the Western Cape, South Africa

Naomi S. Levitt and Krisela Steyn
Faculty of Health Sciences, Department of Medicine, University of Cape Town, South Africa

Elijah Marangu, Natisha Sands and John Rolley
School of Nursing and Midwifery, Deakin University, Australia

David Ndetei
Africa Mental Health Foundation and University of Nairobi, Kenya

Fethi Mansouri
Centre for Citizenship and Globalization, Deakin University, Australia

Claire van Deventer
Department of Family Medicine and Rural Health, University of the Witwatersrand, South Africa

Bob Mash
Division of Family Medicine and Primary Care, Stellenbosch University, South Africa

Oathokwa Nkomazana
Faculty of Medicine, Department of Surgery, University of Botswana, Botswana

Wim Peersman
Faculty of Medicine and Health Sciences, Department of Family Medicine and Primary Health Care, Ghent University, Belgium

Merlin Willcox
Division of Medical Sciences, Department of Primary Care Health Sciences, University of Oxford, United Kingdom

Robert Mash
Division of Family Medicine and Primary Care, Faculty of Medicine and Health Sciences, Stellenbosch University, South Africa

Nthabiseng Phaladze
School of Nursing, Faculty of Health Sciences, University of Botswana, Botswana

Tania Steyl and Julie Phillips
Department of Physiotherapy, University of the Western Cape, South Africa

Kate Rees and Virginia Zweigenthal
Faculty of Health Sciences, School of Public Health and Family Medicine, University of Cape Town, South Africa

Kate Joyner
Division of Nursing, Faculty of Medicine and Health Sciences, Stellenbosch University, South Africa

Leslie London and Sabela Petros
School of Public Health and Family Medicine, Division of Public Health Medicine, University of Cape Town, South Africa
Health Department, Western Cape Government, South Africa

Tracey Naledi
School of Public Health and Family Medicine, Division of Public Health Medicine, University of Cape Town, South Africa

Oladoyinbo O. Samuel and Pierre J.T. de Villiers
Division of Family Medicine and Primary Care, Stellenbosch University, South Africa